The Science and Safety of Beverages

The Science and Safety of Beverages

Edited by

Roji Waghmare
Department of Food Engineering and Technology,
Institute of Chemical Technology, Mumbai, Maharashtra, India

Manoj Kumar
Chemical and Biochemical Processing Division, ICAR-Central Institute for Research on Cotton Technology, Mumbai, Maharashtra, India

ELSEVIER

ACADEMIC PRESS
An imprint of Elsevier

Academic Press is an imprint of Elsevier
125 London Wall, London EC2Y 5AS, United Kingdom
50 Hampshire Street, 5th Floor, Cambridge, MA 02139, United States

ISBN: 978-0-443-36536-2

For information on all Academic Press publications visit our website at
https://www.elsevier.com/books-and-journals

Publisher: Mara Conner
Acquisitions Editor: Kelsey Connors
Editorial Project Manager: Kritika Sharma
Production Project Manager: Anitha Sivaraj
Cover Designer: Raman Kumar

Typeset by TNQ Tech

Dedicated to all students, researchers, and food professionals.

Contents

Contributors

Ayele Assefa Adugna
Department of Food Technology and Process Engineering, Haramaya Institute of Technology, Haramaya University, Dire Dawa, Ethiopia

Hirpha Adugna Areti
Department of Chemical Engineering, Haramaya Institute of Technology, Haramaya University, Dire Dawa, Ethiopia

Zanoor Ul Ashraf
School of Bioengineering and Food Technology, Shoolini University, Solan, Himachal Pradesh, India

Jesus Fernando Ayala-Zavala
Secretariat of Science, Humanities, Technology and Innovation, Center for Research in Food and Development (CIAD), Sonora, Mexico

K. Aysha Sherin
Department of Food Engineering and Technology, Institute of Chemical Technology, Mumbai, Maharashtra, India

Gleyde Anny Cruz Barros
Postgraduate Program in Food Science and Technology (PPGCTA), Federal University of Ceará (UFC), Fortaleza, Ceará, Brazil

Himanshu Chandelkar
Department of Food Engineering and Technology, Institute of Chemical Technology, Mumbai, Maharashtra, India

Debjit Chowdhury
Department of Food Engineering and Technology, Institute of Chemical Technology, Mumbai, Maharashtra, India

K.S. Darshan
Department of Food Engineering and Technology, Institute of Chemical Technology, Mumbai, Maharashtra, India

Felipe Sousa da Silva
Nucleus of Technology and Industrial Quality of Ceará (NUTEC), Fortaleza, Ceará, Brazil

Andréa Cardoso de Aquino
Postgraduate Program in Food Science and Technology (PPGCTA), Federal University of Ceará (UFC), Fortaleza, Ceará, Brazil

Magnólia Carneiro de Oliveira
Postgraduate Program in Food Technology (PPGTA), Federal Institute of Education, Science and Technology of Ceará (IFCE), Limoeiro do Norte, Ceará, Brazil

Luciana de Siqueira Oliveira
Postgraduate Program in Food Science and Technology (PPGCTA), Federal University of Ceará (UFC), Fortaleza, Ceará, Brazil; Universidade Federal do Ceará, Departamento de Engenharia de Alimentos, Campus do Pici, Fortaleza, Ceará, Brazil

Ronaldo Ferreira do Nascimento
Universidade Federal do Ceará, Departamento de Química Analítica e Físico-Química, Campus do Pici, Fortaleza, Ceará, Brazil

Larissa Graziele Rauber Duarte
Instituto Federal do Sul de Minas, IFSULdeMINAS, Machado, MG, Brazil

Mariana Buranelo Egea
Goiano Federal Institute of Education, Science and Technology, Campus Rio Verde, Rio Verde, GO, Brazil

Lateefat Motunrayo Ewuoso
Department of Science Laboratory Technology, Abeokuta, Ogun State, Nigeria

Sibele Santos Fernandes
Federal University of Rio Grande, School of Chemistry and Food, Rio Grande, Brazil

Tatiana Sainara Maia Fernandes
Universidade Federal do Ceará, Departamento de Química Analítica e Físico-Química, Campus do Pici, Fortaleza, Ceará, Brazil

José Leitão Sena Lima Filho
Postgraduate Program in Food Technology (PPGTA), Federal Institute of Education, Science and Technology of Ceará (IFCE), Limoeiro do Norte, Ceará, Brazil

Andrêssa Maria Medeiros Theóphilo Galvão
University of International Integration of Afro-Brazilian Lusophony (UNILAB), Institute of Rural Development (IDR), Food Engineering Course, Redenção, Ceará, Brazil

Asir Gani
School of Bioengineering and Food Technology, Shoolini University, Solan, Himachal Pradesh, India

Rabira Lemessa Gudeta
Department of Food Technology and Process Engineering, Haramaya Institute of Technology, Haramaya University, Dire Dawa, Ethiopia

Poonam Kanwar
School of Bioengineering and Food Technology, Shoolini University, Solan, Himachal Pradesh, India

Manoj Kumar
Chemical and Biochemical Processing Division, ICAR-Central Institute for Research on Cotton Technology, Mumbai, Maharashtra, India

Ailton Cesar Lemes
School of Chemistry, Federal University of Rio de Janeiro, Rio de Janeiro, RJ, Brazil

Likhitha M.C.
Department of Food Engineering and Technology, Institute of Chemical Technology, Mumbai, Maharashtra, India

Jéssica Roberta Pereira Martins
Postgraduate Program in Food Technology (PPGTA), Federal Institute of Education, Science and Technology of Ceará (IFCE), Limoeiro do Norte, Ceará, Brazil

Luana Guabiraba Mendes
Postgraduate Program in Food Technology (PPGTA), Federal Institute of Education, Science and Technology of Ceará (IFCE), Limoeiro do Norte, Ceará, Brazil; Nucleus of Technology and Industrial Quality of Ceará (NUTEC), Fortaleza, Ceará, Brazil

Maria Aparecida Liberato Milhome
Postgraduate Program in Food Technology (PPGTA), Federal Institute of Education, Science and Technology of Ceará (IFCE), Limoeiro do Norte, Ceará, Brazil

Kelvi Wilson Evaristo Miranda
Laboratory of Research and Innovation in Plant Products and Packaging, Federal University of Ceará (UFC), Fortaleza, Ceará, Brazil

Rebecca Miranda
Department of Food Engineering and Technology, Institute of Chemical Technology, Mumbai, Maharashtra, India

Sabeera Muzzaffar
Department of Food Science and Technology, University of Kashmir, Srinagar, Jammu and Kashmir, India

Dessalegn Legese Negewo
Department of Food Technology and Process Engineering, Haramaya Institute of Technology, Haramaya University, Dire Dawa, Ethiopia

Crisiana de Andrade Nobre
Nucleus of Technology and Industrial Quality of Ceará (NUTEC), Fortaleza, Ceará, Brazil; Postgraduate Program in Food Science and Technology (PPGCTA), Federal University of Ceará (UFC), Fortaleza, Ceará, Brazil; Universidade Federal do Ceará, Departamento de Engenharia de Alimentos, Campus do Pici, Fortaleza, Ceará, Brazil

Tiago Rocha Nogueira
Nucleus of Technology and Industrial Quality of Ceará (NUTEC), Fortaleza, Ceará, Brazil

Fuad Pereira Nogueira Filho
Nucleus of Technology and Industrial Quality of Ceará (NUTEC), Fortaleza, Ceará, Brazil; Graduate Program in Development and Environment, Federal University of Ceará, Fortaleza, Ceará, Brazil

Bukola Funmilola Olatunji
Department of Food Science and Technology, College of Basic and Applied Science, Mountain Top University, Prayer City, Ogun State, Nigeria

Raquel Martins da Silva Fernandes de Oliveira
Federal University of Goiás, Faculty of Agronomy, Goiânia, Brazil

Hilal Ahmad Punoo
Department of Food Science and Technology, University of Kashmir, Srinagar, Jammu and Kashmir, India

Swayamdeep S. Shinde
Department of Food Engineering and Technology, Institute of Chemical Technology, Mumbai, Maharashtra, India

Mayara Salgado Silva
Postgraduate Program in Food Technology (PPGTA), Federal Institute of Education, Science and Technology of Ceará (IFCE), Limoeiro do Norte, Ceará, Brazil

Sunday Samuel Sobowale
Department of Food Science and Technology, College of Basic and Applied Science, Mountain Top University, Prayer City, Ogun State, Nigeria

N. Vamsi Vara Prasad
Department of Food Engineering and Technology, Institute of Chemical Technology, Mumbai, Maharashtra, India

Akriti Verma
Department of Food Engineering and Technology, Institute of Chemical Technology, Mumbai, Maharashtra, India

Vishal
Department of Food Engineering and Technology, Institute of Chemical Technology, Mumbai, Maharashtra, India

Roji Waghmare
Department of Food Engineering and Technology, Institute of Chemical Technology, Mumbai, Maharashtra, India

Tuyiba Nazir Zargar
Department of Food Science and Technology, University of Kashmir, Srinagar, Jammu and Kashmir, India

Preface

The beverage industry is dynamic. The market of beverages is a swiftly expanding segment in the functional food industry. However, their high moisture content, diverse raw materials, and complex processing conditions make beverages particularly vulnerable to microbiological, chemical, and physical hazards. Ensuring safety without compromising quality and sensory attributes remains a major scientific and technological challenge.

Science and Safety of Beverages presents a structured and science-based overview of beverage safety across a wide range of products. The opening chapter introduces fundamental principles of beverage science and safe production practices. Subsequent chapters address quality assurance and microbial safety in fruit, vegetable, dairy, plant-based, alcoholic, and nonalcoholic fermented beverages, highlighting shelf-life enhancement and quality preservation strategies.

Advances in processing technologies for safe beverage production, including conventional and emerging preservation methods, are discussed with respect to their impact on microbial stability and product quality. The role of packaging materials and contaminant migration is critically examined to highlight safety challenges associated with modern distribution systems. Dedicated chapters on analytical techniques for beverage analysis provide insight into quality control, safety assessment, and regulatory compliance.

This edited book is intended to serve as a comprehensive reference for undergraduate and postgraduate students of food science, food technology, food engineering, and nutrition, as well as researchers, quality assurance professionals, and beverage industry practitioners. The editors hope that this book will contribute meaningfully to food safety education and strengthen scientific understanding in the rapidly evolving beverage sector.

Editors

Dr. Roji Waghmare
Institute of Chemical Technology, Mumbai

Dr. Manoj Kumar
ICAR-CIRCOT, Mumbai

Acknowledgments

The editors would like to express their sincere gratitude to all the contributing authors for their valuable inputs, technical expertise, and timely cooperation, which were essential in bringing this edited volume to completion. The diversity of perspectives and depth of research presented in the chapters have significantly enriched the scientific value of this book.

The editors also acknowledge the support extended by their respective institutions and departments for providing the necessary academic environment and facilities. Special appreciation is extended to research scholars and students who assisted in literature compilation, organization, and technical discussions during the preparation of this book.

We sincerely appreciate the guidance and cooperation of the publishing team for their professional handling of the editorial process and production of this book.

Finally, the editors would like to thank their families for their patience, encouragement, and unwavering support throughout the development of this edited work.

Editors
Dr. Roji Waghmare
Dr. Manoj Kumar

CHAPTER

Introduction to beverage science: Principles and practices for safe production 1

Likhitha M.C.[1], Debjit Chowdhury[1], Swayamdeep S. Shinde[1], Roji Waghmare[1] and Manoj Kumar[2]
[1]*Department of Food Engineering and Technology, Institute of Chemical Technology, Mumbai, Maharashtra, India;*
[2]*Chemical and Biochemical Processing Division, ICAR-Central Institute for Research on Cotton Technology, Mumbai, Maharashtra, India*

1.1 Introduction

Beverages in all forms of liquid foods, including alcoholic (beers, wines, and spirits) and non-alcoholic (water, soft drinks, cola, fruit juices and smoothies, tea, coffee, dairy products, and carbonated and noncarbonated drinks) beverages compose a significant portion of the food industry. Any beverage production system's quality is correlated with the efficiency of its quality management system, which includes raw material quality, processing design, equipment quality, and customer satisfaction. Customers will reject the goods of these companies if any one of the requirements is not met. Numerous beverages are recalled for a variety of food safety concerns, including packaging contamination risk, microbial outbreaks, and declining product quality attributes like off tastes, an unpleasant taste, smell and textural deformities (Aadil et al., 2019).

Over the last 11,000 years, water and breast milk were the primary beverages consumed, with breast milk considered a 'complete beverage' due to its balanced content of protein, fat, carbohydrates, and water. Alcoholic beverages like beer and wine emerged around 8000 BCE. Archeological evidence confirms beer production between 4000 and 3500 BCE and wine from domesticated grapes in Iran dates to 5400–5000 BCE (Kiple & Ornelas, 2000). Distillation, first developed around 4000 BCE in Mesopotamia for perfumes, later enabled higher alcohol concentrations in spirits (Standage, 2005). In 1872, pasteurization of beer was initiated by Anheuser-Busch along with refrigerated train cars to distribute across the U.S (Plavchan, 1976). Tea is a product of Camellia sinensis traditionally drank in Thailand, Burma, Assam, and southwest China (Macfarlane and Macfarlane. 2003). The practice of drinking tea is believed to have been initiated by Chinese emperor Shen Nung about 2700 BCE. Coffee is native to Africa, specifically Ethiopia or Yemen (Ukers, 1948). Juice is defined as liquid derived from plants; the early version was lemonade that emerged in the 16th century in Italy, and by mid-17th century, orange juice became popular. There are also more recent value additions: calcium and vitamin D added that by 2002, 30% of sales of Minute Maid were fortified orange juice (Kiple and Ornelas, 2000). Others include Spirulina, echinacea and other herbs (Nicholls, 1998). Diversity of Beverages: Over 5000 years, foods have continued to evolve. Mostly in the last 50 years, there has been an

The Science and Safety of Beverages. https://doi.org/10.1016/B978-0-443-36536-2.00012-0

explosion in diversity, going from milk, wine, beer, tea, coffee to sports drinks, energy drinks, and high-calorie alcoholic drinks. Other newer categories belong to the plant-based beverages prepared from legumes, oilseeds, grains, pseudo-cereals and nuts (Walther et al., 2022). With urbanization and changes in lifestyles, health-oriented consumers increasingly look toward beverages rich in essential nutrients, vitamins, minerals, fiber, and phytochemicals (Slavin & Lloyd, 2012).

Health awareness amongst people and an increase in lifestyle diseases have forced people to turn to healthier drinks with lower alcohol content (Rajan et al., 2024). Conventional drinks are also made using cereal grains, herbs, calyces, fruits, water, and sugars with techniques passed down through generations (Sengev et al., 2012). Fermented drinks are over 5000 varieties found across the world. It is of immense cultural significance and is made using cereals like rice, wheat, and millets to give an enhanced taste and nutritional value to the drink. Such procedures are believed to have originated in India as one of the first examples of low-cost biotechnology. Fermentation using beneficial microorganisms like lactic acid bacteria helps to increase nutrient values and solubility of proteins. Plant-based fermented drinks that are quite common in Europe and the US are prized for their bioactive components (Nazir et al., 2019). Cereals help to facilitate the survival of yeast as well as Lactobacilli under trying conditions found in the human gut to bring about beneficial effects of fermentation (Maja and Sharareh, 2017). Along with these functions, cereals also have prebiotic effects for increasing Lactobacillus and Bifidobacterium (Mbuagbaw & Noorduyn, 2012).

This book offers a detailed introduction to beverage science, addressing the basic processing requirements, microbiological hazards, and safety issues associated with these processes. The book delves into the various new developments in food safety, particularly concerning spoilage microorganisms, pathogens, and techniques of pasteurization and sanitization pertaining to different types of beverages. The book analyses fruit/vegetable juice, dairy products, and plant-based beverages—safest methods, processes, and natural preservatives specifically adapted to these unique types of beverages—such as HPP, UHT treatment, and natural preservatives. The book delves into the different types of fermented (alcoholic and non-alcoholic) beverages, concentrating specifically on microbial quality, processes, various fermentation processes, and potential chemical hazards associated with such products. The book reviews the advanced processing techniques such as UV, PEF, and HPP processing methods, while emphasizing the importance of GMPs and international food safety specifications (ISO, FSSAI, and Codex, FDA) to secure proper food hygiene and beverage quality.

1.2 Basics of beverage science

1.2.1 Key steps in beverage production

Drinks are produced with the aid of water, sweeteners, acids, flavors, colors, preservatives, and stabilizers (Furia, 1973). Water is the key ingredient that comprises about 90% of the total volume of the drink. Water is processed for treatment through filtration, softening, and pH adjustment. Sweeteners provide sweetness, and calories; common ones include sugar and glucose syrup. Low-calorie drinks use artificial sweeteners like saccharin and aspartame. Acids like citric and malic acid add tartness and help preserve beverages. Coloring and flavoring agents enhance the look and taste of beverages. These agents may be natural, synthetic, or nature-identical and must follow safety limits (Khatri & Shalini, 2008). Preservatives such as benzoic acid and sorbic acid inhibit microbial growth. Stabilizers and emulsifiers prevent separation and maintain texture. Fruit-based drinks contain juice or pulp, which add natural flavor and color. Plant extracts are added for both flavor and health benefits. Carbonated drinks use carbon dioxide for fizziness and improved mouthfeel. Clouding agents like gum acacia give drinks a cloudy appearance. Foaming agents such as saponins produce foam in carbonated beverages.

1.2.2 Basic terminologies and general processing steps involved in beverage production

The general processing steps in beverage production can vary depending on the type of beverage being produced (e.g., soft drinks, alcoholic beverages, juices, etc), but they generally follow a sequence of steps to ensure the final product is safe, flavorful, and of high quality.

1.2.2.1 Pulping

Pulping is a crucial unit operation in the processing of fruit-based beverages. It involves extracting or separating the pulp from the seeds and skin of pulpy fruits such as papaya, mango, apple, and guava. At a small-scale or cottage level, pulping can be done manually using simple tools like a pestle and mortar, hand-operated pulpers, or blenders. On an industrial scale, pulping is typically performed using power-operated pulper-finishers, which are equipped with brushes, beaters, screens, and sieves. The fruit is first brushed and then pushed through a screen, followed by sieving to remove seeds and skin, leaving the pulp separated for further processing (Ashurst, 2007, pp. 35–67).

1.2.2.2 Juice extraction

Juice extraction is an essential operation in the juice production of juicy fruits like citrus fruits, pineapple, and litchi. It can be done in various presses such as a roller press, a plunger press, or a continuous screw type expeller press. In the roller press, the fruits are crushed by wooden rollers made of granite. In a plunger press, the fruits are kept in an inverted cup in which a mechanical system presses the fruits against a metallic cone fixed in the cup. In a continuous screw type expeller press, fruits are fed into a hopper which leads to a rotating screw fixed in a conical part with perforations. The perforations help extract the juice, which collects in juice collection tanks (Mushataq, 2018).

1.2.2.3 Clarification

Beverage clarification today is normally done simply by filtration, centrifugation in decanting centrifuges, finishers with fine screens, or by modern membrane processing techniques. In other instances, enzymatic processing can also be performed as a means of clarification. This process is particularly essential for cloudy juices and is normally done after pasteurization. Cloudy fruit juices contain such substances as pectin, starch, gums, polyphenols, proteins, and lipids that may result in haze during storage; hence, these must be removed.

1.2.2.4 Pasteurization

The pasteurization procedure has a significant role to play in consumer safety (Parish, 1997). This procedure follows a common practice in preparing a variety of beverages such as fruit and veg juices, soft beverages, carbonated beverages, beverages, and dairy beverages. However, different beverage types require different combinations of temperature and time for pasteurization. The main aim of pasteurization in any beverage is to eliminate microorganisms (pathogens and spoilage-causing bacteria) and to inactivate enzymes, especially in fruit and veg juices. Common pathogens for beverages include Salmonella, E. coli, and Alicyclobacillus. Pectin methyl esterase, an enzyme in orange juice, catalyzes the action of pectin de-esterification, which forms soft gels in the presence of divalent ions, resulting in precipitation of juice cloud, a defect. Tubular and plate heat exchanger pasteurizers are employed for beverage pasteurization purposes. At present, researchers are engaged in finding a non-heat pasteurization technique for fruit juices (Keyser et al., 2008).

1.2.2.5 Carbonation

Carbonation is applied in soft drinks and other sort of flavored drinks such as beers and champagnes. Carbonation has become widely demanded owing to the distinct taste and 'sensation' triggered by both the mechanical action of the CO2 bubbles and the chemical action of the resulting carbonic acid (Chandrashekar et al., 2009). Carbonation basically entails the use of high pressure to inject carbon dioxide gas into a beverage, with a resulting increase in the solubility of the gas with increasing pressure levels. The gas is mostly injected continuously using a venturi in the liquid base of the beverage, with the prepared beverage collected in a pressurized container or a retail bottle directly after injection with carbon dioxide gas. The major equipment involved in a carbonation apparatus comprises a venturi, a stainless-steel container, pumps, refrigerated baths, sensors, and liquid as well as gas ducts. Carbonated drinks in sparkling wine are normally prepared using natural fermentation in which the resultant gas in fermented drinks is retained utilizing a mechanism to suppress escape of the gas.

1.2.2.6 Fermentation

Fermentation is the operation that involves the conversion of Carbohydrates into alcohol or acid. It is a prudent step in the preparation of alcohol as well as some milk-based drinks (Paul Ross et al., 2002). This fermentation requires a controlled environment in terms of fermentation time, fermentation temperature, pH levels, agitation, and nutrient availability. The microbes involved as fermentation starters include some special bacteria and a type of yeast. The type of yeast Saccharomyces cerivesiae is dominant during the fermentation stage in the production of malt and wine. It is pertinent that the fermentation medium becomes warmer during the fermentation stage. This necessitates the use of cooling facilities to prevent the resultant destruction of the yeast. This fermentation takes place under aerobic conditions until the sugars are exhausted (Paul Ross et al., 2002).

1.2.2.7 Brewing

Brewing is the process of hot water extraction of components from plant materials. Brewing is an important unit operation used in the manufacturing of tea, coffee, and beer. The wort obtained after the mashing process in the production of beer is brewed by boiling with hops in a brewing tank. The brewing step has contributions to the concentration of wort, sterilization, enzyme inactivation, protein precipitation, sugar caramelization, and preservatives and flavor compounds extraction from hops. In the production of coffee, brewing is the critical stage, and optimization can be achieved by regulating factors like coffee-to-water ratio, particle size, water temperature, and mixing time. It is also a significant process used in the production of instant tea.

1.2.2.8 Distillation

Distillation is a crucial process in the production of distilled alcoholic beverages, such as whiskey, brandy, and vodka. In this process, fermented materials (like grains, fruits, or vegetable extracts) are heated to separate alcohol and other components based on their different boiling points. Distillation can be carried out in two main ways: batch distillation and continuous column distillation. In batch distillation, multiple distillations are performed, with the distillate being returned to the same still or a different still for re-distillation. Coffey stills are the most commonly used continuous column stills, specifically designed for the continuous distillation of pure spirits from wine or beer (Altay et al., 2025).

1.2.2.9 Maturation and aging

Aging and maturation comprise winemaking's important processes, often used synonymously. Typically, this certain phase lasts for a duration from months up to years and is associated with changes in the wine that are desirable. It may also involve additional steps like racking with fining. Filtration can be required if it depends on the type of wine that is produced. Phenolic compounds oxidize, aldehydes as well as esters form, also glycosides hydrolyze during maturation. Physical changes cause salts to precipitate volatile substances to be lost and carbon dioxide gas to escape. Brightness reduction along with color changes and even taste profile alterations in wine with tannin softening do result from each of these physical and chemical changes (Wang et al., 2023).

1.2.2.10 Packaging

Packaging is the final step in the processing of all types of beverages. Its primary functions include protection, containment, and convenience. Packaging also plays a significant role in the marketing of beverages, often being referred to as a "silent salesman." Beverages are packaged in a variety of materials and forms, including glass bottles, PET bottles, plastic cups, metal cans, and pouches. Certain packaging methods are specifically designed for particular beverages, such as casking, kegging, bottling, and canning for beer (Ramos et al., 2015).

1.3 Health benefits and nutritional qualities

Beverages play a vital role in human nutrition, which contain essential vitamins, minerals, and phytochemicals, which are beneficial to health. Fruits and vegetables, whether consumed whole or as beverages, are valued for their rich content of essential vitamins, minerals, fiber, and bioactive phytochemicals like antioxidants, phytoestrogens, and anti-inflammatory agents, which help support overall health and reduce the risk of obesity and cardiovascular diseases (Butu & Rodino, 2019).

Though fruit juices are nutrient-rich, their sugar content might create some issues for those with diabetes, obesityes, or dental problems. For example, vegetable juices or mixtures of fruit juices and vegetables can serve as healthier alternatives. They reduce sugar consumption yet retain essential nutrients. Other benefits of vegetable juices include metabolism regulation. Moreover, they act as detoxifiers as well as regenerators. If these juices are processed for separation through the use of a centrifuge juicer while drawn from fresh materials without the use of preservatives, they will provide the body with amino acids, minerals, enzymes, salts, and vitamins. The fiber content in those juices increases feelings of fullness. It also helps in the proper regulation of the body's digestive system (Wang et al., 2014). Certain juices extracted from beets, carrots, celery, currants, spinach, grapes, cherries, and watermelons added with garlic and ginger juice have proved useful in the strengthening of the body's immune system as well as in the lowering of blood pressures as well as levels of cholesterol. Antioxidant functions of those juices make them effective (Binia et al., 2015; Zheng et al., 2017). Melon juices, apricots, peaches, or broccoli juices serve as effective agents in the treatment of conditions of potassium deficiency in the body. An absence of either magnesium or calcium in the body is also treated with the aforementioned juices. Pineapple juices, added with those of ginger, pear, or parsley juices, act as effective agents in the prevention of heart diseases. Orange juices are the most important natural sources of vitamin C. Additionally, juices of cranberries act as effective natural sources of the stated vitamin (Nelson, 2005, pp. 1–213). Most interestingly, their study proposes that the availability of vitamin C is the same even while synthesized (Mangels et al., 1993).

Fermented drinks like wines, teas, ciders, herbal infusions, and cocoa add nutritious tannins to the diet at a daily intake of 0.1–0.5 g (Serrano et al., 2009). Polyphenolic compounds mainly derive from plant beverages and dried fruits that add antioxidant, antimicrobial, and anti-inflammatory properties (Fabbrini et al., 2022). Whole red grape juice containing seeds, pulp, and skin is most affluent with resveratrol and flavonoids being potent antioxidants that display anticancer and therapeutic activities for numerous diseases (Aubert & Chalot, 2018). However, the nature and utility of grape juice remain dependent upon numerous variables like the type of grapes used (variety), methods of growth (conventional or organic or biodynamic), and geographic location. Research on these juices analyzing the quantitative and qualitative aspects of the presence of chemical constituents like phenolic compounds has reportedly generated substantial variations affecting their substantial activity under in vitro and in vivo analyses (Granato et al., 2016). In this way, these fermented juices and plant beverages act as excellent carriers of active molecules contributing toward preventive health care and managing chronic diseases (Angelino et al., 2020).

TFBs are considered functional foods that promote various physiological functions, enhance health, and improve quality of life; they may also contribute to the reduction of chronic disease risks. Studies conducted in all continents have established clear connections between fermented foods and beverages and their resident beneficial microorganisms with various health benefits. These include potential weight management, the prevention of CVD, and antidiabetic properties, including improvement in glucose and lipid profiles and reduction in the risk of T2D (McGovern et al., 2004). In a placebo-controlled trial where prehypertensive patients consumed milk fermented with Lactococcus lactis NRRL B-50,571, there was a significant reduction in SBP, DBP, triglycerides, total cholesterol, and LDLs as compared to controls (Beltrán-Barrientos et al., 2018). More importantly, fermented foods and beverages have been inversely related to all-cause mortality (McGovern et al., 2004). Health properties exerted by TFB are mainly attributed to the presence of both prebiotics and probiotics, which regulate immune response, metabolic activity, body composition, and blood pressure (Xiang et al., 2019). TFB may have other potential benefits on brain health promotion through stress reduction and improvement of memory and also reduce the risk of anxiety disorders, depression, and behavioral changes.

1.4 Classification of beverages

As depicted in Fig. 1.1 below, the beverage market consists of two types of categories: “alcoholic” and “non-alcoholic drinks.” The non-alcoholic drinks market consists of juices, bottled water, “still drinks,” and Carbonated Soft Drinks (CSDs). The CSD market is defined as “carbonated drinks made with pure water, sugar, and natural flavorings.” The idea of adding carbon dioxide in drinks lies in the “inspiration derived from naturally carbonated mineral waters.” This innovation dates back to the 18th century by a man named Jacob Schweppe, who developed the world’s first CSD, establishing the

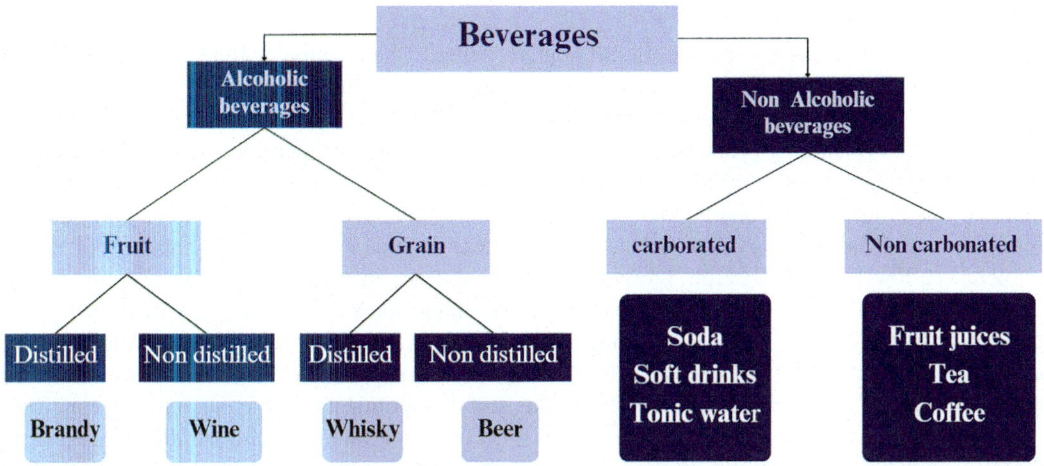

FIGURE 1.1

Classification of beverages.

Redrawn from Vasudevan and Chengaiyan, 2024 Copyright Jeevitha Gada Chengaiyan et al.

Schweppes Company in the process (Ashurst, 2016, pp. 1–405). Still drinks include fruit nectars, flavored waters, non-alcoholic beers, and ready-to-drink (RTD) teas and coffees. Juices refer to packaged beverages containing 100% fruit or vegetable juice, such as orange, apple, pineapple, grape, and blended smoothies. Bottled water is produced for direct human consumption and is classified into natural mineral water, spring water, and other drinking waters in the industrial context (Aadil et al., 2019).

1.4.1 Fruit and vegetable-based beverages

Fruits are essential parts of the human diet. A fruit-based beverage is a non-fermented beverage made by combining sugar, water, fruit, and additions that can be consumed straight. When compared to synthetic beverages, natural beverages have superior nutritional and antioxidant qualities. Astringency and bitterness limit the usage of some fruits with high nutritional content. Blending two or more fruit and vegetable juices in the right mix to make RTS beverages is the greatest substitute for this. According to a number of studies, combining fruits improves their flavor, aroma, taste, nutritional value, and shelf life (Bhardwaj & Pandey, 2011). As an alternative to pasteurization, other processing techniques including as high hydrostatic pressure, high intensity pulse electric field, and ultrasound have been developed with encouraging outcomes. Fruits are characterized by high sugar content and thus are a raw material particularly suitable for alcoholic fermentation and other fermentations, such as acetic or lactic fermentation. Numerous examples can be mentioned for both alcoholic and non-alcoholic fermented fruit-based beverages, such as vinegar, fruit beer, water kefir, cider, wine (both conventional wine and wines from fruits other than grape) (Laureys et al., 2014).

1.4.2 Dairy-based beverages

The market for dairy-based beverages is still relatively small when compared to the sales of plain milk and yogurt, and the market for functional dairy beverages is dominated by dairy products that contain probiotics and/or prebiotics. Whey-based beverages (both fruit juice-type and dairy-type) and fortified dairy beverages (including probiotics, prebiotics, fibers, polyphenols, peptides, sterol/stanols, minerals, vitamins, and fish oil) are the two main categories into which functional dairy beverages can be divided. Restoring gut microbiota balance is best achieved by consuming probiotic bacteria through food products (Macfarlane & Macfarlane, 2003). These include reducing the symptoms of lactose intolerance, lowering cholesterol, preventing intestinal tract infections, preventing colon cancer, controlling rotavirus, preventing Helicobacter pylori-related ulcers, improving the immune system, preventing irritable bowel syndrome, curing antibiotic-associated diarrhea, and preventing hypertension (Park & Chen, 2009; Reid et al., 2003) The survival of probiotic bacteria in fermented milk depends critically on the choice of probiotic strains and the optimization of manufacturing conditions (both formulation qualities and storage conditions) (Martínez-Villaluenga et al., 2006; Saarela et al., 2003). Commercially, probiotic drinks made from fruit juice, cereal items and daily dosage dairy drinks have gained popularity in recent years. Customers can now choose from a large variety of probiotic products on the market (Hilliam, 2004, pp. 52–54) Fig. 1.2.

1.4.3 Plant based beverages

Plant-based fermented beverages are generally beverages with nutritional value developed by fermenting plant-based raw materials with lactobacillus or yeast. Plant-based fermented beverages are generally considered as nutritious and sustainable functional drinks, which can be used as substitutes for milk and other dairy products (Das & Deka, 2012). Cereals like rice, wheat, and millet are staple foods rich in nutrients and have health benefits, especially when fermented. Fermentation enhances their nutritional value and supports the growth of probiotics. Grain-based fermented beverages are gaining popularity due to health trends. The beverage industry in North America has taken advantage of this opportunity and developed a series of nutritious, healthy and natural functional beverages. Among them, plant-based beverages is regarded as the backbone to drive the market development and competitiveness (Yang & Dharmasena, 2021). Most consumers are influenced by the main selection criteria in terms of consumption behavior, and pay attention to the sensory acceptance of plant-based beverages. Therefore, how to improve the nutrition and flavor of plant-based drinks is an urgent problem to be solved in the beverage industry. Studies have shown that fermentation has been used by the beverage industry to improve the taste, flavor, and functional properties of products (Cardinali et al. 2021) used 23 strains of lactic acid bacteria as fermentation agents to ferment specially formulated cereals and pseudo-cereal substrates, found that the nutritional components of the beverage fermented by compound strains were richer, and its biological development value was significantly increased.

1.4.4 Alcoholic beverages

The oldest and most significant technological advancement is the use of yeast to produce alcoholic beverages from fermentable carbon sources. All alcoholic beverages are produced using yeast, and

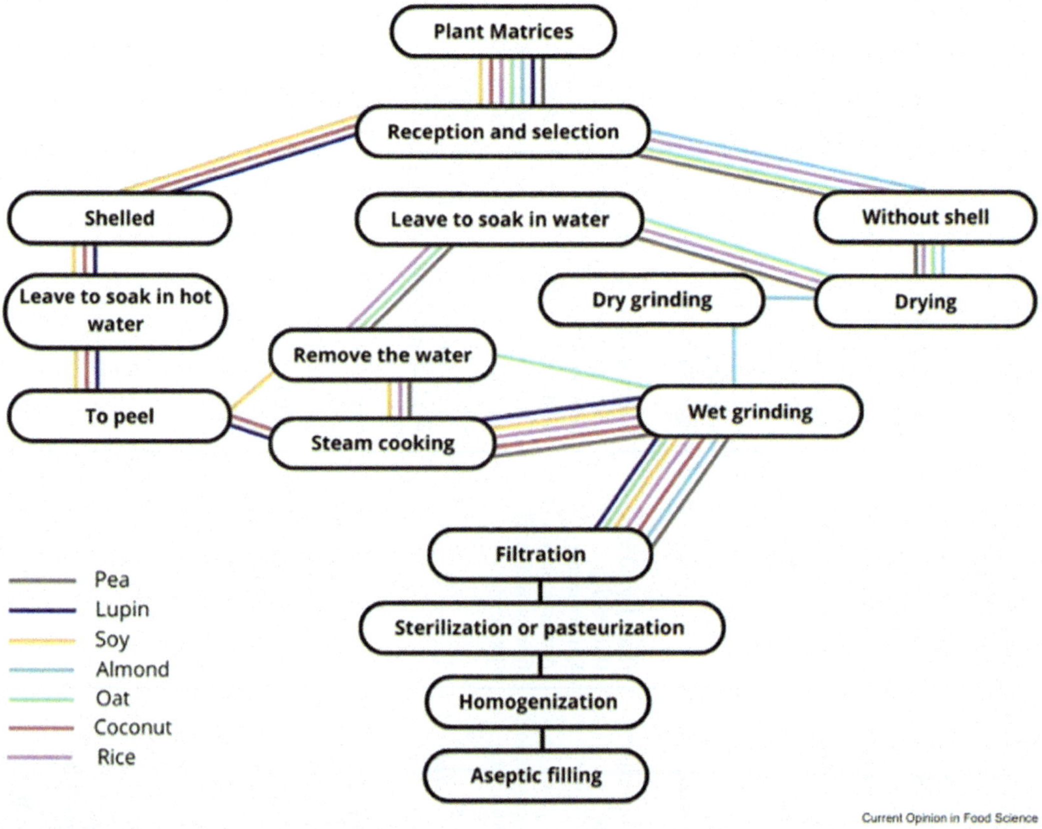

FIGURE 1.2

Steps involved in the preparation of plant-based beverages.

Reproduced with the permission from Marafon et al. (2025), Copyright 2025, Elsevier.

choosing the right strains of yeast is crucial for maintaining the sensory quality of the final product as well as maximizing alcohol yield.

Saccharomyces cerevisiae is the yeast species that is most commonly used in the manufacturing of alcoholic drinks globally, and the specific strains of this species that are used in fermentation have a significant impact on the flavor and fragrance qualities of various beverages (Walker et al., 2019, pp. 477–512). In addition to having beneficial health effects (such as preventing cardiovascular disease, having antiaging or antioxidant qualities, and promoting bone formation), alcoholic beverages also include important nutrients (such as nitric oxide, resveratrol, and other polyphenolic substances). Alcoholic beverages are widely acknowledged to be microbiologically safe because of their low pH (4.5) and high ethanol content (0.4%) (Kourtis & Arvanitoyannis, 2007). According to Menz et al. (2010) *Salmonella typhimurium* and *Escherichia coli* can develop during the first 24 h of fermentation of hopped wart, a semi beer product, and they can survive for up to 60 h Table 1.1.

Table 1.1 Microbial safety challenges and preservation approaches in beverages.

Beverages	Main microbial risk		Source of contamination	Typical preservation method	References
(Fruit beverages)	(Bacteria)	*E. coli strains (especially O157:H7, known for low infective doses and acid tolerance) and Salmonella (associated with poor hygiene and acid-tolerant serovars)*	(Soil is the main source for Alicyclobacillus and heat-resistant Molds) (Fecal contamination)	Pasteurization (e.g., 74°C/16 s), High Hydrostatic Pressure (HHP) (effective against vegetative cells), Pulsed Electric Fields (PEF) (effective against pathogens, often combined with mild heat), UV radiation/Gamma-ray irradiation (effective against pathogens)	Murphy et al. (2006); Mosqueda-Melgar et al. (2008); Lima Tribst et al. (2009)
	(Protozoa & Mycotoxins)	*C. parvum (highly infectious), C. cayetanensis (resistant to disinfectants).* *Patulin (in apple juice) and Ochratoxin A (in grape juice) are the most important fruit juice-associated mycotoxins*			
(Vegetable beverages)	(Gram-negative bacteria associated with vegetable soft rot)	(vegetable soft rot - Pseudomonas, Enterobacteriaceae such as Pectobacterium) (Alicyclobacillus spoilage – associated with off flavors production in over in 78% of juice processors)	(Raw Ingredients) (Processing Environment) Airborne Spores of filamentous fungi (like molds)	Thermal Pasteurization (Heat treatment is typically between 75 and 90 °C or higher for 25–30 s) Electro plasmolysis (effective destruction of the cell membrane matrix using high electric current. Applied to apple and carrot tissue).	Toropilová and Bystricky (2015); The European Parliament and the Council (2004a)
	Heat Resistant Molds (HRM)	*(Paecilomyces Byssochlamys, Aspergillus - primarily associated with visual defect)*			
(Dairy beverages)	(Bacterial Pathogens)	*Listeria monocytogenes (Major concern for ready-to-eat (RTE) dairy like soft cheeses and ice cream)* *Escherichia coli* (e.g., *O157:H7 STEC) - raw milk and cheeses made from raw milk.* *Coxiella burnetii - Pasteurization parameters* (e.g., *72°C for 15s in the UK) are designed to inactivate this organism.*	(Fecal contamination from animal; improper human handling; post-pasteurization environmental contamination)	Pasteurization (72°C for 15 s). Ultra-High Temperature (UHT) processing and sterilization used for specific products.	Cerf and Condron (2006); Nwakoby et al. (2025)
	(Yeasts and Molds)	*(Penicillium, Mucor, Candida - spoilage in yogurt, sour cream, and cheese – off flavors)* *Mycotoxins* (e.g., *Aflatoxin M1) - Aspergillus* spp			

• (Plant based beverages) • (Cereal beverages) • (Fruit & vegetable beverages) • (Cereal beverages, by-product beverages)	(Bacterial Spore-formers) Heat Resistant Molds (HRM)	(*Alicyclobacillus*, Enterobacteriaceae, *Lactobacillus*) *(Molds like Paecilomyces/ Byssochlamys)*	Contamination can arise from the raw ingredients and processing environment (e.g., bottling/filling areas) and packaging	Thermal destruction (pasteurization), High-pressure processing technique effectively inhibited lipoxygenase and trypsin activities. (Enzymatic Digestion: Improves efficiency, viscosity, and quality) Fermentation: Use of active strains (lactobacillus or yeast) is intended to improve taste, flavor, and functional properties	Munekata et al. (2020)
(Alcoholic beverages)	(Pathogenic Bacteria) Coliforms (Indicator of sanitation quality) *Bacillus cereus (Spore-former)*	*(E. coli, Salmonella, Listeria) LAB account for 60% to 70% of beer spoilage incidents)*	Raw materials contain abundant sugars and starches (nutrients for bacteria), and fermentation temperature (18–35°C) is favorable for bacterial growth.	Pasteurization (e.g., beer sterilized by heating to 71–75°C, yakju heating to 65°C for 30 min). Filtration (e.g., beer filtration using membranes with 0.2–0.5 mm pore size). Identifying critical control points (CCPs) is necessary to identify persistent organism like Bacillus cereus.	Bartowsky et al. (2003); Jeon et al. (2015); Torres-Guardado et al. (2022)
(Non-alcoholic fermented beverages)	(Acetic Acid Bacteria) (Yeasts and Off-Flavors) (Molds and Mycotoxins)	*(Acetobacter liquefaciens Acetobacter hansenii, Acetobacter pasteurianus, and Alcaligenes)* (*Pichia* spp) (Molds such as Rhizopus stolonifer, Aspergillus flavus, and Aspergillus niger)	(Raw materials, utensils, and tap water used during the mixing process)	Fermentation: Use of active strains (lactobacillus or yeast) is intended to improve taste, flavor, and functional properties. (Antimicrobial-Producing Strains: LAB generates antibiotics and bacteriocins that inhibit spoilage and pathogenic microorganisms)	Baschali et al. (2017); Mashau et al. (2021)

1.5 Processing and preservation method

1.5.1 Thermal processing

Thermal processing inactivates the enzymes that cause spoiling and eliminates pathogenic and spoiling microorganisms from foods and beverages, it has long been one of the most widely used and authorized techniques for preventing foodborne illnesses and guaranteeing food safety. The combination of treatment duration and temperature determines the heat treatment's intensity (Soni et al., 2022).

1.5.1.1 Traditional thermal pasteurization

The most popular method for pasteurizing fruit juices and other liquids is thermal processing. A 5-log decrease of the most resistant bacteria of public health importance is the foundation of juice pasteurization Various combinations of temperature and time could be used to complete the procedure.

Low temperature long time (LTLT): According to D'Amico et al. (2006), fruit juice has historically been pasteurized by batch heating it to 63–65°C for a considerable amount of time. Because of the unfavorable quality changes that occur during this process, high temperature short-term treatment has taken place of this approach.

High temperature short time (HTST): Because HTST treatment takes a lot shorter time to complete, it may minimize the unwanted quality changes caused by batch heating. The most popular technique for heat treating fruit juice at the moment is HTST pasteurization. For instance, HIST processes orange juice for 15–30 s at 90–95°C. Additionally, HTST treats apple juice for 25–30 s at 77–88°C (Charles-Rodríguez et al., 2007).

1.5.2 Non thermal processing

Temperature is not the primary role in the inactivation of microbes and enzymes in non-thermal preservation technologies, although a little rise in temperature may occur during the treatment (Barba et al., 2018, pp. 1–315). Consequently, there are less quality-degradative processes that can occur during heat processing (Barba et al., 2014). High-pressure homogenization (HPH), ultraviolet (UV) irradiation, pulsed electric fields (PEF) processing, and high-pressure processing (HPP) are some of the most promising new non-thermal methods to increase shelf life (Barba et al., 2014).

1.5.2.1 Pulsed electric field

Pulsed electric field processing (PEF) applies short bursts of high voltage electricity for microbial inactivation and causes no or minimum effect on food quality attributes. Briefly, PEF is a legitimate technology for producing high-value, safe beverage products (Dubey et al., 2023). Biological membranes permeabilize as a result of PEF pulse application. After being exposed to an electric field, cells' plasma membranes become permeable to tiny molecules. This permeability causes swelling and ultimately ruptures the cell membrane, which lowers or eliminates the microbial load (Bevilacqua et al., 2018). *Zygosaccharomyces bacilli* (MTCC 257) was reduced by 5.1 logarithmic units in amla juice, whereas ascorbic acid and antioxidant capacity were retained by 63% and 88.9%, respectively, according to Bansal et al. (2015). The native microbiota in the coconut water-nanori blended beverage was decreased by 3 log CFU/mL (Rethinam & Krishnakumar, 2022) Additionally Mosqueda-Melgar et al. (2012), mentioned that the PEF-treated samples had a 120-day shelf life at 27–30 °C. Pear juice's naturally existing microorganisms were completely inactivated without affecting the juice's sensory qualities. Up to 93% of the initial peroxidase activity (POD) in carrot juice was found by Vorobiev and Lebovka (2020). PEF effect decreased about 26.92% and 20.93% polygalacturonase in a juice blend including whole or skim milk. PEF inactivated POD and lipoxygenase (LOX) by 17.5%–29% and 34%–39%, respectively, in a juice blend containing soymilk (Morales-de la Peña et al., 2018).

1.5.2.2 High hydrostatic pressure

Many juices, such as apple, orange, asparagus pomegranate, strawberry, mango and pomegranate have shown that HHP is an effective technology for extending their shelf life (Bevilacqua et al., 2018). The following variables affect how microbes react to high pressures: While Gram-positive bacteria are the most resistant and their spores need extremely high pressures to be inactivated, Molds and yeasts are the most susceptible microorganisms. Gram-negative bacteria are mediumly sensitive. In general, challenges arise when spoilage enzymes in juices are inactivated since enzyme sensitivity varies depending on the type of product. In general, challenges arise when spoilage enzymes in juices are inactivated since enzyme sensitivity varies depending on the type of product (Chakraborty et al., 2015). However Martínez-Villaluenga et al. (2006), confirmed that Pectin Methyl Esterase PME in apple juice can be inactivated by HHP treatment under the right circumstances. Pressure may cause partial or full unfolding of the enzyme's native structure, which can be either irreversible or reversible.

1.5.2.3 Ultrasound processing

Recent years have seen the introduction of ultrasonic processing, a new technique in the food business that not only lowers the quantity of microorganisms but also minimizes product loss and prevents quality degradation (Dolas et al., 2019). The typical frequency range for ultrasound sterilizing is 20–100 kHz. Ultrasound's cavity impact has the potential to sterilize plant-based beverages by causing damage to the cell walls of microorganisms and producing free radicals (Abid et al., 2013).

Ultrasound's cavitation effect alters intracellular micro dynamics and disturbs intracellular constituents, which in turn prevents or deactivates the cell's enzymes. The beverage's utilization of ultrasonic sterilization Research is still being conducted by industry. Ultrasound has been demonstrated to lower harmful germs in fruit and vegetable juices, including carrot juice and citrus juice Compared to conventional thermal processing, ultrasonic processing has been shown to increase beverage shelf life and lower processing costs, resulting in a 16% and 55% reduction in processing temperature and time, respectively (Koshani et al., 2015).

1.6 Safety challenges in beverage production

1.6.1 Microbial safety concerns (pathogens, spoilage organisms)

Spoilage in beverages refers to the metabolic processes caused by microorganisms that make the drink undesirable or unsafe for human consumption (Nychas & Panagou, 2011, pp. 3–28). This is because deterioration leads to changes in the sensory attributes of the drink, for instance, changes to appearance, aroma, and taste (Stratford, 2006). The microbial contamination of soft drinks is normally carried out during processing, with possible causes being raw materials, factory environment conditions, equipment and packaging cleanliness, as well as poor sanitation procedures (Mbuagbaw & Noorduyn, 2012). Soft drinks as well as alcoholic drinks remain highly consumed despite being susceptible to microbial contamination as well as pathogens that might result in health risks to the population. It is imperative to have an understanding of microorganisms present, conditions favorable for their development, as well as control mechanisms needed for ensuring quality (Shankar et al., 2021).

For soft drinks, the main concern microbes are associated with the fermentation of sugars into ethanol and the production of carbon dioxide that results in swelling/rupture of bottles. Yeast species like Zygosaccharomyces, Saccharomyces, and Pichia ferment sugars into ethanol and carbon dioxide (resulting in swelling/rupture of bottles) and give rise to off-flavors. Though less prevalent because they are aerobic microbes, acetic acid bacteria (AAB) like Acetobacter and Gluconobacter generate off-flavors, hazes, and swelling of packages, especially so if the package material permits the diffusion of oxygen (Bartowsky et al., 2003). Aspergillus and Penicillium species of molds can also contaminate soft drinks and generate off-flavors, hazes, and potential production of toxic mycotoxins (Boeira et al., 1999). For the production of alcoholic drinks, the major concern microbes are associated with the fermentation of sugars in the drink into ethanol and the production of off-flavors like volatile phenols and the development of turbidity. *Saccharomycodes ludwigii* is known for its resistance to sulfites, while *Dekkera/Brettanomyces* species can produce mousy flavors (Malfeito-Ferreira et al., 2009, pp. 615–645). Lactic acid bacteria (LAB), such as *Lactobacillus* and *Pediococcus*, can lead to spoilage, causing ropiness, bitterness and off-flavors like diacetyl and volatile phenols (Jarvis, 2003; Ibarburu et al., 2010). Acetic acid bacteria (AAB), including *Gluconobacter* and *Acetobacter*, can oxidize ethanol to acetic acid, resulting in a vinegar-like flavor, often referred to as "cider sickness" (Shankar et al., 2021).

A number of methods, such as using tainted raw materials during harvest and cleaning water from processing equipment can contaminate fruit and vegetable juices with microorganisms or harmful bacteria. This could result in foodborne illnesses (Huang et al., 2015). Notable pathogenic microorganisms that cause outbreaks associated to juice include *Salmonella* spp. and *Escherichia coli* O157: H7. *Salmonellaenterica* serovar Typhimurium, *E. coli* O157:H7, *Cryptosporidium parvum, and Campylobacter jejuni* have all been implicated in foodborne infections due to unpasteurized apple juice and cider in the US and Canada. Additionally, *Salmonella enteritidis* from orange, grape and lemonade juices and *Salmonella* spp. from homemade watermelon juice were documented in the United States in 1993 (Raybaudi-Massilia et al., 2009).

Maintaining the safety and quality of beverages demands an efficient monitoring protocol. Prevention relies on strict hygiene, cleanliness of equipment and sanitation. Some heat-resistant spores may still remain present; however, pasteurization destroys the majority of microorganisms (Stratford, 2006; Park & Chen, 2009). Preservative chemicals such as sorbates, benzoates and DMDC are commonly used to prevent microbial growth. Filtration and altered packing of the atmosphere, apart from increasing CO_2 levels, reduce the probability of the presence of microorganisms, particularly fungi (Shankar et al., 2021). Safety procedures are further strengthened by putting HACCP and GMP frameworks into practice (Sikora, 2005, pp. 41–48). The use of natural antimicrobials, such as plant extracts and essential oils, to reduce spoilage organisms is one of the emerging trends in beverage preservation (Shankar et al., 2021). Additionally, because of their synergistic benefits and capacity to minimize the usage of individual agents, combination preservation systems which combine various preservation techniques such low pH, preservatives, and modified atmosphere are gaining popularity. Better detection techniques are also crucial because they assist preserve product safety by accurately and quickly identifying infections and spoiling organisms. Manufacturers can preserve the quality of their beverages and secure the public's health by comprehending microbiological dangers and putting these management methods into place.

1.6.2 Chemical safety concerns

Chemical contamination in food refers to the presence of different classes of contaminants in food, such as veterinary drugs and pesticides used in agriculture, acrylamides used in processing, mycotoxins that form during storage, environmental pollutants like dioxins, inorganic contaminants, processing contaminants and packaging migrants. Everything, including tools, containers and packaging, that is intended to come into touch with food. Although humans can be exposed to many dangerous substances through their diet. The effects are usually less obvious than those brought on by biological threats. Even though chemical-induced acute toxicity is now very rare, chronic exposure to low levels of dangerous chemicals through diet is quite problematic because of their ability to cause cancer, mutagenesis and teratogenicity. The exposure can also result in chronic sickness (Borchers et al., 2010; Lawley et al., 2012).

1.6.2.1 Migrants from packaging

Food contact material (FCM) are any items or materials such as equipment, containers, and packaging that are meant to come into contact with food. An FCM should be inert and not cause the addition of chemical compounds to the food (Magnuson et al., 2013). According to Bach et al. (2012) there have been reports of chemical migration in polyethylene terephthalate (PET)bottled water. Although their origin is unclear, plasticizers, formaldehyde, acetaldehyde, and antimony are linked to migration from PET into bottled water. The chemicals may originate from recycled PET bottles, background contamination, cap-sealing resins, PET containers, and water processing procedures. After exposing bottled fluids to sunshine for 2–10 days, it was discovered that the kind of water affected migration (Bach et al., 2014). Also, phthalates and (Bis Phenol A) BPA are always concerning compounds that may leach into foods through containers.

1.6.2.2 Food additives

Benzene can occur in vitamin C drinks as a result of the reaction between benzoic acid and ascorbic acid (vitamin C) (Ju et al., 2008). Fresh palm wine naturally contains ascorbic acid (Priti & Paul, 2016), and plant material might contain benzoic acid at any stage of the winemaking process. This gives both substances the chance to mix and create benzene, which may be harmful to human health. Further research is necessary to determine the precise source of benzene in palm wine. An analysis of more than 100 samples of soft drinks and other beverages, with an emphasis on those that contain ascorbic or erythorbic acid in addition to benzoate salts, according to research conducted in the US (NTP—National Toxicology Program, 2014). Additionally, it was stated that the producers had reformulated these high-benzene items, and after a retest, samples of the reformulated products revealed that the levels of benzene were below 1 ppb. Because benzoates are frequently used as preservatives, the amount of benzene in bottled and canned goods matters. If the levels are discovered to be higher than permissible criteria, corrective measures ought to be implemented (Nwaiwu & Itumoh, 2017).

1.6.2.3 Heavy metals

Heavy metals may also be present in drinking water at amounts higher than those that make the water unsafe to drink. Elements weighing four to five times the water's weight are considered heavy metals. Because of their toxicity and biological buildup, heavy metals like lead, chromium, and cadmium are harmful to humans (Fakhri et al., 2015). Lead, chromium, and cadmium have maximum allowable limits of 0.01, 0.05, and 0.003 mg/L, respectively (WHO, 2011; ZABS, 2000). The neurological, circulatory, digestive and other bodily systems are physiologically impacted by elevated heavy metal concentrations (Priti & Paul, 2016). Over time, lead and cadmium build up in soft tissues and bone as strong neurotoxins that can cause cancer. Chromium targets the iron- and two-oxoglutarate-dependent dioxygenase family enzymes and other histone modifying enzymes to mediate the toxicity and carcinogenicity (Chervona et al., 2012). Even though packaged water is believed to be one of the safest sources of water, if it is unsafe, it can cause water-borne diseases.

1.6.3 Physical hazards

Physical hazards are extraneous materials or foreign substances that are not typically present in food products and can harm, sicken, or traumatize those who consume them (Aladjadjiyan, 2006). When physical contaminants like glass, metal, or plastic are present in food goods, consumers may suffer severe injuries or health risks (Alamri et al., 2021). From sourcing raw materials to processing, packaging, and distribution, these risks can arise at any point in the food manufacturing and supply chain (Mahalik, 2014; Pettoello-Mantovani et al., 2021). Injury brought on by these items is seen right away or shortly after food consumption, and the causes of the issue are readily apparent. Some of these ingredients have the potential to seriously harm the consumer's health, including asphyxiation, internal bleeding, discomfort in the throat, dysphagia, regurgitation, death, and damage to the teeth and oral cavity (European Commission, 2015; Waltzman, 2006).

From September 2012 to December 2016, a total of 515 consumer complaints about the presence of physical hazards in dairy products were gathered from the website Reclame Aqui (www.reclameaqui.com.br). The most common complaints were about a foreign object (42.4%), followed by insects (23.3%), hair (15.2%), plastic (11.1%), metal (6.2%), and fabric (1.8%). When there is broken glass in the product, there is a risk of harm to the consumer. These complaints can be caused by broken bulbs in the milking environment or by damaged pressure or temperature gauges used in the industrial process (Le et al., 2014).They may also originate from glass drinking milk marketing containers that sustain damage during handling or processing (cleaning or filling). Complaints listed on the website related to insects, including flies, cockroach fragments, ants, and larvae constitute up to 23 percent. In addition to potentially causing biological contamination, food contamination by insects can result in choking and customer suffocation because these insects can transport pathogens like *Salmonella* and *E. coli*, among others (Aguiar et al., 2018). Filtration makes it simple to get rid of tiny insects when milk is being received. Dirt, including hair, on the finished product is a sign that fundamental hygiene standards have not been fulfilled. Metal objects are regarded as physical hazards with a high potential for seriousness since they might result in injuries such lacerations to the mouth and throat (Oslen, 1998). For the elimination of metals inadvertently present in dairy products, magnets or milk powder sieving can be effective substitutes (Maja & Sharareh, 2017). Since easy opening lids are frequently made of plastic, the presence of plastic components in the finished dairy product accounted for 11.1% of 515 complaints. This could be related to packaging. Additionally, UHT milk comes in plastic bottles (van Asselt et al., 2017). The goods with the most complaints were UHT milk and yogurt or milk drinks, suggesting that the choice of chemicals employed for flavoring and foreign object removal may have been flawed (Ashurst et al., 2017).

1.6.4 Key factors influencing beverage safety: Water quality, raw material handling and production environment

The effectiveness of a beverage manufacturing system is closely linked to the effectiveness of its quality management system (QMS), encompassing factors such as the quality of raw materials, processing layout, equipment standards, health of workers, ambience in which product is prepared. Failure to meet any of these aspects can lead to consumer rejection of the products. Beverages are often recalled due to food safety issues, including packaging contamination risks, microbial outbreaks, and deteriorative product characteristics like unpleasant tastes and odors, or textural irregularities. Some of the factors are.

1.6.4.1 Water

Conventional soft drinks comprise 90% water. Traces of several ions are present in drinking water which changes the flavor. Softened water is typically used by soft drink manufacturers to avoid off-tastes from chlorine residues (Ashurst et al., 2017). Soft drink water should meet the physical, chemical, and microbiological standards for drinking water in accordance with the World Health Organization (WHO), US Environmental Protection Agency (EPA), and European Directive EC 98/1983. Regulation's criteria also apply to the creation of ice that comes into contact with food. Drinking water must be the source of the ice. It needs to be produced and kept in storage in a way that prevents contamination of any kind (Juvonen et al., 2011).

1.6.4.2 Raw material

A food industry cannot accept a raw material, ingredient, or other item used in food processing if it is or likely will be contaminated with parasites, pathogenic microbes, toxins, etc., even if the appropriate procedures are followed. Even after sorting and other processing steps, the final product will not be suitable for human consumption. The quality of the juice is mostly determined by the quality of its ingredients or raw materials, which include fruits, water, sugars, flavors, additions, preservatives, etc. High-grade raw fruits that are unharmed or contaminated are necessary for the manufacturing of premium quality products. These must be clear of any pathogenic microorganisms that could jeopardize the product's ultimate quality and safety, such as yeast, mold, or other microbial hazards (Ashurst et al., 2017). As soon as raw fruits are received at a juice plant, the fruit skins are cleaned with chlorinated water to remove surface microbes and disinfect the fruit. To get rid of dirt and other contaminants, cleaning chemicals then thoroughly rinse the fruits with clean water. Additionally, fruit extract or before making juices or smoothies, pulp needs to be sterilized. Quality of the water have to be filtered, neutralized, disinfected, and cold lime soft. Certain chemicals used in juices have been shown to be harmful to health because they contain radioactive materials, heavy metals, or mycotoxin strains.

The visual qualities of tea are mostly used to assess its quality because it should be devoid of any obvious materials like fiber, soil, stones, and stalks. Raw tea leaves are cleaned of foreign contaminants using magnetic separators and screening or sifting devices. Tea dust is also promptly removed from the production area using dust extractors. Because of its low water activity, tea is a shelf-stable product; yet, because of its unsanitary handling, packing, and storage practices, it is susceptible to bacterial or mold attack. It has been claimed that *A. acidiphilus, A. acidoterrestris, A. herbarius, and A. pomorum* cause tea and herbal teas to spoil (Cladière et al., 2018; Goto et al., 2003; Matsubara et al., 2002).

1.6.4.3 Premise sanitation

Sanitary areas and facilities must adhere to the same general standards as other types of properties. A sufficient number of clean restrooms with an effective sewage system should be available at food enterprise locations. Food preparation areas cannot be directly connected to restrooms. It is necessary to keep hand washing basins and food washing stands apart (Regulation (EC) No 852/2004 of the European Parliament and of the Council of April 29, 2004). Floor construction materials should make cleaning and disinfection simple, if needed. It's also important to maintain the walls' technical integrity so that they may be easily cleaned and disinfected when needed. The way windows and other openings are constructed must avoid allowing dirt to collect. Insect-repellent mesh must be installed on windows that can be opened. The mesh must to be simple to clean and disassemble.

Other surfaces in food handling rooms, such as gadget surfaces and particularly surfaces in contact with food, need to be in good shape and simple to clean and sanitize. Once more, materials that are nontoxic, washable, and resistant to corrosion must be used ("Regulation (EC) No 852/2004 of the European Parliament and of the Council of April 29, 2004"). Equipment in touch with food should be cleaned and disinfected as needed to reduce the risk of contamination, in compliance with the guidelines in Chapter 5 of Annex II to Regulation (EC) No. 852/2004. The design and materials used to manufacture equipment that comes into direct contact with food, as well as its technical state, must not raise the possibility of food contamination and must enable precise cleaning and disinfection as required.

1.6.4.4 Equipment sanitation

Fruit juices attract a range of microorganisms because they are a rich source of nutrients and important components. To guarantee the safety of the finished product, 99% of germs must be removed from equipment surfaces and contact areas by meticulous monitoring of sanitary operations. Hygienic conditions are crucial in a tea processing facility because any neglect in this area would result in bacterial infections and tea tainting, which will lower the quality of the product. In order to hygiene production, the tea business has implemented several hygienic measures, such as using potassium permanganate to clean floors and other surfaces that come into contact. Cleaning tools and equipment is crucial because failing to do so would result in a bacterial harbor.

Generally, alcoholic drinks possess low pH values and attract harmful bacteria in a restricted manner. Among other causes, poor equipment and area cleaning to remove germs to form biofilms may weaken the quality parameters of the drinks and eventually compromise product safety (Horsáková et al., 2009). Among the quality issues that may relate to the production of wines, it is essential to mention soil deposits that will change the wine's texture and sensory characteristics.

This soil deposition in storage tanks is accelerated during wine fermentation and may become a site for the attraction of microorganisms. Thus, besides the other hygienic operations, the removal of dirt is one of the most important steps. Cleaning followed by disinfection of the processing location and touch sites regularly will avoid the collection of biofilms.

All equipment and utensils coming in direct contact with the product, the milk delivery vehicles, and the storage tanks should be cleaned properly before receiving milk. The routine visual inspections of tanks and evaluation of their cleaning performance have to be documented or tracked.

The quality of the equipment is another important matter as it may contain foreign particles or even harmful bacteria, which may degrade the quality of the finished product. A quality management group should, therefore ensure that all the equipment and other materials coming into direct contact with the product, like the bottle, packaging containers, jars etc. are sterilized. Non-returnable bottles, or caps should be cleaned using an adequate cleaning agent before use, and the main packaging material of the product has to be sterile (Aadil et al., 2019).

1.6.4.5 Personal hygiene

It is important to ensure that personal hygiene is maintained by individuals participating in food handling to avoid contamination. The use of gloves and masks by employees is also important during food preparation. The establishment should be equipped with equipment necessary for the determination of individual body temperatures (Ridho et al., 2022). It should be noted that anyone who may cause direct or indirect contamination of food products, such as people suffering from wounds, skin conditions, ulcers, diarrhea, or other communicable diseases, should not be allowed in food processing rooms. Food establishment employees should inform management of their conditions in the event of an illness or its symptoms (Błaszczyk, 2020).

1.6.4.6 Production environment

Clean air inside work environments must also be kept clean, together with the use of harmless and appropriate disinfectants and agents for cleaning. The use of clean water and energy must also be done effectively and responsibly. Waste and wastewater must then be properly treated, hygienically and environmentally (Ridho et al., 2022).

Beverages, being sources of essential nutrients, at the same time provide a favorable environment for the growth of microorganisms associated with food spoilage like molds, yeast, and bacterial growth. Various extrinsic (Relative humidity, temperature, package type, storage and transport conditions, general environment) and intrinsic (pH value, water activity value, presence of nutrients, antimicrobial activity, food physical characteristics) factors influence the growth of these microbes. According to Nychas et al. (2008) and Pothakos et al. (2014). Inhibition of microbial growth may be achieved through the incorporation of antimicrobial compounds, packaging materials that minimize contact with microorganisms, non-thermal processes such as high-pressure processing, heat-based processes such as pasteurization and sterilization, and bio-preservatives. Such approaches are geared toward increasing the shelf life and safety of beverage products. In 2016, Tamime et al. stated that in the food and beverage sector, temperature management is a basic technique for managing microorganisms. This includes controlling the temperature at various points in the production chain, including handling and processing settings. Any breach in hygiene might affect the quality of the final product, hence cleanliness is crucial in tea manufacturing facilities. As lower humidity levels can promote fungal infection, maintaining humidity levels above 90% is essential to preventing such deterioration (Aadil et al., 2019). In dairy farms, raw milk is conveyed in cans or tankers and stored in cold storage tanks ($<10°C$), the environment of the storage affects the population of mesophilic bacteria, which dramatically increase both with time and temperature, causing milk spoilage. In dairy farms, in order to maintain the quality of milk, it is cooled below 6°C as soon as possible after collection which increases the shelf life by about 1–2 days. This highlights the significance of a hygienic processing environment in ensuring and enhancing the quality of the final product (Aadil et al., 2019).

1.6.4.7 Training

In India, the FSSAI's FoSTaC program aims to strengthen food safety by training Food Safety Supervisors (FSS). Licensed food businesses must appoint one certified FSS per 25 food handlers. These supervisors promote hygiene, good manufacturing practices, and internal training. In the EU, Regulation (EC) 852/2004 (Chapter 12) mandates food hygiene training for all food industry workers, which can be formal or informal, depending on job roles. Training must be job-specific and designed based on the company's needs and employee skills. Proper training is crucial across the entire food chain from procurement to delivery to ensure awareness of hazards, hygiene, CCPs, and protocols for monitoring, documentation, and corrective actions. Tailored training improves food quality, such as in raw milk production, by addressing contamination risks and hygienic practices (Dzwolak, 2014; Murphy, 2013).

1.7 Regulatory and ethical considerations

The beverage market functions in a highly regulated environment governed by international, regional, and national standards. Such standards are critical in ensuring the safety of beverages and maintaining a positive relationship with consumers. International standards such as ISO 22,000 and Codex Alimentarius offer a basic requirement for food safety and quality management systems, including HACCP (ISO, 2023; FAO/WHO, 2020). National agencies such as the FDA in the US, EFSA in Europe, and Health Canada ensure compliance with standards and regulations through legislations dealing with labeling, additives, and traceability.

Regulation (EC) No 852/2004 states that appropriate conditions must be guaranteed in regard to storing food in a manner that inhibits spoilage. In this case, the regulation highlights that ensuring food quality preservation is, in theory, impossible and depends entirely on the type of food. In this regard, one can say that despite providing appropriate conditions, food can only be kept safe and fresh for a specific period of time. In this case, this regulation highlights that food must be protected throughout the course of production, processing, distribution, and storing (The European Parliament and the Council, 2004a). Another area that is extremely important in consideration is food labeling regulation. For example, EU Regulation (EU) 1169/2011 has made it compulsory to list allergens and nutritional values openly, and in the US, beverage packaging is required under FDA guidelines regarding health claims and nutrition transparency (European Commission, 2021; FDA, 2023).

From an ethical perspective, the drink industry is facing ever more demands concerning safety but also social and environmental accountability. Such issues that relate to the ethicality of the industry include transparency in production procedures, the treatment of employees, and less harm toward the environment via sustainable packages and waste materials (Haseli et al., 2024). Government agencies, for instance, in Chile and Mexico, have established restrictions on front-of-package marketing that relate to the ever-rising concern of health among the public, especially about obesity and alcohol-related risks (WHO, 2021; Taillie et al., 2020). For the industry to remain responsible, there is a connection between government restrictions and ethicality.

1.7.1 Overview of international and regional regulations

Many nations across the world have issued guidelines to ensure that liquids are safe for consumption and labeled properly (WHO, 2021).Internationally, bodies such as World Health Organization (WHO) and Codex Alimentarius have issued basic food hygiene and food safety guidelines (FAO/WHO, 2020). ISO 22,000 is one key international regulation to ensure food safety and hygiene at a production level (ISO, 2023). ISO 22,000 functions alongside other systems such as ISO 9001 to provide enhanced food quality and food safety (ISO, 2023). In the European Union, Regulation (EU) 2019/787 deals with the definition, labeling, and packaging guidelines for alcohol-containing liquids such as spirits. A generic regulation called Regulation (EC) No 178/2002 is entirely equipped to ensure that food is always safe and traced within all EU member states (European Commission, 2002). In the United States, the FDA regulates the labeling guidelines of non-alcoholic beverages (FDA, 2023). On the regulation of alcohol-containing liquids such as beer and liquor, the alcohol-containing liquids are supervised by the FDA's sister department called Alcohol and Tobacco Tax and Trade Bureau which also regulates labeling requirements including the definition of "alcohol-free" (TTB, 2023). In Canada, the Canadian Food Inspection Agency (CFIA, 2023) regulates the labeling requirements for food including liquids. There are guidelines on the labeling requirements for labeling "alcohol-free". In Asia, China has adopted National Food Safety Standards (GB/GB-T) as a means of regulating quality and beverage safety (NHC China, 2023). On the other hand, countries such as Australia and New Zealand make laws on allergens, residues of chemicals, and microbes found in beverages (FSANZ, 2023). Some Latin American countries, such as Mexico and Chile, have gone further by adding sugar taxes and putting warning labels on sugary drinks to reduce health risks (Taillie et al., 2020). Even though these laws differ from place to place, they all work toward the same goal-keeping beverages safe for people to drink (WHO, 2021).

1.7.2 Codex regulations

There's a surge in beverage consumption worldwide and thus enforcing legislations to become stringent with beverage manufacturers to ensure safe consumption and fair, smoother trade within countries. Food and Agriculture Organization (FAO) and the World Health Organization (WHO) collectively formed Codex Alimentarius Commission (CAC) in 1962, which adopted the Codex Alimentarius or "Food Code" comprising of standards and guidelines (Mukherjee et al., 2022). It is noteworthy that soft drinks and non-carbonated beverages do not yet have any published Codex standards. However, food hygiene is covered in the Codex Recommended International Code of Practice General Principles of Food Hygiene, which is applicable to the production of soft drinks, for instance (Dransfield, 1999).

Several guidelines for fruit juices, concentrated fruit juices, and nectars have been released by the Codex Alimentarius Commission. Products like tomato juice and nectars like apricot, pear, and peach are covered by these requirements. In 1989, general guidelines for fruit nectars and juices that weren't covered by specific guidelines were released. These standards are comprehensive and include product definitions, important composition and quality criteria, regulations concerning food additives, pollutants, cleanliness, container fill weights, and certain labeling requirements. They also cover methods of analysis and sampling (Dransfield, 1999). Fruit juices, fruit nectars, fruit purée, and mixed fruit juices, nectars, and purées must be labeled as "concentrated" if the product is made by physically removing water from the fruit juice in an amount that raises the Brix level to a value at least 50% higher than the Brix value established for reconstituted juice from the same fruit. When concentrated fruit juice, concentrated fruit purée, concentrated fruit nectar, or mixed concentrated fruit juice/nectar/purée must be reconstituted before being consumed as fruit juice, fruit purée, fruit nectar, or mixed fruit juices/nectars/purées, the label must include the necessary instructions for reconstitution on a volume/volume basis with water to the applicable Brix value in the Annex for reconstituted juice. The current FAD/WHO Codex Alimentarius limit for iron in orange juice is 15 mg/kg (Southgaten et al., 1995). In 1992, the various standards for fruit juices and nectars were re-issued in Volume six of the new Codex Alimentarius format (Dransfield, 1999). The fourth edition of the Codex Alimentarius Standard for Fermented Milks (CXS 243–2003), released in 2018, outlines uniform guidelines for several fermented or cultured dairy products, including acidophilus milk, kefir, and kumys (koumiss). The Codex Standard also specifies a minimum of 10^7 colony forming units (CFU)/g of starter culture and 10^6 CFU/g of microorganisms mentioned as viable bacteria for both sterilized and non-sterilized fermented milks (in labeling) (Mukherjee et al., 2022).

1.7.3 Ethical considerations: Clean label claims, sustainability, and transparency

Modern consumers want more than a guarantee that beverages will not harm them; they seek beverages that can appeal to their values, as shown in the modern trend of clean label beverages. These products are inspired by simplicity, using natural ingredients and excluding artificial additives and synthesized chemicals. For example (Inguglia et al., 2023), say, "The clean label concept generally refers to formulated products whose declared ingredients are either traditionally consumed or perceived as less processed, without known side effects, thus highlighting a lack of synthetic preservatives, colourants, and flavor enhancers." However, there is no specific universal definition for the term "clean label," meaning this consumer understanding may differ. Transparency about ingredients and sourcing builds trust, while the words "organic," "non-GMO," and "no added sugar" make up the three most influential terms on store shelves today, according to Grande C. Consumers are increasingly opting for "free from" products-additives such as cleaner labels that boast functional ingredients like vitamins and prebiotics for additional health benefits. Many said they would pay more for clean label products, particularly if claims are backed by trusted or official sources. Beverages have the highest price premium, with an average of $3.50 for clean label versions, compared to a conventional $2.00-which highlights a 75% increase in price–as the value of an offering in this space at a premium positioning.

The other major ethical focus in the beverage industry regards sustainability. Nowadays, companies are expected to reduce waste, utilize eco-friendly packaging, and lower their carbon footprint. Sustainability labels, which also may include carbon footprint or eco-certification, are on the rise. The approach of these labels, however, is to assist consumers in making choices that are better for the environment. In practice, third-party certifications, such as Fair Trade and organic labels, commonly help support the ethical or sustainability claims of companies. Evidence indicates that many shoppers do not read or act on these labels. There is crystal clear evidence, however, that people will pay more for items that show sustainable and ethical practices, assuming the information provided to them comes from a trusted source or from government-backed sources. Clean label and sustainability claim also act as marketing tools. While they raise brand appeal, there's growing concern about "greenwashing" that is, when claims go beyond genuine practice which can erode consumer trust if exposed.

This study showed how using biodegradable or recyclable materials and managing the return through some kind of incentive or recycling programs helps to reduce pollution. Another way in which beverage makers are taking more sustainable approaches involves circular supply chains, in which waste is reused or transformed into useful products.

Transparency binds it all together. A very central consumer trend in the food and beverage market today is an increasing preference for natural, barely processed goods, amidst escalating consumer needs linked to transparency, simplicity, and sustainability. People now expect companies to be fully accountable for their supply chains and to communicate about them openly in ways that are honest and socially responsible (Kovalchuk, 2024). Ethical brands share where it comes from, how it was made, and the impact on people and the planet quite upfront. This openness builds consumer loyalty and holds companies accountable for their actions (Innova Market Insights. (2025). In a nutshell, clean labels, sustainability, and transparency are not just marketing trends but are becoming core expectations in ethical beverage production (Haseli et al., 2024).

1.7.4 Navigating certifications and compliance

When it comes to beverage manufacturing, food safety is not merely an issue involving hygiene but also requires an organized system to secure safety before it becomes an issue. To ensure this, one such system used is the HACCP system. Even with HACCP, though, this system does not include the management and record-keeping needed for modern supply chains currently used throughout the global food industry. To incorporate all these factors, the broader food safety management system ISO 22,000 is used instead. ISO 22,000 essentially incorporates an important system that uses HACCP with management system elements such as risk management, traceability, and document organization (https://www.dnv.com). Another part of ISO 22,000 could include prerequisite program (PRP) and operational prerequisite program (OPRP) concepts, both relating to the management of production environment conditions (Baurina & Amirova, 2021). Certifications essentially help the beverage industry prove its products are safe, of high quality, and meet food safety standards. A standard such as ISO 22,000:2018 provides an organizational way for managing food safety risks throughout the food manufacturing process (Rihawi, 2024). This will help companies with ISO 22,000 enhance their performance, fight contamination, and build customer trust. ISO 22,000 implementation not only increases safety controls but will aid companies with better market access, especially for companies exporting beverages (Karaman, 2014).

However, research indicates that organizations that implement ISO 22,000 enjoy the overall advantage of enhanced production control, reduced safety occurrences, and enhanced adherence to national and international legislations—mainly within the food/beverage industry, where it is critical to maintain consistency. In addition to adhering to international requirements, food organizations must comply with their country's food laws and legislations. In the Indian setting, for example, the Food Safety and Standards Authority of India (FSSAI) dictates that every food business, including those that produce beverages, must abide by the food law, which states Food Safety and Standards Act, 2006, and theFood Safety and Standards (Licensing and Registration of Food Businesses) Regulations, 2011 (FSSAI). To facilitate enhanced adherence to these requirements, FSSAI initiated the implementation of the Food Safety Training and Certification (FoSTaC), a systematic level of training for food handlers ranging from basic, advanced, to specialized (FSSAI). Under this scheme, food business operators are expected to engage a minimum of one certified Food Safety Supervisor (FSS) for every 25 food handlers to oversee the adherence to hygiene and food safety processes within the organization (FSSAI). In conformity with the scheme, FoSTaC TRAINING is anchored to the hygiene standards listed within Schedule four of the regulation, which includes notions of good manufacturing practice (GMP), good hygiene practices (GHP), and sanitation (FSSAI). The FoSTaC Training is obligatory for particular food business operators to ensure that their staff members are equipped with the knowledge to handle food safely, especially when engaged in beverage processing (FSSAI, 2023).

Further expanding on this point, many organizations choose to follow FSSC 22,000, which is in essence an upgraded version of ISO 22,000. This standard takes into account industry-specific criteria such as the handling of allergens, the protection from food fraud, and the development of food defensive plans. Furthermore, FSSC 22,000 is approved by the Global Food Safety Initiative (GFSI), which explains its widespread acceptance by those organizations seeking to market their products internationally (FSSC Foundation). The current version of FSSC 22,000, Version 6, came out in April 2024 and emphasizes tougher guidelines on issues such as the maintenance of equipment in organizations, the traceability of raw materials sourcing, and even unannounced audits (SGS, 2024).

For organizations that have already been certified in ISO 22,000, transitioning into FSSC 22,000 is relatively easy. For example, Danone's beverage company in China found transitioning into FSSC 22,000 quite easy with only a minor glitch in their first FSSC audit (Danone China, 2021). In Brazil, packaging firms that have employed FSSC 22,000 have not only improved their food safety management but have become more competitive, have greater employee knowledge, and have a good public image (Cantanhede et al., 2018). These national trainings and certification standards have been made in accordance with various standards across the globe, such as ISO 22,000:2018, a globally accepted Food Safety Management System that is based on hazard analysis and critical control points (HACCP) (Karaman, 2014). Organizations' activities have also been inspected and checked by national regulatory bodies such as FSSAI, FDA, and EFSA in relation to whether they act in accordance with food legislation. Organizations must act in accordance with both FoSTaC and ISO 22,000 if they are in the beverage industry, ensuring they remain compliant with food safety legislation and thus retaining a good public image and ensuring safe food is offered (FSSAI; Karaman, 2014). Not acting in accordance with these rules and standards means organizations can pay fines or have their operating licenses withdrawn. In these organizations, acting in accordance with these food safety and standards rules means investing in employee education and safety system update (Nyarugwe et al., 2020). In recent times, organizations have been encouraged to ensure their food safety standards and certification fit well with their objectives of sustainability. Many organizations in the beverage industry have employed Circular Supply Chain Management together with standards like FSSC 22,000. By doing this, waste is reduced but no safety or quality is reduced (Haseli et al., 2024). In conclusion, these standards such as HACCP, ISO 22,000, and FSSC 22,000 are not optional but have become useful tools in organizations and firms for being compliant with these rules and standards and for obtaining public acceptance and loyalty in organizations in these various sectors (Baurina & Amirova, 2021).

1.8 Practices for safe beverage production

1.8.1 GMP

The World Health Organization approximates that food contamination makes 600 million individuals sick and kills 420,000 annually (WHO, 2022). Workers, machinery, raw materials, processing, and the environment affect food safety, with the majority of foodborne disease resulting from preventable errors (Uçar et al., 2016). Good Manufacturing Practices (GMP) are meant to manage these factors through high-quality and safe foods and drinks (De Oliveira et al., 2016, pp. 129–139). GMP offers good practices for controlling conditions for operations in food plants based on four pillars: exclusion, removal, inhibition, and destruction of contaminants (Bagchi, 2014, pp. 1–549; De Oliveira et al., 2016, pp. 129–139). Successful execution is dependent on training employees, management, motivation, resources, and communication, which result in safer products, cleaner facilities, increased productivity, reduced complaints, and enhanced working conditions (da Cruz et al., 2006). First adopted in 1969 by Codex Alimentarius in its 'General Principles of Food Hygiene' and then revised in 1997, 2003, and 2020, GMP is a response to developments in science and technology (Sikora, 2015; FAO, 2021). Optional in most countries, GMP is compulsory in the US, Japan, and EU as the basis of HACCP (Farid et al., 2019; Karnieli, 2016, pp. 141–160). Despite this, the cost and complexity of adoption are hurdles to compliance for small, medium enterprises (SMEs), leading to low compliance and increased risks of foodborne illness (Dzwolak, 2019; Sun & Wang, 2019). Noncompliance is even greater in low- and middle-income countries (Munasinghe et al., 2015; Nyokabi et al., 2021), where SMEs are over 90% of the food industry have difficulties in complying with requirements, compromising competitiveness, constraining market access, and posing a threat to food security by elevating dependence on imports (Baregheh et al., 2012; Hasnan & Mohd Ramli, 2020).

The FDA regulates GMP in food, drugs, devices, and supplements, and in the manufacture of food, it provides support for safe global production (Błaszczyk, 2020). Existing GMPs, documented in Title 21 U S. Code of Federal Regulations (CFR) Part 110, specify 10 fundamental rules such as documentation, validation, facility design and cleaning, employee expertise, contamination avoidance and audit (Kołożyn-Krajewska & Sikora, 2010). Repeated offenses include poor sanitary design (85%), poor hygiene (55%), poor documentation (55%), poor cleaning (50%), poor training (35%) and poor worker health control (15%).

Many people in Ghana are starting their own businesses to produce locally manufactured traditional beverages like "Sobolo" which is made from dried calyces of the bissap plant.

(*Hibiscus sabdariffa*) and "Asaana" a drink made from fermented corn and sweetened with sugar to taste, as a result of their growing popularity (Aboagye et al., 2020). There are worries that these suppliers produce the drinks in unsanitary conditions and with inferior raw ingredients and contaminated water, thereby endangering the product's as well as consumers safety (Musah et al., 2014). Additionally, some "Sobolo" and "Asaana" sellers sell their drinks to customers packaged in polythene bags and used drinking water bottles. As these contaminated beverage products put consumers at risk of bacterial infection, leading to potentially fatal food-borne diseases like salmonellosis and typhoid, it is important to apply the standardized HACCP approach in processing these products so as to guarantee "Sobolo" and "Asaana" products' safety and quality standards for the consumer. For health safety, methods such as washing raw materials, heating water to 100°C, sanitizing equipment, personal hygiene, and processing beverage products in an enclosed environment are recommended (Aboagye et al., 2020). Finally, "the implementation of GMP is performed according to the diagnosis, PDCA road map planning, re-evaluation, and correction of nonconformities, driven by inspection and checklist activities, with priorities based on company resources" (Costa Dias et al., 2012).

1.8.2 GHP

Good Hygienic Practices (GHP) guarantee the production of food and beverages in a clean environment free from contamination risk, including the cleaning of equipment, proper use of clean water, disposal of waste, and hygiene practices like hand washing and protective clothing (FAO). Regulation (EC) 852/2004 Annex II lays down the minimum mandatory hygienic standards for all food businesses within the European Union and serves as the basis offood safety management. GHP keeps contaminants from entering or propagating at any point during manufacturing and is the backbone of food safety schemes (FAO, 2009). Two of the most important GHP-based interventions in food factories are ensuring hand hygiene, which avoids cross-contamination of cooked and raw food (Uçar et al., 2016) and the provision of personal protective equipment (PPE) in the form of hair covers, gloves, protective garments and masks to ensure hygienic food production facilities (Chen et al., 2025). Research indicates that the bigger food companies in Poland have more GHP/GMP regulation awareness than smaller companies; for example, 75% of beverage companies use GMP/GHPsystems, with very high compliance for personal hygiene (83%), disinfection practices (91%–100%) and medical examination of employees (100%) (Konecka-Matyjek et al., 2005). Food handlers control food safety directly through personal cleanliness and thus education and training are important despite the fact that mobile and street vendors lack formal training in many cases (FAO, 2009).

According to Regulation (EC) 852/2004, hygiene levels also cover buildings, facilities, and storage. Food premises need to be supplied with sufficient workspace, pest harborage prevention, and processing and storage under appropriate temperatures (Błaszczyk, 2020). Measures include sanitary sewage systems, toilets separate from food preparation areas, changing rooms, secure storage of cleaning chemicals, and workspaces in compliance with GHP requirements. Surfaces and equipment must be nontoxic, washable, corrosion-resistant, and easy to disinfect, while water and ice used in food production must be potable. Workers with infectious diseases or symptoms such as diarrhea, ulcers or skin infections must report to supervisors to avoid contamination risks (Błaszczyk, 2020). Food enterprises should also practice proper storage to avoid spoilage, keep raw materials separate from finished goods, and mark unfit food and keep it away. Packaging materials should be reusable, simple to sterilize, and safe for food contact. Staff supervision and food hygiene training are also required by regulation, which can be in the form of formal courses, in-workplace instruction, or in-house training (European Commission, 2012). Training must be tailored to workers' jobs and skill levels, HACCP principles, and all phases of the production continuum from raw material receipt to the final product delivery (Martins et al., 2012; European Commission, 2012).

1.8.3 HACCP

Hazard Analysis and Critical Control Point (HACCP) is a form of anticipatory process control system aimed to secure food and consumers from chemical, physical, and biological risks by identifying, or controlling, critical control points (CCPs) systematically. Employed globally as the.

"Standard for food safety management, there has been verification that it is effective in preventing and controlling" hazards (Wang et al., 2024). HACCP works through implementing control measures at points of production where "The health risk is most likely to emerge." Food enterprises are required to set up prerequisite programs. Such programs will help in controlling health risks (PRPs) such as Good Manufacturing Practices (GMP) and Sanitation Standard Operating Procedures (SSOP) values before using a system (Stanley et al., 2011; Toropilová and Bystricky, 2015) The regulation (EC) 852/2004 stipulates that procedures in the HACCP system should follow principles must be specific for all food business's products & processes & revised according to new technology in order to avoid new risks (Błaszczyk, 2020). The seven fundamental principles of HACCP are hazard analysis, CCP identification, establishing critical limits, monitoring, corrective action, verification and documentation (Regulation (EC) 852/2004). Implementation is a matter of managerial dedication, employee training, and multidisciplinary action to guarantee the safe identification and control of hazards (De Oliveira et al., 2016, pp. 129–139).

Field applications of HACCP in the beverage sector show its indispensable contribution to food safety. Some examples of CCPs are pasteurization, sterilization, distillation, filtration, and the use of sifters or magnets to remove contaminants (Trafiałek et al., 2015). Special studies illustrate its applicability: in "Traven," a nettle-infused fermented drink, CCPs were found in raw material preparation, wort production, fermentation, filtration, and packaging (Krukovich & Masanskiy, 2018). Likewise, Soy-kununzaki, Nigerian traditional drink, showed CCPs at soaking, milling, fermentation and packaging for concerns of microbial growth and physical impurities (Nahemiah et al., 2014). In beer and wine making, CCPs occur during raw material inspection, fermentation, filtration, packaging and sanitizing equipment (Kourtis & Arvanitoyannis, 2001), whereas in soft drinks and juices, water treatment, washing fruits, pasteurization, and hygienic filling are critical (Kourtis & Arvanitoyannis, 2001). In coffee milk drinks, risks encompass acrylamide production in roasting, metal contamination upon grinding, and microbiological risk, all regulated by roasting temperature, pasteurization, homogenization, packaging cleanliness, and cold-chain storage (Wang et al., 2024).

Every CCP must have evidence-based critical limits, which separate acceptable from not acceptable conditions according to measurable parameters like time, temperature, pH, water activity, and additive levels (Mortimore & Wallace, 2013; Stanley et al., 2011). For instance, EU rules place upper limits on Ochratoxin A (2.0 μg/kg for wine), patulin (50 μg/kg for juices), inorganic tin (100 mg/kg for canned drinks), and lead (0.15–0.20 mg/kg for wines and products thereof) (Regulation (EC) 1881/2006; (Błaszczyk, 2020). CCPs are kept under control through monitoring, with corrections when deviations occur, such as in coffee milk production, which involves roasting, sterilization, metal detectors, and packaging to required standards (Wang et al., 2024). Validations of system functions ensure that everything works as expected, and records confirm traceability for required compliance, such as risk analysis, CCPs, monitoring, corrective actions, and audits (Dzwolak, 2014; Stanley et al., 2011); (Commission Notice on FSMS, 2016). However, implementation might be hindered through constraints such as ignorance, resistance to change, and inequal implementation. To mitigate such challenges, there should be maintenance techniques and systems supported and led by top management with a push for continuous education and assistance. This includes staff education and practice sessions periodically and checking periodically for continued success (Oluwasegun Uzoigwe & Kongolo, 2024).

1.8.4 Cleaning and sanitation

"Sanitation lays the basis for beverage and food safety in food and beverage facilities," starting with proper procedures and attention to cleanliness and sanitization (Marriott & Gravani, 2006). "Cleaning involves the removal of visible soil, grease, and oxidative soil," making surfaces clean to the eye, in contrast to sanitizing surfaces to be "free from most harmful bacteria and spoilage microorganisms"

(Marriott & Gravani, 2006). Proper sanitation should "reduce or eliminate" microbial contaminants with little to no "effect upon product quality or consumer safety" (Pan et al., 2006). Involvement and commitment of the highest management level are necessary because "consumer safety and product quality can be compromised if sanitation and proper handling practices are not followed," potentially leading to "name and product recalls and consequent lawsuits and loss of public image and brand recognition" (Marriott & Gravani, 2006). "International food safety laws require a food safety system to be compatible with the principles of HACCP," and as such, "the need to sanitize becomes a fact and a responsibility" (Błaszczyk, 2020) for facilities globally to ensure compliance with proper food safety standards and prevent any eventual "adverse effects on consumer safety" (Marriott & Gravani, 2006). In pursuing a proper and workable sanitation program for the dairy and beverage industry facility's continuous goal of preventing microbial contamination as a necessary aspect of ensuring proper product quality and public safety through proper storage and preparation techniques in its facilities and respective procedures for continuous "reduction or elimination of microbial contamination with little to no effect upon product quality or consumer safety" (Pan et al., 2006) in its facilities through clean in place and clean out-of-place technology and procedures in pursuit of proper sanitation in any facility to benefit public safety as well as product and facility well-being in terms of continuous microbial and product contamination prevention and elimination. For a workable and continuous sanitation program to be accomplished in its facilities to benefit public safety as well as product and facility well-being in terms of microbial and product contamination prevention and elimination through clean in place and clean out-of-place technology and procedures in pursuit of proper sanitation in.

CIP is very effective in closed food processing systems with vessels, pumps, valves, and pipes, where fluid movement provides adequate shear force to remove soil and microorganisms, thus preventing surface reinfection, especially on previously sanitized surfaces (Tomas & Tiwari, 2013). Biofilms usually accumulate on joints, gaskets, and other crevices, where the design may be protective against excessive flow forces, making calculations on biofilm formation relatively more conservative in complex pipes. To resist contaminants, food-growing crops usually utilize detergents like NaOH solution, together with an acid, while chemical sanitizers like chlorine are very effective, acting by interfering with biological membranes, as well as blocking enzymes crucial for metabolism (Tomas & Tiwari, 2013). From a processing point of view, the CIP sequence would require a pre-rinse to remove all debris, followed by caustic detergent washing, followed by an intermediate or second final rinse, an optional step with an acid solution to flush out mineral residues, sanitize by means of heat or chemicals, with final rinses to leave residues asymptotic (Alembong, 2024). They require tremendous monitoring observations on their performance. Their effectiveness is noted by means of on-stream bulk analysis (e.g., flow, pressure, temperature, conductivity, pH), on-stream surface analysis, and microbiological analysis like bio-proving swabs, analysis of water rinses, or most rapid bioluminic methods (ATP bioluminiscing) (Lodolo, 2020).

1.9 Challenges and opportunities

The food and beverage service industry is a dynamic industry because it is usually associated with a rapidly changing environment shaped by consumer attitudes and behaviors. The study of consumer behavior allows companies to tailor their offerings, promotional strategy, and service formats to better fit the changing needs of their target market. This essay reviews the key drivers of consumer behavior affecting the food and beverage sector and reviews the impact these drivers have upon management strategy. Demographic characteristics including age, gender, level of income, education, and lifestyle are essential to determine consumer behavior in this particular industry (Mavrogiannis et al., 2008). The beverage sector makes an important contribution to the environmental issues of the world such as plastics, water, and carbon pollution. With the world facing the depletion of natural resources, the sector has reached a crossroads, playing an increasingly important role in environmental agendas. Innovation in food and beverage management plays an important role in promoting sustainable growth in organizations and helping to address consumer needs. By making use of the current trends and some approaches, organizations can manage difficulties and make the most of innovation opportunities despite the risks. However, along with opportunities, innovation brings some risks of complexity in risk management, resource issues, and cultural changes (Bowden, 2008).

"Sustainability practices have become more and more imperative in the food & beverage industry because of the immense pressure being received from the industry to address concerns pertaining to the environment, society, and economics." The food & beverage industry has started focusing on sustainability due to certain global issues that have emerged in front of the industry in terms of the environment, climate change, and social inequality (Mavrogiannis et al., 2008). "Sustainability refers to a combination of social responsibility, environmental stewardship, and economic viability. This refers to the triple bottom line approach—managing for People & Planet & Profit." Organizations are following sustainable practices in order to fulfill their social responsibility toward society & the environment & the economy & to derive innovation & competitive advantages. But following sustainable practices in the industry is challenging due to the complex legal framework & operational issues.

The management of the beverage industry focuses on the integration of profit, the planet, and people because it is under the triple bottom line concept. The sustainability of the industry is a result of government regulations, consumer demands, investor demands, and the need to mitigate the risk of climate change. Organizations can adopt green approaches because of government legislations on the matter, meet the demands of ethical consumers, and attract investors who consider ESG factors. Sustainability increases the resilience of organizations as it minimizes the use of scarce resources. Climate change and resource scarcity accelerate the green revolution of the industry. The sustainability of the industry increases the reputation of the business.

Issues pertaining to the environment, across the global beverages sector, can be very complex and are interconnected. This necessitates an integrated approach.

Triple Bottom Line Approach in Focus: The beverage industry has to be based on an approach that considers profit, people, and planet simultaneously.

Promote Green Innovation: The industry should actively engage in research and developments of green innovations such as recyclable materials, environmentally friendly production processes, and green product offerings.

Improve Green Supply Chains: It is important to adopt a supply chain process that is more sustainability-focused through ethical procurement, efficient logistics, and environmentally conscious distribution.

Advancement in Reverse Logistics: Effective systems for return, reuse, and recycling of items will be established to decrease any wastage of resources.

Implement Circular Economy Practices: Circular economy practices can help reduce wastage and allow for more optimal use of resources throughout the entire product life cycle. (George, 2024)

Optimal use of the production process with a broader, more encompassing perspective means following proactive, preventive, environmentally responsible measures focused on minimizing water, emissions, and wastage—and ultimately, the overall sustainability of the production process. On a general perspective, the implementation of Cleaner Production (CP) practices in the food and beverage sector can potentially result in a 35% cost savings strategy. As the environmentally responsible market is growing at an ever-increasing rate, it is increasingly important for businesses to follow CP practices, as per their requirements, in order to be able to successfully compete in a market where environmental responsibility is set on the critical balance scale (Espinosa et al., 2021).

In order to cater to the rising requirements from both consumers and retailers, medium-scale food production companies must spend on new product development. The demand pattern for products keeps fluctuating; thus, innovation and movement beyond existing products become critical. One of the most important factors is whether or not a product is useful to both markets and production companies. Pricing is a critical aspect that must be considered from a consumer perspective in order for good value to be offered. Protection of production margins must also be ensured from a company perspective. Cost knowledge is critical in ensuring accurate product pricing and contributing toward maintaining production margins. Enterprise Resource Planning is a major aspect in new product launches. Enterprise Resource Planning, with its inherent processes and functionality with a user-friendly interface, helps optimize these processes.

1.10 Conclusion

The beverage industry is a dynamic sector in the global food system, integrating science, technology, culture, and safety as a way of delivering products that can meet both consumer needs and societal expectations. Besides ingredients and equipment, beverage manufacture encompasses sourcing of raw materials, processing, preservation, and safety systems and regulatory compliance. Good practices such as pasteurization, fermentation, and carbonation, and frameworks for safety like GMP, GHP, SOPs, and HACCP ensure quality and hygiene. Food safety remains central; microbial, chemical, and physical hazards demand strict sanitation, high-quality raw materials, trained staff, and innovative technologies such as high-pressure processing and pulsed electric fields. At the same time, consumer demand for healthier, low-sugar, natural, plant-based, and functional beverages is driving the industry toward change, while expectations around clean labels, traceability, sustainable packaging, and ethical sourcing are also high. Adherence to global and national standards-Iso 22,000, Codex, FSSAI, among others-reinforces safety and builds trust. Sustainability, fair trade, and labeling truthfulness stresses the ethical responsibility of producers. In essence, success in the beverage sector calls for striking a balance between innovation, safety, health trends, and social responsibility. Thus, the beverage industry represents one unique intersection: tradition with innovation, regulation with creativity, responsibility with opportunity. As the beverage sector keeps growing, it must do so under firm commitment to safety, scientific integrity, and social responsibility. The future of beverages is not just about creating new flavors or functional ingredients but about producing goods that are safe, transparent, ethical, and green. It is this holistic approach which will characterize the next generation of beverage science, shaping a healthy and more sustainable food future.

References

Aadil, R. M., Madni, G. M., Roobab, U., Ur Rahman, U., & Zeng, X. A. (2019). *Quality control in beverage production: An overview quality control in the beverage industry: Volume 17: The science of beverages* (pp. 1–38). Pakistan: Elsevier, Pakistan Elsevier. https://doi.org/10.1016/B978-0-12-816681-9.00001-1. Available from: http://www.sciencedirect.com/science/book/9780128166819.

Abid, M., Jabbar, S., Wu, T., Hashim, M. M., Hu, B., Lei, S., Zhang, X., & Zeng, X. (2013). Effect of ultrasound on different quality parameters of apple juice. *Ultrasonics Sonochemistry, 20*(5), 1182–1187. https://doi.org/10.1016/j.ultsonch.2013.02.010

Aboagye, G., Gbolonyo-Cass, S., Korley Kortei, N., & Annan, T. (2020). Microbial evaluation and some proposed good manufacturing practices of locally prepared malted corn drink ("asaana") and Hibiscus sabdarifa calyxes extract ("sobolo") beverages sold at a university cafeteria in Ghana. *Scientific African, 8*, Article e00330. https://doi.org/10.1016/j.sciaf.2020.e00330

Aguiar, R. S., Esmerino, E. A., Rocha, R. S., Pimentel, T. C., Alvarenga, V. O., Freitas, M. Q., Silva, M. C., Sant'Ana, A. S., Silva, A. C. O., & Cruz, A. G. (2018). Physical hazards in dairy products: Incidence in a consumer complaint website in Brazil. *Food Control, 86*, 66–70. https://doi.org/10.1016/j.foodcont.2017.11.020

Aladjadjiyan, A. (2006). Physical hazards in the agri-food chain. In P. A. Luning, F. Devlieghere, & R. Verh_e (Eds.), *Safety in the agri-food chain* (p. 209e222). Wageningen: Wageningen Academic.

Alamri, M. S., Qasem, A. A. A., Mohamed, A. A., Hussain, S., Ibraheem, M. A., Shamlan, G., Alqah, H. A., & Qasha, A. S. (2021). Food packaging's materials: A food safety perspective. *Saudi Journal of Biological Sciences, 28*(8), 4490–4499. https://doi.org/10.1016/j.sjbs.2021.04.047

Alembong, H. A. (2024). *Clean-in-place processes for food and beverage industries using systems engineering principles*. University of Johannesburg (South Africa).

Altay, Ö., Aydın, Ö. K., Öner, H. B., Filiz, Ö., & Ertekin, F. K. (2025). Principles of distillation process. In *Mass transfer operations in the food industry* (pp. 45–81). https://doi.org/10.1016/B978-0-12-819536-9.00008-4

Angelino, D., Rosi, A., Vici, G., Russo, M. D., Pellegrini, N., & Martini, D. (2020). Nutritional quality of plant-based drinks sold in Italy: The food labelling of Italian products (FLIP) study. *Foods, 9*(5), 682. https://doi.org/10.3390/foods9050682

Ashurst, P., Hargitt, R., & Palmer, F. (2017). *Soft drink and fruit juice problems solved*. Oxford, UK: CRC Press, Woodhead Publishing.

Ashurst, P. R. (2007). *Fruit and juice processing chemistry and technology of soft drinks and fruit juices*. Wiley. https://doi.org/10.1002/9780470995822.ch3

Ashurst, P. R. (2016). *Chemistry and technology of soft drinks and fruit juices chemistry and technology of soft drinks and fruit juices*. United Kingdom: wiley. https://doi.org/10.1002/9781118634943

Aubert, C., & Chalot, G. (2018). Chemical composition, bioactive compounds, and volatiles of six table grape varieties (Vitis vinifera L.). *Food Chemistry, 240*, 524–533. https://doi.org/10.1016/j.foodchem.2017.07.152

Bach, C., Dauchy, X., Chagnon, M. C., & Etienne, S. (2012). Chemical compounds and toxicological assessments of drinking water stored in polyethylene terephthalate (PET) bottles: A source of controversy reviewed. *Water Research, 46*(3), 571–583. https://doi.org/10.1016/j.watres.2011.11.062

Bach, C., Dauchy, X., Severin, I., Munoz, J. F., Etienne, S., & Chagnon, M. C. (2014). Effect of sunlight exposure on the release of intentionally and/or non-intentionally added substances from polyethylene terephthalate (PET) bottles into water: Chemical analysis and in vitro toxicity. *Food Chemistry, 162*, 63–71. https://doi.org/10.1016/j.foodchem.2014.04.020

Bagchi, D. (2014). *Nutraceutical and functional food regulations in the United States and around the world: Second edition nutraceutical and functional food regulations in the United States and around the world: Second edition*. United States: Elsevier Inc. https://doi.org/10.1016/C2012-0-00335-3

Bansal, V., Sharma, A., Ghanshyam, C., Singla, M. L., & Kim, K. H. (2015). Influence of pulsed electric field and heat treatment on Emblica officinalis juice inoculated with Zygosaccharomyces bailii. *Food and Bioproducts Processing, 95*, 146–154. https://doi.org/10.1016/j.fbp.2015.05.005

Barba, F. J., Criado, M. N., Belda-Galbis, C. M., Esteve, M. J., & Rodrigo, D. (2014). Stevia rebaudiana Bertoni as a natural antioxidant/antimicrobial for high pressure processed fruit extract: Processing parameter optimization. *Food Chemistry, 148*, 261–267. https://doi.org/10.1016/j.foodchem.2013.10.048

Barba, F. J., SantAna, A. S., Orlien, V., & Koubaa, M. (2018). *Innovative technologies for food preservation: Inactivation of spoilage and pathogenic microorganisms innovative technologies for food preservation: Inactivation of spoilage and pathogenic microorganisms*. Spain: Elsevier. Available from: http://www.sciencedirect.com/book/9780128110317.

Baregheh, A., Rowley, J., Sambrook, S., & Davies, D. (2012). Innovation in food sector SMEs. *Journal of Small Business and Enterprise Development, 19*(2), 300–321. https://doi.org/10.1108/14626001211223919

Bartowsky, E. J., Xia, D., Gibson, R. L., Fleet, G. H., & Henschke, P. A. (2003). Spoilage of bottled red wine by acetic acid bacteria. *Letters in Applied Microbiology, 36*(5), 307–314. https://doi.org/10.1046/j.1472-765x.2003.01314.x

Baschali, A., Tsakalidou, E., Kyriacou, A., Karavasiloglou, N., & Matalas, A. L. (2017). Traditional low-alcoholic and non-alcoholic fermented beverages consumed in European countries: A neglected food group. *Nutrition Research Reviews, 30*(1), 1–24. https://doi.org/10.1017/S0954422416000202

Baurina, S. B., & Amirova, R. I. (2021). FSSC 22000 certification as a food security tool. *IOP Conference Series: Earth and Environmental Science, 666*(3), Article 032060. https://doi.org/10.1088/1755-1315/666/3/032060

Beltrán-Barrientos, L. M., González-Córdova, A. F., Hernández-Mendoza, A., Torres-Inguanzo, E. H., Astiazarán-García, H., Esparza-Romero, J., & Vallejo-Cordoba, B. (2018). Randomized double-blind controlled clinical trial of the blood pressure–lowering effect of fermented milk with Lactococcus lactis: A pilot study2. *Journal of Dairy Science, 101*(4), 2819–2825. https://doi.org/10.3168/jds.2017-13189

Bevilacqua, A., Petruzzi, L., Perricone, M., Speranza, B., Campaniello, D., Sinigaglia, M., & Corbo, M. R. (2018). Nonthermal technologies for fruit and vegetable juices and beverages: Overview and advances. *Comprehensive Reviews in Food Science and Food Safety, 17*(1), 2–62. https://doi.org/10.1111/1541-4337.12299

Bhardwaj, R. L., & Pandey, S. (2011). Juice blends-a way of utilization of under-utilized fruits, vegetables, and spices: A review. *Critical Reviews in Food Science and Nutrition, 51*(6), 563–570. https://doi.org/10.1080/10408391003710654

Binia, A., Jaeger, J., Hu, Y., Singh, A., & Zimmermann, D. (2015). Daily potassium intake and sodium-to-potassium ratio in the reduction of blood pressure: A meta-analysis of randomized controlled trials. *Journal of Hypertension, 33*(8), 1509–1520. https://doi.org/10.1097/HJH.0000000000000611

Błaszczyk, I. (2020). The management of food safety in beverage industry. In *Safety issues in beverage production* (pp. 1–38). Academic Press.

Boeira, L. S., Bryce, J. H., Stewart, G. G., & Flannigan, B. (1999). Inhibitory effect of fusarium mycotoxins on growth of brewing yeasts. 1 Zearalenone and Fumonisin B1*. *Journal of the Institute of Brewing, 105*(6), 366–375. https://doi.org/10.1002/j.2050-0416.1999.tb00027.x

Borchers, A., Teuber, S. S., Keen, C. L., & Gershwin, M. E. (2010). Food safety. *Clinical Reviews in Allergy and Immunology, 39*(2), 95–141. https://doi.org/10.1007/s12016-009-8176-4

Bowden, M. M. (2008). *An assessment of the world wine auction marketplace* (p. 432). UNLV Theses, Diss. Prof. Pap. Capstones.

Butu, M., & Rodino, S. (2019). Fruit and vegetable-based beverages—nutritional properties and health benefits. In A. M. Grumezescu, & A. M. Holban (Eds.), *Natural beverages* (pp. 303–338). Academic Press.

Cantanhede, V., Pereira, K. S., & Weingart Barreto, D. (2018). FSSC 22000 packaging implementation: A plastics industry research. *Polímeros, 28*(1), 38–43. https://doi.org/10.1590/0104-1428.06816

Cardinali, F., Osimani, A., Milanović, V., Garofalo, C., & Aquilanti, L. (2021). Innovative fermented beverages made with red rice, barley, and buckwheat. *Foods, 10*(3), 613. https://doi.org/10.3390/foods10030613

Cerf, O., & Condron, R. (2006). Coxiella burnetii and milk pasteurization: An early application of the precautionary principle? *Epidemiology and Infection, 134*(5), 946–951. https://doi.org/10.1017/s0950268806005978

CFIA. (2023). *Food labeling for industry.* Canadian Food Inspection Agency. https://inspection.canada.ca.

Chakraborty, S., Rao, P. S., & Mishra, H. N. (2015). Effect of combined high pressure-temperature treatments on color and nutritional quality attributes of pineapple (Ananas comosus L.) puree. *Innovative Food Science and Emerging Technologies, 28*, 10–21. https://doi.org/10.1016/j.ifset.2015.01.004

Chandrashekar, J., Yarmolinsky, D., Von Buchholtz, L., Oka, Y., Sly, W., Ryba, N. J. P., & Zuker, C. S. (2009). The taste of carbonation. *Science, 326*(5951), 443–445. https://doi.org/10.1126/science.1174601

Charles-Rodríguez, A. V., Nevárez-Moorillón, G. V., Zhang, Q. H., & Ortega-Rivas, E. (2007). Comparison of thermal processing and pulsed electric fields treatment in pasteurization of apple juice. *Food and Bioproducts Processing, 85*(2), 93–97. https://doi.org/10.1205/fbp06045

Chen, I. C., Chi, C. H., & Ku, H. H. (2025). Deep learning for the detection of good hygienic practices control measures for food handlers. *Food Control, 171*. https://doi.org/10.1016/j.foodcont.2024.111041

Chervona, Y., Arita, A., & Costa, M. (2012). Carcinogenic metals and the epigenome: Understanding the effect of nickel, arsenic, and chromium. *Metallomics*. https://doi.org/10.1039/c2mt20033c. http://www.rsc.org/Publishing/Journals/MT/index.asp 4

Cladière, M., Delaporte, G., Le Roux, E., & Camel, V. (2018). Multi-class analysis for simultaneous determination of pesticides, mycotoxins, process-induced toxicants and packaging contaminants in tea. *Food Chemistry, 242*, 113–121. https://doi.org/10.1016/j.foodchem.2017.08.108

Costa Dias, M. A., Sant'Ana, A. S., Cruz, A. G., Faria, J.d. A. F., Fernandes de Oliveira, C. A., & Bona, E. (2012). On the implementation of good manufacturing practices in a small processing unity of mozzarella cheese in Brazil. *Food Control, 24*(1–2), 199–205. https://doi.org/10.1016/j.foodcont.2011.09.028

da Cruz, A. G., Cenci, S. A., & Maia, M. C. A. (2006). Quality assurance requirements in produce processing. *Trends in Food Science and Technology, 17*(8), 406–411. https://doi.org/10.1016/j.tifs.2006.03.003

D'Amico, D. J., Silk, T. M., Wu, J., & Guo, M. (2006). Inactivation of microorganisms in milk and apple cider treated with ultrasound. *Journal of Food Protection, 69*(3), 556–563. https://doi.org/10.4315/0362-028X-69.3.556

Danone China. (2021). https://www.fssc.com/insights/danones-smooth-transition-from-iso-22000-to-fssc-22000/

Das, A. J., & Deka, S. C. (2012). Fermented foods and beverages of the North-East India. *International Food Research Journal, 19*(2), 377–392.

De Oliveira, C. A. F., Da Cruz, A. G., Tavolaro, P., & Corassin, C. H. (2016). *Food safety: Good manufacturing practices (GMP), sanitation standard operating procedures (SSOP), hazard analysis and critical control point (HACCP) antimicrobial food packaging*. Brazil: Elsevier Inc. https://doi.org/10.1016/B978-0-12-800723-5.00010-3. Available from: http://www.sciencedirect.com/science/book/9780128007235

Dolas, R., Saravanan, C., & Kaur, P. (2019). Emergence and era of ultrasonic's in fruit juice preservation: A review. *Ultrasound Sonochemistry, 58*(58).

Dransfield, J. S. (1999). Legislation controlling production, labelling and marketing of fruit juices and fruit beverages. In *Production and packaging of non-carbonated fruit juices and fruit beverages* (pp. 360–385). Boston, MA: Springer US.

Dubey, P. K., Kumar, K. S., Rawson, A., Anandakumar, S., Baskaran, N., & Thamburaj, S. (2023). Effect of pulsed electric field on physicochemical properties of rice and black gram fermented batter. *Journal of Food Process Engineering, 46*(9), e14411.

Dzwolak, W. (2014). HACCP in small food businesses – The polish experience. *Food Control, 36*(1), 132–137. https://doi.org/10.1016/j.foodcont.2013.07.043

Dzwolak, W. (2019). Assessment of HACCP plans in standardized food safety management systems – The case of small-sized Polish food businesses. *Food Control, 106*, Article 106716. https://doi.org/10.1016/j.foodcont.2019.106716

Espinosa, R. V., Soto, M., Garcia, M. V., & Naranjo, J. E. (2021). *Challenges of implementing cleaner production strategies in the food and beverage industry: Advances in intelligent systems and computing, 1307.*

European Commission. (2012). *Guidance document on the implementation of certain provisions of regulation (EC) no 852/2004 on the hygiene of foodstuffs.*

European Commission. (2015). *RASF for safer food - The rapid alert system for food and feed 2014 annual report.* Luxembourg: Publications Office of the European Union. Retrieved. from: http://ec.europa.eu/food/safety/rasff/docs/rasff_annual_report_2014.pdf.

European Commission. EU guidelines on good manufacturing practices (GMP) for food products. https://food.ec.europa.eu/.

Fabbrini, M., D'Amico, F., Barone, M., Conti, G., Mengoli, M., Brigidi, P., & Turroni, S. (2022). Polyphenol and tannin nutraceuticals and their metabolites: How the human gut microbiota influences their properties. *Biomolecules, 12*(7), 875. https://doi.org/10.3390/biom12070875

Fakhri, Y., Mohseni, S. M.o., Jafarzadeh, S., Langarizadeh, G., Moradi, B., Zandsalimi, Y., Rahimizadeh, A., & Mirzaei, M. (2015). Assessment of carcinogenic and non-carcinogenic risk lead in bottled water in different age groups in Bandar Abbas Ciry, Iran. *Global Journal of Health Science, 7*(4), 286–294. https://doi.org/10.5539/gjhs.v7n4p286

FAO. (2021). *Food hygiene and sanitation.* https://www.fao.org.

FAO/WHO. (2020). *Codex Alimentarius: General principles of food hygiene.* https://www.fao.org.

FSANZ. (2023). *Food standards code. Food standards Australia New Zealand.* https://www.foodstandards.gov.au.

FSSAI. (2023). Food safety and standards authority of India: Regulations and guidelines. https://www.fssai.gov.

FDA. (2023). *Food labeling & nutrition.* U.S. Food and Drug Administration. https://www.fda.gov.

Farid, M., Kodama, K., Arato, T., Okazaki, T., Oda, T., Ikeda, H., & Sengoku, S. (2019). Comparative study of functional food regulations in Japan and globally. *Global Journal of Health Science, 11*(6), 132-132.

Food and Agriculture Organizations of the United Nations (FAO). (2021). *Code of practice by codex Alimentarius on general principles of food hygiene 1969.* Retrieved from www.fao.org/fao-who-codexalimentarius/sh-proxy/en/?lnk=1.

Furia, T. E. (1973). *CRC handbook of food additives, 1.* CRC press.

George, A. S. (2024). Economics and environmental responsibility in the global beverage industry: A critical analysis of sustainability challenges and opportunities. *Partners Universal Multidisciplinary Research Journal (PUMRJ), 2*(1).

Goto, K., Mochida, K., Asahara, M., Suzuki, M., Hiroaki, K., Yokota, A., & Alicyclobacillus, pomorum sp (2003). Nov., a novel thermo-acidophilic, endospore-forming bacterium that does not possess ω-alicyclic fatty acids, and emended description of the genus Alicyclobacillus. *International Journal of Systematic and Evolutionary Microbiology, 53*(5), 1537–1544. https://doi.org/10.1099/ijs.0.02546-0

Granato, D., de Magalhães Carrapeiro, M., Fogliano, V., & van Ruth, S. M. (2016). Effects of geographical origin, varietal and farming system on the chemical composition and functional properties of purple grape juices: A review. *Trends in Food Science and Technology, 52*, 31–48. https://doi.org/10.1016/j.tifs.2016.03.013

Haseli, G., Nazarian-Jashnabadi, J., Shirazi, B., Hajiaghaei-Keshteli, M., & Moslem, S. (2024). Sustainable strategies based on the social responsibility of the beverage industry companies for the circular supply chain. *Engineering Applications of Artificial Intelligence, 133*, Article 108253. https://doi.org/10.1016/j.engappai.2024.108253

Hasnan, N. Z. N., & Mohd Ramli, S. H. (2020). Modernizing the preparation of the Malaysian mixed rice dish (MRD) with cook-chill central kitchen and implementation of HACCP. *International Journal of Gastronomy and Food Science, 19.* https://doi.org/10.1016/j.ijgfs.2019.100193. Available from: www.journals.elsevier.com/international-journal-of-gastronomy-and-food-science.

Hilliam, M. (2004). *Healthier dairy.* World Food Ingredients.

Horsáková, I., VoldGˆich, M., ýHg̃, ovský, Sedláþková, P., Šicnerová, P., & Ulbrich, P. (2009). Asaia sp. as a bacterium decaying the packaged still fruit beverages. *Czech Journal of Food Science, 27*, S362–S365.

Huang, X. C., Yuan, Y. H., Guo, C. F., Gekas, V., & Yue, T. L. (2015). Alicyclobacillus in the fruit juice industry: Spoilage, detection, and Prevention/Control. *Food Reviews International, 31*(2), 91–124. https://doi.org/10.1080/87559129.2014.974266

Ibarburu, I., Aznar, R., Elizaquível, P., García-Quintáns, N., López, P., Munduate, A., Irastorza, A., & Dueñas, M. T. (2010). A real-time PCR assay for detection and quantification of 2-branched (1,3)-β-d-glucan producing lactic acid bacteria in cider. *International Journal of Food Microbiology, 143*(1–2), 26–31. https://doi.org/10.1016/j.ijfoodmicro.2010.07.023

Inguglia, E. S., Song, Z., Kerry, J. P., O'Sullivan, M. G., & Hamill, R. M. (2023). Addressing clean label trends in commercial meat processing: Strategies, challenges and insights from consumer perspectives. *Foods, 12*(10), 2062. https://doi.org/10.3390/foods12102062

Innova Market Insights. (2025). *Global clean label trends*. https://www.innovamarketinsights.com.

ISO. (2023). ISO 22000:2018—Food safety management systems—Requirements. https://www.iso.org

Jarvis, B. (2003). Chemistry and microbiology of cider making. *Science*, 1318–1323.

Jeon, S. H., Kim, N. H., Shim, M. B., Jeon, Y. W., Ahn, J. H., Lee, S. H., Hwang, I. G., & Rhee, M. S. (2015). Microbiological diversity and prevalence of spoilage and pathogenic bacteria in commercial fermented alcoholic beverages (beer, fruit wine, refined rice wine, and yakju). *Journal of Food Protection, 78*(4), 812–818. https://doi.org/10.4315/0362-028X.JFP-14-431

Ju, H. K., Park, J. H., & Kwon, S. W. (2008). Evaluation of headspace-gas chromatography/mass spectrometry for the analysis of benzene in vitamin C drinks; pitfalls of headspace in benzene detection. *Biomedical Chromatography, 22*(8), 900–905. https://doi.org/10.1002/bmc.1008. Available from: http://onlinelibrary.wiley.com/journal/10.1002/(ISSN)1099-0801.

Juvonen, R., Virkajärvi, V., Priha, O., & Laitila, A. (2011). *Microbiological spoilage and safety risks in non-beer beverages produced in a brewery environment, VTT Tiedotteita-Research*. Finland: Espoo.

Karaman, A. D. (2014). Implementation of a food safety management system according to ISO 22000: A case study of a Turkish dairy company. *Food Control, 43*, 1–8. https://doi.org/10.1016/j.foodcont.2014.02.035

Karnieli, O. (2016). *Bioreactors and downstream processing for stem cell manufacturing stem cell manufacturing*. Israel: Elsevier Inc. https://doi.org/10.1016/B978-0-444-63265-4.00006-6

Keyser, M., Muller, I. A., Cilliers, F. P., Nel, W., & Gouws, P. A. (2008). Ultraviolet radiation as a non-thermal treatment for the inactivation of microorganisms in fruit juice. *Innovative Food Science and Emerging Technologies, 9*(3), 348–354. https://doi.org/10.1016/j.ifset.2007.09.002

Khatri, P., & Shalini, R. (2008). Additives used in soft drinks. *Beverage and Food World, 7*, 30–34.

Kiple, K. F., & Ornelas, K. C. (2000). *The Cambridge world history of food*. Cambridge, UK; New York: Cambridge University Press.

Kołożyn-Krajewska, D., & Sikora, T. (2010). *Food safety management. Theory and practice*. Warsaw (in Polish): C.H. Beck.

Konecka-Matyjek, E., Turlejska, H., Pelzner, U., & Szponar, L. (2005). Actual situation in the area of implementing quality assurance systems GMP, GHP and HACCP in Polish food production and processing plants. *Food Control, 16*(1), 1–9. https://doi.org/10.1016/j.foodcont.2003.10.007

Koshani, R., Ziaee, E., Niakousari, M., & Golmakani, M. T. (2015). Optimization of thermal and thermosonication treatments on Pectin Methyl esterase inactivation of sour Orange juice (citrus aurantium). *Journal of Food Processing and Preservation, 39*(6), 567–573. https://doi.org/10.1111/jfpp.12262

Kourtis, L. K., & Arvanitoyannis, I. S. (2001). Implementation OF hazard analysis critical control point (HACCP) system to the alcoholic beverages industry. *Food Reviews International, 17*(1), 1–44. https://doi.org/10.1081/fri-100000514

Kourtis, L. K., & Arvanitoyannis, I. S. (2007). Implementation of hazard analysis critical control point (HACCP) system to the NON-alcoholic beverage industry. *Food Reviews International, 17*(4), 451–486. https://doi.org/10.1081/FRI-100108533

Kovalchuk, Y. (2024). Clean label movement: Redefining consumer expectations and product development. *IJCRT, 12*(7), 95–108.

Krukovich, O., & Masanskiy, S. (2018). *Development of the food safety management system for fermented beverages with special appointments based on HACCP principles*, 65(1).

Laureys, D., De Vuyst, L., & Griffiths, M. W. (2014). Microbial species diversity, community dynamics, and metabolite kinetics of water kefir fermentation. *Applied and Environmental Microbiology, 80*(8), 2564–2572. https://doi.org/10.1128/aem.03978-13

Lawley, R., Curtis, L., & Davis, J. (2012). Chemical hazards in food – A food safety watch guide. *Food Safety Info*.

Le, S., Bazger, W., Hill, A. R., & Wilcock, A. (2014). Awareness and perceptions of food safety of artisan cheese makers in Southwestern Ontario: A qualitative study. *Food Control, 41*(1), 158–167. https://doi.org/10.1016/j.foodcont.2014.01.007

Lima Tribst, A. A., & de Souza Sant'Ana, A. (2009). Pilar Rodriguez de Massaguer, Review: Microbiological quality and safety of fruit juices—past, present and future perspectives. *Critical Reviews in Microbiology, 35*(4), 310–339. https://doi.org/10.3109/10408410903241428

Lodolo, E. J. (2020). Sustainability through management of water, process and product hygiene on food and beverage sites. *Journal of the American Society of Brewing Chemists, 78*(1), 1–15. https://doi.org/10.1080/03610470.2019.1683707

Macfarlane, A., & Macfarlane, I. (2003). *Green gold: The empire of tea*. London: Ebury Press.

Magnuson, B., Munro, I., Abbot, P., Baldwin, N., Lopez-Garcia, R., Ly, K., McGirr, L., Roberts, A., & Socolovsky, S. (2013). Review of the regulation and safety assessment of food substances in various countries and jurisdictions. *Food Additives & Contaminants: Part A, 30*(7), 1147–1220. https://doi.org/10.1080/19440049.2013.795293

Mahalik, N. (2014). Advances in packaging methods, processes and systems. *Challenges, 5*(2), 374–389. https://doi.org/10.3390/challe5020374

Maja, W., & Sharareh, H. (2017). Lactobacillus Rhamnosus GR-1 in fermented rice pudding supplemented with short chain inulin, long chain inulin, and oat as a novel functional food. *Fermentation, 3*(4), 55.

Malfeito-Ferreira, M., Barata, A., & Loureiro, V. (2009). *Wine spoilage by fungal metabolites wine chemistry and biochemistry*. New York: Springer. https://doi.org/10.1007/978-0-387-74118-5_27

Mangels, A. R., Block, G., Frey, C. M., Patterson, B. H., Taylor, P. R., Norkus, E. P., & Levander, O. A. (1993). The bioavailability to humans of ascorbic acid from oranges, orange juice and cooked broccoli is similar to that of synthetic ascorbic acid. *Journal of Nutrition, 123*(6), 1054–1061.

Marafon, K., Prestes, A. A., de Souza, C. A. F., & Prudencio, E. S. (2025). Bioactive compounds' importance in plant-based beverages: a review. *Current Opinion in Food Science, 63*, 101304.

Marriott, N. G., & Gravani, R. B. (2006). *Principles of food sanitation*. UK: Springer.

Martínez-Villaluenga, C., Frías, J., Gómez, R., & Vidal-Valverde, C. (2006). Influence of addition of raffinose family oligosaccharides on probiotic survival in fermented milk during refrigerated storage. *International Dairy Journal, 16*(7), 768–774. https://doi.org/10.1016/j.idairyj.2005.08.002

Martins, R. B., Hogg, T., & Otero, J. G. (2012). Food handlers' knowledge on food hygiene: The case of a catering company in Portugal. *Food Control, 23*(1), 184–190. https://doi.org/10.1016/j.foodcont.2011.07.008

Mashau, M. E., Maliwichi, L. L., & Jideani, A. I. O. (2021). Non-alcoholic fermentation of maize (Zea mays) in Sub-Saharan Africa. *Fermentation, 7*(3). https://doi.org/10.3390/FERMENTATION7030158. Available from: https://www.mdpi.com/2311-5637/7/3/158.

Matsubara, H., Goto, K., Matsumura, T., Mochida, K., Iwaki, M., Niwa, M., & Yamasato, K. (2002). Alicyclobacillus acidiphilus sp. nov., a novel thermo-acidophilic, omega-alicyclic fatty acid-containing bacterium isolated from acidic beverages. *International Journal of Systematic and Evolutionary Microbiology, 52*(5), 1681–1685. https://doi.org/10.1099/00207713-52-5-1681

Mavrogiannis, M., Bourlakis, M. A., Dawson, P. J., & Ness, M. R. (2008). Assessing export performance in the Greek food and beverage industry: An integrated structural equation model approach. *British Food Journal, 110*(7), 638–654. https://doi.org/10.1108/00070700810887130

Mbuagbaw, L., & Noorduyn, S. G. (2012). The palm wine trade: Occupational and health hazards. *The International Journal of Occupational and Environmental Medicine, 3*(4), 157–164.

McGovern, P. E., Zhang, J., Tang, J., Zhang, Z., Hall, G. R., Moreau, R. A., Nuñez, A., Butrym, E. D., Richards, M. P., Wang, C.-shan, Cheng, G., Zhao, Z., & Wang, C. (2004). Fermented beverages of pre- and proto-historic China. *Proceedings of the National Academy of Sciences, 101*(51), 17593–17598. https://doi.org/10.1073/pnas.0407921102

Menz, G., Vriesekoop, F., Zarei, M., Zhu, B., & Aldred, P. (2010). The growth and survival of food-borne pathogens in sweet and fermenting brewers' wort. *International Journal of Food Microbiology, 140*(1), 19–25. https://doi.org/10.1016/j.ijfoodmicro.2010.02.018

Morales-de la Peña, M., Martín-Belloso, O., & Welti-Chanes, J. (2018). High-power ultrasound as pre-treatment in different stages of soymilk manufacturing process to increase the isoflavone content. *Ultrasonics Sonochemistry, 49*, 154–160. https://doi.org/10.1016/j.ultsonch.2018.07.044

Mortimore, S. E., & Wallace, C. A. (2013). *HACCP – A practical approach* (3rd ed.). New York: Springer Publications.

Mosqueda-Melgar, J., Raybaudi-Massilia, R. M., & Martín-Belloso, O. (2008). Non-thermal pasteurization of fruit juices by combining high-intensity pulsed electric fields with natural antimicrobials. *Innovative Food Science and Emerging Technologies, 9*(3), 328–340. https://doi.org/10.1016/j.ifset.2007.09.003

Mosqueda-Melgar, J., Raybaudi-Massilia, R. M., & Martín-Belloso, O. (2012). Microbiological shelf life and sensory evaluation of fruit juices treated by high-intensity pulsed electric fields and antimicrobials. *Food and Bioproducts Processing, 90*(2), 205–214. https://doi.org/10.1016/j.fbp.2011.03.004

Mukherjee, A., Gómez-Sala, B., O'Connor, E. M., Kenny, J. G., & Cotter, P. D. (2022). Global regulatory frameworks for fermented foods: A review. *Frontiers in Nutrition, 9*. https://doi.org/10.3389/fnut.2022.902642

Munasinghe, J., de Silva, A., Weerasinghe, G., Gunaratne, A., & Corke, H. (2015). Food safety in Sri Lanka: Problems and solutions. *Quality Assurance and Safety of Crops & Foods, 7*(1), 37–44. https://doi.org/10.3920/qas2014.x007

Munekata, P. E. S., Domínguez, R., Budaraju, S., Roselló-Soto, E., Barba, F. J., Mallikarjunan, K., Roohinejad, S., & Lorenzo, J. M. (2020). Effect of innovative food processing technologies on the physicochemical and nutritional properties and quality of non-dairy plant-based beverages. *Foods, 9*(3). https://doi.org/10.3390/foods9030288. Available from: https://www.mdpi.com/2304-8158/9/3/288.

Murphy, P. A., Hendrich, S., Landgren, C., & Bryant, C. M. (2006). Food mycotoxins: An update. *Journal of Food Science, 71*(5), R51. https://doi.org/10.1111/j.1750-3841.2006.00052.x

Murphy, S. C. (2013). Evaluation of HACCP training under the grade "A" dairy HACCP core curriculum. *Journal of Extension, 51*. Available from: https://joe.org/joe/2013august/rb7.php.

Musah, B. O., Nii-trebi, N. I., Nwabugo, M. A., & Asmah, R. H. (2014). Microbial quality of locally prepared hibiscus tea in accra. *IOSR Journal of Environmental Science, Toxicology and Food Technology, 8*(11), 23–27. https://doi.org/10.9790/2402-081122327

Mushtaq, M. (2018). Extraction of fruit juice: An overview. *Fruit Juices*, 131–159.

Nahemiah, D., Solomon Bankole, O., Tswako, M. A., Nma-Usman, K. I., Hassan, H., & Isa Fati, K. (2014). Hazard analysis critical control points (Haccp) in the production of *soy-kununzaki*: A traditional cereal-based fermented beverage of Nigeria. *American Journal of Food Science and Technology, 2*(6), 196–202. https://doi.org/10.12691/ajfst-2-6-5

Nazir, M., Arif, S., Khan, R. S., Nazir, W., Khalid, N., & Maqsood, S. (2019). Opportunities and challenges for functional and medicinal beverages: Current and future trends. *Trends in Food Science and Technology, 88*, 513–526. https://doi.org/10.1016/j.tifs.2019.04.011

Nelson, M. (2005). *The barbarian's beverage: A history of beer in ancient Europe the Barbarian's beverage: A history of Beer in Ancient Europe*. Canada: Routledge Taylor & Francis Group. https://doi.org/10.4324/9780203309124

NHC China. (2023). National food safety standards of China (GB/GB-T). *National Health Commission of the People's Republic of China*. https://www.nhc.gov.cn.

Nicholls, W. (1998). *Drinking your vitamins (and minerals)*. The Washington Post. USA.

NTP—National Toxicology Program. (2014). *Report on carcinogens* (13th ed.). Department of Health and Human Services, Public Health Service: Research Triangle Park, NC, USA. Available online: http://ntp.niehs.nih.gov/pubhealth/roc/roc13/.

Nwaiwu, O., & Itumoh, M. (2017). Chemical contaminants associated with palm wine from Nigeria are potential food safety hazards. *Beverages, 3*(1), 16. https://doi.org/10.3390/beverages3010016

Nwakoby, I. P., Iheukwumere, I. H., Iheukwumere, C. M., Nwakoby, N. E., Idigo, M. A., & Ike, V. E. (2025). Microbial contamination in dairy products and its legal implications. *African Journal of Nutrition and Applied Research, 1*(1), 9–16. https://doi.org/10.54117/j2hx1174

Nyarugwe, S. P., Linnemann, A. R., Hofstede, G. J., Fogliano, V., & Luning, P. A. (2020). Integrating food safety culture in food safety management systems: A systematic review. *Food Control, 111*, Article 107075. https://doi.org/10.1016/j.foodcont.2019.107075

Nychas, G. J. E., & Panagou, E. (2011). *Microbiological spoilage of foods and beverages food and beverage stability and shelf life*. Greece: Elsevier Ltd. https://doi.org/10.1533/9780857092540.1.3. Available from: http://www.sciencedirect.com/science/book/9781845697013.

Nychas, G. J. E., Skandamis, P. N., Tassou, C. C., & Koutsoumanis, K. P. (2008). Meat spoilage during distribution. *Meat Science, 78*(1–2), 77–89. https://doi.org/10.1016/j.meatsci.2007.06.020

Nyokabi, S., Luning, P. A., de Boer, I. J. M., Korir, L., Muunda, E., Bebe, B. O., Lindahl, J., Bett, B., & Oosting, S. J. (2021). Milk quality and hygiene: Knowledge, attitudes and practices of smallholder dairy farmers in central Kenya. *Food Control, 130*. https://doi.org/10.1016/j.foodcont.2021.108303. Available from: https://www.journals.elsevier.com/food-control.

Oluwasegun Uzoigwe, D., & Kongolo, D. (2024). Integration of hazard analysis and critical control points HACCP with maintenance practices: Enhancing food safety in the food and beverage industry; A review. *International Journal of Latest Technology in Engineering, Management & Applied Science, XIII*(IV), 88–101. https://doi.org/10.51583/ijltemas.2024.130411

Oslen, A. R. (1998). Regulatory action criteria for filth and other extraneous materials - I. Review of hard or sharp foreign objects as physical hazards in food. *Regulatory Toxicology and Pharmacology, 28*, 181e189.

Pan, Y., Breidt, F., & Kathariou, S. (2006). Resistance of Listeria monocytogenes biofilms to sanitizing agents in a simulated food processing environment. *Applied and Environmental Microbiology, 72*(12), 7711–7717. https://doi.org/10.1128/aem.01065-06

Parish, M. E. (1997). Public health and nonpasteurized fruit juices. *Critical Reviews in Microbiology, 23*(2), 109–119. https://doi.org/10.3109/10408419709115132

Park, Y. J., & Chen, J. (2009). Microbial quality of soft drinks served by the dispensing machines in fast food restaurants and convenience stores in Griffin, Georgia, and surrounding areas. *Journal of Food Protection, 72*(12), 2607–2610. https://doi.org/10.4315/0362-028X-72.12.2607

Pettoello-Mantovani, M., Mestrovic, J., Namazova-Baranova Md PhD, L., Giardino, I., Somekh, E., & Vural, M. (2021). Ensuring safe food for infants: The importance of an integrated approach to monitor and reduce the risks of biological, chemical, and physical hazards. *Journal of Pediatrics, 229*, 315. https://doi.org/10.1016/j.jpeds.2020.10.074

Plavchan, R. J. (1976). *A history of Anheuser-Busch, 1852–1933*. New York: Arno Press.

Pothakos, V., Snauwaert, C., De Vos, P., Huys, G., & Devlieghere, F. (2014). Psychrotrophic members of Leuconostoc gasicomitatum, Leuconostoc gelidum and Lactococcus piscium dominate at the end of shelf-life in packaged and chilled-stored food products in Belgium. *Food Microbiology, 39*, 61–67. https://doi.org/10.1016/j.fm.2013.11.005

Priti, P., & Paul, B. (2016). Assessment of heavy metal pollution in water resources and their impacts: A review. *Journal of Basic and Applied Engineering Research, 3*, 671–675.

Rajan, R., Vinutha, N. V., Brindha, L., Shukla, S., & Mishra, S. (2024). Exploring global expansion trends and strategies in the food and beverage industry: A comprehensive analysis. *School of Commerce, JAIN, 6*(1).

Ramos, M., Valdés, A., Mellinas, A. C., & Garrigós, M. C. (2015). New trends in beverage packaging systems: A review. *Beverages, 1*(4), 248–272. https://doi.org/10.3390/beverages1040248

Raybaudi-Massilia, R. M., Mosqueda-Melgar, J., Soliva-Fortuny, R., & Martín-Belloso, O. (2009). Control of pathogenic and spoilage microorganisms in fresh-cut fruits and fruit juices by traditional and alternative natural antimicrobials. *Comprehensive Reviews in Food Science and Food Safety, 8*(3), 157–180. https://doi.org/10.1111/j.1541-4337.2009.00076.x

Regulation (EC) no 852/2004 of the European Parliament and of the Council of 29 April 2004 on the hygiene of foodstuffs https://faolex.fao.org/docs/pdf/eur63426.pdf.

Reid, G., Jass, J., Sebulsky, M. T., & McCormick, J. K. (2003). Potential uses of probiotics in clinical practice. *Clinical Microbiology Reviews, 16*(4), 658–672. https://doi.org/10.1128/CMR.16.4.658-672.2003

Rethinam, P., & Krishnakumar, V. (2022). Processing of coconut water. In *Coconut water: A promising natural health drink-distribution, processing and nutritional benefits* (pp. 139–239). Cham: Springer International Publishing.

Ridho, S. L. Z., Sabli, H. B. H. M., Ibrahim, K. B. C., Detmuliati, A., Alfitriani, A., & Jauhari, H. (2022). Internal factor analysis of cleanliness, health, safety, and environment sustainability implementation in food and beverage services. *Journal of Business on Hospitality and Tourism, 8*(1), 114. https://doi.org/10.22334/jbhost.v8i1.322

Rihawi, B. (2024). The impact of ISO 22000: 2018 on food facilities performance with multiple production lines. *CyTA - Journal of Food, 22*(1). https://doi.org/10.1080/19476337.2024.2431281

Ross, R. P., Morgan, S., & Hill, C. (2002). Preservation and fermentation: Past, present and future. *International Journal of Food Microbiology, 79*(1–2), 3–16. https://doi.org/10.1016/s0168-1605(02)00174-5

Saarela, M., Hallamaa, K., Mattila-Sandholm, T., & Mättö, J. (2003). The effect of lactose derivatives lactulose, lactitol and lactobionic acid on the functional and technological properties of potentially probiotic Lactobacillus strains. *International Dairy Journal, 13*(4), 291–302. https://doi.org/10.1016/S0958-6946(02)00158-9

Sengev, I. A., Akpapunam, M. A., & Ingbian, E. K. (2012). Physicochemical and sensory properties of instant Kunun-Zaki flour blends from Sorghum and Mango mesocarp flours. *Nigerian Food Journal, 30*(2), 8–16. https://doi.org/10.1016/s0189-7241(15)30028-x

Serrano, J., Puupponen-Pimiä, R., Dauer, A., Aura, A. M., & Saura-Calixto, F. (2009). Tannins: Current knowledge of food sources, intake, bioavailability and biological effects. *Molecular Nutrition & Food Research, 53*(2), Article S310. https://doi.org/10.1002/mnfr.200900039

SGS. (2024). *Understanding FSSC 22000 version 6: Key changes and transition. SGS technical brief.* Retrieved from https://www.sgs.com/en.

Shankar, V., Mahboob, S., Al-Ghanim, K. A., Ahmed, Z., Al-Mulhm, N., & Govindarajan, M. (2021). A review on microbial degradation of drinks and infectious diseases: A perspective of human well-being and capabilities. *Journal of King Saud University - Science, 33*(2), Article 101293. https://doi.org/10.1016/j.jksus.2020.101293

Sikora, T. (2005). *Methods and systems of food quality and safety assurance.*

Sikora, T. (2015). Good manufacturing practice (GMP) in the production of dietary supplements. In *Dietary supplements* (pp. 25–36). Woodhead Publishing.

Slavin, J. L., & Lloyd, B. (2012). Health benefits of fruits and vegetables. *Advances in Nutrition, 3*(4), 506–516. https://doi.org/10.3945/an.112.002154

Soni, A., Bremer, P., & Brightwell, G. (2022). A comprehensive review of variability in the thermal resistance (D-Values) of food-borne Pathogens—A challenge for thermal validation trials. *Foods, 11*(24), 4117. https://doi.org/10.3390/foods11244117

Southgate, D. A. T., Johnson, I. T., & Fenwick, G. R. (1995). Nutritional value and safety of processed fruit juices. In *Production and packaging of non-carbonated fruit juices and fruit beverages* (pp. 331–359). Boston, MA: Springer US.

Standage, T. (2005). *A history of the world in 6 glasses.* New York: Walker & Co.

Stanley, R., Knight, C., & Bodnar, F. (2011). Experiences and challenges in the development of an organic HACCP system. *NJAS - Wageningen Journal of Life Sciences, 58*(3–4), 117–121. https://doi.org/10.1016/j.njas.2011.01.006

Stratford, M. (2006). Food and beverage spoilage yeasts chapter 11. In H. Querol, & G. Fleet (Eds.), *Yeasts in food and beverages* (pp. 335–379). Berlin, Germany: Springer-Verlag.

Sun, S., & Wang, X. (2019). Promoting traceability for food supply chain with certification. *Journal of Cleaner Production, 217*(4), 658–665. https://doi.org/10.1016/j.jclepro.2019.01.296

Taillie, L. S., Reyes, M., Colchero, M. A., Popkin, B., & Corvalán, C. (2020). An evaluation of Chile's law of food labeling and advertising on sugar-sweetened beverage purchases from 2015 to 2017: A before-and-after study. *PLoS Medicine, 17*(2). https://doi.org/10.1371/JOURNAL.PMED.1003015. Available from: https://dx.plos.org/10.1371/journal.pmed.1003015.

The European Parliament and the Council. (2004a). Regulation (EC) no 852/2004 on the hygiene of foodstuffs. *Official Journal of the European Union L, 139.*

Tomas, N., & Tiwari, B. K. (2013). Sustainable cleaning and sanitation in the food industry. In B. K. Tiwari, T. Norton, & N. M. Holden (Eds.), *Sustainable food processing* (1st ed., pp. 363–376). Wiley. https://doi.org/10.1002/9781118634301.ch15

Toropilová, J., & Bystricky, P. (2015). Why HACCP might sometimes become weak or even fail. *Procedia Food Science, 5*, 296–299.

Torres-Guardado, R., Esteve-Zarzoso, B., Reguant, C., & Bordons, A. (2022). Microbial interactions in alcoholic beverages. *International Microbiology, 25*(1), 1–15. https://doi.org/10.1007/s10123-021-00200-1

Trafiałek, J., Lehrke, M., Lücke, F. K., Kołozyn-Krajewska, D., & Janssen, J. (2015). HACCP-based procedures in Germany and Poland. *Food Control, 55*, 66–74. https://doi.org/10.1016/j.foodcont.2015.01.031

TTB. (2023). Alcohol labeling and formulation. In *Alcohol and tobacco tax and trade bureau.* https://www.ttb.gov.

Uçar, A., Yilmaz, M. V., & Çakiroglu, F. P. (2016). *Food safety–problems and solutions.*

Ukers, W. H. (1948). *The romance of coffee: An outline history of coffee and coffee-drinking through a thousand years* (1st ed.). New York, USA: Tea and Coffee Trade Journal Co.

van Asselt, E. D., van der Fels-Klerx, H. J., Marvin, H. J. P., van Bokhorst-van de Veen, H., & Nierop Groot, M. (2017). Overview of food safety hazards in the European dairy supply chain. *Comprehensive Reviews in Food Science and Food Safety, 16*(1), 59–75. https://doi.org/10.1111/1541-4337.12245

Vasudevan, S., & Chengaiyan, J. G. (2024). Ensuring beverage excellence: A quality control guide. Food Science and Engineering, 38–53.

Vorobiev, E., & Lebovka, N. (2020). Potato and carrot crops. In *Processing of foods and biomass feedstocks by pulsed electric energy* (pp. 277–297).

Walker, G. M., Lappe-Oliveras, P., Moreno-Terrazas, R. C., Kirchmayr, M., Arellano-Plaza, M., & Gschaedler-Mathis, A. C. (2019). *Yeasts associated with the production of distilled alcoholic beverages yeasts in the Production of wine.* United Kingdom: Springer New York. https://doi.org/10.1007/978-1-4939-9782-4_16

Walther, B., Guggisberg, D., Badertscher, R., Egger, L., Portmann, R., Dubois, S., Haldimann, M., Kopf-Bolanz, K., Rhyn, P., Zoller, O., Veraguth, R., & Rezzi, S. (2022). Comparison of nutritional composition between plant-based drinks and cow's milk. *Frontiers in Nutrition, 9.* https://doi.org/10.3389/fnut.2022.988707

Waltzman, M. L. (2006). Management of esophageal coins. *Current Opinion in Pediatrics, 18*(5), 571–574. https://doi.org/10.1097/01.mop.0000245361.91077.b5

Wang, Y., Zhang, S., Iqbal, S., Chen, Z., Wang, X., Wang, Y. A., Liu, D., Bai, K., Ritenour, C., Kucuk, O., & Wu, D. (2014). Pomegranate extract inhibits the bone metastatic growth of human prostate cancer cells and enhances the in vivo efficacy of docetaxel chemotherapy. *The Prostate, 74*(5), 497–508. https://doi.org/10.1002/pros.22769

Wang, L., Chen, S., & Xu, Y. (2023). Distilled beverage aging: A review on aroma characteristics, maturation mechanisms, and artificial aging techniques. *Comprehensive Reviews in Food Science and Food Safety, 22*(1), 502–534.

Wang, Z., Zabed, H. M., Singh, A. K., Ibrahim, M. A., & Chen, N. (2024). Research on risk control in coffee milk beverage production based on HACCP and FMEA. *BIO Web of Conferences, 142*, Article 01020. https://doi.org/10.1051/bioconf/202414201020

WHO. (2011). *Guidelines for drinking-water quality, 38* (pp. 104–108).

WHO. (2021). *Food safety and international standards*. https://www.who.int.

WHO. (2022). *Food safety and good manufacturing practices*. https://www.who.int.

Xiang, Y., Guo, Z., Zhu, P., Chen, J., & Huang, Y. (2019). Traditional Chinese medicine as a cancer treatment: Modern perspectives of ancient but advanced science. *Cancer Medicine, 8*(5), 1958–1975. https://doi.org/10.1002/cam4.2108

Yang, T., & Dharmasena, S. (2021). U.S. Consumer demand for plant-based milk alternative beverages: Hedonic metric augmented Barten's synthetic model. *Foods, 10*(2), 265. https://doi.org/10.3390/foods10020265

ZABS. (2000). *Zambian standards bottled drinking water: Specifications*. Private Report. Lusaka.

Zheng, J., Zhou, Y., Li, S., Zhang, P., Zhou, T., Xu, D.-P., & Li, H.-B. (2017). Effects and mech anisms of fruit and vegetable juices on cardiovascular diseases. *International Journal of Molecular Sciences, 18*, 555.

CHAPTER

2 Quality assurance in fruit beverages for microbial safety and best practices

Sabeera Muzzaffar, Tuyiba Nazir Zargar and Hilal Ahmad Punoo
Department of Food Science and Technology, University of Kashmir, Srinagar, Jammu and Kashmir, India

2.1 Introduction

The development of functional foods, which are foods with specific biological activities and functions, has been facilitated by the increasing consumer awareness of the potential health benefits of food items (Topolska et al., 2021). In addition to having a good effect on the economy through increased food sector earnings and international exports, the growth in fruit and fruit juice production and consumption can also have a negative influence when foodborne illness outbreaks and spoiling issues arise. Reports of fruit and/or fruit juice-borne illness outbreaks or spoiling issues have mostly occurred in the past 20 years. Foodborne pathogens such as *Salmonella* spp., *Cryptosporidium parvum*, and *Escherichia coli* 0157:H7 (Yoder & Beach, 2007) as well as spoilage bacteria like *Alicyclobacillus acidoterrestris*, Tribst et al. (2009) were implicated in these instances. Both the fruit juice business and public health authorities face significant obstacles as a result of this. National food standard authorities have released a number of guidelines as a result of these issues, which prompted an attempt to create stricter methods and controls to regulate the microbiological purity and safety of fruit juices. The 5-log reduction procedures for juices and the HACCP regulation for processed juices are pertinent examples (FDA, 2001). Additionally, a number of farm-to-fork management strategies have been researched to prevent or lessen outbreaks of foodborne illness or incidents of spoiling (Buzrul et al., 2008).

Beverages provide a rich tapestry of human experience in addition to meeting water demands. Beyond just being enjoyable, they are also necessary to human nutrition, with fermented items supporting intestinal health and milk giving children the nutrition they need. Essential vitamins, minerals and health-promoting phytochemicals can be found in beverages. Juices are more convenient to drink than entire fruits for both small children and the elderly. Juices' ease of production and transportation is another advantage over entire fruits and vegetables (Rivankar et al., 2019). The beverage sector may be separated into two main categories: alcoholic and non-alcoholic. Alcoholic industries produce both distilled and nondistilled beverages, whilst non-alcoholic industries produce soft drinks, syrups, fruit juices, and fruit-based goods (Vasudevan & Chengaiyan, 2025). The fruit-based beverages are classified into various categories as seen in Fig. 2.1.

Fruits have long been a vital part of human diet. However, until the turn of the twentieth century, only a select few were permitted to drink freshly squeezed fruit juices. In America, Welch was the first

The Science and Safety of Beverages. https://doi.org/10.1016/B978-0-443-36536-2.00011-9

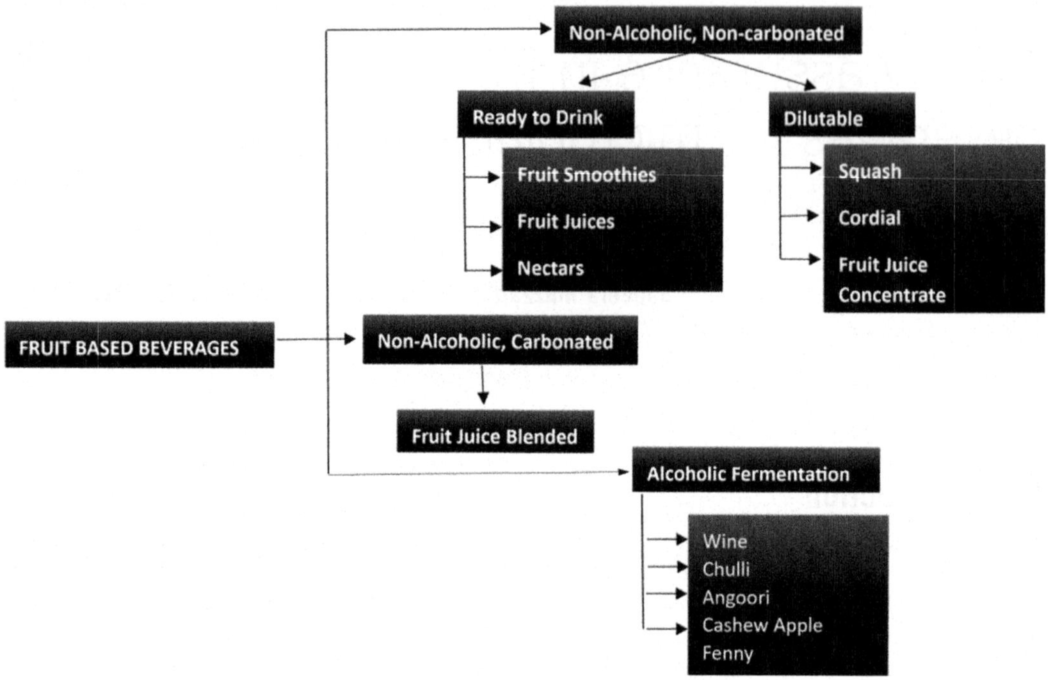

FIGURE 2.1

Fruit based beverages classification.

to use heat treatment to preserve grape juice in 1869. MüllerThurgan did the same in Switzerland in 1896 (Kardos, 1962). The manufacturing of fruit juices that had been kept thus started, and the 20th century saw a significant advancement in this field. Significant dietary changes resulted from the discovery of the importance of vitamins and minerals in the human body at that time. As a result, eating fruit has become a must. There are innumerable fruit juice products available in marketplaces throughout the world today. Their raw materials, composition, quality, nutrient content, sensory characteristics, and packaging can all vary significantly. In certain instances, the brand name is the most significant distinction. Drinks made with fruit juice are often categorized based on the amount of fruit they include. As a result, three categories can be established: fruit nectars, juices, fruit musts, and fruit-based soft drinks. Fruit musts and juices are produced mechanically. They are similar to the original fruit in terms of content and have the same color, flavor, and perfume. Vitamin enrichment and sugar addition are permitted in some goods, but they must be disclosed on the label. Food industry additives, such as coloring agents, fragrances, and preservatives, are prohibited in juices and fruit musts. As a result, it is rapidly consumed fresh or preserved by heat treatment (Horváth-Kerkai, 2006). This chapter examines the evolution and implementation of quality assurance practices in the fruit beverage industry, with emphasis on microbial safety, regulatory frameworks, and best practices such as HACCP and GMPs to ensure consumer protection and product integrity.

2.2 Quality characteristics of beverages

Drink quality is determined by a number of factors, including positive attributes like color and overall appearance: taste characteristics like mouthfeel, flavor, and aftertaste; olfactory characteristics like odor, aroma, retro-nasal; and ortho-nasal, and tactile characteristics like body, mouth feel, and lack of contaminants (tastes and odd flavors). Discoloration, sedimentation, foaming, gas, an unpleasant odor (especially of vinegar or ketone), astringency and bitterness are some of the drawbacks (Pinto et al., 2022; Fig. 2.2).

The attributes of the finished product are significantly altered as a result of the fruit juice heat treatments. When processing fruit juice, microbiological and chemical safety are crucial and so are the sensory qualities. Both initial acceptance and recurring purchases of the items depend heavily on characteristics like color or tactile qualities. Thus, a key factor in customer satisfaction with fruit juices is their sensory quality. The most popular method for processing fruit juices is thermal treatment, however this method often results in detrimental alterations to the liquids' nutritional value and flavor (Lee et al., 2013). In terms of overall flavor, color, cloudiness, acidity, odor, and resemblance, the pasteurized samples were noticeably less appealing. Thus, new nonthermal methods are used to preserve the quality; nonetheless, processing parameters must be optimized to minimize color deterioration and browning in fruit juice. For instance, high pressure treatment is a non-thermal method that has been shown to inactivate microorganisms by disrupting their membranes. It also maintains nutritional value while having less of an impact on the quality and sensory qualities of fruit juices because lower molecular weight compounds, like pigments, volatile compounds, and certain vitamins,

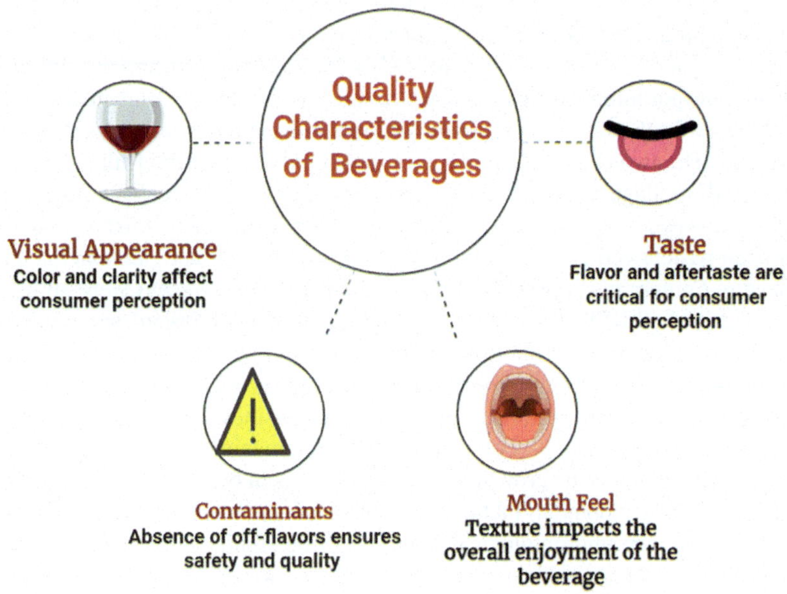

FIGURE 2.2

Quality characteristics of beverages.

remain unchanged because pressure has no effect on covalent bonds (Kasikçi & Bağdatlioğlu, 2016). Additionally, pulsed electric field (PEF) processing (4 μs, 35 kV/cm, and 1200 pps) preserved the volatile compounds that give apple juice its flavor and color better than heat treatment (Aguilar-Rosas et al., 2007). According to sensory tests, PEF-treated fruit juices have a better flavor and tests than thermally processed juices. Khandpur and Gogate (2015) conducted an evaluation of the taste, smell, and mouth experience of ultrasound treated orange juice. They discovered that the juice treated with ultrasound was the most palatable to customers and was the same as the fresh, unprocessed fruit juices. The elimination of oxygen is thought to be the reason for the beneficial effects of ultrasound treatment. According to Santhirasegaram et al. (2015), juices that underwent non-thermal treatments had the least amount of fluctuation in hedonic ratings when compared to the untreated juice.

2.3 Microbial contamination: Source and control

The primary challenges facing the beverage industry are chemical, microbiological, and physical hazards. Many pathogens are present at various levels throughout the food chain because of their high degree of adaptability and capacity to persist, thrive, and create potentially hazardous substances in the microbiological environment (Ranadheera et al., 2020, pp. 187–221). Low quality raw materials raise the risk of exposure since fresh fruits naturally contain microbial populations (Harris et al., 2003). Nutrients for the development of microbes may be found in most meals. Apart from microorganisms, metabolic materials such as enzymes are responsible for contamination, rotting, and degradation. Antimicrobials have been used extensively to fight pathogenic microorganisms and spoiling in a number of sectors that affect the health of humans and animals, including the food chain. Generally, issues with the supply and processing chain might alter the food's environmental conditions and encourage the development of these microorganisms (Lopez et al., 2018).

A microflora that is often found on the surface of fruits throughout harvest and postharvest processing, such as transportation, storage, and processing, is present in fruit juices. They serve as a substrate for the growth of several microorganisms, including fungi (molds, yeasts) and bacteria that can withstand acid. The two categories of microorganisms that affect the fruit-based beverage sector are pathogenic and spoilage bacteria. There are very few pathogenic bacteria in the fruit-based beverage sector. However, unpasteurized fruit juices have often been linked to outbreaks. Juices that have not been pasteurized are uncommon on the European market. *Salmonella species*, *Cryptosporidium parvum*, *Escherichia coli O157:H7*, and *Listeria monocytogenes* were all involved in these outbreaks (Ahmed et al., 2018). When we talk about spoilage microorganisms, we are talking about those that, by growing, deteriorate the product and lower the beverage's quality. However, harmful microbes would contaminate and cause food poisoning, which would lower the product's safety in this situation. Fortunately, pathogenic outbreaks are rare in this business because of the high acidity of the goods, although microbial spoiling is very widespread (Subramaniam & Wareing, 2016). Both internal and external variables influence the growth of microorganisms in fruit-based drinks. Intrinsic variables that inhibit microbial development include the presence of antimicrobials, carbonation, or the distinctive high acidity. The microbiological quality will be significantly impacted by external variables such as packing, storage, and cleanliness during processing (Avîrvarei et al., 2023). Because they can grow in acidic environments, yeasts and molds are the groups linked to the majority of spoiling in fruit-based beverages. The largest cause of spoiling in the fruit-based beverage sector is yeast. Furthermore, it is known that the goods are also impacted by bacteria that can withstand acid.

Bacteria such as *Acetobacter, Alicyclobacillus, Bacillus, Clostridium, Gluconobacter, Lactobacillus, Leuconostoc, Saccharobacter, Zymobacter, and Zymomonas* are frequently responsible for spoiling. The majority of spoilage bacteria are exclusively found in still, uncarbonated liquids and cannot thrive in carbonated items. This guideline does not apply to lactic acid bacteria, which can be found in any carbonated product. *Leuconostoc* and *Lactobacillus* are the most prevalent LAB. Fruit juices are also regularly spoiled by Acetic Acid Bacteria, including *Acetobacter* and *Gluconobacter.* Vegetable juices are often spoiled by spore-forming genera such *Clostridium* and *Bacillus*, which are often hindered by pH (Juvonen et al., 2011). One of the most hazards in the business is the genus Alicyclobacillus, which can thrive after processing because it can withstand the heat treatment used on pasteurized juices. It is a spore-forming, heat-resistant, acidophilic bacterium. A distinctive phenolic or antiseptic off-flavor and aroma, containing guaiacol, are signs of rotting. Ascorbic acid and sorbate benzoate both function to stop its development. *A. acidocaldarius, A. acidoterrestris, and A. cycloheptanicus* are the three species of Alicyclobacillus spoilage (Subramaniam & Wareing, 2016).

Yeasts are the most common spoilage microorganisms in fruit-based beverages due to their high acidity and carbonation tolerance, as well as their propensity to grow in high-sugar drinks. Around 100–150 yeasts are known to degrade foods or drinks, and approximately 40% of commercially available fruit juices have been shown to be infected with yeasts. An abundance of yeast indicates poor cleanliness in an industrial facility (Zara et al., 2020). *Brettanomyces, Candida, Cryptococcus, Debaryomyces, Dekkera, Saccharomyces, Schizosaccharomyces, Sporobolomyces, Torulopsis*, and *Zygosaccharomyces* are the most common spoilage fungi in the fruit-based beverage business. The most frequent spoilage yeast is *Zygosaccharomyces*, which causes significant economic losses in the fruit-based beverage sector (Avîrvarei et al., 2023).

Molds are naturally occurring contaminants in fresh fruits, but they can also enter the goods via airborne pollution. They are often aerobic and hence develop near the surface. Mycelium formation distinguishes molds. Its spoiling generates unpleasant flavors and odors, as well as a reduction in the product's sugar content. Some produce degradative enzymes. Poor hygiene in the production process can allow molds to get access to goods, particularly xerophilic ones that can survive high sugar concentrations (Snyder et al., 2019). *Acremonium, Aspergillus, Alternaria, Botrytis, Byssochlamys, Cladosporium, Eupenicillum, Fonseceae, Fusarium, Geotrichum, Humicola, Monilia, Mucor, Neosartorya, Paecillomuces, Penicillum, Rhizopus*, and *Talaromyces* are the most abundant in fruit juices (Avîrvarei et al., 2023). Some spoilage molds may withstand heat treatments on drinks, such as 72–80 degrees for 10–20 min. Heat-Resistant Molds (HRM) comprise the *genera Byssochlamys, Paecilomyces, Neosartorya, Talaromyces, and Eupenicillum. Ascospores, chlamydospores*, and *sclerotia* are all heat-resistant spores that can be discharged Table 2.1.

Fruit drinks may become contaminated by microorganisms from a variety of sources throughout the supply and demand chains. Understanding these sources is crucial to guaranteeing the safety and quality of the beverages. The main causes of microbial contamination in fruit drinks are described in the sections that follow.

Table 2.1 Microbial contamination sources in fruit beverages.

Contamination sources	Explanation	Effect of safety and quality	References
Mycotoxins	Fruit and fruit juice could be contaminated by the toxins produced by fungi, especially in unfavorable climatic conditions	Foodborne illnesses caused by mycotoxins are a significant food safety concern.	Nan et al. (2022)
Pathogens	Severe threats of microorganisms are *Salmonella* species, *Escherichia coli* O157:H7, and *Cryptosporidium parvum*.	Pathogens endanger public health and consumer confidence by producing serious foodborne illnesses.	Lamichhane et al. (2024).
Heavy metals	During manufacturing and storage processes contamination can come from both industrial and environmental sources.	Fruit beverage safety can be threatened by heavy metals, which can also provide major health	Scutarasu and Trincă (2023).
Environmental conditions	The incidence of biogenic amines and mycotoxins is influenced by several factors, including soil types, composition, and climate.	Such conditions may result in higher concentrations of dangerous chemicals in fruit drinks, which might compromise their safety.	Gardini et al. (2016).

2.4 Preharvest contamination

It is generally established that a variety of physicochemical, microbiological, and organoleptic markers, together with stability throughout time, define the quality of food. First and foremost, the unique qualities and attributes of the primary and secondary raw materials are among the elements that significantly affect the quality of food items. However, it is well recognized that environmental elements like temperature, relative humidity, lighting, pressure, and so on can have a detrimental effect on food goods' quality while they are being stored.

One of the top priorities for producers to guarantee the safety and superior quality of their goods is the investigation of the effects of different external influences on the shelf life and quality of drinks made from fruit raw materials (Kuz'mina et al., 2023). One of the main reasons of contamination in fruit drinks is environmental conditions. These have an impact on factors of quality and safety. Climate, soil composition, and soil types are important factors that influence the occurrence of biogenic amines and mycotoxins.

Production and storage operations may potentially be contaminated by heavy metals from industrial and environmental sources. Floods and droughts are examples of extreme weather events that promote the growth of toxic fungus, which raises the amounts of mycotoxins in the goods. This is the situation in Serbia, where drought led to floods, highlighting the issue, and raising the possibility of mycotoxin contamination in agricultural goods (Dragan et al., 2019). The microbial community and potential for mycotoxin formation are determined by the kind of soil. Hazardous metabolites can be produced by some fungus species that are found in particular types of soil (Abdel-Sater et al., 2001).

Fruit beverages may include heavy metal pollution from the soil, which might have negative health effects (Garvey, 2019). Although these environmental elements are crucial for understanding contamination, they also need to be incorporated into technological and regulatory procedures for monitoring and controlling these pollutants in order to guarantee food safety.

2.5 Harvest and postharvest handling

Pathogens that might infect fresh fruit are primed by water, particularly those used for irrigation, washing, and chilling. Consuming tainted fruits and vegetables is linked to several outbreaks of foodborne illnesses, putting public health at risk. Waterborne pathogens such as *Salmonella enterica* and *Listeria monocytogenes*, which Gu et al. (2021) have shown to be significantly prevalent in agricultural water sources (19.4% and 27.1%, respectively), are also found to be present in water collected from ponds and wells. Water used for hydrocooling and washing can potentially infect fruits and vegetables if it has come into contact with feces or other microbiological dangers (Gerba, 2009). If a fluid medium is utilized for both irrigation and postharvest processing, edible portions of fruits and vegetables may get contaminated. The use of a basement water medium greatly raises the possibility of pathogen translocation (Gerba & Choi, 2006). According to other research, the risk is very high since one hepatitis A virus per 10 L is more than enough to put a person at danger. This suggests that the risk of infection grows uniformly even with low quantities of pathogens like viruses (Gerba & Choi, 2006).

2.6 Storage and distribution

Extrinsic and intrinsic variables are among the many crucial components that influence the growth of microbes in both alcoholic and nonalcoholic drinks. Antimicrobials, nutritional supplements, carbonation, and acidity are examples of intrinsic elements. However, the product's microbiological quality will be impacted by raw components, production methods, packaging, storage conditions, and the cleanliness of the manufacturing facility (Shankar et al., 2021). Although many microorganisms may live in an acidic and low-oxygen environment, only a small number of them can grow in drinks (Pop et al., 2016). The metabolic process of spoiling, which alters the sensory qualities of drinks to the point that they are unsuitable or undesirable for human consumption, is frequently associated with these microorganisms, which include a broad range of bacteria, yeasts, and molds (Kregiel, 2015). The accumulative process of mold development and mycotoxin generation can occur at several stages of the food chain, starting in the field and intensifying throughout later stages including harvest, drying, and storage. Water activity (aw), Temperature, relative humidity (RH), pH, fungal strain, and substrate are the primary variables influencing the development of mycotoxins (Mandappa et al., 2018).

The methods to control the spoilage microorganism include preserving UV irradiation, applying surface waxes, surfactants, and chemical sanitizers, submerging the products in hot water, regulating storage temperature, filtering, and maintaining clean equipment. The microbial burden has been decreased by cold-pasteurizing the fruit juices with the preservative dimethyl dicarbonate. Additional techniques include processing the items under high pressure, applying a pused electric field, and employing UV radiation. An efficient method of preventing spoiling is to simulate the growth of the bacteria and yeast (Shearer et al., 2002). Fruit residues and items that contain sticky sugar are particularly vulnerable to mold and yeast infestation. Excellent sterile practices and adherence to

GMPs are the soda pop industry's best defenses against microbiological contamination, especially with regard to yeasts. The Hazard Analysis and Critical Control Point (HACCP) methodology has been adopted by sustainment processors worldwide. Natural product juice producers in the US must follow HACCP, and a successful HACCP framework is created using excellent rural practices (FDA, 2001).

2.7 Safety management practices

Numerous attributes that are ascribed to a food product during its production process are ultimately determined by its quality. One component of food health quality is food safety. A thorough response to this problem is linked to effective food safety management in a food company operator, which involves a variety of tasks completed at various levels inside a food industry. Food safety may be achieved through two distinct methods: Quality Assurance (QA) and Quality Control (QC). Although the tools used in both systems are similar, the focus is entirely different. Both the strategies have laws, they need very different organizations, structures, resources, abilities, and methods of operation (Wahab et al., 2024). QC is a reactive strategy that is impacted by outside forces. A QC company places a strong emphasis on measurement, which must be reliable and statistically significant, as well as on business and legal matters. QA, on the other hand, is a preventative strategy motivated by internal business norms. The consumer is the main focus, and operational processes need to be strong and frequently evaluated (Blackburn, 2003). Relying only on testing to ensure product safety has a number of drawbacks (Van Schothorst & Jongeneel, 1992) (Any statistical interpretation of the data requires that the contaminant be dispersed evenly across the batch. The microbiological state of the batch and the findings of the microbial test frequently differ significantly because microbiological dangers are typically distributed heterogeneously (ICMSF, 1986). It could still be prohibitive to test enough sample units for all the pertinent dangers to provide useful information, even if the microbial distribution is homogenous. Most importantly, microbiological testing does not identify or control the causes; it simply detects the consequences. As a result, the management of microbiological hazards in food has irrevocably shifted from OC to QA, with an emphasis on preventative control methods rather than evaluating the final product. Even though microbiological analysis has since been the target of a lot of criticism, it still plays a crucial function in a QA framework, albeit with a change in focus and application (Awuchi, 2023; Blackburn, 2003) states that food safety management depends on the interaction of several essential components, such as knowledge, instruments (like risk assessment), and procedures (like HACCP). Providing safe food is based on a food safety objective, which specifies the frequency or maximum concentration of a microbiological hazard in a product considered adequate for consumer protection. The FSO is accomplished by the implementation of many techniques that have been embraced by the food sector and are utilized in a coordinated manner. These consist of the Hazard Analysis Critical Control Point system, Good Hygiene Practice (GHP), and Good Manufacturing Practice (GMP) (Blackburn, 2003). The minimal hygienic and processing standards required to guarantee the manufacture of nutritious food are known as good manufacturing practices, or GMPs. The criteria pertaining to circumstances and operations in a food plant are covered in further detail by the precursor programs. The goal of many GMPs and other preparatory programs is to make sure that the conditions required to avoid possible food contamination and cross contamination are established. Many hygienic and food safety procedures are considered good manufacturing practices that prevent undesirable levels of hazards or remove health risks from meals. To meet particular food safety criteria, food processing and handling facilities must create and implement their own GMP programs in addition to the ones mandated by national food laws and regulations. In order to guarantee the safety of processed goods, the food processing industry has historically depended on following GMPs. Safety in the food processing industry was later addressed more thoroughly with the advent of the Hazard Analysis and Critical Control Point system. However, there should be a few fundamental conditions or needs to meet the HACCP system's structure in order to construct an effective HACCP system.

The idea of HACCP (Hazard Analysis and Critical Control Points) is to prevent issues by identifying hazards, establishing critical control points, and creating procedures for monitoring, preventing, and correcting them. It is a straightforward and logical control system. When developing it, seven fundamental concepts should be taken into consideration:

1. Conduction of possible hazards analysis;
2. Identification of Critical Control Points (CCPs).
3. Determination of Critical Limits for CCPs.
4. Establishment of a monitoring system for control on CCPs.
5. Setting of corrective actions.
6. Fixing of verification procedures.
7. Establishment of principles for maintaining records and documentation (Torres-Monroy et al., 2025)

The HACCP system must recognize and evaluate any potential hazardous elements that could be present in the manufacturing processes, as well as biological, physical, and chemical dangers Fig. 2.3.

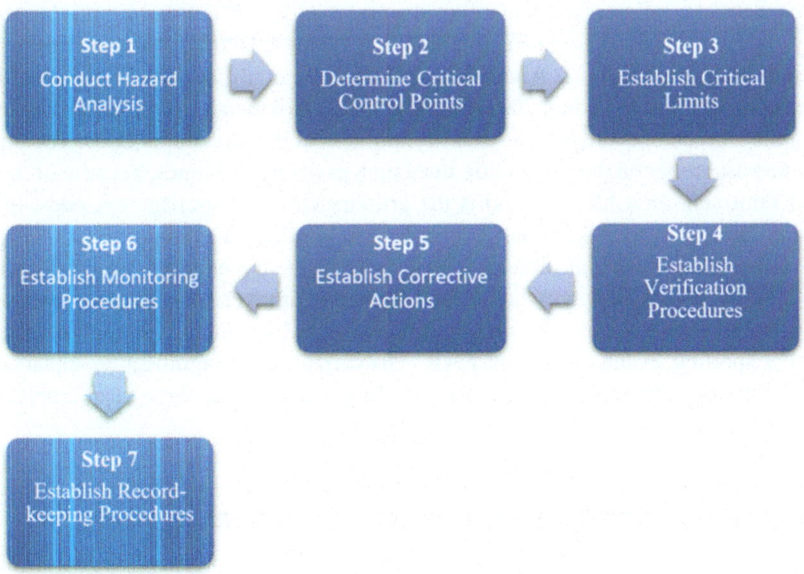

FIGURE 2.3

HACCP implementation in fruit beverages.

In addition to a few other requirements, GMPs that cover all food safety and sanitary procedures that are not covered by the HACCP plan are now considered precondition programs for putting a HACCP system into place. Therefore, taking into account the GMPs that are presently in use, food processing firms that intend to implement HACCP systems must define certain extra needs. Standard operating procedures must be documented for the GMP or HACCP precursor program activities created in food processing facilities. By examining the discrepancies between the efficacy of the present GMPs and their anticipated levels, these SOPs assist in identifying the HACCP requirements that require additional development (Mendis & Rajapakse, 2009).

2.8 Sanitation and hygiene practices

Fruit juices can become contaminated by pathogenic microbes and spoilage in a number of ways. Contamination of fruit and fruit juice may arise from field-adapted procedures and processing conditions. Fruits are thought to be the primary source of pathogenic and spoiling microorganisms that enter processing lines. Equipment used to prepare fruit juice, such as presses, grinders, extractors, pipelines, filling machines, and packaging materials, can also cause contamination (Jay & Anderson, 2001; Narciso & Parish, 1997). Juice recontamination during pasteurization and the potential for microorganisms to establish themselves inside the plant are the outcomes of improper sanitation practices. Due to their ability to withstand acid, three kinds of fruit juice spoiling microorganisms—aciduric bacteria, molds, and yeasts—have been identified as the most significant throughout time (Sourri et al., 2022) According to Keller and Miller (2005), this microbial group— particularly the genera *Lactobacillus* and *Leuconostoc*—was formerly thought to be the most significant category of spoilage bacteria for acidic foodstuffs (Winniczuk & Parish, 1997). Acetylmethyl carbinol and diacetyl, two Lactic Acid Bacterial metabolites, can give juices off aromas reminiscent to buttermilk. Additionally, these microbes can create carbon dioxide, ethanol, lactic, acetic, and formic acids, which can change the juice's flavor (Jay & Anderson, 2001). LAB can utilize some of these acids as markers of fruit juice spoiling (Shui & Leong, 2002; Sellnow, 2020; Gökmen & Acar, 2004). One of the biggest issues facing the fruit and beverage industries' cleanliness at the moment is LAB. The equipment that comes after the pasteurizer on the production line (such as filling machines, because of the difficulty of cleaning and sanitizing their filler valves) is the primary cause of spoilage episodes, in which these microorganisms are involved. Additionally, according to Martínez-Viedma et al. (2008), LAB have the capacity to release exopolysaccharides, which can lead to the development of biofilms and raise the dangers of spoiling and postcontamination. A significant number of fruit juice packs with a high percentage of spoilt samples from the start of production (which implies sanitation issues) are often indicative of a spoiling event caused by LAB. Pasteurization, a significantly enhanced sanitation system, and the use of sanitizers during the fruit washing stage are the three most crucial steps used to reduce LAB in fruit juice facilities (Bastos et al., 2005).

2.9 Emerging technologies for quality assurance

Food and beverage safety, particularly with regard to food quality and cleanliness, has become a widespread global health concern in recent years. Food is a daily essential for development, vitality, health, and illness prevention on a worldwide scale. Therefore, it is crucial to guarantee that customers are provided with only safe and certified food items. Though, customers are having trouble selecting legal food products because of a variety of problems, including inadequate food quality, food impurities, food adulteration, poor cleanliness, outdated food, and others. Since food adulteration directly affects human health, it is one of the main consumer concerns in developing nations. Because the food has been blended or swapped with other approved or forbidden ingredients, it is impossible for consumers to identify tainted food using their senses and can only be detected by laboratory equipment. Therefore, in order to guarantee food safety and public health, the creation of food and beverage evaluations is crucial and need to be a top priority. For evaluating food and beverages, a number of methodological techniques and technologies have been developed, such as electromagnetic sensing, taste, odor, and imaging (Abasi et al., 2018). Conventional techniques for evaluating beverage quality entail laborious and time-consuming laboratory analysis, which often calls for a number of pricey pieces of equipment, consumables, and trained operators. These techniques generally involve equipment such as high-performance liquid chromatography (HPLC), gas chromatography, spectrometers for UV-visible and near-infrared, viscometers, and colorimeters among others (Wang et al., 2017). Additionally, the intensities of organoleptic descriptors, including flavor, fragrance, mouthfeel, and tastes, are evaluated by sensory evaluation. A fixed panel of eight to 16 people and many training sessions for the particular product are necessary for this kind of sensory test, which results in time-consuming and expensive procedures for executing the sessions, processing data, and doing statistical analysis (Piper & Scharf, 2004). Certain industries, like brewing, rely on one or two individuals, like the master brewer, to evaluate the product's sensory quality. However, this approach lacks objectivity, accuracy, and reliability because it does not adhere to any systematic, quantitative methodology and does not incorporate statistical analysis (Viejo *et al.*, 2018). Depending on the number of samples to be evaluated and the desired mean values anticipated for liking findings, the acceptability test is another kind of sensory test that requires assembling at least 30 to 100 consumers. Along with the lengthy questionnaires that are usually given to participants, this makes the techniques subjective and time-consuming because they rely on responses from consumers that may be biassed for a variety of reasons, including cultural effects. For instance, Asians have demonstrated a tendency to be courteous and refrain from using the extremes of the scales (Stone et al., 2020).

To evaluate some of those quality characteristics in food and drinks, certain innovative approaches have been developed that combine automated analytic techniques with artificial intelligence, such as computer vision (CV). These techniques are less time-consuming and more economical, enabling more accurate, consistent, dependable, and objective outcomes (Gill et al., 2011). These methods utilize various data sources, like pictures or videos, which are subsequently processed by computer-based algorithms. These algorithms can be fully automated by combining them with robotics, and they are combined with machine learning modeling to forecast the final product's quality based on various measured parameters. These approaches may also involve the use of arrays of sensors or multisensor systems, which are typically combined with other AI techniques to evaluate certain quality characteristics, including tastes, odors, flaws, and processing conditions, among others (Viejo et al., 2019a; Viejo et al., 2019b). Some of the most exciting new technologies being used in the beverage business are discussed in the sections that follow.

2.9.1 Artificial intelligence

John McCarthy developed the idea of automating machines and established an artificial intelligence lab at Stanford University in the 1960s, which is when the notion of AI first emerged (Joshi, 2019). Apart from their capacity for self-learning, artificial intelligence generally refers to robots that are built and programmed to think, act, solve issues, and make judgments similarly to humans (Viejo & Fuentes, 2020). It may be divided into two categories: (i) weak or applied AI, which is only able to carry out certain tasks like identifying, searching, or analyzing particular components; and (ii) strong or generalized AI, which is able to comprehend, improve, and solve issues, often via machine learning. Although only weak or applied AI has been achieved thus far, generalized AI is theoretically possible (Joshi, 2019). The general idea of AI can comprise any combination of its several subfields, including machine learning, computer vision, robots, sensors, and biometrics. AI has been applied in the beverage sector for a variety of purposes, including decision making, product creation, quality assurance, and monitoring (Mohammadi & Minaei, 2019).

2.9.2 Robotics

Robots once programmed by a computer can carry out their own (Ceccarelli, 2022). These tasks can be adaptive and increasingly sophisticated, requiring the integration of other AI techniques like CV and ML to continuously retrain and learn to do more complicated processes, or they can be basic and repetitive (Chen & de Luca, 2021). Because robotics are dependable, don't get bored or fatigued, and can complete jobs quickly while maintaining high accuracy and precision, their application in the food and beverage sectors has grown (Nayik et al., 2015). Packaging, palletizing, pick and place, and manufacturing are among the primary uses of robots in the beverage sector (Iqbal et al., 2017). However, for more automated applications like quality control, inspection, and as the most frequent beverage pourers or dispensing machines, several businesses and research organizations have combined them with AI divisions (Caldwell, 2012). When it comes to robotics development for product creation, production, and quality evaluation, the alcoholic beverage area has been the most studied. Using artificial intelligence, Makr Shakr is a robotic cocktail mixer that uses a mobile application to let users create their own cocktail drink from a variety of 60 spirits. Two robotic arms then produce the drink (Condé et al., 2017; Viejo et al., 2019a; Viejo et al., 2019b) created a robot (FIZZeyeRobot, The University of Melbourne, Melbourne, Victoria, Australia) that can pour sparkling wine uniformly and can serve up to 50 mL from a single bottle up to three times. It is equipped with servo motors and Arduino boards (Arduino Computing platform, Ivrea, Italy), and it can be adjusted by changing the delay times and bottle position angle. Two robotic arms have been used to create a beer dispenser that is controlled by RobotStudio (ABB Robotics, Zürich, Switzerland). One arm is programmed to hold the glass, while the second arm may handle the tap (Peano, 2018).

2.9.3 Computer vision technology

According to Awwad et al. (2019), the CV approach is a subset of artificial intelligence that involves automatically extracting information from photos or videos by mimicking the capabilities of the human eye. To completely automate the process as an AI system, it may be combined with robots, certain equations or algorithms, fundamental statistics, and machine learning algorithms. This might enable the process to function independently and categorize or forecast the product's quality attributes.

Compared to some traditional procedures like visual inspection and sensory analysis, which have human error as a potential drawback, this method is considered to be faster, more accurate, and more reliable due to its nondestructive, noncontact, replicable, and automatic nature (Wu & Sun, 2013). The three primary processes in the CV process are (i) acquisition, (ii) preprocessing, and (iii)analysis and interpretation for the picture or video.

A camera or scanner and a steady, consistent illumination source are required pieces of equipment for acquisition (Lukinac et al., 2019). For preprocessing and analysis and interpretation, the use of a computer and software with image analysis capabilities (Solem, 2012). Specific algorithms need to be developed according to the type of visual assessment and the parameters to evaluate Fig. 2.4.

Few CV techniques have been created specifically for spirits. Nevertheless, a technique for evaluating color from image analysis was created for drinks like cachaça, a Brazilian distilled beverage made from sugarcane. This method used a digital camera above the glass and a lighting source below it as a background, yielding results in both RGB and CIELab color scales (Rodrigues et al., 2014). In order to identify copper in sugarcane spirits, Pessoa et al. (2017) created a color assessment method using photos taken with a digital camera equipped with a Bayer RGB mosaic filter, which is made up of a grid of color filters and photosensors, a charge-coupled device, a porcelain plaque, and an illuminated black box. In order to evaluate the safety and quality of the finished product at the end of the manufacturing line, Wang et al. (2012) provided a method for detecting foreign matter in Chinese health wine.

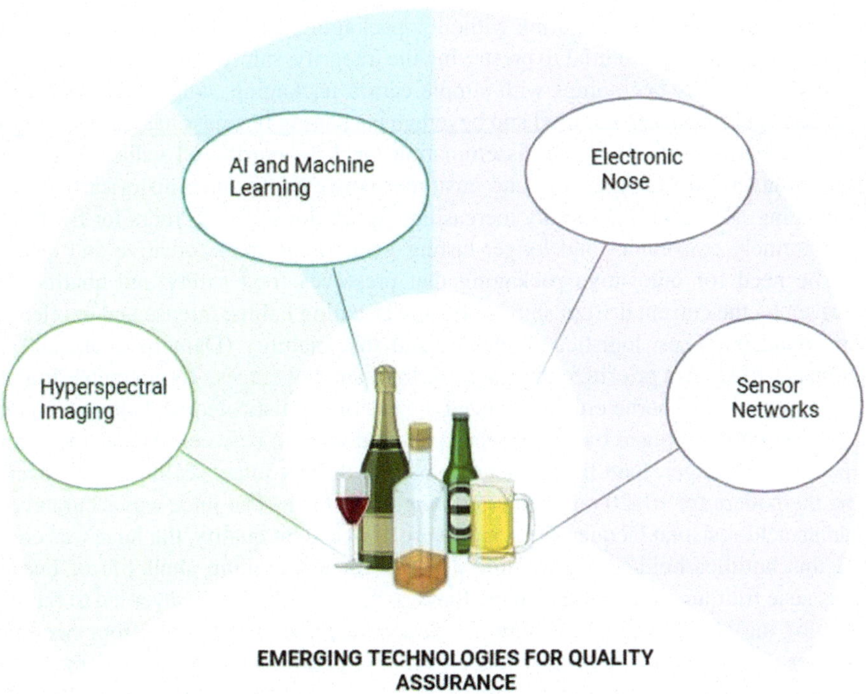

FIGURE 2.4

Emerging technologies for quality assurance.

2.9.4 Machine learning

A computer-based system that can be trained to identify patterns in a dataset in order to categorize or forecast particular parameters is known as machine learning (ML), a subfield of artificial intelligence. By being fed fresh data, ML may become more proficient (Viejo et al., 2019a; Viejo et al., 2019b). The two categories of learning algorithms supervised and unsupervised can also be further subdivided into other categories. The capacity of machine learning to enhance production and evaluate quality in a quicker, more accurate, objective, and economical manner has led to an increase in its application in the food and beverage sector in recent years. Approximately 95% of food and beverage products fail within 3 years after debut, which has led to the industry's demand for ML adoption. To help create better products that consumers will accept, machine learning models have been created to forecast consumer needs, sensory descriptors of the products, acceptability, and physicochemical composition, among other quality attributes (Buss, 2018). Particularly in the past 10 years, ML has been widely used to alcoholic beverages. Using Ramah spectra (600–1800 cm1) as inputs, models have been developed in the spirits industry to classify whisky (whisky) samples according to (i) age, (ii) cask material, (iii) distillery and (iv) variety. The authors compared various machine learning algorithms and found that relevance radial basis function networks produced the best results, with an accuracy >95% (Backhaus et al., 2012).

2.10 Packaging effects on quality and safety

It is impossible to imagine food and drink without a packaging. Thus, from the farm or facility to the final consumer, packaging is essential to preserving the integrity, safety, and quality of agricultural and processed goods. From its beginnings with simple carton packaging, which was done primarily for containment and transportation, the food and beverage packaging business has come a long way. Food confinement, protection, informational dissemination (such as nutritional value, usage instructions, manufacturer contact information, etc.) and customer convenience have historically been the main goals of packaging. However, the rapidly increasing expectations of customers for fresher, safer, less processed, extremely convenient and longer-lasting goods have made creative and safe packaging necessary. The need for innovative packaging that preserves food safety and quality attributes is primarily driven by the current drift of shifting lifestyles, eating habits, intense and unrelenting market competition, retail practices, logistics efficiency, and sustainability (Dainelli et al., 2008). Furthermore, the present food laws prioritize the safety of food and beverages. To guarantee food safety, the problems of previous food-borne epidemics need the use of sophisticated packaging techniques. Fruit juices are traditionally packaged by heating the deaerated juice to between 90 and 95°C in a plate- or tubular type heat exchanger, then filling metal cans with the hot juice, sealing them, inverting them, and keeping them there for 10–20 min before cooling them down. The juice was accurately deaerated, the cans had an acid-resistant lacquer, the seams were of excellent quality, the juice was commercially sterile, and this hotfilled/hold/cool procedure allowed for a minimum shelf life of one to 2 years. However, because fruit juices are acidic, many flaws or scratches in the tin layer led to rapid corrosion, metal dissolving into the juice, hydrogen gas formation, and container failure from swelling. As long as the container closure, which is usually made of metal, is impervious to juice damage, using glass containers solves these issues. Fruit juices were also frequently packaged in glass bottles, however the hotfilled/hold/cool method had to be used carefully to prevent glass containers from breaking. The preferred packing material for premium fruit juices is still glass. However, a growing number of fruit juices and concentrates have been aseptically packed in recent years, usually in laminates made of paperboard, aluminum foil, and plastic film. These items are kept at room temperature, and the barrier qualities of the carton, the way the juice interacts with the carton, and the external storage environment all have a big impact on the keeping quality in terms of nutritional contents, shelf life, etc. (Ghoshal, 2019, pp. 21–50).

2.11 Regulatory framework and guidelines

Despite being high in vitamins and minerals, drinking fruit juices might increase your chance of contracting a microbial illness. The type of fruit, where it comes from, and whether or not it was preserved all affect the microbiota in juices. The majority of bacteria seen on fruit surfaces originate in the soil. Additionally, germs can be transported to the fruit surface by air and water (Matthews, 2014). Juice microbiological safety is a result of both manufacturing cleanliness and the raw materials' microbiological purity. Numerous types of bacteria that are also present under refrigerated storage settings have the capacity to proliferate, which is linked to the risk of microbial contamination.

Fruit is most frequently infected by the following microflora:

- Acid-tolerant fungi, such as molds and yeasts;
- Bacteria resistant to environmental acidification, arising from soil or air;
- Lactobacilli;
- Acid-tolerant bacteria (Biadała et al., 2024).

The goal of sustainability in juice production is to reduce negative effects on the environment while maintaining positive social and economic effects. The procurement of raw materials (fair trade methods, local and organic farming), sensible water management, energy efficiency, supply chain transparency, waste management, and social responsibility are important factors to take into account for a sustainable juice manufacturing process (Hales et al., 2024). Retail and wholesale merchants have been forced to assume more responsibility for guaranteeing food quality and safety in the age of rapidly increasing consumer demands, the globalization of the product market, and the necessity to comply with regulatory requirements (Tanwar et al., 2022). The International Food Standard was therefore created by members of the German Retail Federation, French Retail Federation, the Italian retail trade union CONAD (Consorzio Nazionale Dettaglianti), Federdistribuzione and COOP (Coop società cooperativa) (Nowicki & Kafel, 2021). The risk assessment methodology that underpins the IFS standard gives users some latitude in operations and products. The Global Food Safety Initiative, which is founded on broad principles of food safety and quality management systems, has recognized the IFS worldwide (Biadała et al., 2024).

However, the primary focus is on establishing trust in products and procedures; that is, onsite evaluation, documentation review, and control are used to guarantee safety, quality, legality, and compliance with particular-client needs (Tanwar et al., 2022). It is possible to gather proof that the production process is conducted in compliance with the established assumptions and procedures by keeping track of the tests performed on semi and final products. In turn, this is essential for increasing the manufacturer's reputation and winning over customers. In the manufacturing of juice, ESG (Environmental, Social, and Governance) principles are closely linked with food quality requirements.

High-quality goods are ensured by using fruit from farms free of plant protection treatments, minimizing production waste and losses, using fewer chemicals during the manufacturing process, being transparent, and supporting the local community. Additionally, manufacturing in compliance with the IFS standard is ensured by this sustainable strategy to production (Hales et al., 2024).

National laws establish the rules for juice labeling, nutritional content, and marketing strategies in addition to international standards. As an illustration of how public health recommendations impact juice manufacturing methods, the 2015–20 Dietary Guidelines for Americans place a strong emphasis on the necessity of fortification in response to consumer health concerns. In order to ensure product safety, quality, and sustainability, it is imperative that juice production conform to both regional and international norms (Sellnow, 2020).

2.12 Food traceability and recall system

Modern consumers are well conscious of the effects that the production and distribution of the food they eat have on the environment and society. The steady rise in food-borne diseases caused by tainted food supplies, whether from plant or animal sources, has raised a lot of concerns during the last 10 years. Food safety is essential for both consumers and food businesses, and it has emerged as the cornerstone of sustainable development. Traceability of food supply chains has been acknowledged globally by both industry and regulatory authorities as a means of attaining food safety. By supplying the necessary data at every stage of the supply chain, a well-designed traceability system gives food companies complete transparency about the product. Traceability has been widely used as a risk management strategy to stop the supply of contaminated food from moving through the supply chain by allowing producers and regulators to remove or recall food goods (Rao & Shukla, 2022; Regattieri et al., 2007).

Traceability describes as "the ability to follow the movement of a food through specified stage(s) of production, processing, and distribution" by the Codex Alimentarius Commission (Balkrishna et al., 2021, pp. 311–343). Product identity, data to track, product routing, and traceability tools are the four basic pillars around which a food traceability system is built (Sandhu et al., 2011). Product identification begins with physical attributes including weight, volume, dimensions, and packaging. Data collection, which can be accomplished by barcoding, radio frequency identification (RFID), Quick Response capture, or the most sophisticated technique, DNA analysis, is the second pillar for efficient traceability (Ilie-Zudor et al., 2011). Link management, the third pillar, essentially involves controlling identification from the manufacturing location to the point of sale or care. Data transmission, the fourth and final pillar of a good traceability system, is the most crucial as it links the information flow with the actual movement of items. It has been stated that the expensive expense of the infrastructure needed to deploy a tracking system has prevented food firms in India from putting in place an efficient traceability system throughout the food supply chain. Additionally, one of the other relevant factors has been ignorance and a general disdain for the food safety culture (Rao & Shukla, 2022; Regattieri et al., 2007). As a result, it's critical to inform all parties involved about the advantages of a strong traceability system for emergency management and recall. Furthermore, it is important to determine the forward and backward traceability of the food goods as well as the control points at the receiving and dispatching phases in order to support an efficient recall procedure. Besides, an efficient traceability system requires data recording and information management. Improved control points and improved tracing and monitoring of damaged items provided within the supply chain may be achieved by more thorough and precise record keeping before, during, and after processing. High infrastructure costs and the complexity of farmers' group adoption processes, such as entering data into computers or mobile devices, are the reasons for the inadequate deployment of IT-enabled traceability systems (Rao & Shukla, 2022; Regattieri et al., 2007).

2.13 Conclusion

By and large, the concern for microbiological safety of fruit beverages would be paramount for the public health department and future sustainability of the fruit juice industry. Well, shifting from reactive testing toward a broader framework of Quality Assurance underscores the importance of preventive measures in managing food safety. These provide the groundwork for even advanced systems like HACCP, providing structured methods in finding and controlling all potential hazards of the food through each level of production. However, success in the actual implementation of the systems means a food processing house has to be able to set up their program tailored according to specific requirements while ensuring all their operation practices are made as SOPs. The discussion above also highlights the need for constant further research and updating of safety measures to stay up with changing situations in the field. In the face of evolving foodborne pathogens, the fruit juice sector needs to be on the alert to improve microbiological quality and safety in every effort. A society of safety and compliance can help the industry avoid risks while creating trust with consumers on fruit beverages. Ultimately, the integration of innovative technologies and methodologies will play an important role in advancing food safety practices, so that the sought after benefits of fruit and fruit juice consumption are realized without compromising public health.

References

Abasi, S., Minaei, S., Jamshidi, B., & Fathi, D. (2018). Dedicated non-destructive devices for food quality measurement: A review. *Trends in Food Science & Technology, 78*, 197–205. https://doi.org/10.1016/j.tifs.2018.05.009

Abdel-Sater, M. A., Zohri, A. A., & Ismail, M. A. (2001). Natural contamination of some Egyptian fruit juices and beverages by mycoflora and mycotoxins. *Journal of Food Science and Technology, 38*(4), 407–411.

Aguilar-Rosas, S. F., Ballinas-Casarrubias, M. L., Nevarez-Moorillon, G. V., Martin-Belloso, O., & Ortega-Rivas, E. (2007). Thermal and pulsed electric fields pasteurization of apple juice: Effects on physicochemical properties and flavour compounds. *Journal of Food Engineering, 83*(1), 41–46. https://doi.org/10.1016/j.jfoodeng.2006.12.011

Ahmed, T., Das, K. K., & Uddin, M. A. (2018). The microbiological quality of commercial fruit juices-current perspectives. *Bangladesh Journal of Microbiology, 35*(2), 128–133.

Avîrvarei, A. C., Salanţă, L. C., Pop, C. R., Mudura, E., Pasqualone, A., Anjos, O., & Coldea, T. E. (2023). Fruit-based fermented beverages: Contamination sources and emerging technologies applied to assure their safety. *Foods, 12*(4), 838.

Awuchi, C. G. (2023). HACCP, quality, and food safety management in food and agricultural systems. *Cogent Food & Agriculture, 9*(1). https://doi.org/10.1080/23311932.2023.2176280. Available from: www.tandfonline.com/action/journalInformation?journalCode=oafa20

Awwad, S., Tarvade, S., Piccardi, M., & Gattas, D. J. (2019). The use of privacy-protected computer vision to measure the quality of healthcare worker hand hygiene. *International Journal for Quality in Health Care, 31* (1), 36–42. https://doi.org/10.1093/intqhc/mzy099

Backhaus, A., Ashok, P. C., Praveen, B. B., Dholakia, K., & Seiffert, U. (2012). Classifying scotch whisky from near-infrared Raman spectra with a radial basis function network with relevance learning. In , *411. ESANN 2012 proceedings, 20th European symposium on artificial neural networks, computational intelligence and machine learning* (p. 416).

Balkrishna, A., Rupala, P., Jyoti, D., & Arya, V. (2021). *Global food traceability: Current status and future prospects.* Informa UK Limited. https://doi.org/10.1201/9781003242543-12

Bastos, M.d. S. R., de Fátima Ferreira Soares, N., José de Andrade, N., Cristina Arruda, A., & Elesbão Alves, R. (2005). The effect of the association of sanitizers and surfactant in the microbiota of the Cantaloupe (Cucumis melo L.) melon surface. *Food Control, 16*(4), 369–373. https://doi.org/10.1016/j.foodcont.2004.04.002

Biadała, A., Szablewski, T., Cegielska-Radziejewska, R., Tomczyk, Ł., & Budych, D. (2024). Utilizing the IFS standard for the implementation of sustainable development practices in juice production. *Sustainability, 16* (20), 9123. https://doi.org/10.3390/su16209123

Blackburn, C.d. W. (2003). *Microbiological analysis and food safety management: GMP and HACCP systems detecting pathogens in food* (pp. 3–19). United Kingdom: Elsevier. https://doi.org/10.1533/9781855737044.1.3. Available from: https://www.sciencedirect.com/book/9781855736702

Buss, D. (2018). Food companies get smart about artificial intelligence. *Food Technology, 72*(7), 26–41.

Buzrul, S., Alpas, H., Largeteau, A., & Demazeau, G. (2008). Inactivation of Escherichia coli and Listeria innocua in kiwifruit and pineapple juices by high hydrostatic pressure. *International Journal of Food Microbiology, 124*(3), 275–278. https://doi.org/10.1016/j.ijfoodmicro.2008.03.015

Caldwell, D. (2012). *Robotics and automation in the food industry: Current and future technologies* (pp. 1–503). Italy: Elsevier Ltd. https://doi.org/10.1533/9780857095763. Available from: http://www.sciencedirect.com/science/book/9781845698010

Ceccarelli, M. (2022). *Fundamentals of mechanics of robotic manipulation, 112* (pp. 1–381). Cham, Switzerland: Springer.

Chen, Y., & de Luca, G. (2021). Technologies supporting artificial intelligence and robotics application development. *Journal of Artificial Intelligence and Technology, 1*(1), 1–8. https://doi.org/10.37965/jait.2020.0065

Condé, B. C., Fuentes, S., Caron, M., Xiao, D., Collmann, R., & Howell, K. S. (2017). Development of a robotic and computer vision method to assess foam quality in sparkling wines. *Food Control, 71*, 383–392. https://doi.org/10.1016/j.foodcont.2016.07.020

Dainelli, D., Gontard, N., Spyropoulos, D., Zondervan-van den Beuken, E., & Tobback, P. (2008). Active and intelligent food packaging: Legal aspects and safety concerns. *Trends in Food Science & Technology, 19*(1), Article S103. https://doi.org/10.1016/j.tifs.2008.09.011

Dragan, M., Brankica, L., Radivoj, P., Zoran, P., Jelena, J., Srdjan, S., & Sasa, J. (2019). Climate change: Impact on mycotoxins incidence and food safety. *Теория и практика переработки Мяса, 4*(1), 9–16.

FDA. (2001). Hazard analysis and critical control point (HACCP): Procedures for the safe and sanitary processing and importing of juice, final rule. *Federal Register, 66*(13), 6137–6202.

Gardini, F., Özogul, Y., Suzzi, G., Tabanelli, G., & Özogul, F. (2016). Technological factors affecting biogenic amine content in foods: A review. *Frontiers in Microbiology, 7*. https://doi.org/10.3389/fmicb.2016.01218

Garvey, M. (2019). Food pollution: A comprehensive review of chemical and biological sources of food contamination and impact on human health. *Nutrire, 44*(1). https://doi.org/10.1186/s41110-019-0096-3

Gerba, C. P. (2009). *Indicator microorganisms environmental microbiology* (pp. 485–499). United States: Elsevier Inc.. https://doi.org/10.1016/B978-0-12-370519-8.00023-7. Available from: http://www.sciencedirect.com/science/book/9780123705198

Ghoshal, G. (2019). *Recent development in beverage packaging material and its adaptation strategy.* Elsevier BV. https://doi.org/10.1016/b978-0-12-816683-3.00002-5

Gill, G. S., Kumar, A., & Agarwal, R. (2011). Monitoring and grading of tea by computer vision - A review. *Journal of Food Engineering, 106*(1), 13–19. https://doi.org/10.1016/j.jfoodeng.2011.04.013

Gökmen, V., & Acar, J. (2004). Fumaric acid in apple juice: A potential indicator of microbial spoilage of apples used as raw material. *Food Additives and Contaminants, 21*(7), 626–631. https://doi.org/10.1080/02652030410001712501

Gu, G., Strawn, L. K., Ottesen, A. R., Ramachandran, P., Reed, E. A., Zheng, J., Boyer, R. R., & Rideout, S. L. (2021). Correlation of Salmonella enterica and Listeria monocytogenes in irrigation water to environmental factors, fecal indicators, and bacterial communities. *Frontiers in Microbiology, 11*. https://doi.org/10.3389/fmicb.2020.557289. Available from: https://www.frontiersin.org/journals/microbiology#

Hales, J., Kemper, J., White, S. K., & Veer, E. (2024). Reflections on food policy in the context of healthy and sustainable diets. *Food Policy, 128*. https://doi.org/10.1016/j.foodpol.2024.102708. Available from: https://www.sciencedirect.com/science/journal/03069192

Harris, L. J., Farber, J. N., Beuchat, L. R., Parish, M. E., Suslow, T. V., Garrett, E. H., & Busta, F. F. (2003). Outbreaks associated with fresh produce: Incidence, growth, and survival of pathogens in fresh and fresh-cut produce. *Comprehensive Reviews in Food Science and Food Safety, 2*(s1), 78–141. https://doi.org/10.1111/j.1541-4337.2003.tb00031.x

Horváth-Kerkai, E. (2006). *Manufacturing fruit beverages. Handbook of fruits and fruit processing* (pp. 205–215).

Ilie-Zudor, E., Kemény, Z., Van Blommestein, F., Monostori, L., & Van Der Meulen, A. (2011). A survey of applications and requirements of unique identification systems and RFID techniques. *Computers in Industry, 62*(3), 227–252.

Iqbal, J., Khan, Z. H., & Khalid, A. (2017). Prospects of robotics in food industry. *Food Science and Technology, 37*(2), 159–165. https://doi.org/10.1590/1678-457x.14616

Jay, S., & Anderson, J. (2001). Fruit juice and related products. In *Spoilage of processed foods: Causes and diagnosis* (pp. 187–198).

Joshi, N. (2019). How far are we from achieving artificial general intelligence. *Forbes*.

Juvonen, R., Virkajärvi, V., Priha, O., & Laitila, A. (2011). Microbiological spoilage and safety risks in non-beer beverages. *VTT Tiedotteita - Valtion Teknillinen Tutkimuskeskus, 2599*, 1–107.

Kardos, E. (1962). Gyümölcs-és zöldséglevek, üdıtöitalok (fruit and vegetable juices SoftDrinks). *Müszaki Könyvkiadó, Budapest, Hungary*, 17–18.

Kasikçi, M. B., & Bağdatlioğlu, N. (2016). High hydrostatic pressure treatment of fruit, fruit products and fruit juices: A review on phenolic compounds. *Food and Health, 2*(1), 27–39.

Keller, S. E., & Miller, A. J. (2005). Microbiological safety of fresh citrus and apple juices. In *Microbiology of fruits and vegetables* (pp. 211–230). United States: CRC Press. https://doi.org/10.1201/9781420038934.ch9. Available from: https://www.taylorfrancis.com/books/e/9781420038934

Khandpur, P., & Gogate, P. R. (2015). Understanding the effect of novel approaches based on ultrasound on sensory profile of orange juice. *Ultrasonics Sonochemistry, 27*, 87–95. https://doi.org/10.1016/j.ultsonch.2015.05.001

Kregiel, D. (2015). Health safety of soft drinks: Contents, containers, and microorganisms. *BioMed Research International, 2015*, 1–15. https://doi.org/10.1155/2015/128697

Kuz'mina, E. I., Egorova, O. S., Akbulatova, D. R., & Sviridov, D. A. (2023). *Research of the impact of external factors on changes in consumer properties of beverages from fruit raw materials*.

Lamichhane, A., Regmi, S., Pandit, K., Upadhaya, S., Acharya, J., Koirala, S., Aryal, S., Gurung, K., Thapa, J., Adhikari, S., Sharma, S., Poudel, P., & Sharma, S. (2024). Identification of fungal pathogens among COVID-19 and non COVID-19 cases in Bhaktapur hospital, Nepal. *BMC Research Notes, 17*(1). https://doi.org/10.1186/s13104-024-07010-4

Lee, H., Kim, H., Cadwallader, K. R., Feng, H., & Martin, S. E. (2013). Sonication in combination with heat and low pressure as an alternative pasteurization treatment-effect on Escherichia coli K12 inactivation and quality of apple cider. *Ultrasonics Sonochemistry, 20*(4), 1131–1138. https://doi.org/10.1016/j.ultsonch.2013.01.003

Lopez, M. E., Gontijo, M. T., Boggione, D. M., Albino, L. A., Batalha, L. S., & Mendonça, R. C. (2018). Microbiological contamination in foods and beverages: Consequences and alternatives in the era of microbial resistance. In *In Microbial contamination and food degradation* (pp. 49–84). Academic Press.

Lukinac, J., Mastanjević, K., Mastanjević, K., Nakov, G., & Jukić, M. (2019). Computer vision method in beer quality evaluation—A review. *Beverages, 5*(2), 38. https://doi.org/10.3390/beverages5020038

Mandappa, I. M., Basavaraj, K., & Manonmani, H. K. (2018). Analysis of mycotoxins in fruit juices. In *Fruit juices: Extraction, composition, quality and analysis* (pp. 763–777). India: Elsevier Inc.. https://doi.org/10.1016/B978-0-12-802230-6.00036-9. Available from: http://www.sciencedirect.com/science/book/9780128022306.

Martínez-Viedma, P., Abriouel, H., Omar, N. B., Valdivia, E., López, R. L., & Gálvez, A. (2008). Inactivation of exopolysaccharide and 3-hydroxypropionaldehyde-producing lactic acid bacteria in apple juice and apple cider by enterocin AS-48. *Food and Chemical Toxicology, 46*(3), 1143–1151. https://doi.org/10.1016/j.fct.2007.11.010

Matthews, K. R. (2014). *Microorganisms associated with fruits and vegetables microbiology of fresh produce* (pp. 1–19). United States: wiley. https://doi.org/10.1128/9781555817527.ch1. Available from: https://onlinelibrary.wiley.com/doi/book/10.1128/9781555817527

Mendis, E., & Rajapakse, N. (2009). GMP and HACCP. In *The ceylon chamber of commerce.*

Mohammadi, V., & Minaei, S. (2019). Artificial intelligence in the production process. In *Engineering tools in the beverage industry* (pp. 27–63). Woodhead Publishing.

Nan, M., Xue, H., & Bi, Y. (2022). Contamination, detection and control of mycotoxins in fruits and vegetables. *Toxins, 14*(5), 309. https://doi.org/10.3390/toxins14050309

Narciso, J. A., & Parish, M. E. (1997). Endogenous mycoflora of Gable-top Carton paperboard used for packaging fruit juice. *Journal of Food Science, 62*(6), 1223–1239. https://doi.org/10.1111/j.1365-2621.1997.tb12249.x

Nayik, G. A., Muzaffar, K., & Gull, A. (2015). Robotics and food technology: A mini review. *Journal of Nutrition & Food Sciences, 5*(4), 1–11.

Nowicki, P., & Kafel, P. (2021). *IFS food standard V7: Evolution or revolution.*

Peano, D. (2018). *Innovative beer dispenser based on collaborative robotics (Doctoral dissertation, Politecnico di Torino).*

Pessoa, K. D., Suarez, W. T., dos Reis, M. F., de Oliveira Krambeck Franco, M., Moreira, R. P. L., & dos Santos, V. B. (2017). A digital image method of spot tests for determination of copper in sugar cane spirits. *Spectrochimica Acta - Part A: Molecular and Biomolecular Spectroscopy, 185*, 310–316. https://doi.org/10.1016/j.saa.2017.05.072

Pinto, T., Vilela, A., & Cosme, F. (2022). Chemical and sensory characteristics of fruit juice and fruit fermented beverages and their consumer acceptance. *Beverages, 8*(2), 33. https://doi.org/10.3390/beverages8020033

Piper, D., & Scharf, A. (2004). Descriptive analysis: State of the art and recent developments. In *ForschungsForum eV.*

Pop, O. L., Vodnar, D. C., Suharoschi, R., Mudura, E., & Socaciu, C. (2016). L. plantarum ATCC 8014 entrapment with prebiotics and Lucerne green juice and their behavior in simulated gastrointestinal conditions. *Journal of Food Process Engineering, 39*(5), 433–441. https://doi.org/10.1111/jfpe.12234

Ranadheera, C. S., Prasanna, P. H. P., Pimentel, T. C., Azeredo, D. R. P., Rocha, R. S., Cruz, A. G., Vidanarachchi, J. K., Naumovski, N., McConchie, R., & Ajlouni, S. (2020). *Microbial safety of nonalcoholic beverages.* Elsevier BV. https://doi.org/10.1016/b978-0-12-816679-6.00006-1

Rao, E. S., & Shukla, S. (2022). Food traceability system in India. *Measurement: Food, 5*, Article 100019.

Regattieri, A., Gamberi, M., & Manzini, R. (2007). Traceability of food products: General framework and experimental evidence. *Journal of Food Engineering, 81*(2), 347–356.

Rivankar, S. N., Walke, G. A., Patil, A. N., & Nigalye, A. (2019). Beverage industry in India & scope for medium scale juice extraction units in Goa. *Goa: IOSR Journal of Engineering.*

Rodrigues, B. U., Da Costa, R. M., Salvini, R. L., Da Silva Soares, A., Da Silva, F. A., Caliari, M., Cardoso, K. C. R., & Ribeiro, T. I. M. (2014). Cachaça classification using chemical features and computer vision. *Procedia Computer Science, 29*. https://doi.org/10.1016/j.procs.2014.05.186. http://www.sciencedirect.com/science/journal/18770509

Santhirasegaram, V., Razali, Z., George, D. S., & Somasundram, C. (2015). Effects of thermal and non-thermal processing on phenolic compounds, antioxidant activity and sensory attributes of Chokanan Mango (Mangifera indica L.) juice. *Food and Bioprocess Technology, 8*(11), 2256–2267. https://doi.org/10.1007/s11947-015-1576-y

Scutarasu, E. C., & Trincă, L. C. (2023). Heavy metals in foods and beverages: Global situation, health risks and reduction methods. *Foods, 12*(18). https://doi.org/10.3390/foods12183340. Available from: www.mdpi.com/journal/foods

Sellnow, C. (2020). *Socioeconomic determinants of expenditures on fortified and unfortified fruit juice*. South Dakota State University.

Shankar, V., Mahboob, S., Al-Ghanim, K. A., Ahmed, Z., Al-Mulhm, N., & Govindarajan, M. (2021). A review on microbial degradation of drinks and infectious diseases: A perspective of human well-being and capabilities. *Journal of King Saud University - Science, 33*(2), Article 101293. https://doi.org/10.1016/j.jksus.2020.101293

Shearer, A. E. H., Mazzotta, A. S., Chuyate, R., & Gombas, D. E. (2002). Heat resistance of juice spoilage microorganisms. *Journal of Food Protection, 65*(8), 1271–1275. https://doi.org/10.4315/0362-028X-65.8.1271

Shui, G., & Leong, L. P. (2002). Separation and determination of organic acids and phenolic compounds in fruit juices and drinks by high-performance liquid chromatography. *Journal of Chromatography A, 977*(1), 89–96.

Snyder, A. B., Churey, J. J., & Worobo, R. W. (2019). Association of fungal genera from spoiled processed foods with physicochemical food properties and processing conditions. *Food Microbiology, 83*, 211–218. https://doi.org/10.1016/j.fm.2019.05.012

Solem, J. E. (2012). *Programming computer vision with Python: Tools and algorithms for analyzing images*. O'Reilly Media, Inc.

Sourri, P., Tassou, C. C., Nychas, G. J. E., & Panagou, E. Z. (2022). Fruit juice spoilage by alicyclobacillus: Detection and control methods—A comprehensive review. *Foods, 11*(5). https://doi.org/10.3390/foods11050747. Available from: https://www.mdpi.com/2304-8158/11/5/747/pdf

Stone, H., Bleibaum, R. N., & Thomas, H. A. (2020). *Sensory evaluation practices*. Academic press.

Subramaniam, P., & Wareing, P. (Eds.). (2016). *The stability and shelf life of food*. Woodhead Publishing.

Tanwar, S., Parmar, A., Kumari, A., Kumar Jadav, N., Hong, W.-C., & Sharma, R. (2022). Blockchain adoption to secure the food industry: Opportunities and challenges. *Sustainability, 14*(12), 7036. https://doi.org/10.3390/su14127036

Topolska, K., Florkiewicz, A., & Filipiak-Florkiewicz, A. (2021). Functional food— consumer motivations and expectations. *International Journal of Environmental Research and Public Health, 18*(10), 5327.

Torres-Monroy, K. C., Menjura-Rojas, E. M., Arévalo-Arévalo, H. A., Vásquez-Mejía, S. M., & Barragán-Fonseca, K. B. (2025). *Enhancing safety through implementation of HACCP plan for black soldier fly (Hermetia illucens) larvae meal as animal feed*.

Tribst, A. A. L., de Souza Sant'Ana, A., & de Massaguer, P. R. (2009). Microbiological quality and safety of fruit juices—past, present and future perspectives. *Critical Reviews in Microbiology, 35*(4), 310–339.

Van Schothorst, M., & Jongeneel, S. (1992). HACCP, product liability and due diligence. *Food Control, 3*(3), 122–124.

Vasudevan, S., & Chengaiyan, J. G. (2025). Ensuring beverage excellence: A quality control guide. *Food Science and Engineering*, 38–53.

Viejo, C. G., & Fuentes, S. (2020). Beer aroma and quality traits assessment using artificial intelligence. *Fermentation, 6*(2), 56.

Viejo, C. G., Fuentes, S., Torrico, D. D., Howell, K., & Dunshea, F. R. (2018). Assessment of beer quality based on a robotic pourer, computer vision, and machine learning algorithms using commercial beers. *Journal of Food Science, 83*(5), 1381–1388. https://doi.org/10.1111/1750-3841.14114

Viejo, C., Torrico, D. D., Dunshea, F. R., & Fuentes, S. (2019a). Emerging technologies based on artificial intelligence to assess the quality and consumer preference of beverages. *Beverages, 5*(4), 62.

Viejo, C., Torrico, D. D., Dunshea, F. R., & Fuentes, S. (2019b). Development of artificial neural network models to assess beer acceptability based on sensory properties using a robotic pourer: A comparative model approach to achieve an artificial intelligence system. *Beverages, 5*(2), 33.

Vinny Sandhu, A. K., Thind, S. S., & Minhas, K. S. (2011). Traceability in food supply chain from "farm to fork". *Indian Food Industry, 30*, 23–31.

Wahab, Y. A., Al-Ani, L. A., Khalil, I., Schmidt, S., Tran, N. N., Escribà-Gelonch, M., Woo, M. W., Davey, K., Gras, S., Hessel, V., & Muhd Julkapli, N. (2024). Nanomaterials: A critical review of impact on food quality control and packaging. *Food Control, 163*. https://doi.org/10.1016/j.foodcont.2024.110466. Available from: https://www.sciencedirect.com/science/journal/09567135

Wang, Y., Zhou, B., Zhang, H., & Ge, J. (2012). A vision-based intelligent inspector for wine production. *International Journal of Machine Learning and Cybernetics, 3*(3), 193–203. https://doi.org/10.1007/s13042-011-0051-y

Wang, L., Sun, D. W., Pu, H., & Cheng, J. H. (2017). Quality analysis, classification, and authentication of liquid foods by near-infrared spectroscopy: A review of recent research developments. *Critical Reviews in Food Science and Nutrition, 57*(7), 1524–1538. https://doi.org/10.1080/10408398.2015.1115954

Winniczuk, P. P., & Parish, M. E. (1997). Minimum inhibitory concentrations of antimicrobials against microorganisms related to citrus juice. *Food Microbiology, 14*(4), 373–381. https://doi.org/10.1006/fmic.1997.0103

Wu, D., & Sun, D. W. (2013). Colour measurements by computer vision for food quality control - A review. *Trends in Food Science and Technology, 29*(1), 5–20. https://doi.org/10.1016/j.tifs.2012.08.004

Yoder, J. S., Beach, M. J., & Centers for Disease Control and Prevention (CDC). (2007). Cryptosporidiosis surveillance–United States, 2003–2005. *MMWR Surveill Summ, 56*(7), 1–10.

Zara, G., Budroni, M., Mannazzu, I., Fancello, F., & Zara, S. (2020). Yeast biofilm in food realms: Occurrence and control. *World Journal of Microbiology and Biotechnology, 36*(9), 134.

CHAPTER

Microbiological safety and quality evaluation of vegetable beverages

3

Lateefat Motunrayo Ewuoso[1], Bukola Funmilola Olatunji[2], Sunday Samuel Sobowale[2] and K. Aysha Sherin[3]

[1]*Department of Science Laboratory Technology, Abeokuta, Ogun State, Nigeria;* [2]*Department of Food Science and Technology, College of Basic and Applied Science, Mountain Top University, Prayer City, Ogun State, Nigeria;* [3]*Department of Food Engineering and Technology, Institute of Chemical Technology, Mumbai, Maharashtra, India*

3.1 Introduction

The global consumption of vegetable beverages has increased markedly over the last 2 decades, driven by consumer preference for natural, nutritious, and minimally processed products that contribute to a healthy diet. Vegetable beverages, which include juices, extracts and blends derived from raw vegetables, have been promoted for their functional benefits, including rich supplies of vitamins, minerals, phytochemicals, and antioxidants. With all the nutritional benefits come the major problem of microbiological safety, in that the vegetable beverages are usually consumed fresh or with minimum heating, which renders the products susceptible to microbial contamination. As the fresh juice industry, especially cold-pressed and minimally processed juice products marketed as raw, continues to expand, there is an increased need to maintain consumer demand in fresh juice products and guarantee microbiological safety. The growing use of the HACCP in the process of juice production is also indicative of moods toward this issue at the industrial and regulatory level (Food Safety and Standards (Fortification of Foods) Regulations, 2018). As a result, the microbiologic appraisal of safety has obtained a central position in the field of academic work and industry production of vegetable beverages globally, as it influences regulations pertinent to the production, preservation, and circulation of food products.

Microbiological safety and quality of vegetable beverages are important because the products are widely consumed, and the raw materials used are at high risk. In contrast to foods that are uniformly subjected to harsh thermal processing, most vegetable beverages are minimally or not processed at all, thereby leaving microorganisms relatively unharmed and capable of growing during storage and shipment. Such issues predispose them to be vectors for foodborne pathogens that may result in severe gastrointestinal infections, or in worst-case scenarios, life-threatening diseases. Providing proper control over the use of the juices (Rahman et al., 2021), showed that fresh produce obtained in Dhaka had significant microbial loads that may be maintained in the juice preparation processes. The discovery of findings like these leads to the conclusion that microbiological safety cannot be made synonymous to shelf life itself but it is a determinant which has serious health consequences on the

The Science and Safety of Beverages. https://doi.org/10.1016/B978-0-443-36536-2.00006-5

whole population. Although the microbes that occur in the juice may not be harmful, their existence may still have a detrimental effect on the appearance, taste and smell of the product (Usaga and Worobo, 2018). reported that although UV treatment has been observed to lower the level of microorganisms in cucumber, spinach, and carrot juices, the treatment is not always effective at destroying all microorganisms. Some of the remaining microbes might continue to multiply when stored and such gradual growth rate can damage the overall quality of the juice. Vegetable drinks comprise an extensive variety of merchandizing of fresh vegetables as solitary-ingredient juices or in mixes. It is emerging that the drinks are healthy since they contain vital nutrients such as carotenoids, polyphenols, flavonoids, vitamin, and minerals (Usaga and Worobo, 2018). The popularity of cold-pressed juices, smoothies and extracts may be understood as the desire of consumers to use more plant-based food that can be branded as functional food. Nevertheless, these products are highly perishable and are highly susceptible to microbial contamination despite their attractive nutritional properties. Pasteurization, refrigeration, and natural preservatives are the techniques that should be used in order to decrease the number of microbes and increase the shelf life.

The chapter discusses the safety and quality of vegetable beverages including the key microbial hazards, microbes associated with product spoilage and how the products may become contaminated. It explains the inherent aspects of vegetable juices including pH, nutrient composition, and water activity, which influence the behavior of microbes and product shelf life (Schuh et al., 2020). Another aspect that the chapter analyzes is the effect of the processing such as washing, extraction, pasteurization, high-pressure processing, and non-thermal processing on reducing microbes and preserving quality (Safwa et al., 2024). It dwells on indicators of microbes that are widely utilized in the industry, their roles in safety evaluation, and the role of these measurements in regulatory matters and quality management (Shahbaz and Shahbaz, 2022). Since vegetable beverages are increasingly promoted as fresh, natural and functional foods, this chapter highlights the need to balance maintaining nutritional quality with ensuring microbial safety during processing and storage. The chapter does not cover fruit juices or fermented vegetable beverages, focusing only on non-fermented vegetable drink products.

3.2 Nutritional profile vegetables used in beverage industry

Vegetable-derived beverages such as from carrot, tomato, beetroot and leafy greens tend to be low in fat and protein but offer substantial amounts of water, carbohydrates (mainly natural sugars), vitamins, minerals, and bioactive compounds (e.g., carotenoids, phenolics).Carrot juice, for instance, provides significant amounts of β-carotene (a provitamin A), various minerals such as potassium, magnesium, iron, copper, manganese, and smaller quantities of B-group vitamins, vitamin E and K. In many carrot-juice samples, the content of β-carotene (and other carotenoids) can exceed the adult Recommended Daily Intake in a typical serving size. Tomato juice is a very important vegetable juice in the world market, not only used as a drink, but also as a raw material in combination with other beverages and most food applications. It is highly appreciated for its nutritious value, especially its elevated level of lycopene, 3-carotene, vitamin C, potassium, and other antioxidants, which help ensure cardiovascular health or prevent cancer and immune modulation (U.S. Department of Agriculture, 2018). Tomato juice has also gained popularity as an attractive functional drink due to its nutritional richness, delicious taste, and the fact that it is acceptable among different markets. In conclusion, tomato juice can be defined as a highly accepted vegetable drink with a vast functional capability.

Beetroot juice is another prominent vegetable beverage, distinguished by its content of phenolic compounds, betalain pigments, and inorganic nitrates all contributing to its antioxidant potential and possible vascular benefits (Mudgal et al., 2022). It is especially abundant in dietary nitrates, betalain pigments, phenolics, folate, vitamin C, potassium, and iron, and therefore, carries a heavy dose of antioxidants and bioactive components that help in cardiovascular health, increased blood circulation, and better exercise performance (USDA, 2018). Occurring betalains also impart the beetroot juice with its deep red color thereby making it have a greater appeal over other vegetable juices. In short, beetroot juice is nutritious and an attractive commercial product as an individual or mixed beverage. However, its production and retail handling are susceptible to microbiological hazards. To maintain the safety of consumers, global microbiological standards (Hong Kong Center for Food Safety., 2018; FSSAI, 2018) and the incorporation of cost-effective decontamination systems are needed.

The leafy green extracts made out of vegetables (spinach: *Spinacia oleracea*, kale: *Brassica oleracea* var. sabellica, lettuce: *Lactuca sativa*, moringa: *Moringa oleifera*, and others) rich in chlorophyll are a new type of functional drinks. The juices are extensively advertised to be densely composed of nutrients, including vitamins A, C, and K, folates, iron, calcium, phytonutrients (carotenoids and flavonoids) to fight antioxidant, anti-inflammatory and immune-enhancing activities (Wadamori et al., 2017; USDA, 2018). Rising consumer awareness about the natural, detoxifying, and plant-based drinks has increased the popularity of the leafy green drinks in both first- and third-world countries. Such attempts of combating contamination can be done through washing with potable water, chlorine rinses, and the usage of advanced sanitizers like electrolyzed water, which have demonstrated the ability to inactivate microbial pathogens without important sensory alterations (Rahman et al., 2019; Bhilwadikar et al., 2019). The use of ultraviolet (UV) to treat fresh juices has also been approved by regulatory agencies such as the (Food Safety and Standards (Fortification of Foods) Regulations, 2018), and biological controls using lactic acid bacteria are under investigation to be used in leafy extracts (Tarifa et al., 2023).

Table 3.1.

3.3 Factors influencing microbial growth

The growth and survival of microorganisms depend on various internal and external factors that affect how quickly they grow, change or die in different environments. Knowing these factors is important in food science, environmental microbiology, and public health because even minor changes in conditions can significantly impact microbial behavior. One of these factors is temperature. There is a range of growth of each microorganism: minimum, optimal and maximum. Indicatively, psychrotrophic bacteria such as *Listeria monocytogenes* have the ability to grow at refrigerator temperatures, whereas mesophilic species such as *Escherichia coli* can reproduce at a temperature of about 30–37°C. Proteins anesthetically damaged by high temperatures, membranes disrupted by high temperatures resulting in difficulty to survive as well as low temperatures slowing down cellular processes. Water activity (a_w) is also another important factor. Microbes require the presence of water to perform enzyme activities, transport nutrients and to divide their cells. Majority of bacteria demand a_w of over 0.90 and yeasts and molds can work with less. Water activity reduction by drying, salting or solutes inhibits microbial growth as it slows down the mobility of water and forms osmotic pressure. pH also plays a significant role in the development of microbial communities. Most of the harmful bacteria can be inhibited by

Table 3.1 Nutritional profile of some of the vegetables used in beverage industry.

Vegetable	Macro nutrients (%)	Minerals (g)	Vitamins (g)	References
Carrot	Moisture- 88.8 Protein- 0.7 Fat- 0.5 Carbohydrate- 6 Total sugars −5.6 Crude fiber- 2.4	Ca - 34 mg/100 Fe - 0.4 mg/100 P- 25 mg/100 Na- 40 mg/100 K- 240 mg/100 Mg - 9 mg/100 Cu - 0.02 mg/100 Zn- 0.2 mg/100	Carotenes- 5.33 mg/100 Thiamine- 0.04 mg/100 Riboflavin- 0.02 mg/100 Niacin- 0.2 mg/100 Vitamin C - 4 mg/100	Sharma et al. (2012)
Tomato	Moisture- 91.18 Protein- 17.71 Fat- 4 0.96 Carbohydrates- 5.96 Total sugar- 50.60 Ash- 8.75	Na- 56.9–80.65 mg/100 K- 16.63–1097 mg/100 Ca- 48.47–162.07 mg/100 Mg- 76.87–265.93 mg/100 Al- 1241.38 μg/100 Cr- 60–327.59 μg/100	Vitamin A- 267.33–833 IU/100 Vitamin E– 14.02–16.13 μg/100 Vitamin K- 98.28 μg/100 Vitamin C- 10.86–85 mg/100 Vitamin B$_6$-1.29–1.72 mg/100 Folate- 13–15 mg/100 Niacin- 9.68 mg/100	Ali et al. (2021)
Beet root	Moisture- 85.56 Fat- 0.21 Protein- 1.04 Carbohydrate- 9.05 Dietary fiber- 2.2 Ash- 1.18	Fe- 1.11 mg/100 Zn- 0.21 mg/100 Cu- 0.06mg/100 Mn - 0.23 mg/100	Vitamin C- 4.9 mg/100 Thiamine- 0.032 mg/100 Riboflavin- 0.05 mg/100 Total phenolic content- 255 mg GAE/100 Total flavonoid content- 260 mg RE/100	Mirmiran et al. (2020)
Spinach	Moisture- 92.1 Protein- 2.0 Fat- 0.7 Carbohydrate- 2.90	Ca- 73 mg/100 P- 21 mg/100 Fe- 1140 μg/100	Thiamine- 30 mg/100 Riboflavin- 260 mg/100 Niacin- 500 mg/100 Ascorbic acid- 28 mg/100	Kumar et al. (2020)
Cucumber	Water- 95.23 Protein- 0.65 Fat- 0.11 Carbohydrate- 3.63	Ca- 16 mg/100 Fe- 0.28 mg/100 Mg- 13 mg/100 P- 24 mg/100 Na- 2 mg/100	Vitamin C- 2.8 mg/100 Vitamin K- 16.6 μg/100 Vitamin A- 105 IU/100 Thiamine- 0.03 mg/100 Riboflavin- 0.03 mg/100	Butnariu and Butu (2015)

acidic conditions, which interfere with enzyme activities and transport at the membrane. As an example, fermented vegetables contain lactic acid that reduces the pH to an extent that inhibits the growth of spoilage bacteria. Bacteria usually live well in a near-neutral pH, and fungi can tolerate lower pH, so they have an advantage in low-pH foods and beverages (Willey et al., 2020). The availability of nutrients influences the rate and extent of the growth of microorganisms. They require carbon, nitrogen, minerals and factors of growth in usable forms. The rich nutrient habitats result in rapid growth whereas the nutrient poor habitats slow metabolism and drive microorganisms into the survival or starvation phases. The species that do well are also determined by the types of nutrients such as lactic acid bacteria in juices that have high carbohydrates.

There is also availability of oxygen that dictates which groups of microbes prevail. Aerobes require oxygen, anaerobes do not, and facultative anaerobes are able to adjust to each. Oxygen influences the redox potential that influences the metabolism of microbes and production of toxins. As an example, *Clostridium botulinum* is an anaerobic (low-oxygen) organism that flourishes in improperly cans food (Wilkins, 2022). The activities of microbes can be curtailed through the presence of antimicrobial agents that may be naturally occurring or added intentionally. Plant phenolics and essential oils, organic acids and bacteriocins may interfere with cell membranes and metabolism. Sorbates and nitrates are two examples of food-grade preservatives, which are typically employed to prevent spoilage and pathogens (Willey et al., 2020). Finally, interrelations between microorganisms within a food system or environment may either encourage or inhibit growth. Commensal microbes can also secrete acids, hydrogen peroxide, or bacteriocins which repress other microbes. Conversely, the interactions may stimulate augmentation of survival that is, in mixed microbial communities in fermented foods. All these factors interact with each other, and the outcome of microbial growth relies on their combined effects rather than a single factor. Understanding these interactions is essential for developing effective food safety strategies and managing microbial risks in sensitive products like fresh vegetable beverages.

3.4 Sources of contamination in vegetable beverages

Microbiological safety of vegetable beverages (e.g.., carrot juice, cucumber) is greatly affected by factors such as quality of raw materials, handling practices and processing conditions. This contamination can occur at the various levels of the supply chain such as during cultivation and harvesting, during preparation in retail and then on the producer level. Among the contaminants, the most significant ones are bacteria, yeasts, molds and parasites, which can cause serious effects on the health of the consumers of those drinks that have not been treated enough, or due to the inability to preserve the products (Erhirhie et al., 2020; WHO, 2008). There is also too much supply of water, irrigation of wastewater, animal manure and contaminated soils are all contributing factors to microbial risks to fresh vegetables during their initial production.

In a case in point, the tomatoes and leafy greens grown using contaminated water were detected to harbor the *Escherichia coli*, *Salmonella* spp. and intestinal parasites in a study conducted in Nigeria and Ghana (Auta et al., 2017; Nasiru et al., 2015). On the same note, Adekunle et al. reported that there was a wide variation of the microbial concentration in produce depending on the season and post-harvest treatment. The process of beverage preparation, especially in small and informal units, is prone to contamination due to dirty utensils, poor sanitation, and the use of unsafe water. In Ethiopia, it has been found that there are high coliform, yeast, and mold counts in fresh juices produced in cafes mainly due to improper washing of produce and poor handling by the vendors (Wondimagegn and Mohammed, 2025).

3.4.1 Raw material contamination

Every ingredient's cleanliness matters a lot when making plant-based drinks safe. Since vegetables are typically consumed without cooking, they carry higher risk of carrying harmful germs. Spoilage happens fast, which adds to the problem (Erhirhie et al., 2020; WHO, 2008). Mixing various parts of vegetables like green leaves, tubers, fruit etc in one drink increases the chance for many kinds of bacteria to come together. This mix makes checking everything much harder. Rules like GAP and HACCP guide producers to keep things under control. Sticking closely to those steps lowers possible dangers along the way (Lee et al., 2023; Food Safety and Standards (Fortification of Foods) Regulations, 2018).

3.4.2 Water used in processing

Water is often used in making vegetable drinks. It serves many purposes, such as washing, diluting, blending and packaging. However, it can also be a major source of microbial contamination. Pathogens can easily enter food if the water used during processing is untreated or unsafe (Moses et al., 2016; WHO, 2008). To prevent waterborne contamination and ensure product safety, it is important to improve drinking water systems, provide better hygiene training, and implement HACCP-based water monitoring (Rahman et al., 2019; Bhilwadikar et al., 2019).

3.4.3 Processing environment and equipment

The microbiological safety of vegetable beverages is highly influenced by the facilities and equipment applied in the processing. Although raw materials and water are safe, bad sanitation, machines that are not well maintained, and contaminated surfaces may introduce pathogens (Lee et al., 2023; WHO, 2008). Smaller processors are also at a higher risk of being exposed to airborne microbes, insects, dusts and poor waste management because they lack sufficient hygiene facilities. Unless tools like knives, blenders, tanks and dispensing equipment are cleaned correctly, biofilms may form, and therefore the quality of ingredients will be compromised. This is in view of the fact that certain types of beverages being processed require rigid cleaning, sanitation and maintenance practices.

3.4.4 Personnel hygiene

Microbial safety of vegetable juices such as carrot juice depends on personal hygiene. Even in cases where the raw materials, water, and equipment are safe, food handlers can be a direct cause of contamination by failing to wash their hands clean or carelessly handling food products. The problem is more common with small and informal processing facilities, where there is little food safety training and control (Boakye et al., 2023; Lee et al., 2023). Therefore, there is a challenge and opportunity of improving the hygiene of the workers. To improve the microbial quality of vegetable beverages worldwide, consumers should be safe and extensive training, constant assessment, and increased implementation of hygiene should be performed to guarantee consumer safety (Rahman et al., 2019; Bhilwadikar et al., 2019).

3.4.5 Transportation and market handling

The beverages and vegetables that are prepared out of the vegetables are greatly influenced by transportation as well as the way they are handled by the market. An even high-quality produce can be contaminated during transportation, display at the market or during on-site processing, particularly in places with weak cold chains and sanitation systems (Wadamori et al., 2017; WHO, 2008). The microbial load is usually added by the market surfaces, hands, and wash water. In Ghana, Nigeria, and Korea, the studies revealed that vegetables harbored parasites, coliforms, and spoilage organisms (Brooks, 2014; Tango et al., 2018). Small and medium-sized enterprises do not have enough resources and infrastructure to meet international regulations regarding clean transport and appropriate temperatures (Food Safety and Standards (Fortification of Foods) Regulations, 2018; FSSAI, 2018), which may be a significant issue.

3.4.6 Post-processing contamination of vegetable beverages

Contamination of microbiological safety of vegetable juices such as cabbage and carrot juice is a serious threat that is caused during post-processing. The pathogens and microorganisms that cause spoilage may re-enter the product even after undergoing either thermal or non-thermal treatments since these beverages form favored conditions because they contain nutrients, have a neutral pH, and have water activity (Usaga and Worobo, 2018; Food Safety and Standards (Fortification of Foods) Regulations, 2018). Poor hygiene and laxity in enforcing regulations increase this risk in developing countries. Safe consumption is necessary across the world through improved hygienic packaging, training of the vendors, and strong microbiological monitoring (Bhilwadikar et al., 2019; Rahman et al., 2021).

3.4.7 Storage and packaging

The storage and the packaging process is important in ensuring the microbial safety and the quality of vegetable beverages. Their weak alkali pH, presence of nutrients, and high content of water render them highly perishable thus they grow microorganisms when their storage or packaging is poor (Wazed et al., 2023). Refrigeration is slower than keeping at room temperature, which accelerates spoilage (Jimma et al., 2022; Obasi et al., 2019). The containers that are poorly closed (which are typical of informal markets) also increase the chances of contamination (Afolabi et al., 2015).

3.5 Microorganisms of concern in vegetable beverages

The microbial contamination, bacteria, fungi and parasites, is very prone in vegetable drinks, which can compromise its safety and quality (Bhilwadikar et al., 2019). Examples of critical bacterial pathogens are *Escherichia coli* (particularly, O157:H7), *Salmonella* spp., *Listeria monocytogenes, Staphylococcus aureus, Klebsiella pneumoniae, and Clostridium botulinum* (Marr and Russo, 2019; Moses et al., 2016; WHO, 2008). *E. coli O157:H7* has the ability to penetrate improperly handled, contaminated, manure-treated soil, or water and can survive in cold-pressed, low-acid juices (Obasi et al., 2019; Rahman et al., 2021). *Salmonella* is known to survive in beverages with low pH, whereas *Listeria* is able to proliferate in refrigeration. *S. aureus* also releases heat stable enterotoxins which mainly occur due to poor handling, *C. botulinum* spores are also potentially severe under anaerobic, low-acid conditions (e.g., sealed juices that are not properly acidified or refrigerated) and are caused by fungal contaminants (e.g., *Candida, Saccharomyces, Rhodotorula*) and molds (e.g., *Aspergillus, Penicillium, Fusarium, Alternaria*). Sugars may be fermented by yeasts, resulting in off-flavors and turbidity and may be fermented by molds that can form mycotoxins and spoilage (Akpan et al., 2020). These fungi can survive at low pH conditions, high sugar and low temperature. Good farming practices, comprehensive washing and sanitization, hygienic handling, and advanced preservation techniques that have been developed, including UV-C treatment or high-pressure processing, are all needed in prevention. FDA, FSSAI, and FSA regulate microbials and mycotoxin concentration of beverages by establishing a maximum limit (FDA, 2020).

Table 3.2.

A significant issue with vegetables in vegetable drinks is the presence of organisms that cause spoilage, which affects the safety, shelf-life, and the sensory properties without necessarily posing immediate health risks (Usaga and Worobo, 2018; Wondimagegn and Mohammed, 2025). Their action leads to the unpleasant alteration in the flavor, odor, texture, color, and acceptability. Among the most important microbes that cause spoilage, one can single out lactic acid bacteria (LAB), yeasts, acetic acid bacteria (AAB), and *Pseudomonas* spp., which are present in raw materials, processing settings, and equipment surfaces (Erhirhie et al., 2020; Rahman et al., 2021). LAB is Gram-positive, facultative anaerobic fermenters covert sugars to lactic acid resulting in rapid acidification, sourness, turbidity, gas and off-flavors. They are acid-tolerant and can withstand mild levels of preservation techniques, and thus are common in the unsanitary handling in harvesting, washing, and cutting. *Candida, Saccharomyces, Pichia, Hanseniaspora, and Rhodotorula* are the yeasts grow in low-oxygen acidic conditions to provide ethanol, CO_2, pigments and volatile products causing off-flavors, frothing and turbidity, good indicators of poor hygiene. Sugars and ethanol are oxidized by AAB to acetic acid which causes souring, off-flavors and turbidity of oxygenated drinks. *Pseudomonas* spp. have a wide range of nutrients and produce cloudiness, off-odors and surface biofilms and can survive low-sugar low-pH and neutral-pH beverages in refrigeration (Wondimagegn and Mohammed, 2025). The management needs hygienic handling of raw materials and sanitization, optimum processing and proper storage.

3.6 Microbiological assessment of vegetable beverages

Microbiological analysis is also crucial in the safety and quality of the vegetable drinks, particularly freshly made or minimally processed juices, which are of health advantage (Uddin et al., 2021; Wondimagegn and Mohammed, 2025). Some of these critical analyses are total viable counts (TVC), coliforms, yeasts and molds, and which when combined imply the microbial load and the general hygienic quality. The presence of high levels of microbes may result in food-related diseases, unpleasant odor, and undesirable flavor and color modification which decreases consumer acceptance. The evaluation strategies are the combination of the general assessment, for example, TVC, with the definite numbers of coliforms and yeasts/molds to get the overall image of the safety, quality, and

Table 3.2 Microorganisms of concern in vegetable-based beverages.

Vegetable-based beverages	Microorganisms	Significance in beverage	References
Carrot juice	*Alicyclobacillus acidoterrestris*	Thermo-acidophilic spoilage organism producing off-odors such as guaiacol	Silva and Gibbs (2001)
	Lactobacillus spp.	Involved in controlled fermentation and acidification	
	Escherichia coli	Potential foodborne pathogen associated with contamination during processing	
Tomato juice	Lactic acid bacteria (e.g., *Leuconostoc mesenteroides*	Involved in spontaneous or uncontrolled fermentation, leading to acid production and quality deterioration.	Ray (2004)
	Clostridium botulinum	Capable of toxin production if pH and thermal processing are inadequately controlled.	
	Molds such as *Penicillium* and *Aspergillus* species.	Responsible for off-flavors, discoloration, and reduced shelf life.	
Cucumber juice/ Smoothies	*Pseudomonas* spp.	Responsible for off-odors, slime formation, and reduced shelf life.	Beuchat (1996)
	Yeasts such as *Saccharomyces cerevisiae*	Cause unwanted fermentation leading to gas formation and flavor deterioration.	
	Listeria monocytogenes	Potential foodborne pathogen associated with raw and minimally processed vegetables.	
Beetroot juice	*Lactobacillus plantarum*	Commonly involved in controlled fermentation and acidification.	Rembiałkowska et al. (2007)
	Candida spp.	Spoilage yeasts responsible for fermentation defects and off-flavors.	
	Coliforms	Indicators of poor hygiene and inadequate handling practices.	

Continued

Table 3.2 Microorganisms of concern in vegetable-based beverages.—cont'd

Vegetable-based beverages	Microorganisms	Significance in beverage	References
Spinach or kale green juices	*Salmonella* spp.	Major foodborne pathogens frequently linked to leafy green vegetables.	Olaimat and Holley (2012)
	E. coli O157:H7	Pathogenic strain commonly associated with raw vegetables and contaminated irrigation water.	
	Enterobacter spp.	Indicator organisms reflecting poor sanitation or post-harvest contamination.	
Celery juice	*Listeria monocytogenes*	Potential pathogen associated with raw celery and refrigerated storage conditions.	Francis et al. (1999)
	Pseudomonas fluorescens	Spoilage organism contributing to sensory deterioration during storage.	
	Enterobacter cloacae	Indicator of poor handling and inadequate hygiene during processing.	
Mixed vegetable smoothies (e.g., kale, spinach, carrots)	*Salmonella* spp.	Pathogen commonly introduced through contaminated leafy vegetables.	Piagentini and Güemes (2002)
	Bacillus cereus	Spore-forming bacteria can survive when pasteurization is done incorrectly.	
	Yeasts and molds	These spoilage organisms grow during refrigeration, which causes a loss of quality.	
Pumpkin juice	*Aspergillus flavus*	Potential mycotoxin-producing mold affecting product safety.	Akinyele and Adetuyi (2005)
	Lactic acid bacteria	Can initiate fermentation, altering acidity and sensory quality.	

Table 3.2 Microorganisms of concern in vegetable-based beverages.—cont'd

Vegetable-based beverages	Microorganisms	Significance in beverage	References
	E. coli	Possible contaminant indicating poor hygiene and unsafe handling.	
Cabbage juice (fermented or raw)	*Lactobacillus brevis*, *Lactobacillus plantarum*	Involved in fermentation and acidification, which helps with microbial stability and product quality.	Di Cagno et al. (2015)
	Candida spp.	Spoilage yeasts can lead to unwanted fermentation, off-flavors, and a shorter shelf life.	
	Staphylococcus aureus	They can be contaminants if there is improper handling and poor personal hygiene.	

possible health hazard. It is essential to maintain all the production chain of raw materials to the final packaged beverage to make sure that they do not violate the international food safety standards (Bhilwadikar et al., 2019; Obasi et al., 2019).

3.6.1 Total viable count (TVC)

Aerobic plate count or total viable count (TVC) is an important quantitative approach to measuring the level of microorganisms in vegetable beverages (Uddin et al., 2021). It determines the total culturable heterotrophic microorganisms, which is an indicator of hygiene, degree of processing and possibility of spoilage. Vegetable drinks are rich in nutrients, and water, which is conducive to the growth of microbes unless preserved well. TVC plays a vital role in research and regulation where it is used to anticipate the shelf life and assess health hazards. Research of in-house prepared fruit and vegetable juices shows the correlation of TVC with storage conditions, handling practices and source of contamination (Bulti and Melkam, 2018; Al Amin et al., 2018). The benefits of this method are that the health of consumers is preserved by avoiding spoilage and food poisoning, and these are also useful and trustworthy method in quality management during the production, distribution and storage of foods.

3.6.2 Coliform test

Coliforms are Gram-negative and rod-shaped microorganisms that perform the role of fecal contamination and degradation indicators of poor hygiene in vegetable beverages (Erhirhie et al., 2020; Tango et al., 2018). Their existence can be a danger of safety and the necessity of adherence to the rules. The quality of the products is also affected by coliforms because high numbers are associated with reduced shelf life and more spoilage because of the other microorganisms coexisting. Frequent analysis of coliforms, combined with the total viable count (TVC) and yeast/mold count, is an effective solution to microbiological surveillance, as it can guarantee the safety and quality of vegetable drinks, as well as protect human health (Bhilwadikar et al., 2019; Obasi et al., 2019).

3.6.3 Yeast and mold count

Eukaryotic microorganisms that occur in vegetable beverages include yeasts and molds, which have both positive and negative impacts (Bulti & Melkam, 2018; Wondimagegn and Mohammed, 2025). Some yeasts help to ferment, however, majority of yeasts and molds bring about spoilage, such as affecting taste, aroma and effervescence. Molds will be able to form visible colonies, and mycotoxins are dangerous to human health. Environmental factors include the temperature, humidity, and hygienic handling that affect their development. Microbial surveillance is a vital part of vegetable beverage manufacturing as it is necessary to monitor yeasts and molds regularly in order to guarantee the quality of the product, increase its shelf life, avoid spoilage, and guarantee the safety of consumers.

3.6.4 Rapid detection techniques

The rapid detection methods are more advanced as compared to the traditional methods, which offer faster results, without sensitivity or specificity loss. Such methods are applicable in detecting contamination in the course of production, handling of raw materials up to storage. They contribute to the prevention of spoilage and reduce the possibility of product recalls (Bhilwadikar et al., 2019; Uddin et al., 2021). Immunological, for example, ELISA and lateral flow, nucleic acid-based, biosensor, microfluidics, and automated culture or fluorescence techniques have become important rapid methods of detection. Combining them with traditional culture techniques provides an effective framework of safety and quality monitoring related to the vegetable drinks of beverages (Tarifa et al., 2023). The culture-based approaches are still essential to determining the micro-biological safety of vegetable beverages since it is accurate, simple and economical. These include culturing of microorganisms on selective or different media under controlled conditions, which permits counting, isolation as well as identification of the bacteria. Although molecular and rapid detection methods have advanced, the culture method remains essential in determining microbial control, regulation, and microbial ecology in vegetable-based beverages (Erhirhie et al., 2020; Wondimagegn and Mohammed, 2025).

3.7 Regulatory standards and guidelines for vegetable beverages

In the case of juices prepared by means of vegetables, such as purees and concentrates, the processors must adhere to the provisions of HACCP, provided in 21 CFR Part 120. This is where the product is offered in the form of juice or employed in making drinks. The rule demands that there is a documented hazard analysis. In the case of microbial hazards, the processors should set up critical control points (CCPs) to address dangers such as pathogens (FDA, 2021). One of the conditions is a five log pathogen reduction, the juice should be treated with methods like pasteurization or some non-thermal approved method, which should result in a reduction of the most resistant relevant pathogens, like *E. coli O157:H7*, *Salmonella* and *Listeria*, to achieve 100 thousand-fold (10^5) before or after packaging. Exemptions can be made on further controls of pathogen reduction where the additional pathogen-reduction control is necessary and the processing parameters are recorded, including shelf-stable juices and certain concentrates processed properly. The HACCP system consists of the hazard analysis, identification of CCPs, determination of critical limits, monitoring procedures, correction actions, record keeping and verification. This systematic preventive measure is used to control microbial hazards throughout the processing, packaging, and distribution (Food and Drug Administration., 2003). GMP and GHP make sure that all the activities in handling the raw materials, cleaning equipment, personnel hygiene and transporting products are done in sanitary conditions and reduce chances of contamination before and after production. Processing treatments, packaging, storage temperature and handling are of significant importance to the shelf life and microbial safety of unpasteurized or minimally processed juices. A case in point, an experiment on high hydrostatic pressure (HHP) treated vegetable juices revealed that the sub-lethally damaged pathogens had a chance to recover throughout the storage. This result supports the necessity of proven processing and storage procedures (Kaddumukasa et al., 2017). The other research on fresh unpasteurized vegetable juices related physicochemical parameters (pH, acidity and °Brix) with storage parameters (ambient and refrigeration) in influencing the growth of microorganisms, spoilage and shelf life of fresh fruits and vegetables. According to this study, the correct storage temperature and packaging are crucial as they ensure the safety and quality of the product (Nasiłowska et al., 2018). The regulatory structures such as the five log reduction by FDA are implicitly employed to maintain shelf-stable or safe short-shelf-life products through the application of pathogen reduction, hygienic processing, sampling and batch acceptance criteria.

The standards for evaluating the microbiological safety of ready-to-consume vegetable beverages are outlined in Table 3.3. The microbiological quality of ready-to-consume vegetable beverages is assessed using indicator organisms that reflect product safety, hygiene, and spoilage potential. Aerobic plate count (APC) provides an overall estimate of viable microorganisms and serves as a general indicator of processing and handling conditions. Acceptable APC levels indicate good manufacturing practices, while higher values suggest poor sanitation or improper storage. Total coliform count (TCC) is used to evaluate sanitary quality and possible contamination from water, raw materials, or equipment. The presence of *Escherichia coli* indicates fecal contamination and poses a direct health risk, making strict limits essential. *Staphylococcus aureus* is commonly linked to human handling and reflects personal hygiene during processing. The absence of *Salmonella* spp. is mandatory due to its high pathogenicity. Yeast and mold counts are important spoilage indicators, as excessive growth leads to sensory deterioration and reduced shelf life. Together, these standards support effective quality control and ensure consumer safety.

3.8 Strategies to improve safety and quality of vegetable beverages

Maintaining strict hygiene during processing is crucial to improve the safety and quality of vegetable beverages. Cleaning and sanitizing equipment, processing areas and contact surfaces helps prevent microbial contamination from raw materials, handlers, or the environment. Consistent sanitation procedures, together with proper manufacturing and hygiene practices, play a key role in limiting spoilage and preventing the entry of harmful microorganism. This is especially important in making

Table 3.3 Standards for evaluating the microbiological safety of ready-to-consume vegetable beverages.

Indicators	Microbiological quality levels	
	Satisfactory	Unsatisfactory
Aerobic plate count	5.0×10^3–4.0×10^4 (cfu/mL)	>4.0×10^4 (cfu/mL)
Total coliform count	10–100(cfu/mL)	>100 (cfu/mL)
Escherichia coli	<100 MPN/mL	>100 (cfu/mL)
Staphylococcus aureus	<100 (cfu/mL)	>100 (cfu/mL)
Salmonella spp.	Not detected in 25 mL	Detected in 25 mL
Yeasts and molds	2–3 (cfu/mL)	>3 (cfu/mL)

fresh or minimally processed vegetable beverages, where limited processing creates fewer barriers to microbial growth. Traditional thermal pasteurization kills pathogens and spoilage organisms, but it can also lower some nutrients and sensory traits like vitamins, aroma, and color (Petruzzi et al., 2017). Non-thermal and mild preservation methods are gaining interest to tackle these problems. High Pressure Processing (HPP) at 300–600 MPa effectively targets bacteria, yeasts, and molds while better preserving flavor, nutrients, and texture compared to heat treatment (Anderson and Anderson, 2025). UV-C Treatment, with or without mild heat, can achieve a five log reduction of common pathogens and spoilage microbes in turbid or cold-pressed vegetable juices. This method extends shelf life while maintaining better color, cloudiness, and overall quality than standard pasteurization (Gouma et al., 2020). Other new non-thermal methods, such as cold plasma, pulsed electric fields, and ultra-sonication, are being studied for their ability to kill microbes while minimizing damage to nutrients and sensory qualities (Gulzar et al., 2024). Using these technologies alone or together can improve microbial safety while keeping nutritional and sensory quality intact. Proper packaging, including aseptic filling, sterile containers, and secure seals, along with cold chain storage, is vital to preventing contamination after processing and suppressing microbial growth during storage and transport. Non-thermal methods like HPP or UV-C work best when proper packaging follows hygiene standards. Human factors, such as staff hygiene, equipment cleanliness, and monitoring sanitation practices, greatly affect microbial safety. Regular staff training, strict monitoring of hygiene practices, and adherence to good manufacturing and hygiene practices help maintain control from handling raw materials to processing, filling, and storage, reducing the risk of contamination.

3.9 Conclusion

The quality and safety of microbes in vegetable beverages largely depend on the complex interactions of production processes, preservatives and control measures. Pathogenic and spoilage microorganisms present the most significant risk, especially for perishable products. Proper risk evaluation and a HACCP system are crucial for ensuring safety throughout production. Both domestic and international regulations provide guidelines on microbiological, chemical and physical risks, outlining critical control areas and compliance criteria. Implementing these standards along with training on good manufacturing practices and hygiene ensures that vegetable beverages meet consumer expectations and market demands. Future efforts should focus on harmonizing national and international standards, strengthening the cold chain system, raising awareness and ensuring that vegetable drinks remain safe, high-quality, and competitive in the global market.

References

Afolabi, O., Oloyede, A., Abibu, W., & Adeyanju, A. (2015). Microbial safety of polyethylene packaged sliced fruits sold in abeokuta, south-west Nigeria. *Journal of Natural Sciences Research, 5*(Issue 13). www.iiste.org.

Akinyele, B. J., & Adetuyi, F. C. (2005). Effect of processing methods on the nutritive value of pumpkin (Cucurbita pepo linn.) seed flour. *Journal of Food Technology, 3*(3), 336–341.

Akpan, G. A., Enwere, N. J., & Ubong, E. J. (2020). Microbial spoilage and safety concerns associated with fruit and vegetable juices: A review. *Asian Food Science Journal, 18*(3), 30–43.

Al Amin, M., Mamun, M. R., & Das, K. K. (2018). Microbiological quality analysis of commercial fruit juice in Dhaka city, Bangladesh. *Stamford Journal of Microbiology, 8*, 15–18. https://doi.org/10.3329/sjm.v8i1.42432

Ali, M. Y., Sina, A. A. I., Khandker, S. S., Neesa, L., Tanvir, E. M., Kabir, A., Khalil, M. I., & Gan, S. H. (2021). Nutritional composition and bioactive compounds in tomatoes and their impact on human health and disease: A review. *Foods, 10*(1). https://doi.org/10.3390/foods10010045

Anderson, L., & Anderson, L. (2025). Role of high-pressure processing in enhancing juice safety and quality. *Journal of Food Processing and Technology, Reviewed*, 1001160–1001161. https://doi.org/10.35248/2157-7110.25.16.1160

Auta, T., Bawa, J. A., & Suchet, C. M. (2017). Parasitic contamination of common fresh fruits and vegetables sold in fresh water markets in Abuja Town, Katsina State, Nigeria. *Journal of Advanced Biology and Biotechnology, 14*, 1–8. https://doi.org/10.9741/JABB.2017(3)300

Beuchat, L. R. (1996). Pathogenic microorganisms associated with fresh produce . IAMFES, United States. *Journal of Food Protection, 59*(2), 204–216. https://doi.org/10.4315/0362-028X-59.2.204

Bhilwadikar, T., Pounraj, S., Manivannan, S., Rastogi, N. K., & Negi, P. S. (2019). Decontamination of microorganisms and pesticides from fresh fruits and vegetables: A comprehensive review from common household processes to modern techniques. *Comprehensive Reviews in Food Science and Food Safety, 18*(4), 1003–1038. https://doi.org/10.1111/1541-4337.12453

Boakye, M. K., Tornyi, J. M., Dzubey, I., Adzoyi, P., Ayimah, J. C., Boakye, D. S., & Wiafe, E. D. (2023). Assessment of food hygiene and safety knowledge, attitude, and practices of fruit and vegetable vendors in the Ho central market. *Ghana Heliyon, 9*(9). https://doi.org/10.1016/j.heliyon.2023.e19579

Brooks, A. A. (2014). Evaluation of microbial contamination of street-vended fruit salad in Calabar, Nigeria. *International Journal of Current Microbiology and Applied Sciences, 3*(Issue 7). http://www.ijcmas.com.

Bulti, M. F., & Melkam, M. D. (2018). Microbiological quality and safety of street-vended fresh fruit juices in Jimma Town, Southwest Ethiopia. *Journal of Food Quality, 2018*, Article 1389751.

Butnariu, M., & Butu, A. (2015). *Chemical composition of vegetables and their products handbook of food chemistry* (pp. 627–692). Romania: Springer Berlin Heidelberg. https://doi.org/10.1007/978-3-642-36605-5_17

Di Cagno, R., Filannino, P., & Gobbetti, M. (2015). *Fermented foods: Fermented vegetables and other products encyclopedia of food and health* (pp. 668–674). Italy: Elsevier Inc. https://doi.org/10.1016/B978-0-12-384947-2.00284-1

Erhirhie, E. O., Omoirri, M. A., Chikodiri, S. C., Ujam, T. N., Emmanuel, K. E., & Oseyomon, J. O. (2020). Evaluation of microbial quality of vegetables and fruits in Nigeria: A review. *International Journal of Nutrition Sciences, 5*(3), 99–108. https://doi.org/10.30476/IJNS.2020.86034.1065

FDA. (2021). Juice HACCP and the FDA food safety modernization act: Guidance for Industry. http://www.regulations.gov.

Food and Drug Administration. (2003). *Small entity compliance guide: Juice HACCP.* U.S. Department of Health and Human Services.

Food safety and standards (fortification of foods) regulations. (2018).

Food Standards Agency. (2020). *Guidance on microbiological criteria and food safety.* Food Standards Agency.

Francis, G. A., Thomas, C., & O'Beirne, D. (1999). The microbiological safety of minimally processed vegetables. *International Journal of Food Science and Technology, 34*(1), 1–22. https://doi.org/10.1046/j.1365-2621.1999.00253.x

Gouma, M., Álvarez, I., Condón, S., & Gayán, E. (2020). Pasteurization of carrot juice by combining UV-C and mild heat: Impact on shelf-life and quality compared to conventional thermal treatment. *Innovative Food Science & Emerging Technologies, 64*, Article 102362. https://doi.org/10.1016/j.ifset.2020.102362

Gulzar, S., Martín-Belloso, O., Elez-Martínez, P., & Soliva-Fortuny, R. (2024). The application of non-thermal technologies for the production of healthier high-quality fruit/vegetable juices and beverages – A revisit. *Acta Horticulturae, 1387*, 1–10. https://doi.org/10.17660/actahortic.2024.1387.1

Hong Kong Centre for Food Safety. (2018). *Microbiological guidelines for food.*

Jimma, F. I., Mohammed, A., Adzaworlu, E. G., Nzeh, J., Quansah, L., & Dufailu, O. A. (2022). Microbial quality and antimicrobial residue of local and industrial processed fruit juice sold in Tamale, Ghana. *Springer Nature, Ghana Discover Food, 2*(1). https://doi.org/10.1007/s44187-022-00028-2

Kaddumukasa, P. P., Imathiu, S. M., Mathara, J. M., & Nakavuma, J. L. (2017). Influence of physicochemical parameters on storage stability: Microbiological quality of fresh unpasteurized fruit juices. *Food Science and Nutrition, 5*(6), 1098–1105. https://doi.org/10.1002/fsn3.500

Kumar, D., Kumar, S., Gochar, C. S., Rampur, M., Saharanpur, M., Pradesh, U., Corresponding, I., & Shekhar, C. (2020). Nutritional components in green leafy vegetables: A review. *Journal of Pharmacognosy and Phytochemistry, 9*(5). www.phytojournal.com.

Lee, J. C., Neonaki, M., Alexopoulos, A., & Varzakas, T. (2023). Case studies of small-medium food enterprises around the world: Major constraints and benefits from the implementation of food safety management systems. *Foods, 12*(17), 3218. https://doi.org/10.3390/foods12173218

Marr, C. M., & Russo, T. A. (2019). Hypervirulent Klebsiella pneumoniae: A new public health threat. *Expert Review of Anti-Infective Therapy, 17*(2), 71–73. https://doi.org/10.1080/14787210.2019.1555470

Mirmiran, P., Houshialsadat, Z., Gaeini, Z., Bahadoran, Z., & Azizi, F. (2020). Functional properties of beetroot (beta vulgaris) in management of cardio-metabolic diseases. *Nutrition and Metabolism, 17*(1). https://doi.org/10.1186/s12986-019-0421-0

Moses, A. E., James, R. A., & Ekanem, U. S. (2016). Prevalence of *Escherichia coli* O157 in fruits, vegetables and animal feacal waste used as manure in farms of some communities of Akwa Ibom state-Nigeria. *Central African Journal of Public Health, 2*(1), 22–27. https://doi.org/10.11648/j.cajph.20160201.14

Mudgal, D., Singh, S., Deepali Mudgal, C., & Singh, B. (2022). Nutritional composition and value added products of beetroot: A review. *Journal of Current Research in Food Science, 3*(1). www.foodresearchjournal.com.

Nasiłowska, J., Sokołowska, B., & Fonberg-Broczek, M. (2018). Long-term storage of vegetable juices treated by high hydrostatic pressure: Assurance of the microbial safety. *BioMed Research International*, 1–12. https://doi.org/10.1155/2018/7389381

Nasiru, M., Auta, T., & Bawa, J. A. (2015). Geohelminth contamination of fruits and vegetables cultivated on land irrigated with waste water in Gusau local government area, Zamfara state, Nigeria. *Zoological Society of Nigeria, 13*, 7–10.

Obasi, B. C., Whong, C. M. Z., Ameh, J. B., & Ella, E. E. (2019). Microbiological quality assessment of commercially and laboratory prepared Orange juice. *Journal of Bio-Technology and Research, 52*, 19–27. https://doi.org/10.32861/jbr.52.19.27

Olaimat, A. N., & Holley, R. A. (2012). Factors influencing the microbial safety of fresh produce: A review. *Food Microbiology, 32*(1), 1–19. https://doi.org/10.1016/j.fm.2012.04.016

Petruzzi, L., Campaniello, D., Speranza, B., Corbo, M. R., Sinigaglia, M., & Bevilacqua, A. (2017). Thermal treatments for fruit and vegetable juices and beverages: A literature overview. *Comprehensive Reviews in Food Science and Food Safety, 16*(4), 668–691. https://doi.org/10.1111/1541-4337.12270

Piagentini, A. M., & Güemes, D. R. (2002). Shelf life of fresh-cut spinach as affected by chemical treatment and type of packaging film. *Brazilian Journal of Chemical Engineering, 19*(4), 383–389. https://doi.org/10.1590/s0104-66322002000400005

Rahman, M. M., Azad, M. O. K., Uddain, J., Adnan, M., Ali, M. C., Al-Mujahidy, S. M. J., Roni, M. Z. K., Rahman, M. S., Islam, M. J., Rahman, M. H., Choi, K. Y., & Naznin, M. T. (2021). Microbial quality assessment and efficacy of low-cost disinfectants on fresh fruits and vegetables collected from urban areas of Dhaka, Bangladesh. *Foods, 10*(6). https://doi.org/10.3390/foods10061325

Rahman, S., Khan, I., & Oh, D. H. (2019). Electrolyzed water as a novel sanitizer in the food industry: Current trends and future perspectives. *Foods, 8*(11), 580. https://doi.org/10.3390/foods8110580

Ray, B. (2004). *Fundamental food microbiology* (3rd ed.). CRC Press.

Rembiałkowska, E., Srednicka, D., Czerwinski, J., & Wojcik, A. (2007). Organic versus conventional beetroot juice: Microbiological quality. *Food Control, 18*(6), 632–638.

Safwa, S. M., Ahmed, T., Talukder, S., Sarkar, A., & Rana, M. R. (2024). Applications of non-thermal technologies in food processing Industries-A review. *Journal of Agriculture and Food Research, 18*. https://doi.org/10.1016/j.jafr.2023.100917

Schuh, V., Schuh, J., Fronza, N., Bortolini Foralosso, F., Verruck, S., Vargas Junior, A., & Mello da Silveira, S. (2020). Evaluation of the microbiological quality of minimally processed vegetables. *Food Science and Technology, 40*(2), 290–295. https://doi.org/10.1590/fst.38118

Shahbaz, M., & Shahbaz, M. (2022). Microbiological safety of fresh-cut produce and salads served at quick service restaurants. *Biomedical Journal of Scientific and Technical Research, 47*(4). https://doi.org/10.26717/BJSTR.2022.47.007536

Sharma, K. D., Karki, S., Thakur, N. S., & Attri, S. (2012). Chemical composition, functional properties and processing of carrot-A review. *Journal of Food Science and Technology, 49*(1), 22–32. https://doi.org/10.1007/s13197-011-0310-7

Silva, F. V. M., & Gibbs, P. A. (2001). Alicyclobacillus acidoterrestris spoilage of fruit and vegetable juices. *Food Research International, 34*(5), 449–471.

Tango, C. N., Wei, S., Khan, I., Hussain, M. S., Kounkeu, P. F. N., Park, J. H., Kim, S. H., & Oh, D. H. (2018). Microbiological quality and safety of fresh fruits and vegetables at retail levels in Korea. *Journal of Food Science, 83*(2), 386–392. https://doi.org/10.1111/1750-3841.13992

Tarifa, M. C., Agustín, M.d. R., & Brugnoni, L. I. (2023). Biological control of foodborne pathogens by lactic acid bacteria: A focus on juice processing industries. *Revista Argentina de Microbiología, 55*(4), 378–386. https://doi.org/10.1016/j.ram.2023.04.001

Uddin, T. M., Chakraborty, A. J., Khusro, A., Zidan, B. R. M., Mitra, S., Emran, T. B., Dhama, K., Ripon, M. K. H., Gajdács, M., Sahibzada, M. U. K., Hossain, M. J., & Koirala, N. (2021). Antibiotic resistance in microbes: History, mechanisms, therapeutic strategies and future prospects. *Journal of Infection and Public Health, 14*(12), 1750–1766. https://doi.org/10.1016/j.jiph.2021.10.020

Usaga, J., & Worobo, R. W. (2018). Microbial safety and quality evaluation of UV-treated, cold-pressed colored and turbid juices and beverages . International association for food protection. *Costa Rica Journal of Food Protection, 81*(9), 1549–1556. https://doi.org/10.4315/0362-028X.JFP-18-085

U.S. Department of Agriculture. (2018). All about the fruit group. Available at: https://www.choosemyplate.gov/fruit. (Accessed 1 February 2018).

Wadamori, Y., Gooneratne, R., & Hussain, M. A. (2017). Outbreaks and factors influencing microbiological contamination of fresh produce. *Journal of the Science of Food and Agriculture, 97*(5), 1396–1403. https://doi.org/10.1002/jsfa.8125

Wazed, M. A., Abdul Momin Sheikh, M., Akhtaruzzaman, M., Shihabul Awal, M., & Rubel Mozumder, N. H. M. (2023). Quality evaluation and shelf life analysis of fruit juice cocktail containing mango (Mangifera indica) and pineapple (Ananas comosus). *Journal of Agriculture and Food Research, 14*, Article 100773. https://doi.org/10.1016/j.jafr.2023.100773

Wilkins, M. R. (2022). Factors influencing microbial growth and its kinetics. In *Current developments in biotechnology and bioengineering* (pp. 373–395). Elsevier. https://doi.org/10.1016/B978-0-323-91167-2.00014-9

Willey, J. M., Sherwood, L. M., & Woolverton, C. J. (2020). *Prescott's microbiology* (11th ed.). McGraw-Hill Education.

Wondimagegn, M. K., & Mohammed, S. A. (2025). Microbiological quality of some selected fresh fruit juices served in dessie town's charming cafes and restaurants, nestled in the heart of north-eastern Ethiopia. *Discover Food, 5*(1). https://doi.org/10.1007/s44187-025-00479-3

World Health Organization. (2008). *Microbiological hazards in fresh leafy vegetables and herbs: Meeting report.* World Health Organization.

Further reading

Ali, I., Rasheed, A., Ahmad Khan, A., Khan, R., Ahmad, M., Bashir, R., & Mohamed, H. M. (2024). Exploring the health benefits and utility of carrots and carrot pomace: A systematic review. *International Journal of Food Properties, 27*(1), 180–193. https://doi.org/10.1080/10942912.2023.2301569

Asma, A., Ahmed, Z., Ahmad, H., & Khalid, N. (2019). Estimates and burden of foodborne pathogens in RTE beverages in relation to vending practices. *Food Quality and Safety, 3*(2), 107–115. https://doi.org/10.1093/fqsafe/fyz007

Food and Drug Administration. (2007). *Guidance for industry: Juice hazard analysis critical control point hazards and controls guidance – First edition.* U.S. Department of Health and Human Services.

Fufa Bulti, K., & Melkam, D. L. (2018). Microbiological quality of fruit juices sold in cafes and restaurants of shewarobit town, Amhara, Ethiopia. *African Journal of Microbiology Research, 12*(26), 623–628. https://doi.org/10.5897/ajmr2018.8868

Kaur, G., Sandhya, Kaur, M., Challana, V., & Kaur, S. (2025). Application of cold plasma, a novel nonthermal method on fruit juices: A review on quality and safety. *Quality Assurance and Safety of Crops and Foods, 17* (1), 163–189. https://doi.org/10.15586/qas.v17i1.1527

Martin, S. (2025). High-pressure processing for extending the shelf life of fresh juices. *Journal of Food Processing and Technology Reviewed*, 1001163–1001164. https://doi.org/10.35248/2157-7110.25.16.1163

U.S. Food and Drug Administration (FDA). (2018a). *Code of Federal regulations (CFR). Title 21. Chap. I. Subchap. B. Part 120. Hazard analysis and critical control point (HACCP) systems.* Available at: http://www.accessdata.fda.gov/scripts/cdrh/cfdocs/cfcfr/CFRSearch.cfm?CFRPart=120. (Accessed 19 December 2017) Accessed.

U.S. Food and Drug Administration (FDA). (2018b). *Code of federal regulations (CFR). Title 21. Chap. I. Subchap. B. Part 179. Sec. 179.39. Ultraviolet radiation for the processing and treatment of food.* Available at: http://www.accessdata.fda.gov/scripts/cdrh/cfdocs/cfcfr/CFRSearch.cfm?fr=179.39. (Accessed 1 February 2018) Accessed.

Zoglopiti, E., Roufou, S., Psakis, G., Okafor, E. T., Dasenaki, M., Gatt, R., & Valdramidis, V. P. (2025). Unravelling the hydrodynamic cavitation potential in food processing: Underlying mechanisms, crucial parameters, and antimicrobial efficacy. *Food Engineering Reviews.* https://doi.org/10.1007/s12393-025-09419-4

CHAPTER

4 Dairy beverages: Enhancing shelf life and improving the food safety

Zanoor Ul Ashraf[1], Hilal Ahmad Punoo[2], Asir Gani[1] and Poonam Kanwar[1]
[1]*School of Bioengineering and Food Technology, Shoolini University, Solan, Himachal Pradesh, India;* [2]*Department of Food Science and Technology, University of Kashmir, Srinagar, Jammu and Kashmir, India*

4.1 Introduction

Milk has long been regarded as one of nature's most complete foods, sustaining human diets for thousands of years. Today, it continues to be a vital dietary component for more than six billion people worldwide (Górska-Warsewicz et al., 2019). Milk, a white liquid secreted by the mammary glands of mammals, serves as the primary nutritional source for young mammals, including human infants. It is abundant in proteins, lactose, saturated fats, and other vital elements including calcium. Furthermore, milk consists of immune-modulating and immune-promoting agents. Colostrum, the first milk made during early lactation, is very high in antibodies and immuno-modulating compounds that strengthen the immune system and provide protection against a number of illnesses. Growing demand for products made from milk has led to a steady increase in the nation's milk production (Drewnowski, 2011). Since dairy products are rich in vital proteins, vitamins, and minerals, they are consumed in large quantities all over the world. They may be quite effective in transporting extra nutrients. Certain populations' nutritional demands can be met by fortifying or enriching these beverages with functional substances, which may also have positive health effects (Singh et al., 2017). Furthermore, incorporating non dairy components, including vegetable or fruit juices, with milk components can improve the nutracutical, property and cost-effectiveness (Gallo et al., 2019, pp. 1–35) (Krupa et al., 2011). Moreover, dairy-based drinks are light, refreshing, and healthy since they have a naturally nourishing base. Also, essential elements like calcium are provided in a palatable form especially to youngsters via fortified milk beverages, which are boosted with flavor, color, and sugar to make them more appealing (Matsuyama et al., 2017). Despite these benefits, the dairy products are susceptibility to physicochemical deterioration and microbiological contamination posing a serious challange for food safety and shelf life. Since dairy-based beverages are perishable, it is necessary to use efficient preservation techniques to guarantee product stability while preserving its nutritional and sensory qualities. Thus, a combination of thermal and non-thermal processing methods, innovative packaging, and the use of natural preservatives are needed to extend the shelf life of dairy products. Although traditional techniques like pasteurization and ultra-high temperature (UHT) treatment are good at lowering the microbial burden, they can cause unintended changes in the nutritional makeup and flavor (Silva & Gibbs, 2010). In addition, food safety is still a major concern in the manufacturing of dairy

The Science and Safety of Beverages. https://doi.org/10.1016/B978-0-443-36536-2.00002-8

beverages because of the possibility of contamination from harmful microbes such *Salmonella* species, *Escherichia coli, and Listeria monocytogenes* (Oliveira & Fraqueza, 2020). These risks can be reduced by using antimicrobial agents, adhering strictly to good manufacturing standards (GMP), and doing hazard analysis and critical control points (HACCP). Additionally, new developments in smart packaging technologies, such oxygen-scavenging and antimicrobial coatings, offer even more defense against contamination and spoiling. Thus, this chapter examines the most current developments in preservation techniques meant to improve the safety and shelf life of dairy products. The use of bioactive substances, creative processing methods, and clever packaging solutions that support safe and sustainable dairy production are highlighted.

4.2 Historical evolution and cultural significance

4.2.1 Historical evolution

For thousands of years, dairy products have been an integral component of human nutrition and culture, demonstrating its usefulness and symbolic significance in communities all over the world. The domestication of livestock, improvements in food preservation, and shifting dietary patterns are all intricately linked to their evolution ancient (Stock & Wells, 2023). It is known that buttermilk, whey, and other early dairy based drinks were manufactured by ancient societies in Mesopotamia, Egypt, and the Indus Valley. Rural groups were the main consumers of milk and its byproducts during the Middle Ages. As fermentation evolved into an important preservation technique, it produced nutrient-dense, like kefir and kumis which had longer shelf lives. Due to their portability and long-term preservation, these drinks were especially useful in commerce (McCormick, 2012). Further in the 19th century dairy beverage production saw a dramatic shift throughout the Industrial Revolution. The large-scale production and distribution of fresh milk and flavored dairy drinks were made possible by technological developments like cooling and pasteurization, by Louis Pasteur (Steele, 2000). As food processing advancements like homogenization and aseptic packaging increased the shelf life and accessibility of dairy products over time, making them a staple of the world's diet. Over time, innovations in food processing, including homogenization and aseptic packaging, further extended the shelf life and accessibility of dairy beverages, allowing them to become a global dietary staple. In the current era, due to advancements in flavoring and fortification, dairy beverages have moved beyond their historical origins to become international commodities. For consumers who are health conscious, the dairy products are being marketed as functional foods enhanced with vitamins, minerals, and probiotics (Jang et al., 2024). Dairy drinks, which offer nutritional advantages as well as a link to cultural heritage, continue to unite innovation with tradition. Their development demonstrates how inventively humans have transformed a basic resource into a wide range of goods that satisfy both utilitarian and cultural demands (Jang et al., 2024).

4.2.2 Cultural significance

Dairy drinks have significant cultural importance in many different regions and have become a staple of the worldwide diet. In Europe, fermented milk products like buttermilk and whey have become essentials, especially in northern Europe, and milk-based beverages are frequently associated with strength and vitality (Sani et al., 2019). In South Asia, milk-based drinks like lassi and spiced milk are essential to the cuisine, serving as a source of nutrition as well as a function in religious festival rituals. Also, the nomadic lifestyle of Central Asia is reflected in the region's long history of ingesting fermented dairy products like kumis, which are prepared from mare's milk (Sani et al., 2019). In Africa, milk is culturally and socially significant, especially to the Maasai people of East Africa, who use milk and its derivatives as a symbol of sustenance and purity in their ceremonies and diet (Sani et al., 2019). Due to their convenience and nutritional advantages, flavored milk drinks and dairy based smoothies have gained popularity in North America. Furthermore, warm beverages like horchata and atole have traditionally been made in Latin American civilizations by combining milk with spices like chocolate and cinnamon. Dairy products like laban and ayran, which are refreshing drinks typically paired with meals and are particularly prized in hot regions, are native to the Middle East.

4.3 Composition and nutritional value of dairy products

Milk and dairy products contribute significantly to the average Polish diet, supplying 9.1% of the total energy, equating to 205 kcal out of an average daily intake of 2261 kcal (Drewnowski, 2025). These dairy products also play an important role in protein supply, contributing 18.1% of the daily protein intake, with branched-chain amino acids like leucine, isoleucine, and valine supplied at 19%–21%. Essential amino acids such as methionine and lysine are provided in varying amounts, from 18.4% for methionine to 21.5% for lysine, while non-essential amino acids like tyrosine and proline are supplied at 23.6% and 24.8%, respectively. In terms of fat, milk and dairy products account for 11.3% of total fat intake, with a significant focus on saturated fatty acids (SFA) at 18.4%, and a smaller share of mono- and polyunsaturated fatty acids (MUFA and PUFA) at 8.8% and 2.1%, respectively (Górska-Warsewicz et al., 2019). Dairy products play a vital role in the human diet, contributing significantly to nutrient intake. They account for about 11.6% of the total cholesterol consumed, with cheese alone responsible for nearly half of this amount. In terms of carbohydrates, dairy products provide around 5%, mainly from yoghurts, milk-based drinks, and other fermented dairy items (2.4%), followed closely by milk itself (2.3%). Moreover, milk and dairy foods are key sources of essential minerals, particularly calcium, supplying nearly 55% of the daily intake where both milk and cheese each contribute over 20%. They also deliver close to one-fourth of the total phosphorus intake, with cheese providing more than 10% and milk about 9.4% (Górska-Warsewicz et al., 2019). Additionally, dairy products make a meaningful contribution to the intake of potassium, magnesium, and zinc, ranging from 10% to 14%, with milk serving as the main source of potassium (6.8%) and magnesium (5.6%), while cheese is the primary contributor of zinc (6.7%). Finally, dairy products provide key vitamins, especially riboflavin and vitamin B12, with milk providing 13.5% of riboflavin and 10.3% of vitamin B12. Vitamin A intake from dairy is at 11%, with cheese providing 5.2% and milk 4.4%. Other vitamins are supplied by dairy at levels below 10% (Górska-Warsewicz et al., 2019).

4.4 Types of dairy beverages

4.4.1 Traditional dairy beverages

Traditional beverages have historically been prepared at the household level using time-honored techniques passed down through generations. Deeply intertwined with local customs and cultural practices, these beverages not only serve as refreshing drinks but also play a vital role in daily nutrition. Rich in essential nutrients such as proteins, vitamins, minerals, and bioactive compounds, traditional beverages often contribute significantly to dietary balance and overall health. Many of them contain probiotics, natural enzymes, and fermentation-derived metabolites that support gut health, digestion, and immunity. In recent years, these beverages have gained increasing popularity in urban settings due to their distinctive taste, cultural identity, and perceived health benefits. As consumer demand has grown, traditional preparation methods once confined to domestic kitchens are now being adapted and scaled up for industrial production (Minz & Singh, 2016, pp. 161–174). However, household preparation remains a labor-intensive and time-consuming process. The techniques involved are often intricate, requiring considerable skill and effort, making them unsuitable for large-scale manufacturing. Consequently, home-based production typically yields limited quantities and variable product quality, which does not align with the needs of modern consumers seeking convenience and consistency. To meet evolving market demands, producers have increasingly adopted industrial-scale production techniques that ensure standardization, safety, and efficiency while preserving the sensory, nutritional, and cultural authenticity of traditional beverages. Through the use of modern technologies such as pasteurization, controlled fermentation, and carbonation, manufacturers can replicate the unique characteristics of traditional recipes on a commercial scale. This transition from household to industrial production has made these beverages widely accessible to urban populations, transforming them into a vital segment of the global food and beverage industry. Today, they continue to provide both nutritional and cultural value to consumers, bridging the gap between traditional heritage and modern lifestyles.

4.4.1.1 Lassi

Lassi also called chhach or matha is a traditional fermented dairy beverage with cultural and nutritional significance in many regions of India (Deshpnde et al., 2020). It is a rich source of essentional amino acids, high quality protein, and readily digested carbohydrates, mostly lactose. Additionally, lassi contains vital minerals including calcium, potassium, phosphorus, and magnesium that support muscle function, electrolyte balance, and bone health. It also has significant levels of B complex vitamins, such as vitamin B12 and riboflavin, which promote metabolism and general health. Its probiotic effect is increased by the live lactic acid bacteria, which also helps with digestion and intestinal health. This beverage is typically enjoyed with either sugar or salt, depending on personal preference, and is commonly referred to as sweet or salted lassi. To make lassi, dahi is churned and water is added until butter granules form. Additionally, it can be customized with flavors and colors to accommodate personal preferences and tastes (Sarkar et al., 2015).

4.4.1.2 Butter milk beverages

Buttermilk is often utilized as an essential ingredient in traditional dairy products to maintain the flavor, appearance and nutritional value of dairy products. Traditional drinks that use buttermilk are discussed below.

4.4.1.3 Ambali

Ambali is a traditional buttermilk-based porridge, popular in India. The preparation involves combining 1 L of water, 250 g of sorghum flour, salt to taste, and buttermilk. Sorghum flour is first mixed with cold water, and then gradually added to boiling water while continuously stirring to prevent lump formation. The mixture is cooked until it thickens into a paste, which is then allowed to ferment overnight. Before serving, buttermilk is added, and the mixture is thoroughly stirred.

4.4.1.4 Rabadi

Rabadi is a cereal-based fermented dairy beverage, commonly consumed in rural regions of Haryana, Punjab, and Rajasthan, particularly during the hot summer months as a refreshing, thirst-quenching drink. The beverage is traditionally made by adding cooled, cooked cereal flour (often from underutilized cereals such as pearl millet, barley, wheat, maize, or sorghum) to buttermilk, allowing the mixture to ferment overnight (Meena et al., 2024). Rabadi is a staple food for many rural populations, especially in millet-producing areas, and is typically consumed fresh. However, this traditional method results in a product with a limited shelf life of 1–2 days and unpredictable sensory quality.

4.4.1.5 Aryan

Ayran is a traditional Turkish fermented dairy drink made by diluting yogurt with water and adding a small amount of salt, generally not exceeding 1% (Baruzzi et al., 2016). It is popular in hot seasons because of its cooling and hydrating properties. The presence of lactic acid bacteria (LAB) in yogurt enhances digestive function and supports a healthy gut microbiome. When stored under proper refrigeration, Ayran remains suitable for consumption for about 10–15 days (Baruzzi et al., 2016).

4.4.1.6 Doogh

Doogh is a traditional Iranian yogurt-based drink, typically prepared by mixing yogurt with water, a pinch of salt, and occasionally aromatic herbs such as mint (Soltani et al., 2012). Valued for its cooling and hydrating properties, Doogh is especially popular in warm climates. It contains beneficial lactic acid bacteria from yogurt, which contribute to digestive health. While the addition of salt can slightly extend its shelf life, Doogh is best enjoyed fresh and should be stored in the refrigerator to preserve its quality (Soltani et al., 2012).

4.4.2 Fermented dairy beverages

Fermented milk-based beverages have been an integral component of traditional diets across diverse cultures worldwide. These products often trace their origins to simple, domestic practices designed primarily for the preservation of surplus milk. A widely adopted method involved allowing milk to undergo spontaneous fermentation overnight, leading to the formation of curd. The resulting curd was typically churned and diluted with water to produce buttermilk an approach still practiced in many rural and agrarian communities. Beyond preservation, such fermentation processes enhanced the nutritional quality and digestibility of milk, contributing to their enduring popularity. In contemporary settings, fermentation is carried out under controlled conditions using specific microbial cultures. The purposeful addition of desirable microbes, especially lactic acid bacteria (LAB), induces milk to go through a number of metabolic changes. These microorganisms mostly break down lactose, generating organic acids that reduce pH and enhance the end product's safety, shelf life, and sensory qualities like flavor, texture, and scent. In order eradicate unwanted microbes and denature whey proteins, the milk is usually heated to 90°C for 10 min before cooling to start the fermentation process. The milk is then inoculated with certain starter cultures after being chilled to a temperature that promotes microbial development. Following this, incubation under ideal conditions promotes microbial activity until the required product characteristics are attained. Among the fermented milk products are yogurt, kefir, and buttermilk, which are valued for their improved nutritional bioavailability and microbial content as well as their organoleptic features and health-promoting qualities. Table 4.1 provides an overview of selected traditional and contemporary fermented milk-based beverages, outlining their fermentation processes, dominant microbial cultures, associated health benefits, and shelf-life characteristics.

4.4.3 Yogurt drinks and probiotic beverages

Traditional products derived from fermented milk have given way to many different kinds of functional drinks with added value. Among these, yogurt drinks, probiotic beverages, and whey-based fermented drinks have gained widespread popularity for their health-promoting effects, convenience, and consumer appeal.

Table 4.1 Traditional dairy fermented beverage.

Beverage	Preparation process	Microorganisms	Health benefits	Shelf life (refrigerated conditions)	References
Lassi	Yogurt is mixed with water and optionally fruits or spices.	Mainly Lactobacillus species	Aids digestion, hydrates, and provides beneficial bacteria.	2–3 days	Deshpnde et al. (2020)
Ambali	Cooked sorghum flour is cooled and fermented overnight with buttermilk.	Lactic acid bacteria	Improves grain digestibility and supports gut flora.	1–2 days	Joshi (2016)
Rabadi	Cereal flour is fermented with buttermilk overnight.	Lactobacillus, Streptococcus species	Rich in fiber and probiotics, beneficial for digestion.	1–2 days	Meena et al. (2024)
Ayran	Yogurt is diluted with water and salt.	Yogurt-derived LAB	Cooling effect, aids digestion, and replenishes electrolytes.	5–7 days	Baruzzi et al. (2016)
Doogh	Yogurt is mixed with water and salt, often carbonated.	LAB from yogurt cultures	Refreshing, probiotic-rich, supports hydration and digestive health.	3–5 days	Soltani et al. (2012)

4.4.3.1 Yogurt drinks

Yogurt drinks are fluid or pourable forms of yogurt, often produced by diluting stirred yogurt with milk or water and blending it with flavoring agents, fruit pulps, or sweeteners. Unlike traditional spoonable yogurt, yogurt drinks are classified as fermented dairy beverages due to their lower viscosity and ease of consumption. These products retain the beneficial microbial cultures present in yogurt typically *Lactobacillus delbrueckii* subsp. *bulgaricus* and *Streptococcus thermophilus* and may also include added probiotic strains. Drinkable yogurt is a common carrier for probiotics, calcium, proteins, and bioactive compounds, offering both nutritional value and digestive support (FAO/WHO, 2002).

4.4.3.2 Probiotic beverages

Probiotic beverages encompass a broader category that includes both dairy and non-dairy formulations intentionally enriched with live probiotic strains known to confer health benefits. In dairy-based systems, probiotics such as *Lactobacillus acidophilus*, *Bifidobacterium bifidum*, and *Lactobacillus casei* are added to improve gut microbiota, modulate immune function, and support digestive health. These beverages may or may not undergo fermentation themselves; rather, they act as delivery vehicles for functional microbial cultures. Both yogurt drinks and whey-based beverages can fall under this umbrella if they meet the minimum viable cell count criteria ($>10^6$ CFU/mL) for probiotics.

4.4.3.2.1 Yakult (probiotic drink)

Yakult is a well-known commercial example of a fermented, probiotic milk-based beverage developed using a specific strain, *Lactobacillus casei Shirota*. It is typically produced from skimmed milk that is heat-treated, fermented, and flavored to yield a sweet, acidic drink. Unlike yogurt, Yakult is not classified as a yogurt drink, as it uses a single probiotic strain and does not contain the standard yogurt starter cultures. Instead, Yakult is categorized as a functional probiotic dairy beverage, with a focus on gut health, microbial balance, and immunity (Nagata et al., 2006).

4.4.3.3 Whey based probiotic beverages

Whey based probiotic beverages utilize cheese whey an underutilized by-product of cheese production as the fermentation medium. These products are rich in lactose, minerals, and bioactive peptides, making whey an ideal substrate for probiotic cultivation. The formulation may involve supplementation with fruit juices, cereals, or prebiotics to improve sensory properties and stability. These beverages not only provide a sustainable use of dairy waste streams but also offer nutritional benefits such as improved gut health and protein digestibility. Their increasing popularity lies in their low-fat content, high bioavailability, and potential for flavor innovation (Pescuma et al., 2010).

4.4.4 Plant-based dairy alternatives

The global market for plant-based milk alternatives is expanding rapidly, driven by evolving consumer preferences, increasing urbanization, and growing awareness of dietary and health considerations (Park, 2021; Sethi et al., 2016). While these non-dairy alternatives generally contain fewer nutrients than conventional cow's milk, they are widely accepted due to their functional properties and the potential health risks associated with dairy consumption. Some studies indicate a potential association between excessive dairy consumption and an elevated risk of certain cancers (Sethi et al., 2016; Vanga & Raghavan, 2018). In contrast, plant-based milk alternatives offer functional benefits, contributing to improved health outcomes (Vanga & Raghavan, 2018). The rising popularity of vegan and vegetarian diets has further accelerated demand for these dairy substitutes in both consumer markets and the food industry. One of the key issues associated with cow's milk is the risk of contamination by pathogenic microorganisms such as *Salmonella* and *Escherichia coli*, which are known to cause food borne diseases. Furthermore, milk protein allergy is common among infants and children, while lactose intolerance affects a considerable portion of the global population since lactose is the predominant carbohydrate in dairy milk. Concerns have also been raised about the relatively high energy content of cow's milk and its possible link to elevated cholesterol levels, which may contribute to chronic health problems when consumed excessively. In light of these challenges, plant-based milk alternatives have gained prominence as suitable substitutes, particularly for individuals with allergies, lactose intolerance, or those pursuing healthier dietary options. Consumer choices for such alternatives differ by region. A study conducted by Pritulska et al. (2021) in Ukraine reported that taste was the most influential factor shaping consumer preference, with almond milk being the most favored (20.4%), followed by oat milk (15.3%) and soy milk (12.3%). Rice and buckwheat milk each accounted for 10.1% of preferences, while 16.2% of participants expressed no preference for plant-based milk substitutes. The highest consumption was observed among individuals aged 25–30 years, followed by the 18–24 age group and those over 50 years old.In India, the demand for plant-based dairy alternatives has increased significantly. In the past year, soy milk (56%) and almond milk (54%) were the most frequently consumed plant-based dairy alternatives, followed by plant-based cheese (31%), oat milk (29%), and plant-based yogurt (21%) (Narsaria & Rajyalakshmi, 2020). These trends highlight a growing consumer shift toward plant-based dairy substitutes, primarily driven by health-conscious choices, dietary preferences, and the increasing availability of plant-based options.

4.5 Stability and shelf life concerns of dairy products

The production of dairy beverages presents several challenges, ranging from maintaining product stability to addressing consumer dietary needs and regulatory compliance. The stability and shelf life of dairy products are influenced by several factors, such as enzymatic activity, chemical reactions, microbial contamination, and environmental conditions. The primary reasons for stability and shelflifeconcern in dairy products are.

4.5.1 Microbial contamination and spoilage

Dairy products, because of their great nutritional value, are susceptible to spoiling since they offer the perfect conditions for the growth of molds, yeasts, and bacteria. Milking, storage, shipping, and handling following pasteurization are among the stages of the production process where contamination may arise (Martin et al., 2021). The safety, stability, and sensory qualities of dairy products are adversely affected by the presence of pathogenic and spoiling microorganisms, which can result in off flavors, texture deterioration, and possible health hazards.

4.5.1.1 Sources of microbial contamination

Raw milk is the main source of contamination for dairy products, it might contain bacteria from the animal, the environment, or improper handling and storage conditions (Owusu-Kwarteng et al., 2020). Cross contamination during processing, dirty equipment, and inadequate hygiene procedures might introduce pathogenic bacteria such *Salmonella* spp., *Escherichia coli, Staphylococcus aureus, and Listeria monocytogenes* (Cossettini et al., 2022). Additionally, even in cold storage, milk and dairy products can degrade due to the proliferation of psychrotrophic bacteria such *Pseudomonas* spp. at refrigeration temperatures.

4.5.1.2 Types of microorganisms involved in dairy spoilage

Spoilage microorganisms in dairy products include both bacteria and fungi, which alter the chemical composition of milk components through enzymatic activit (Edenbach & Marshall, 2009). LAB such as *Lactobacillus* spp. and *Streptococcus* spp.are responsible for the fermentation of lactose into lactic acid, which can lead to excessive souring, undesirable texture changes, and gas production (Fusco et al., 2020). Proteolytic bacteria such as *Pseudomonas fluorescens* produce enzymes that break down milk proteins, resulting in bitterness, gelation, and texture defects (Zhang et al., 2019). Lipolytic bacteria, including *Bacillus* spp., produce lipases that degrade milk fats, leading to rancidity and off-flavors.Yeasts and molds also contribute to the spoilage of dairy products, particularly in cheese and fermented dairy items (Erkmen & Bozoglu, 2016).

4.5.1.3 Impact of microbial spoilage on dairy products

Microbial contamination and spoilage lead to various undesirable changes in dairy products (Erkmen & Bozoglu, 2016). Such as, bacterial metabolism produces volatile compounds such as hydrogen sulfide, acetoin, and diacetyl, leading to rancid, putrid, or yeasty odors responsible for off-Flavors and odors. Enzymatic degradation of proteins and fats in dairy beverages results in coagulation, curdling, slime formation, and phase separation resulting in texture and structural changes (Erkmen &Bozoglu, 2016). In addition, fermentative microorganisms produce gases like carbon dioxide and hydrogen, leading to bloating in cheese, yogurt, and packaged milk. Furthermore, molds and pigment-producing bacteria cause discoloration of dairy beverages, leading to blue, green, or pink patches on dairy surfaces (Garnier et al., 2017).

4.5.2 Impact of enzymatic activity on the shelf life of dairy products

Enzymatic activity plays a significant role in determining the shelf life and quality of dairy products. Enzymes, whether naturally present in milk, introduced by microbial contamination, or added during processing, can cause biochemical changes that affect flavor, texture, stability, and spoilage (Martin et al., 2021). To increase shelf life and preserve the nutritional value and sensory appeal of dairy beverages and other dairy products, enzyme activity must be controlled. Enzymes that are naturally present in raw milk may eventually affect its stability.

4.5.2.1 Lipases (fat-degrading enzymes)

Enzymes called lipases catalyze the degradation of triglycerides, or milk fat, into free fatty acids, a process called lipolysis. This breakdown of lipids can cause dairy products to become rancid and develop unwanted off tastes. Poor storage conditions, incorrect handling, or excessive agitation during the processing phases can all greatly accelerate the rate of lipolysis and increase the activity of these enzymes (Erkmen & Bozoglu, 2016). However, most lipases are efficiently rendered inactive by heat treatments like pasteurization or UHT processing, which prolongs the shelf life of dairy products by maintaining their flavor and quality and inhibiting the breakdown of milk lipids.

4.5.2.2 Proteases (protein degrading enzymes)

Enzymes called proteases catalyze the degradation of milk proteins, especially casein, which can result in the formation of undesirable characteristics in dairy products like phase separation, gelation, and bitterness (Erkmen & Bozoglu, 2016). Plasmin, a naturally occurring enzyme in milk is active even after pasteurization and may contribute to spoiling during prolonged storage. Further, the texture and quality of products like UHT milk can be adversely affected by age gelation, a condition where protein aggregation takes place over time due to leftover protease activity (Gaucher et al., 2011). Therefore, proteases in milk are a major concern for preserving the stability and sensory qualities of dairy products, particularly during extended storage.

4.5.2.3 Lactoperoxidase (antimicrobial enzyme)

Lactoperoxidase is a naturally occurring enzyme in raw milk that contributes significantly to its microbial safety. In the presence of hydrogen peroxide and thiocyanate, it generates antimicrobial compounds that suppress the growth of spoilage and pathogenic bacteria. This enzymatic defense mechanism extends the shelf life of raw milk by slowing bacterial proliferation. Nevertheless, the enzyme's activity diminishes upon exposure to heat, as processes such as pasteurization lead to its inactivation, thereby reducing its preservative role in heat-treated dairy products (Barrett et al., 1999).

4.5.3 Oxidation and chemical reactions

Oxidation and chemical reactions in dairy products can significantly impact their quality, safety, and sensory attributes, especially in terms of flavor, texture, and color.

4.5.3.1 Lipid oxidation

One of the primary chemical reactions in dairy products is lipid oxidation, which occurs when milk fats (triglycerides) react with oxygen in the air. This reaction can be accelerated by exposure to light, heat, and the presence of metal ions, resulting in the production of free radicals (Bhat et al., 2024). Lipid oxidation in high-fat dairy products such as butter, cream, and cheese leads to the formation of rancid compounds, which are responsible for undesirable off-flavors and odors (Bhat et al., 2024). These rancid flavors, often described as "soapy" or "stale," make the dairy product less palatable and reduce its consumer appeal. To mitigate lipid oxidation, dairy products are often packaged in opaque containers and stored in cool, dark environments. Additionally, antioxidants may be added to products to delay or prevent oxidation. However, the shelf life of high-fat dairy products remains a concern due to the ongoing potential for lipid oxidation during storage.

4.5.3.2 Maillard browning

The Maillard reaction represents a significant non-enzymatic chemical process that takes place in dairy systems, particularly during thermal processing. It occurs when reducing sugars, such as lactose, react with amino groups of proteins under elevated temperatures (Tamanna & Mahmood, 2015). This reaction results in the formation of brown-colored compounds, which are largely responsible for the characteristic color changes observed in heat-treated products such as milk powder, cheese, and yogurt. Although controlled Maillard browning can impart desirable sensory attributes such as the development of caramel-like flavors in certain cheeses excessive heating may lead to the generation of unwanted off-flavors, often described as burnt or bitter, thereby diminishing the overall sensory appeal of the product. Moreover, this reaction can adversely affect the nutritional quality of dairy by reducing the bioavailability of key amino acids, particularly lysine, which plays a crucial role in protein metabolism. The extent of Maillard browning is notably intensified in treatments such as ultra-high temperature (UHT) processing, where prolonged exposure to heat enhances pigment formation and flavor deterioration (Troise et al., 2014).

4.5.4 Phase separation and physical instability in dairy products

Phase separation and physical instability are critical challenges in dairy systems, as they can markedly influence the texture, visual appeal, and overall sensory perception of the product, ultimately diminishing its quality and consumer acceptance. Such instability is especially concerning in products like yogurt, milk, cream, and ice cream, where maintaining a homogeneous dispersion of ingredients is essential for ensuring consistent texture and desirable sensory characteristics.

4.5.4.1 Syneresis (wheying off)

Syneresis describes the expulsion of liquid, mainly whey, from the gel matrix of dairy products such as yogurt and cheese. In yogurt, this phenomenon occurs when the aqueous phase separates from the protein network during storage or after mechanical disturbance (Gilbert et al., 2020). It is a frequent quality concern in fermented dairy products, particularly when the gel structure formed during fermentation is weak or when the products pH decreases excessively. The release of whey alters the texture and uniformity of yogurt and detracts from its visual appeal, giving it a watery and less cohesive appearance. Several factors contribute to syneresis, including prolonged fermentation, inadequate cooling, and the use of milk or starter cultures of suboptimal quality (Gilbert et al., 2020). A fragile protein network often arises from incomplete or inconsistent coagulation of milk proteins primarily casein which normally stabilizes the liquid fraction within the gel. To reduce this defect, producers can fine-tune fermentation parameters, maintain tighter pH control, or incorporate stabilizing and gelling agents to reinforce the protein network, thus enhancing texture and minimizing whey separation (Guggisberg et al., 2009).

4.5.4.2 Ice crystal formation in frozen dairy products

Ice cream and other frozen dairy products, including frozen yogurt, are highly sensitive to temperature variations that can lead to the formation of large ice crystals under improper freezing or storage conditions. These crystals originate as water in the mix solidifies during the freezing stage (Tan et al., 2021). The size and uniformity of the ice crystals are crucial determinants of texture smaller, evenly distributed crystals impart a smooth and creamy mouthfeel, whereas larger ones produce a coarse or grainy texture that detracts from product quality (Tan et al., 2021). Temperature instability during storage or distribution can cause cycles of melting and refreezing, allowing the crystals to grow larger, a phenomenon referred to as "temperature abuse." Similarly, slow freezing rates and inadequate process control promote excessive crystal growth. Poor emulsification and insufficient aeration, or low overrun, can further worsen the texture and sensory characteristics of frozen dairy products. To counteract these defects, manufacturers adopt several preventive measures. Rapid freezing is one of the most effective strategies, as it facilitates quick solidification of water into fine crystals (Lomolino et al., 2020). Maintaining stable storage conditions typically at or below $-18^{\circ}C$ also helps prevent temperature cycling that encourages recrystallization. Furthermore, hydrocolloid stabilizers such as guar gum and xanthan gum are frequently incorporated to bind free water, inhibit crystal enlargement, and enhance the smoothness and creaminess of the final product.

4.5.5 Temperature sensitivity and storage conditions in dairy products

Dairy products are particularly sensitive to fluctuations in temperature, making proper storage essential for maintaining their safety, quality, and shelf stability. Inadequate temperature control can accelerate microbial proliferation and spoilage, while also causing the deterioration of important nutritional and functional constituents.

4.5.5.1 Cold chain maintenance

Any disruption in the cold chain whether during transport, handling, or storage can result in temperature fluctuations that accelerate microbial activity, leading to undesirable changes in flavor, texture, and overall safety. Given their sensitivity to temperature abuse, dairy products should be maintained consistently below 4°C (39°F) throughout distribution and retail storage. Even brief temperature deviations can compromise product integrity, shorten shelf life, and increase potential health risks (Mercier et al., 2017).

4.5.5.2 Heat sensitivity

Certain dairy products, including pasteurized milk and probiotic-enriched yogurt, are particularly vulnerable to high temperatures. Pasteurization, a standard heat treatment designed to destroy harmful microorganisms, is typically carried out at 72°C for 15 s (Claeys et al., 2013). However, exposure to excessive heat after this process can degrade fats, proteins, and other vital nutrients, adversely influencing flavor, texture, and nutritional value. Therefore, maintaining appropriate storage conditions particularly consistent refrigeration and minimal temperature fluctuations is essential for preserving product quality and ensuring the viability of probiotic cultures.

4.5.6 Packaging and oxygen exposure in dairy products

Dairy products must be packaged well to preserve their quality since various environmental elements, such as oxygen, moisture, and light, can cause degradation.

4.5.6.1 Permeability of packaging materials

The permeability of packaging materials makes dairy products more susceptible to oxidative reactions and spoiling. When oxygen permeates packing materials, fatty dairy products like cheese, cream, and butter undergo lipid oxidation. This procedure shortens the shelf life and produces rancidity and bad flavors. Likewise, unsightly alterations like mold development and texture degradation, particularly in cheese and yogurt products, can result from moisture penetration. Therefore, dairy packaging should be frequently made airtight and moisture resistant to assist reduces these hazards by preventing mold growth and oxidation.

4.5.6.2 Light-induced degradation

Dairy products can also significantly deteriorate when exposed to light, especially when they are packaged in clear or translucent materials. Vitamin B2, or riboflavin, is one of the most light-sensitive nutrients and is included in a lot of dairy products. Furthermore, photo-oxidation, which is caused by exposure to light, particularly ultraviolet (UV) radiation, can break down riboflavin and other sensitive substances, giving them undesirable flavors, discoloration, and decreased nutritional significance. In order to protect the integrity and quality of the product against light-induced deterioration, many dairy products are now wrapped in opaque or UV protective materials, including tinted plastic or cartons.

4.6 Enhancing stability and shelf life in dairy beverages

Dairy drinks are highly perishable because of their high nutritional content, therefore maintaining stability and increasing their shelf life is important for production. Microbial growth, oxidation, phase separation, and protein aggregation are some of the factors that can cause spoiling and unfavorable alterations in texture, flavor, and appearance. To address these issues, manufacturers employ a range of tactics, including advanced package designs, ingredient optimization, and processing procedures.

4.6.1 Processing techniques for improved stability

Thermal and non-thermal treatments are essential methods used in the dairy sector to improve the microbiological safety and shelf stability of dairy products. Among the various thermal treatments applied to dairy products, pasteurization and ultra-high-temperature (UHT) processing are the most commonly used. Both methods are essential for extending shelf life by destroying pathogenic microorganisms; however, they differ significantly in their processing conditions and their impact on the sensory and nutritional qualities of the final product.

4.6.1.1 Thermal treatments

Thermal treatments involve the application of heat to inactivate pathogenic and spoilage microorganisms, and sometimes enzymes, in food and beverages. Some of thermal treatments are discussed below.

4.6.1.1.1 Pasteurization treatment

Pasteurization involves the application of heat to dairy beverages at a specific temperature and for a defined period to effectively kill harmful bacteria and pathogens. In high-temperature short-time (HTST) pasteurization, for example, the product is heated to around 72°C for 15 s. This process is designed to eliminate microorganisms such as *Salmonella*, *Escherichia coli*, and *Listeria* without causing significant damage to the product's nutritional content or sensory properties, including flavor, texture, and color. Despite its effectiveness in eliminating most pathogenic microorganisms, pasteurization does not achieve complete sterilization therefore, products treated by this method must be kept under refrigeration to prevent microbial regrowth. As a result, pasteurized dairy products generally have a limited shelf life, typically lasting between one and 3 weeks depending on storage conditions. This requirement for continuous cold storage poses logistical challenges, particularly in regions with unreliable refrigeration infrastructure (Ranieri et al., 2009). investigated the influence of different storage temperatures (3, 6.5, and 10°C) on the microbial quality of milk. Their findings showed that milk maintained at 3°C remained microbiologically acceptable for approximately 68 days, whereas storage at 10°C reduced its shelf life to about 10 days. In a related assessment, the same authors examined the interaction between storage temperature, microbial growth, and shelf stability, reporting that milk stored at 5°C retained acceptable quality for around 30 days, while samples kept at

13°C deteriorated within 12 days. Collectively, these results emphasize the critical role of maintaining low temperatures and employing predictive models to optimize storage conditions and extend the shelf life of pasteurized dairy products.

4.6.1.1.2 Ultra-high temperature (UHT) treatment

Ultra-high temperature (UHT) processing is one of the most effective thermal treatments used in the dairy industry to extend the shelf life of milk and other dairy-based beverages. In this method, milk is rapidly heated to temperatures ranging from 135 to 150°C for 2–4 s, which ensures complete sterilization by destroying both spoilage and pathogenic microorganisms. This brief yet intense heating process allows UHT-treated milk to remain stable at room temperature for long periods without refrigeration, making it particularly advantageous for distribution and storage in areas where cold chain facilities are limited (Deeth et al., 2010).

Huppertz et al. (2021) assessed the stability and shelf life of UHT milk stored under varying temperature conditions for 1 year. Their findings indicated that samples stored at 4 and 20°C maintained acceptable quality for approximately 34–36 weeks, with sediment formation being the major factor limiting shelf life. Conversely, milk stored at elevated temperatures of 30 and 37°C exhibited notable deterioration after 16–20 weeks, primarily due to increased sedimentation, off-flavor development, and color changes. These results demonstrate the significant influence of storage temperature on the long-term quality and sensory attributes of UHT milk. Rysstad and Kolstad (2006) further highlighted the role of aseptic packaging in preserving the sterility and quality of UHT milk. This technique involves filling sterilized milk into pre-sterilized containers under aseptic conditions, effectively preventing post-processing contamination. When stored at ambient temperature, such packaging can extend the shelf life of UHT milk to 3–6 months, while refrigeration can further prolong it to nearly 1 year. This dual approach enhances both the stability and marketability of UHT dairy products. Additionally, Endara et al. (2023) explored consumer attitudes toward extended shelf life in high-temperature, short-time (HTST) pasteurized milk. The study revealed that consumers placed high value on longer shelf life and were willing to pay more for such products. However, the introduction of smart labeling systems designed to signal spoilage did not significantly improve acceptance. These findings suggest that although product longevity remains a major factor in consumer choice, strategies to effectively communicate freshness and quality still require refinement to align with consumer expectations.

4.6.1.1.3 Sterilization

Sterilization is a thermal preservation technique commonly employed in dairy processing, wherein products are exposed to temperatures above 110°C for extended durations, typically ranging from 15 to 30 min. The primary objective of this treatment is to achieve complete microbial destruction, including the inactivation of heat-resistant bacterial spores, thereby enabling long-term storage without the need for refrigeration. This process can extend the shelf life of dairy products to over a year. However, the application of intense heat often induces noticeable alterations in sensory and nutritional quality, such as flavor modification, texture changes, and degradation of heat-sensitive vitamins and proteins. Despite these drawbacks, sterilization remains an effective method for producing shelf-stable dairy beverages, particularly in regions where reliable refrigeration infrastructure is limited Table 4.2.

Table 4.2 Thermal processing technologies for dairy beverages.

Technique	Temperature range (°C)	Time duration	Target microorganisms	Impact on nutrients	Shelf life Extension	References
Pasteurization	63–72	15–30 min (LTLT) or 15–30 s (HTST)	Non-spore-forming bacteria	Minimal loss (some vitamins)	7–15 days (refrigerated)	Vaghela et al. (2024)
UHT treatment	135–150	2–5 s	All vegetative microbes and spores	Moderate vitamin loss	6–9 months (aseptic pack)	Deeth et al. (2010)
Sterilization	>110	15–30 min	All microorganisms including spores	High nutrient degradation	≥12 months (sealed can)	Vaghela et al. (2024)

4.6.1.2 Non thermal treatments

High-pressure processing (HPP) and pulsed electric field (PEF) treatment are innovative non-thermal technologies that have garnered significant attention in the dairy industry for their ability to enhance product safety and shelf life while preserving sensory and nutritional qualities. High-pressure processing (HPP), cold plasma, UV radiation and pulsed electric field (PEF) are discussed below.

4.6.1.2.1 High-pressure processing

High-pressure processing (HPP) is a non-thermal preservation method in which packaged food products are subjected to extremely high hydrostatic pressures, generally ranging from 100 to 600 MPa (Sehrawat et al., 2021). This intense pressure uniformly affects the entire food product, leading to the inactivation of harmful microorganisms and spoilage agents without the use of heat. In dairy beverages, HPP is particularly effective because it minimizes changes to sensory and nutritional properties. Unlike conventional thermal methods, HPP does not cause protein denaturation or vitamin loss to the same extent, making it ideal for preserving the fresh taste, creamy texture, and bioactive compounds in products like milk and yogurt drinks (Sehrawat et al., 2021). Its effectiveness against a wide range of pathogens, such as *Listeria monocytogenes* and *E. coli*, helps extend shelf life and ensures microbiological safety.

4.6.1.2.2 Pulsed electric field

PEF, is a non-thermal method that uses short bursts of high-voltage electric pulses to inactivate microorganisms in liquid foods. The electric pulses typically in the range of 20–80 kV per centimeter create temporary pores in the microbial cell membranes, a phenomenon known as electroporation (Lytras et al., 2024). This damages the cell's integrity and leads to microbial death. PEF is especially suited for dairy beverages because it operates at or near room temperature, which helps retain volatile compounds, natural flavors, and nutritional components like vitamins and bioactive peptides. In addition to being energy-efficient and rapid, PEF provides a viable alternative to pasteurization, particularly for heat-sensitive or value-added dairy products. Its success in reducing bacterial load without altering quality makes it a promising technology for the future of clean-label dairy processing (Lytras et al., 2024).

4.6.1.2.3 Cold plasma

In the dairy sector, cold plasma serves as an advanced non-thermal preservation approach that employs ionized gas at low temperatures to produce reactive species such as ozone, free radicals, and ultraviolet photons (Sharma & Singh, 2020). These reactive agents act on the surface of packaged or unpackaged dairy beverages, compromising microbial cell membranes and effectively inactivating spoilage organisms, including bacteria and yeasts. Because cold plasma treatment primarily targets surface microorganisms and exhibits limited penetration, it is particularly advantageous for extending the shelf life of products such as packaged milk, flavored dairy drinks, and yogurt-based beverages. Moreover, as the process operates without significant heat generation, it preserves the nutritional composition and sensory characteristics of dairy products, making it well suited for applications where thermal treatments might otherwise cause quality deterioration (Sharma & Singh, 2020).

4.6.1.2.4 UV irradiation

Ultraviolet C (UV–C) light, with wavelengths ranging from 200 to 280 nm, is increasingly utilized in the dairy industry for the decontamination of product surfaces and transparent liquid matrices (Shabir et al., 2020). Its antimicrobial efficacy stems from its ability to damage microbial DNA, thereby inhibiting the growth of spoilage and pathogenic microorganisms. This technique is particularly suited to clear or low-viscosity dairy beverages—such as skim milk, whey-based drinks, and flavored milks where sufficient light penetration can be achieved. Unlike thermal methods, UV-C treatment does not induce heat-related changes in flavor or texture; however, it may lead to minor degradation of light-sensitive nutrients, including riboflavin and vitamin A. Due to its limited penetration depth, UV-C processing is most effective for thin liquid layers or surface exposure and is often employed in combination with refrigeration or other preservation strategies to enhance microbial stability while maintaining product quality (Shabbir et al., 2020) Table 4.3.

4.6.2 Homogenization to prevent phase separation

Homogenization is a critical processing technique employed in the dairy industry to ensure the uniform distribution of fat globules within liquid dairy products, thereby preventing phase separation and ensuring the stability of the final product (Mehta, 2015). This mechanical process is particularly important for products such as milk, cream, yogurt, and dairy beverages, which are prone to physical instability, leading to the separation of fat or formation of a cream layer on top. Phase separation can detrimentally influence the texture, appearance, and overall sensory attributes of dairy products, underscoring the importance of homogenization as a vital step in modern dairy processing. In this process, milk or other dairy liquids are subjected to intense pressure generally between 100 and 300 MPa and forced through a narrow orifice (Goff et al., 2020). The resulting mechanical action disrupts large fat globules, reducing their size to approximately 0.2–2 μm. This marked decrease in globule size increases the surface area of the fat phase, thereby promoting stronger interactions with the surrounding aqueous matrix. Consequently, the smaller and more uniformly dispersed fat globules remain suspended within the liquid, effectively preventing the separation of cream from the rest of the product (Thiebaud et al., 2003). The efficiency of homogenization arises from the combined effects of

Table 4.3 Non-thermal processing technologies for dairy beverages.

Technology	Working principle	Effectiveness	Impact on quality	Shelf life extension	Technology	References
High-pressure processing (HPP)	Uses 400–600 MPa pressure to inactivate microbes	High for vegetative cells	Retains flavor and nutrients	30–60 days (refrigerated)	High-pressure processing (HPP)	Sehrawat et al. (2021).
Pulsed electric field (PEF)	Short bursts of high voltage (20–80 kV/cm) disrupt cell membranes	Effective for liquids	Minimal thermal damage	20–40 days	Pulsed electric field (PEF)	Lytras et al. (2024).
Cold plasma	Ionized gas produces reactive species	Effective against bacteria, yeast	Surface treatment only	Varies (product-specific)	Cold plasma	Sharma and Singh (2020).
UV Irradiation	UV-C (200–280 nm) disrupts	microbial DNA	Surface or thin	Liquids only	No heat	Shabbir et al. (2020)

shear forces, cavitation, and turbulent flow, which collectively fragment and redistribute fat globules throughout the system. In addition, natural surfactants and milk proteins such as caseins and phospholipids rapidly adsorb to the newly formed fat–water interface. This adsorption reduces interfacial tension and enhances emulsion stability, creating a system that resists creaming during storage (Goff et al., 2020). Beyond its structural benefits, homogenization significantly improves the sensory and physicochemical characteristics of dairy beverages. It imparts a smooth, creamy mouthfeel and uniform viscosity, attributes that strongly influence consumer acceptance. Moreover, the fine dispersion of fat globules facilitates an even distribution of flavor compounds, leading to improved taste perception and overall palatability (Goff et al., 2020).

4.6.3 Use of natural preservatives in dairy beverages

Natural preservatives such as antimicrobial peptides like nisin, plant-derived extracts and essential oils, and probiotic-based bioprotective systems have emerged as promising alternatives for improving the safety and extending the shelf life of dairy beverages. These compounds act by inhibiting the growth of spoilage and pathogenic microorganisms, thereby maintaining product quality and reducing the reliance on synthetic additives.

4.6.3.1 Nisin in dairy beverages

Nisin, a naturally occurring lantibiotic synthesized by *Lactococcus lactis*, is extensively applied in dairy beverages due to its potent antimicrobial activity, particularly against Gram-positive bacteria such as *Listeria monocytogenes* and *Staphylococcus aureus* (Gharsallaoui et al., 2016). Its antimicrobial mechanism is based on its affinity for lipid II, an essential intermediate in bacterial cell wall biosynthesis. By binding to this molecule, nisin not only disrupts cell wall formation but also induces pore formation in the cytoplasmic membrane, ultimately resulting in cell lysis and death (T Hart et al., 2016). In dairy matrices like milk, yogurt, and flavored milk beverages, the efficiency of nisin can vary depending on physicochemical factors such as fat content, pH, and the concentration of divalent cations. High-fat environments may sequester nisin through interactions with fat globules, thereby reducing its antimicrobial action, while ions such as calcium and magnesium can interfere with its membrane-binding capacity (Gharsallaoui et al., 2016). To address these challenges, encapsulation technologies have been developed to achieve a controlled and sustained release of nisin within dairy systems, enhancing its stability and prolonging its antimicrobial activity (Davoodi et al., 2018). In a study by (Radha, 2014), the addition of nisin at concentrations ranging from 50 to 300 IU/mL significantly extended the shelf life of pasteurized milk by approximately 1 week under refrigerated storage at 4°C. However, increasing the concentration beyond this range did not yield further antimicrobial benefits and was associated with minor alterations in sensory attributes. These findings suggest that optimized nisin application can effectively retard microbial proliferation and delay the development of acidity, thereby improving the storage stability of pasteurized milk.

4.6.3.2 Plant extracts and essential oils in dairy beverages

Essential oils extracted from plants, such as thyme, oregano, and cinnamon oils, have drawn interest as natural preservatives in dairy products because of their antioxidant and antimicrobial properties (Pandey et al., 2017). These essential oils contain bioactive substances including phenolics and terpenes that may disrupt genetic material, interfere with enzyme activity, and rupture microbial cell membranes to prevent the growth of bacteria (Burt, 2004). However, there are issues with solubility, sensory acceptability, and possible interactions with dairy ingredients when using essential oils in dairy products. Therefore to address this challenge nanoemulsions and liposomal delivery systems have been studied to enhance their dispersion in milk-based beverages while preserving their antibacterial activity (Dima et al., 2014).

Samaddar et al. (2015) explored the use of essential oil constituents, particularly eugenol and trans-cinnamaldehyde, in the formulation of flavored milk. The study demonstrated that the addition of these bioactive compounds enhanced the product's antioxidant capacity, which in turn contributed to an extended shelf life under refrigerated storage conditions. Sensory analysis further revealed that the incorporation of eugenol and trans-cinnamaldehyde not only maintained but also improved the overall acceptability of the flavored milk, with no significant negative effects on its taste or aroma profile.

4.6.3.3 Probiotic-based bioprotection in dairy beverages

Probiotic cultures, particularly lactic acid bacteria (LAB), play a significant role in the biopreservation of dairy beverages through the synthesis of antimicrobial metabolites such as organic acids, hydrogen peroxide, and bacteriocins (Stiles, 1996). These metabolites suppress the growth of spoilage microorganisms and foodborne pathogens, thereby extending the shelf life of products like probiotic yogurt drinks, kefir, and other fermented milk-based beverages. Among LAB strains, *Lactobacillus rhamnosus* and *Lactobacillus plantarum* have received particular attention for their capacity to inhibit microbial contamination in functional dairy formulations (Pintado et al., 2010). Moreover, co-cultivation strategies involving probiotics and nisin-producing *Lactococcus lactis* have been suggested as an effective means of enhancing microbial stability in dairy systems through synergistic antimicrobial action (Settanni & Corsetti, 2008). In a more recent investigation, Aljasir and D'Amico (2021), evaluated the efficacy of commercial dairy-associated protective cultures against *Listeria monocytogenes*. Their findings demonstrated that probiotic strains were capable of surviving simulated gastrointestinal conditions while exerting inhibitory effects on *L. monocytogenes*, underscoring their potential application in improving the microbial safety of dairy beverages Fig. 4.1.

4.6.4 Ingredient optimization for stability

Ensuring desirable stability, texture, and sensory quality in dairy beverages relies heavily on the careful and deliberate use of stabilizers and emulsifiers. These functional ingredients are vital in controlling undesirable physical and chemical changes such as sedimentation, phase separation, and protein aggregation that can otherwise compromise product integrity, consumer perception, and overall shelf life. When properly chosen and used in appropriate proportions, they strengthen the structural network of dairy systems, maintaining consistency and quality throughout processing, storage, and distribution. Among the commonly used stabilizers, hydrocolloids such as pectin, guar gum, and carrageenan are particularly effective because of their capacity to form gel-like matrices. These compounds improve viscosity and mouthfeel while preventing syneresis, the undesirable release of liquid from the dairy matrix. Their stabilizing action results from their interaction with water molecules and milk proteins, which enhances the cohesiveness of the system. For instance, carrageenan associates with casein micelles to form a three-dimensional network that contributes to the uniformity and body of the beverage (Saha & Bhattacharya, 2010). Similarly, pectin and guar gum function as thickening agents that impart smoothness and prevent phase separation during storage

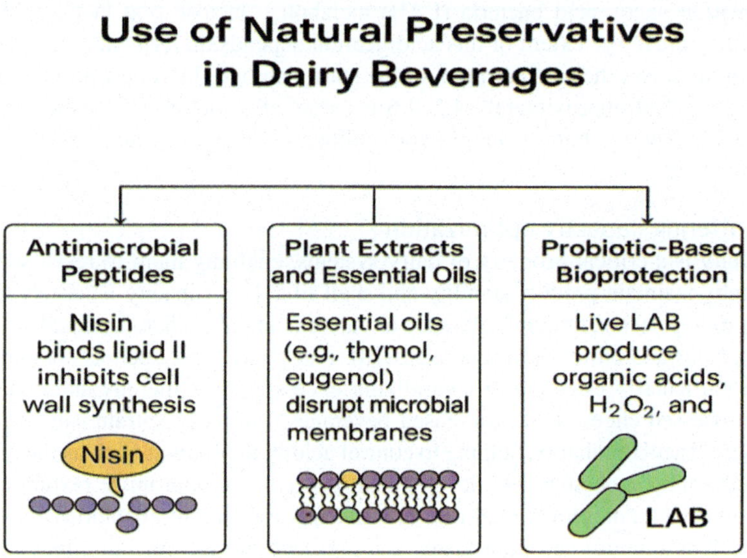

FIGURE 4.1

Natural preservatives in dairy beverages.

(Dickinson, 2003). Emulsifiers such as lecithin and mono- and diglycerides represent another key group of additives that promote physical stability by ensuring even distribution of fat globules. They work by reducing interfacial tension between fat and aqueous phases, thereby preventing coalescence and visible cream separation. Mono- and diglycerides, in particular, enhance the structural and textural stability of emulsions (Adjonu et al., 2014). Lecithin a naturally occurring phospholipid—plays an additional role in improving the heat stability of emulsified dairy systems, making it especially beneficial in ultra-high-temperature (UHT) processed beverages (Berton et al., 2012). In addition to hydrocolloids and emulsifiers, milk-derived proteins such as sodium caseinate and whey protein isolate are also crucial for emulsion stability. These proteins form protective films around fat droplets, which prevent aggregation and phase separation, ensuring homogeneity throughout the product's shelf life. The emulsifying performance of sodium caseinate is well established and can be affected by factors such as protein concentration and ionic strength (Dickinson, 1997). When used together, emulsifiers and proteins often act synergistically, producing enhanced rheological behavior and improved sensory attributes in dairy beverages (Liu et al., 2021).

4.6.4.1 Role of pH

The pH of dairy products plays a vital role in determining their physicochemical stability, microbial safety, and overall sensory characteristics. Maintaining an appropriate pH throughout processing and storage is essential to ensure uniform texture, desirable flavor, and extended shelf life. In fermented dairy products such as yogurt, a gradual decrease in pH occurs as fermentation progresses, effectively suppressing the growth of spoilage and pathogenic microorganisms. However, both excessive acidification and insufficient acidity can lead to undesirable alterations in texture, consistency, and product safety. To maintain product quality, manufacturers closely monitor and regulate pH and buffering capacity, ensuring that the final product remains microbiologically stable and sensorially acceptable. During fermentation, lactic acid bacteria (LAB) metabolize lactose into lactic acid, resulting in a controlled decline in pH. The extent of this acidification depends on fermentation parameters such as temperature, duration, and the concentration of the starter culture. In yogurt production, for instance, achieving a target pH of approximately 4.5–4.6 is essential to obtain the desired gel structure and characteristic tangy flavor, while avoiding over-acidification that can cause excessive gelation, syneresis, or a bitter taste.

4.6.4.1.1 Buffering capacity optimization

Buffering capacity is a critical property of dairy systems, enabling them to resist sudden pH fluctuations and thereby maintain product stability and shelf life. This capacity is largely governed by the composition of milk proteins, mineral salts such as calcium and phosphate, and added buffering agents including phosphates and citrates (Kim et al., 2018). Phosphate salts, such as sodium and potassium phosphate, are particularly effective in neutralizing excess acidity, thereby stabilizing pH levels in products like processed cheese and milk-based beverages. Similarly, citrate salts especially sodium citrate serve as mild acid regulators, helping to control acidity in products such as flavored milk and ice cream while preventing excessive acid development that could compromise texture and flavor. Milk proteins, particularly casein, play a dual role in buffering and structural stability by interacting with mineral ions such as calcium and phosphate. The presence of calcium salts, like calcium chloride, further enhances buffering efficiency, reducing the likelihood of drastic pH shifts during storage or thermal processing. In certain milk- or whey-based beverages, small amounts of sodium bicarbonate are incorporated to counteract acidification that may arise from microbial activity or chemical reactions during storage. The controlled use of these alkaline agents helps manufacturers maintain product freshness, prevent off-flavors, and extend shelf life by ensuring pH stability throughout the product's distribution period.

4.6.5 Antioxidants to reduce oxidation

Antioxidants play a pivotal role in protecting dairy products from oxidative deterioration, thereby preserving their flavor, texture, and nutritional value. Oxidation of lipids and proteins can lead to undesirable sensory changes and reduced shelf life, making antioxidant incorporation essential for product quality. Natural antioxidants such as vitamin E (tocopherols) protect milk fats from peroxidation, while vitamin C (ascorbic acid) mitigates oxidative damage to both proteins and lipids, although it is sensitive to degradation under heat and light exposure.

Plant-derived polyphenols and carotenoids, including β-carotene, offer additional antioxidant protection while enhancing the nutritional profile and color stability of dairy products. In high-fat dairy items such as butter, cheese, and milk powder, synthetic antioxidants like butylated hydroxytoluene (BHT), butylated hydroxyanisole (BHA), and propyl gallate are commonly used to inhibit rancidity and extend product shelf life. Furthermore, enzymatic antioxidants such as superoxide dismutase and catalase provide biological defense against reactive oxygen species, though their stability depends heavily on storage and processing conditions. Collectively, these antioxidant systems contribute to maintaining the freshness, quality, and nutritional integrity of dairy products throughout their shelf life.

4.6.6 Packaging innovations for extended shelf life of dairy products

Packaging plays an important part in the preservation and quality maintenance of dairy products. As customer demands for sustainability, convenience, and longer shelf life increase, creative packaging solutions have been developed to address these issues in the dairy sector. Modern packaging methods aid in shielding dairy products from environmental elements including moisture, light, and oxygen, which can have a big impact on the products nutritional value, stability, flavor, and texture. The main advancements in packaging methods intended to increase the shelf life of dairy products are mentioned in detail below.

4.6.6.1 Modified atmosphere packaging

Modified Atmosphere Packaging (MAP) is an effective method that alters the gas composition inside the container to increase the shelf life of dairy products. The main purpose of MAP is to lower oxygen levels and substitute them with gases that assist slow down oxidative processes and microbial development, such as carbon dioxide or nitrogen (Chowdhury et al., 2017). This method works particularly well for preserving the freshness and avoiding spoiling of foods like fresh cheese, yogurt, and milk. MAP helps prevent the growth of aerobic bacteria that cause microbiological spoiling, such molds and Pseudomonas species, by lowering oxygen levels. It also reduces lipid oxidation, which causes rancidity in dairy products, by decreasing oxygen concentrations. However, raising the amount of carbon dioxide in the packaging has antibacterial properties, especially against mold and bacteria, which further lowers microbial activity and slows down the metabolic reactions that cause spoiling.

The high levels of CO_2 in MAP help preserve dairy products quality without using chemical preservatives. It helps to maintain the taste and nutritional content of milk by reducing the oxidation of milk lipids and the microbial burden. All things considered, MAP successfully maintains the nutritional integrity, freshness, and texture of dairy products, making it a useful method for increasing their shelf life and preserving customer pleasure.

4.6.6.2 Vacuum packaging

The shelf life of dairy products is increased by vacuum packaging, which eliminates air before sealing, inhibits the growth of aerobic microbes, and lowers oxidation. By removing oxygen, this technique helps prevent rancidity, postpone spoiling, and maintain freshness in delicate components (Barukčić et al., 2021). Processed milk, cheese, and butter are among the dairy products that greatly benefit from lower oxygen levels because they limit microbial contamination. While vacuum-sealed butter prevents fat oxidation, retaining taste and avoiding off-flavors, while hard cheeses sustain texture and flavor while undergoing less mold development. Dairy products' quality and stability are successfully improved by this process.

4.6.6.3 Active packaging systems

Active packaging has emerged as an innovative approach in the dairy industry for maintaining product quality and extending the shelf life of beverages. Unlike conventional packaging, which serves mainly as a passive barrier, active packaging interacts with the product or its surrounding atmosphere to control factors such as oxygen, moisture, and microbial activity elements that are critical for preserving freshness and safety. Oxygen scavengers form one of the most effective components of these systems. They absorb residual oxygen trapped inside the package, thereby limiting oxidative reactions that can cause rancidity, off-flavors, and nutrient loss in dairy beverages. This is particularly beneficial for products such as flavored milk, yogurt-based drinks, and milkshakes, where oxidation of fats and proteins can rapidly affect sensory appeal and reduce marketable life. Moisture absorbers also play a crucial role, especially in beverages with relatively high water content, such as yogurt drinks and smoothies. By regulating excess moisture, these agents help prevent microbial spoilage, mold growth, and textural defects like syneresis. This moisture control contributes to maintaining a uniform consistency and stable appearance throughout the product's shelf life. Another significant advancement is antimicrobial packaging, which incorporates compounds that actively suppress microbial growth. Substances such as silver nanoparticles, essential oils (including oregano and thyme oil), and organic acids like lactic acid have been used to inhibit spoilage organisms and foodborne pathogens. Because dairy beverages provide a favorable environment for microbial proliferation due to their high nutrient and moisture content, antimicrobial packaging helps protect against common contaminants such as *Escherichia coli* and *Salmonella*. These systems not only enhance microbiological safety but also preserve sensory characteristics, ensuring that the product remains fresh and stable during storage and distribution.

4.6.6.4 Intelligent packaging and sensors

Packing solutions that use cutting-edge sensors or indications to continually monitor the products quality, safety, and condition throughout the supply chain from manufacture to consumption are referred to as intelligent or smart packaging for dairy beverages. Real-time information on the condition of the product may be obtained from these sensors, which can identify changes in important parameters including temperature, humidity, pH, or microbial activity (Kerry et al., 2006). The temperature history of dairy drinks during storage and transportation is frequently tracked using Time-Temperature Indicators (TTIs). If dairy beverages are not kept properly, they may oxidize, degrade, and spoil since they are extremely sensitive to temperature changes. TTIs assist in maintaining the proper temperature for goods like smoothies, yogurt drinks, and flavored milk, protecting their quality and averting certain health hazards. Furthermore, microbial sensors created to identify the existence of spoilage microorganisms like bacteria, molds, or yeast within the packaging are included into certain intelligent packaging systems. These sensors serve as an early warning system, alerting consumers to any microbial development that might jeopardize the product's freshness or safety. Smart dairy beverage packaging guarantees that consumers obtain safe, high-quality goods by giving real-time data regarding temperature and microbiological activity.

4.6.6.5 Light-barrier packaging

The quality of dairy products can be greatly impacted by light exposure, particularly ultraviolet (UV) radiation, which can degrade sensitive nutrients like riboflavin and result in discoloration and off tastes (Brothersen et al., 2006). Dairy products including milk, yogurt drinks, smoothies, and flavored milk include minerals and chemicals that can be degraded by light, they are especially prone to these problems (Lindmark-Månsson & Åkesson, 2000). In this context light-barrier packaging is necessary to combat this, shielding these goods from damaging light exposure while maintaining their nutritional and sensory qualities.

The dairy beverage sector frequently uses packaging materials designed to block or filter out UV and visible light, such as opaque cartons, laminates made of aluminum foil, or specially coated bottles. By providing a barrier that keeps light out of the packaging, these materials lower the chance of nutritional loss particularly for the light-sensitive vitamin riboflavin and the development of off tastes that can result from oxidation. In addition light-barrier packaging safeguards the nutritional value of the product while also preserving its overall flavor character, guaranteeing that dairy products will continue to taste and be of the desired quality for the duration of their shelf life. Dairy products that are both nutritionally intact and free from undesired alterations brought on by light exposure can be delivered by producers utilizing light-protective packaging, improving the entire experience for customers.

4.7 Future perspectives in dairy beverage development

As consumer preferences change and new scientific discoveries open up new avenues for innovation, the dairy beverage sector is undergoing a dramatic transition. Precision fermentations potential for tailored goods, the incorporation of personalized nutrition into the creation of dairy products, and new research on bioactive chemicals are all set to transform the industry. Along with utilizing cutting-edge technology to produce dairy beverages that satisfy certain dietary and health requirements, these developments are also reacting to the increased consumer demand for useful, health-promoting goods.

4.7.1 Emerging research on bioactive compounds and gut health

Dairy products naturally contain bioactive chemicals, which are gaining increasing amounts of interest owing to their ability to improve gut health and general well-being. Bioactive peptides, oligosaccharides, and other healthy substances found in dairy products particularly fermented drinks like kefir and yogurt are being investigated for their potential to support gut health (Korhonen & Pihlanto, 2006).

4.7.2 Bioactive peptides

Milk casein and whey proteins are abundant in bioactive peptides, which are protein fragments produced during fermentation or digestion. Numerous health advantages, such as antibacterial, antioxidant, antihypertensive, and immune modulatory properties, have been associated with these peptides (Korhonen & Pihlanto, 2006). While certain peptides, like lactotripeptides, can support heart health and blood pressure regulation, others function as prebiotics, encouraging the development of good gut flora. Bioactive peptides are becoming a major emphasis in the creation of dairy drinks targeted at enhancing gut health due to the increasing amount of research on gut microbiota and its connection to illnesses including obesity, inflammatory bowel disease, and even mental health.

4.7.3 Prebiotics and probiotics

Probiotic-fermented dairy products contain live beneficial microbes that can have a beneficial impact on the gut microbiota. Probiotics like Lactobacillus and Bifidobacterium aid in gut health restoration by preserving or reestablishing the balance of the microbiota, which is essential for immune system and digestive function (Lau & Quek, 2024). Furthermore, prebiotic attributes of dairy-derived oligosaccharides, such as galactooligosaccharides or GOS, have gained interest because they provide a food supply for good bacteria in the gut (Gänzle & Follador, 2012). Recent studies are concentrating on finding certain probiotic strains and oligosaccharide types that might offer customized gut health advantages, which could lead to more functional and targeted dairy products (Lau & Quek, 2024).

4.7.4 Gut-brain axis

Research on the gut-brain axis, which explores the two-way link that exists between the gut microbiota and the brain, is currently growing. The gut microbiome has been shown to affect behavior, emotion, and cognition (Santos et al., 2025). Dairy products enhanced with bioactive substances that boost gut health may also benefit mental health as more is known about this relationship. In the future, functional dairy drinks that promote mental and digestive well-being may emerge as a key development area.

4.8 Potential of precision fermentation for customized dairy beverages

Precision fermentation is a groundbreaking technique that uses genetically modified microbes to precisely create particular chemicals. By facilitating the production of highly tailored dairy drinks, this strategy has the potential to completely transform the dairy business and is already having a significant impact on other food industries.

4.8.1 Customization of nutritional content

The manufacturing of dairy products with specific nutritional characteristics is made possible by precision fermentation. In order to increase or decrease particular nutrients including protein, fat, vitamins, and minerals, producers can employ microbes to ferment milk or plant-based substrates (Cho et al., 2025). Moreover, precision fermentation might be used to make dairy products with increased calcium and vitamin D content, which are important for healthy bones, or to make drinks with certain amino acid profiles that help metabolism or muscle repair. According to Cho et al. (2025), this would enable the production of dairy products that address specific health objectives, such better bone health, weight control, or muscular growth.

4.8.2 Lactose-free and hypoallergenic dairy products

Traditional dairy has a lot of drawbacks because of its lactose content, which may lead to people who are lactose intolerant experience gastrointestinal issues. By developing dairy beverages without lactose but with the same nutritional benefits as traditional dairy, precision fermentation can help to address this problem (Cho et al., 2025). Also, precision fermentation could also make it possible to produce dairy-like beverages devoid of casein and whey, the proteins that some consumers may be sensitive to. Furthermore, by producing non-dairy drinks that mimic the flavor, consistency, and nutritional value of conventional dairy, this technology may let customers with dietary restrictions have additional alternatives.

4.8.3 Consumer-centric product development

Personalized nutrition is increasingly recognized as a promising approach to enhance consumer engagement by tailoring food choices to individual health goals and physiological needs. In this context, dairy manufacturers are exploring the development of digital platforms and mobile applications that enable consumers to input personal health data such as age, gender, lifestyle, activity level, and medical history to obtain customized recommendations for dairy-based beverages. This integration of nutritional science with digital technology allows for the formulation of products that better align with specific dietary requirements. Moreover, it fosters a more interactive and informed consumer experience, empowering individuals to make choices that support their overall health and well-being.

4.9 Strategies for improving food safety

4.9.1 Hygienic handling and good manufacturing practices

According to the Food Safety Institute and the guidelines of the U.S. Food and Drug Administration (FDA), maintaining strict hygiene throughout food processing and adhering to Good Manufacturing Practice (GMP) is fundamental to minimizing contamination risks. These practices encompass the hygienic design of processing facilities, routine cleaning and sanitation of equipment, and the safe handling of raw materials. Equally important is the enforcement of personal hygiene standards among food handlers. Maintaining a clean production environment, carefully monitoring each processing stage, and reducing unnecessary human contact with food products collectively help to prevent microbial and chemical contamination. Furthermore, GMP emphasizes proper documentation, traceability, and regular internal audits to ensure process consistency, regulatory compliance, and product safety.

4.9.2 Rapid detection of contaminants

Contemporary food safety systems increasingly depend on rapid and accurate analytical techniques to detect harmful microorganisms and chemical residues in food products (Gao et al., 2024). Among these, biosensor technology and polymerase chain reaction (PCR) have emerged as essential tools for ensuring product safety and quality. Biosensors function by recognizing and quantifying specific biological molecules or toxins, providing real-time monitoring of potential contaminants. In contrast, PCR enables the amplification of trace amounts of microbial DNA, allowing the detection of pathogenic bacteria even when present at very low concentrations (Gao et al., 2024). The integration of these advanced methods into food quality assurance frameworks greatly enhances the ability to identify hazards early, thereby preventing contaminated products from entering the consumer market.

4.9.3 Use of antimicrobial coatings

Antimicrobial coatings are increasingly utilized in food packaging and contact surfaces to suppress microbial proliferation and enhance product safety (Morales-de la Peña et al., 2025, pp. 903–915). These coatings are formulated using either natural or synthetic antimicrobial agents, such as chitosan, silver ions, or essential oils, which act by inhibiting or destroying microorganisms that may compromise food quality. In dairy products and ready-to-eat foods, their application effectively minimizes surface contamination, thereby reducing spoilage and extending shelf life without the need for excessive chemical preservatives. By restricting microbial activity after processing, antimicrobial coatings contribute to maintaining the stability, freshness, and microbiological safety of food products throughout storage and distribution (Morales-de la Peña et al., 2025, pp. 903–915).

4.10 Conclusion

It was concluded that innovative packaging, fermentation, ingredient optimization, and bioactive substances are all utilized to enhance the food safety and shelf life of dairy products. In addition antioxidants, stabilizers, and emulsifiers preserve texture, flavor, and freshness, while fermentation increases nutritional content and prolongs shelf life by preventing microbiological development. Moreover, modern packaging methods, like active systems and modified environment packaging, safeguard the dairy products against oxidation and spoiling. Furthermore, new studies on bioactive peptides, probiotics, and prebiotics may have positive health effects, especially for gut health. These developments will make it possible to create dairy drinks that are more individualized, practical, and handy. These advancements will make it possible to develop dairy beverages that are more convenient, useful, and customized as consumer preferences change.

References

Adjonu, R., Doran, G., Torley, P., & Agboola, S. (2014). Whey protein peptides as components of nanoemulsions: A review of emulsifying and biological functionalities. *Journal of Food Engineering, 122*(1), 15–27. https://doi.org/10.1016/j.jfoodeng.2013.08.034

Aljasir, S. F., & D'Amico, D. J. (2021). Characterization of commercial dairy-associated protective cultures for probiotic potential and inhibition of Listeria monocytogenes. *Food Research International, 143*, Article 110273. https://doi.org/10.1016/j.foodres.2021.110273

Barrett, N. E., Grandison, A. S., & Lewis, M. J. (1999). Contribution of the lactoperoxidase system to the keeping quality of pasteurized milk. *Journal of Dairy Research, 66*(1), 73–80. https://doi.org/10.1017/S0022029998003252

Barukčić, I., Ščetar, M., Lisak Jakopović, K., Kurek, M., Božanić, R., & Galić, K. (2021). Overview of packaging materials for dairy packaging. *Hrvatski časopis za prehrambenu tehnologiju, biotehnologiju i nutricionizam, 16*(3–4), 85–93. https://doi.org/10.31895/hcptbn.16.3-4.5

Baruzzi, F., Quintieri, L., Caputo, L., Cocconcelli, P. S., Borcakli, M., Owczarek, L., Morea, M., et al. (2016). Improvement of Ayran quality by the selection of autochthonous microbial cultures. *Food Microbiology, 60*, 79–88. https://doi.org/10.1016/j.fm.2016.07.001

Berton, C., Ropers, M. H., Viau, M., & Genot, C. (2012). Lipid oxidation in oil-in-water emulsions: Involvement of the interfacial layer. *Comprehensive Reviews in Food Science and Food Safety, 11*(4), 371–390. https://doi.org/10.1111/j.1541-4337.2012.00189.x

Bhat, Z. F., Bhat, H. F., Manzoor, M., Abdi, G., Aadil, R. M., Hassoun, A., & Aït-Kaddour, A. (2024). Enhancing the lipid stability of foods of animal origin using edible packaging systems. *Food Chemistry X, 21*. https://doi.org/10.1016/j.fochx.2024.101185. Available from: https://www.sciencedirect.com/science/journal/25901575.

Brothersen, C., McMahon, D. J., Legako, J., Martini, S., Schwendiman, R., & Broadbent, J. R. (2006). Effect of light exposure on flavor of milk containing 2% milk fat. *Journal of Dairy Science, 89*(6), 1931–1938.

Burt, S. (2004). Essential oils: Their antibacterial properties and potential applications in foods—a review. *International Journal of Food Microbiology, 94*(3), 223–253. https://doi.org/10.1016/j.ijfoodmicro.2004.03.022

Cho, S., Jung, S. Y., Eun, H., & Lee, S. Y. (2025). Precision fermentation for producing food ingredients. *Current Opinion in Food Science, 61*. https://doi.org/10.1016/j.cofs.2024.101242. Available from: https://www.sciencedirect.com/science/journal/22147993.

Chowdhury, T., Chattopadhyay, S. K., & Saha, N. C. (2017). Modified atmosphere packaging (MAP) and the effect of chemical preservative to enhance shelf life of khoa (heat desiccated milk product). *Journal of Packaging Technology and Research, 1*(1), 25–31. https://doi.org/10.1007/s41783-017-0004-3

Claeys, W. L., Cardoen, S., Daube, G., De Block, J., Dewettinck, K., Dierick, K., De Zutter, L., Huyghebaert, A., Imberechts, H., Thiange, P., Vandenplas, Y., & Herman, L. (2013). Raw or heated cow milk consumption: Review of risks and benefits. *Food Control, 31*(1), 251–262. https://doi.org/10.1016/j.foodcont.2012.09.035

Cossettini, A., Vidic, J., Maifreni, M., Marino, M., Pinamonti, D., & Manzano, M. (2022). Rapid detection of Listeria monocytogenes, Salmonella, Campylobacter spp., and Escherichia coli in food using biosensors. *Food Control, 137*, Article 108962. https://doi.org/10.1016/j.foodcont.2022.108962

Davoodi, R., Shahbazi, Y., & Ahmadi, F. (2018). Encapsulation of nisin in liposomes: Characterization, stability, and application in milk. *Food Chemistry, 260*, 194–200. https://doi.org/10.1016/j.foodchem.2018.03.104

Deeth, H. C., Datta, N., Aleong, J. V., & Hamid, I. (2010). Ultra-high-temperature (UHT) treatment of milk and dairy products. In *Heat treatment for insect control* (pp. 227–252). Springer. https://doi.org/10.1007/978-90-481-9464-7_13

Deshpande, H. W., Phulari, S. S., & Katke, S. D. (2020). Studies on process standardization and quality evaluation of flavored lassi. *International Journal of Current Microbiology and Applied Sciences, 9*(9), 2289–2296. https://doi.org/10.20546/ijcmas.2020.909.285

Dickinson, E. (1997). Properties of emulsions stabilized with milk proteins: Overview of some recent developments. *Journal of Dairy Science, 80*(10), 2607–2619. https://doi.org/10.3168/jds.s0022-0302(97)76218-0

Dickinson, E. (2003). Hydrocolloids at interfaces and the influence on the properties of dispersed systems. *Food Hydrocolloids, 17*(1), 25–39. https://doi.org/10.1016/s0268-005x(01)00120-5

Dima, C., Dima, S., & Iordachescu, G. (2014). Encapsulation of essential oils in food products using nanoemulsion techniques. *Food Science and Technology Research, 20*(6), 1091–1096. https://doi.org/10.3136/fstr.20.1091

Drewnowski, A. (2011). The contribution of milk and milk products to micronutrient density and affordability of the U.S. diet. *Journal of the American College of Nutrition, 30*(Suppl. 5), 422S. https://doi.org/10.1080/07315724.2011.10719986

Drewnowski, A. (2025). Perspective: Milk and dairy provide affordable high-quality protein and merit inclusion in the protein foods group. *Current Developments in Nutrition, 9*(1), Article 104539. https://doi.org/10.1016/j.cdnut.2024.104539

Edenbach, L. H., & Marshall, R. T. (2009). Microbiological spoilage of dairy products. In *Compendium of the microbiological spoilage of foods and beverages* (pp. 41–67).

Endara, P., Wiedmann, M., & Adalja, A. (2023). Consumer willingness to pay for shelf life of high-temperature, short-time-pasteurized fluid milk: Implications for smart labeling and food waste reduction. *Journal of Dairy Science, 106*(9), 5940–5957. https://doi.org/10.3168/jds.2022-22968

Erkmen, O., & Bozoglu, T. F. (2016). Spoilage of milk and milk products. In *Food microbiology: Principles into practice, Vol. 1: Microorganisms related to foods, foodborne diseases, and food spoilage* (pp. 307–336). https://doi.org/10.1002/9781119237860.ch19

FAO/WHO. (2002). In *Guidelines for the evaluation of probiotics in food*. London, Ontario, Canada: Joint FAO/WHO Working Group Report.

Fusco, V., Chieffi, D., Fanelli, F., Logrieco, A. F., Cho, G. S., Kabisch, J., Böhnlein, C., & Franz, C. M. A. P. (2020). Microbial quality and safety of milk and milk products in the 21st century. *Comprehensive Reviews in Food Science and Food Safety, 19*(4), 2013–2049. https://doi.org/10.1111/1541-4337.12568

Gallo, M., Ferrara, L., & Naviglio, D. (2019). *An overview of natural beverages natural beverages: Volume 13: The science of beverages*. Italy: Elsevier. https://doi.org/10.1016/B978-0-12-816689-5.00001-8

Gänzle, M. G., & Follador, R. (2012). Metabolism of oligosaccharides and starch in *Lactobacilli*: A review. *Frontiers in Microbiology, 3*, 340.

Gao, R., Liu, X., Xiong, Z., Wang, G., & Ai, L. (2024). Research progress on detection of foodborne pathogens: The more rapid and accurate answer to food safety. *Food Research International, 193*, Article 114767. https://doi.org/10.1016/j.foodres.2024.114767

Garnier, L., Valence, F., & Mounier, J. (2017). Diversity and control of spoilage fungi in dairy products: An update. *Microorganisms, 5*(3), 42. https://doi.org/10.3390/microorganisms5030042

Gaucher, I., Tanguy, G., Fauquant, J., Jardin, J., Rousseau, F., Robert, B., Madec, M.-N., & Gaucheron, F. (2011). Proteolysis of casein micelles by Pseudomonas fluorescens CNRZ 798 contributes to the destabilisation of UHT milk during its storage. *Dairy Science & Technology, 91*(4), 413–429. https://doi.org/10.1007/s13594-011-0019-4

Gharsallaoui, A., Oulahal, N., Joly, C., & Degraeve, P. (2016). Nisin as a food preservative: Part 1: Physicochemical properties, antimicrobial activity, and main uses. *Critical Reviews in Food Science and Nutrition, 56*(8), 1262–1274. https://doi.org/10.1080/10408398.2013.763765

Gilbert, J., Smith, R., & Lee, T. (2020). Syneresis in dairy products: Mechanisms, factors, and control strategies. *Journal of Dairy Science, 103*, 1234–1248. https://doi.org/10.3168/jds.2019-5678

Goff, H. D., Hill, A., & Ferrer, M. A. (2020). *Homogenization of milk and milk products. Dairy Science and Technology Education Series*. University of Guelph.

Górska-Warsewicz, H., Rejman, K., Laskowski, W., & Czeczotko, M. (2019). Milk and dairy products and their nutritional contribution to the average Polish diet. *Nutrients, 11*(8), 1771. https://doi.org/10.3390/nu11081771

Guggisberg, D., Cuthbert-Steven, J., Piccinali, P., Bütikofer, U., & Eberhard, P. (2009). Rheological, microstructural and sensory characterization of low-fat and whole milk set yoghurt as influenced by inulin addition. *International Dairy Journal, 19*(2), 107–115. https://doi.org/10.1016/j.idairyj.2008.07.009

Huppertz, T., Gazi, I., Luyten, H., & Nieuwenhuijse, H. (2021). Changes in stability and shelf-life of ultra-high temperature treated milk during long term storage at different temperatures. *Heliyon, 7*(3), Article e06679. https://doi.org/10.1016/j.heliyon.2021.e06679

Jang, H. J., Lee, N. K., & Paik, H. D. (2024). Overview of dairy-based products with probiotics: Fermented or non-fermented milk drink. *Food Science of Animal Resources, 44*(2), 255–268. https://doi.org/10.5851/KOSFA.2023.E83

Joshi, V. K. (Ed.). (2016). *Cereal-Based Non-Alcoholic Indigenous Fermented Foods. In Ethnic Fermented Foods and Beverages of India.* CRC Press/Taylor & Francis.

Kerry, J. P., O'Grady, M. N., & Hogan, S. A. (2006). Past, current and potential utilisation of active and intelligent packaging systems for meat and muscle-based products: A review. *Meat Science, 74*(1), 113–130. https://doi.org/10.1016/j.meatsci.2006.04.024

Kim, M., Oh, S., & Imm, J. Y. (2018). Buffering capacity of dairy powders and their effect on yoghurt quality. *Korean Journal for Food Science of Animal Resources, 38*(2), 273–281. https://doi.org/10.5851/kosfa.2018.38.2.273

Korhonen, H., & Pihlanto, A. (2006). Bioactive peptides: Production and functionality. *International Dairy Journal, 16*(9), 945–960.

Krupa, H., Jana, A. H., & Patel, H. G. (2011). Synergy of dairy with non-dairy ingredients or products: A review. *African Journal of Food Science, 5*(16), 817–832.

Lau, L. Y. J., & Quek, S. Y. (2024). Probiotics: Health benefits, food application, and colonization in the human gastrointestinal tract. *Food Bioengineering, 3*(1), 41–64. https://doi.org/10.1002/fbe2.12078

Lindmark-Månsson, H., & Åkesson, B. (2000). Antioxidative factors in milk. *British Journal of Nutrition, 84*(S1), S103–S110. https://doi.org/10.1017/S0007114500002324

Liu, F., Ma, C., McClements, D. J., & Gao, Y. (2021). Development of polyphenol-protein-polysaccharide ternary complexes as emulsifiers for beverage emulsions: Impact on formation, stability and bioaccessibility of β-carotene emulsions. *Food Hydrocolloids, 112*, Article 106374. https://doi.org/10.1016/j.foodhyd.2020.106374

Lomolino, G., Zannoni, S., Zabara, A., & Spilimbergo, S. (2020). Current trends in the application of supercritical fluid technologies to fruit and vegetable processing. *Food Engineering Reviews, 12*, 1–18.

Lytras, F., Psakis, G., Gatt, R., Cebrián, G., Raso, J., & Valdramidis, V. (2024). Exploring the efficacy of pulsed electric fields (PEF) in microbial inactivation during food processing: A deep dive into the microbial cellular and molecular mechanisms. *Innovative Food Science & Emerging Technologies, 95*, Article 103732. https://doi.org/10.1016/j.ifset.2024.103732

Martin, N. H., Torres-Frenzel, P., & Wiedmann, M. (2021). Invited review: Controlling dairy product spoilage to reduce food loss and waste. *Journal of Dairy Science, 104*(2), 1251–1261. https://doi.org/10.3168/jds.2020-19130

Matsuyama, M., Harb, T., David, M., Davies, P. S., & Hill, R. J. (2017). Effect of fortified milk on growth and nutritional status in young children: A systematic review and meta-analysis. *Public Health Nutrition, 20*(7), 1214–1225. https://doi.org/10.1017/S1368980016003189

McCormick, F. (2012). Cows, milk and religion: The use of dairy produce in early societies. *Anthropozoologica, 47*(2), 101–113. https://doi.org/10.5252/az2012n2a7

Meena, K. K., Taneja, N. K., Jain, D., & Ojha, A. (2024). Optimization and production of dairy-cereal grain-based probiotic beverage powder and its probiotic survivability under simulated gastric and pancreatic conditions. *Discover Food, 4*(1). https://doi.org/10.1007/s44187-024-00099-3. Available from: https://www.springer.com/journal/44187.

Mehta, B. M. (2015). Chemical composition of milk and milk products. In L. Melton, F. Shahidi, & P. Varelis (Eds.), *Handbook of food chemistry* (pp. 539–564). Springer. https://doi.org/10.1007/978-3-642-36605-5_31

Mercier, S., Villeneuve, S., Mondor, M., & Uysal, I. (2017). Time–temperature management along the food cold chain: A review of recent developments. *Comprehensive Reviews in Food Science and Food Safety, 16*(4), 647–667. https://doi.org/10.1111/1541-4337.12269

Minz, P. S., & Singh, R. R. B. (2016). *Modernization of manufacturing process for traditional Indian dairy products*. Springer Science and Business Media LLC. https://doi.org/10.1007/978-1-4899-7671-0_14

Morales-de la Peña, M., Raybaudi-Massilia, R., Mosqueda-Melgar, J., Soliva-Fortuny, R., & Martín-Belloso, O. (2025). *Recent trends in antimicrobial edible films and coatings*. Elsevier BV. https://doi.org/10.1016/b978-0-323-90747-7.00058-2

Nagata, S., Asahara, T., Ohta, T., et al. (2006). Effect of the continuous intake of fermented milk containing Lactobacillus casei strain Shirota on the intestinal microbial flora and immune system of healthy volunteers. *Journal of Dairy Science, 89*(1), 201–206. https://doi.org/10.3168/jds.S0022-0302(06)72186-1

Narsaria, D., & Rajyalakshmi. (2020). *Insight on the plant-based milk category in India*. GFI India & Ipsos. Available at: https://gfi.org.in/wp-content/uploads/2021/07/Insights-on-the-plant-based-dairy-category-in-India.pdf.

Oliveira, M., & Fraqueza, M. J. (2020). Pathogens in dairy products: Contamination and control methods. In *Foodborne pathogens: Hygiene and safety* (pp. 125–144). Springer. https://doi.org/10.1007/978-3-030-41486-1_6

Owusu-Kwarteng, J., Akabanda, F., Agyei, D., & Jespersen, L. (2020). Microbial safety of milk production and fermented dairy products in Africa. *Microorganisms, 8*(5), 752. https://doi.org/10.3390/microorganisms8050752

Pandey, A. K., Kumar, P., Singh, P., Tripathi, N. N., & Bajpai, V. K. (2017). Essential oils: Sources of antimicrobials and food preservatives. *Frontiers in Microbiology, 7*. https://doi.org/10.3389/fmicb.2016.02161. Available from: http://journal.frontiersin.org/article/10.3389/fmicb.2016.02161/full.

Park, Y. W. (2021). The impact of plant-based non-dairy alternative milk on the dairy industry. *Food Science of Animal Resources, 41*(1), 8–15. https://doi.org/10.5851/KOSFA.2020.E82. Available from: http://www.kosfaj.org/archive/view_article?doi=10.5851/kosfa.2020.e82.

Pescuma, M., Hébert, E. M., Mozzi, F., & de Valdez, G. F. (2010). Functional fermented whey-based beverages. *International Journal of Dairy Technology, 63*(3), 315–323. https://doi.org/10.1111/j.1471-0307.2010.00575.x

Pintado, C. M. B. S., Ferreira, M. A. S. S., & Sousa, I. (2010). Control of pathogenic and spoilage microorganisms from cheese surface by lactobacilli with antimicrobial activity. *Innovative Food Science & Emerging Technologies, 11*(2), 352–357. https://doi.org/10.1016/j.ifset.2010.01.005

Pritulska, N., Motuzka, I., Koshelnyk, A., Motuzka, O., Yashchenko, L., Jarossova, M., Krnacova, P., Wyka, J., Malczyk, E., & Habanova, M. (2021). Consumer preferences on the market of plant-based milk analogues. *Potravinarstvo Slovak Journal of Food Sciences, 15*, 131–142. https://doi.org/10.5219/1485

Radha, K. (2014). Effect of nisin on the shelf life of pasteurized milk. *Indian Journal of Dairy Science, 67*(2), 121–127.

Ranieri, M. L., Huck, J. R., Sonnen, M., Barbano, D. M., & Boor, K. J. (2009). High temperature, short time pasteurization temperatures inversely affect bacterial numbers during refrigerated storage of pasteurized fluid milk. *Journal of Dairy Science, 92*(10), 4823–4832. https://doi.org/10.3168/jds.2009-2144

Rysstad, G., & Kolstad, J. (2006). Extended shelf life milk-advances in technology. *International Journal of Dairy Technology, 59*(2), 85–96. https://doi.org/10.1111/j.1471-0307.2006.00247.x

Saha, D., & Bhattacharya, S. (2010). Hydrocolloids as thickening and gelling agents in food: A critical review. *Journal of Food Science and Technology, 47*(6), 587–597. https://doi.org/10.1007/s13197-010-0162-6

Samaddar, A., Roy, A., Banerjee, S., & Bhattacharya, M. (2015). Role of essential oils as natural preservatives in flavored milk. *Indian Journal of Dairy Science, 68*(1), 56–63.

Sani, A. M., Rahbar, M., & Sheikhzadeh, M. (2019). Traditional beverages in different countries: Milk-based beverages. In *Milk-based beverages, volume 9: The science of beverages* (pp. 239–272).

Santos, J., Maran, P. L., & Rodríguez-Urrutia, A. (2025). Stress, microbiota, and the gut-brain axis in mental and digestive health. *Medicina Clínica, 164*(6), 295–304. https://doi.org/10.1016/j.medcli.2024.11.023

Sarkar, P., Lohith, K. D. H., Dhumal, C., Panigrahi, S. S., & Choudhary, R. (2015). Traditional and ayurvedic foods of Indian origin. *Journal of Ethnic Foods, 2*(3), 97–109. https://doi.org/10.1016/j.jef.2015.08.003

Sehrawat, R., Kaur, B. P., Nema, P. K., Tewari, S., & Kumar, L. (2021). Microbial inactivation by high pressure processing: Principle, mechanism and factors responsible. *Food Science and Biotechnology, 30*(1), 19–35. https://doi.org/10.1007/s10068-020-00831-6

Sethi, S., Tyagi, S. K., & Anurag, R. K. (2016). Plant-based milk alternatives an emerging segment of functional beverages: A review. *India Journal of Food Science and Technology, 53*(9), 3408–3423. https://doi.org/10.1007/s13197-016-2328-3

Settanni, L., & Corsetti, A. (2008). Application of bacteriocins in vegetable food biopreservation. *International Journal of Food Microbiology, 121*(2), 123–138. https://doi.org/10.1016/j.ijfoodmicro.2007.09.001

Shabbir, M. A. B., Ahmed, H., Maan, A. A., Rehman, A., Afzaal, M., Anjum, F. M., & Manzoor, M. F. (2020). Effect of non-thermal processing techniques on pathogenic and spoilage microorganisms of milk and milk products. *Food Science and Technology (Campinas), 40*(Suppl. 2), 20–28. https://doi.org/10.1590/fst.05820

Sharma, S., & Singh, R.k. (2020). Cold plasma treatment of dairy proteins in relation to functionality enhancement. *Trends in Food Science and Technology, 102*, 30–36. https://doi.org/10.1016/j.tifs.2020.05.013

Silva, F. V. M., & Gibbs, P. A. (2010). Non-proteolytic Clostridium botulinum spores in low-acid canned foods and their control through heat processing. *Trends in Food Science & Technology, 21*(2), 95–105. https://doi.org/10.1016/j.tifs.2009.10.004

Singh, B., Khamrui, K., Debnath, A., Lodh, J., Gupta, H. R., & Prasad, W. (2017). Sensory and color profile of milk-coconut sweet as a function of ingredients. *Indian Journal of Dairy Science, 70*(5), 491–495.

Soltani, M., Say, D., & Güzeler, N. (2012). Production and quality characteristics of Doogh. *Akademik Gıda, 10*(4), 50–53.

Steele, J. H. (2000). History, trends, and extent of pasteurization. *Journal of the American Veterinary Medical Association, 217*(2), 175–178. https://doi.org/10.2460/javma.2000.217.175

Stiles, M. E. (1996). Biopreservation by lactic acid bacteria. *Antonie Van Leeuwenhoek, 70*(2–4), 331–345. https://doi.org/10.1007/bf00395940

Stock, J. T., & Wells, J. C. K. (2023). Dairying and the evolution and consequences of lactase persistence in humans. *Animal Frontiers, 13*(3), 7–13. https://doi.org/10.1093/af/vfad022

T Hart, P., Oppedijk, S. F., Breukink, E., & Martin, N. I. (2016). New insights into nisin's antibacterial mechanism revealed by binding studies with synthetic lipid II analogues. *Biochemistry, 55*(1), 232–237. https://doi.org/10.1021/acs.biochem.5b01173

Tamanna, N., & Mahmood, N. (2015). Food processing and maillard reaction products: Effect on human health and nutrition. *International Journal of Food Science, 2015*, 1–6. https://doi.org/10.1155/2015/526762

Tan, M., Mei, J., & Xie, J. (2021). The formation and control of ice crystal and its impact on the quality of frozen aquatic products: A review. *Crystals, 11*(1), 68. https://doi.org/10.3390/cryst11010068

Thiebaud, M., Dumay, E., Picart, L., Guiraud, J. P., & Cheftel, J. C. (2003). High-pressure homogenisation of raw bovine milk. Effects on fat globule size distribution and microbial inactivation. *Innovative Food Science & Emerging Technologies, 4*(3), 259–269. https://doi.org/10.1016/S1466-8564(03)00051-7

Troise, A. D., Dathan, N. A., Fiore, A., Roviello, G. Di F. A., Caira, S., Cuollo, M. De S. G., Fogliano, V., & Monti, S. M. (2014). Faox enzymes inhibited Maillard reaction development during storage both in protein glucose model system and low lactose UHT milk. *Amino Acids, 46*. https://doi.org/10.1007/s00726-013-1497-x

Vaghela, D. R., Parmar, P., Joshi, N. U., Sabhadiya, H. R., et al. (2024). Chapter 9: Pasteurization. In *Unit Operations in Food Processing* (pp. 139–162). Scientific Publishers.

Vanga, S. K., & Raghavan, V. (2018). How well do plant based alternatives fare nutritionally compared to cow's milk? *Canada Journal of Food Science and Technology, 55*(1), 10–20. https://doi.org/10.1007/s13197-017-2915-y

Zhang, C., Bijl, E., Svensson, B., & Hettinga, K. (2019). The extracellular protease AprX from pseudomonas and its spoilage potential for UHT milk: A review. *Comprehensive Reviews in Food Science and Food Safety, 18*(4), 834–852. https://doi.org/10.1111/1541-4337.12452

CHAPTER

Preservation of quality and microbial characteristics of plant-based beverages

5

Mariana Buranelo Egea[1], Sibele Santos Fernandes[2], Raquel Martins da Silva Fernandes de Oliveira[3], Larissa Graziele Rauber Duarte[4] and Ailton Cesar Lemes[5]

[1]*Goiano Federal Institute of Education, Science and Technology, Campus Rio Verde, Rio Verde, GO, Brazil;* [2]*Federal University of Rio Grande, School of Chemistry and Food, Rio Grande, Brazil;* [3]*Federal University of Goiás, Faculty of Agronomy, Goiânia, Brazil;* [4]*Instituto Federal do Sul de Minas, IFSULdeMINAS, Machado, MG, Brazil;* [5]*School of Chemistry, Federal University of Rio de Janeiro, Rio de Janeiro, RJ, Brazil*

5.1 Introduction

Plant-based beverages are colloidal systems that contain liquid and dispersed solid particles derived from plants. These formulations undergo technological processes like homogenization, enzymatic hydrolysis, and ultrafiltration to enhance stability, sensory attributes, and rheological properties. Often enriched with micronutrients, fibers, and bioactive compounds, they are designed to optimize nutritional functionality and bioavailability while serving as sustainable alternatives to dairy-based beverages (Popova et al., 2023; Silva et al., 2024).

Plant-based beverages emerged as an alternative to conventional milk, serving both people with intolerances and allergies and those who prefer to restrict their consumption of dairy products for personal and/or lifestyle reasons, such as vegans or individuals with an aversion to milk (Fructuoso et al., 2021). Initially, the market offered few flavor options, with soy-based beverages standing out. However, over time and with the advancement of nutritional discoveries, other alternatives, such as beverages based on nuts, chestnuts, legumes, and fruits, gained ground, mainly because they provide better nutritional sources (Craig & Fresán, 2021).

In 2024, the global plant-based beverage market was valued at US$18.45 billion, reflecting the growing consumer interest in plant-based alternatives to milk and other traditional beverages. This segment has been experiencing significant growth and is expected to reach US$56.73 billion by 2034, driven by factors such as health concerns, sustainability, and innovation in the sector (Fact.MR., 2024).

Initially, water-soluble plant extracts, known as plant-based milk, were the main plant-based alternative. However, new options emerged as the market evolved, including different plant-based sources and bioactive compounds such as prebiotics and probiotics (Sharma et al., 2024). These alternatives complement the diet and offer nutritional benefits equal to or greater than animal-based milk, reflecting a growing movement in the plant-based universe (Grau-Fuentes et al., 2023).

The Science and Safety of Beverages. https://doi.org/10.1016/B978-0-443-36536-2.00003-X

Preserving the quality and microbial characteristics of plant-based beverages represents a key challenge to ensure that these products meet food safety standards and remain attractive to consumers over time. With the increasing demand for plant-based alternatives, adequate control of these beverages' nutritional, sensory, and microbiological properties has become crucial (Frühauf et al., 2023). Taste, aroma, color, and texture must be maintained. At the same time, the beverages need to be protected against the proliferation that is detrimental to their quality and safety (Sharma et al., 2024).

The nutritional composition of plant-based beverages can vary depending on the total of macro and micronutrients, bioactive compounds, and even anti-nutritional factors, directly influencing consumer choice (Fructuoso et al., 2021). In addition, the importance of personalized nutritional strategies adapted to the population's specific needs, such as correcting nutritional deficiencies, is increasingly highlighted (Maree et al., 2024). A diverse nutritional profile is observed when comparing the nutritional composition of different plant-based beverages, prebiotic and probiotic juices, with cow's milk (Berardy et al., 2022).

Several preservation methods can be used to ensure the durability and safety of plant-based beverages. Pasteurization is a standard method that destroys pathogens and undesirable microorganisms while maintaining the product's sensory properties. Controlled fermentation can be applied to preserve beverages and improve their nutritional profile and flavor. Adding natural preservatives, such as plant extracts and organic acids, is also a proven alternative strategy for consumers seeking more natural and less processed products (Munekata et al., 2020).

Preserving the quality of plant-based beverages is not limited to the industrial process, but also storage and transportation steps. Uncontrolled temperature, humidity, and exposure to light directly influence the stability of the product (Santos et al., 2019). Adopting appropriate storage practices, such as packaging that protects against contamination and degradation, guarantees that plant-based beverages remain safe and high-quality until consumption. Therefore, combined control of all these aspects is essential for commercial success and consumer satisfaction (Grau-Fuentes et al., 2023).

This chapter discusses the nutritional, sensory, and microbiological quality parameters of plant-based beverages and the methods used for their preservation (Fig. 5.1).

5.2 Nutritional and sensory quality characteristics of plant-based beverages

The quality of plant-based beverages is influenced by a series of factors ranging from the raw materials used to the manufacturing and storage processes (Sethi et al., 2016). The plant source, the processing steps performed (such as the type of extraction and fermentation), the addition of complementary ingredients, such as sweeteners or preservatives, and the storage conditions are all determining factors in the quality of the final product. In addition, sensory factors, such as taste, aroma, and texture, play a fundamental role in consumer acceptance (Santana et al., 2020). Understanding how these elements interact is essential for developing high-quality plant-based beverages that meet the nutritional and sensory needs of the marketplace.

Among the most widely consumed plant-based beverages are soy milk, known for its high protein content and nutritional profile similar to cow's milk; almond milk, valued for its light texture and nutty

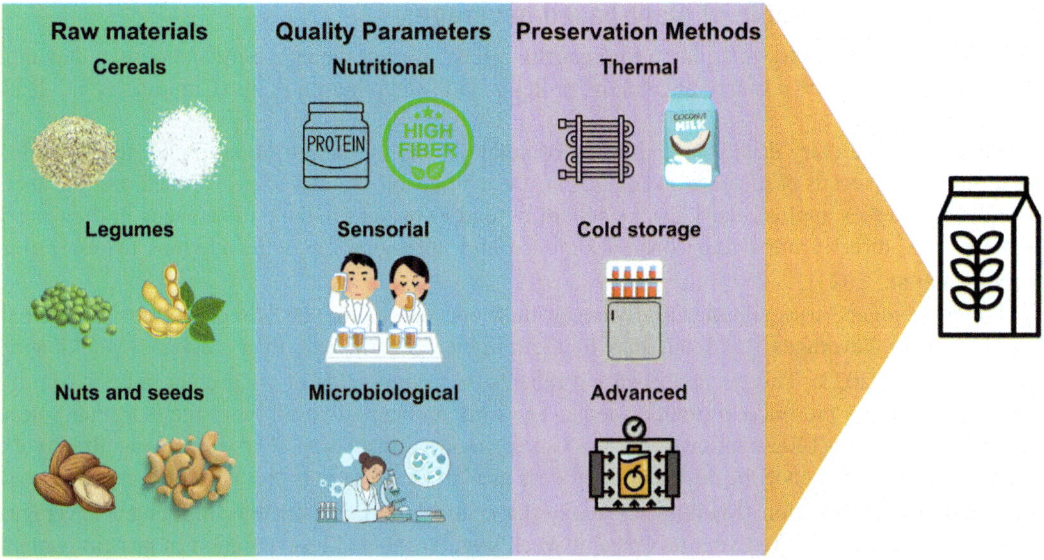

FIGURE 5.1

Main aspects of quality and preservation of plant-based beverages.

flavor; oat milk, which offers a creamy consistency and is rich in beta-glucans; rice milk, typically hypoallergenic and naturally sweet; coconut milk, appreciated for its tropical flavor and richness in medium-chain triglycerides; and pea milk, an emerging option with a neutral taste and high protein content. Each beverage has unique nutritional, functional, and sensory properties, influencing its processing requirements and market acceptance. Exploring their characteristics helps inform strategies for formulation and innovation within the plant-based beverage sector.

A recent study by (Frühauf et al., 2023) analyzed five commercial plant-based beverages in the Brazilian market—soybean, oat, rice, cashew nut, and spelt grain—and identified significant physicochemical and sensory differences. Soy milk stood out with the highest ash content (0.62%), moderate viscosity (11.3 mPa s^{-1}), and the highest acceptability index (71.75%), making it the most preferred. Oat milk had the highest viscosity (16.8 mPa s^{-1}) and fiber content (5.5 g/200 mL), contributing to its creamy texture and favorable sensory ratings by 65%–69% of panelists. Rice milk showed the lowest viscosity (5.0 mPa s^{-1}) but the highest pH (7.42), indicating better chemical stability and hypoallergenic potential. In contrast, cashew nut milk had the lowest ash content (0.15%), low chroma ($C^* = 4.69$), and the lowest acceptability (33.61%), likely due to high sedimentation and poor stability. Spelt grain milk, with moderate viscosity (7.6 mPa s^{-1}) and high hue angle (92.88 degrees), ranked second in preference despite sedimentation. Based on osmolality, soybean, oat, and cashew nut beverages were hypotonic (<270 mOsm/kg), while rice and spelt grain were isotonic (270–330 mOsm/kg), supporting different uses in hydration-oriented formulations.

5.2.1 Nutritional profile of plant-based beverages

Cow's milk and dairy products play a fundamental global role in the economy and human nutrition, mainly because they are a source of calcium, proteins, fats, and other nutrients (Cimmino et al., 2023) (Table 5.1).

Milk and some dairy drinks with simpler formulations contain a nutritional profile that can meet basic nutritional needs (Fructuoso et al., 2021). Depending on the raw material used and the technological processes applied, dairy drinks generally tend to present notable differences in their nutritional profile, directly impacting consumer choice and nutritional recommendations (Mańkiewicz-Żurawska et al., 2023).

Protein content varies significantly between milk and dairy products. Greek yogurts and cereal-enriched dairy beverages stand out due to their higher protein and fiber content (Mańkiewicz-Żurawska et al., 2023). This occurs because it reflects the combination of the protein fraction of milk, associated with the presence of plant proteins. The milk and cereal-based beverage (sorghum) stood out the most (5.17 g/100g), followed by the Greek yogurt formulation. This result was already expected (3.30 g/100g), since the desiccation process used in Greek yogurt production is responsible for increased protein retention (Mańkiewicz-Żurawska et al., 2023). Meanwhile, fermented beverages, pure milk, and fruit-flavored yogurts (except Greek yogurt) showed less variation in protein content,

Table 5.1 Nutritional profile of Popular dairy foods.

Beverages	Carbohydrate (g/100g)	Lipids (g/100g)	Protein (g/100g)	Dietary fiber (g/100g)	Energy (g/100g)	References
Natural yogurt	16.69	3.90	2.58	[a]	112.14	Nole-Jaramillo et al. (2024)
Cow's milk	5.03	3.54	3.26	[b]	215	Walther et al. (2022)
	4.4-5.6	3.3-5.4	3.3-3.9	[c]	270.9	Xie et al. (2025)
	4.78	3.76	3.37	[d]	206	Fructuoso et al. (2021)
Greek plain yogurt	4.40	10.0	3.30	[e]	121.0	Mańkiewicz-Żurawska et al. (2023)
Strawberry yogurt	12.0	2.70	3.50	0.02	90.0	
Smoothie made with milk and cereals	45.27	2.11	5.17	5.46	220.77	Rekha et al. (2024)

[a] *Unevaluated values.*
[b] *Unevaluated values.*
[c] *Unevaluated values.*
[d] *Unevaluated values.*
[e] *Unevaluated values.*

suggesting that some fermentation processes have little effect on protein concentration (Walther et al., 2022).

Carbohydrate content varied widely across dairy products. The milk and sorghum-based beverage presented 45.27 g/100 g, justified by the presence of starch and fibrous contents in its composition, in addition to the milk fraction. This demonstrates that the pulp or sugar addition during formulation and processing also directly influences the increase in carbohydrate content (Mańkiewicz-Żurawska et al., 2023). Another formulation to be highlighted is natural Greek yogurt. After the desiccation process, lactose (primarily found in whey) and other carbohydrates have their contents reduced (Nole-Jaramillo et al., 2024).

Meanwhile, dairy products' low (or absent) dietary fiber content is expected. Because they are derived from plants, unless added as a specific ingredient (Rekha et al., 2024), such as cereal beverages (5.46 g/100 g), conventional dairy formulations do not demonstrate dietary fiber values that are important for human health. Regarding energy value, milk has a higher caloric content (270.9 kcal/100 g), mainly due to its fat content (Xie et al., 2025). Beverages enriched with cereals also tend to have higher energy values due to the carbohydrate content present (Rekha et al., 2024).

The nutritional profile of plant-based beverages is highly variable, especially depending on the type of main ingredient used in their production. Many plant-based beverage formulations have low-calorie and saturated-fat content, considerable fiber, and a wide range of protein content (Grau-Fuentes et al., 2023). As the market evolves, it is important to monitor the nutritional profiles of these beverages, as consumers tend to associate higher-calorie products with less healthy options. Compared with cow's milk, plant-based beverages can be sources of bioactive compounds, proteins, dietary fiber, essential vitamins, and minerals, which directly influence consumer choice (Acquah et al., 2023). Another relevant factor is the dietary energy provided, which may be higher or lower depending on the raw material used and the added ingredients.

As stated earlier, cow's milk is rich in carbohydrates, especially lactose, which contributes to vitamin D and calcium absorption, and is a good source of saturated fats and calcium. However, plant-based beverages can be enriched with calcium carbonate (Craig & Fresán, 2021) and, unlike cow's milk, may have higher levels of micronutrients such as (0,35 mg) (de Oliveira et al., 2024) and varying amounts of magnesium (270–280 mg/100g), potassium (733-1797), sodium (39,85 mg/100g), and zinc (0,45 mg/100g) (Xie et al., 2023). Plant-based beverages rich in dietary fiber have gained prominence, mainly due to their prebiotic action, helping to promote satiety and control appetite, regulate blood glucose levels, prevent glycemic spikes, and reduce LDL-c (Wang et al., 2022).

Many plant-based beverages undergo a fortification process to match the calcium content found in cow's milk (de Oliveira et al., 2024; Roberts & Flaherman, 2022; Silva et al., 2020). When compared to cow's milk, plant-based beverages (except coconut milk) have a lower energy density (140–150 kcal) (Craig & Fresán, 2021), largely due to the lower amount of sugars (especially the absence of lactose), higher fiber content (1–2g/100 g), and predominantly unsaturated lipid composition such as oleic acid (C18:1n-9), linoleic acid (C18:2n-6), and α-linolenic acid (C18:3n-3) (Sharma et al., 2024; Xie et al., 2023). However, (Fructuoso et al., 2021), observed that approximately 27.87% of the plant-based beverage formulations analyzed had a glycemic index similar to cow's milk. This factor is influenced by adding different types of sugars, and beverages predominantly composed of starch, rich in glucose, tend to have a higher glycemic index (Shkembi & Huppertz, 2023).

Protein is the macronutrient that stands out most in plant-based beverages, especially because sources such as soy and peas have protein levels similar to those of cow's milk (3,1 g/100g and 3.3 g/100g to soy and peas, respectively) (Craig & Fresán, 2021; Sharma et al., 2024) Protein sources with a balanced amino acid profile (with high levels of essential amino acids) are classified as proteins with a more balanced amino acid pattern (Liu et al., 2019). The main sources of plant-based proteins include oilseeds, legumes, nuts, and cereals. However, green leaves, such as spinach and kale, should also be mentioned (Tan et al., 2023). Each plant-based protein has unique characteristics; most contain high level of lean protein (Matos et al., 2024). The Digestible Indispensable Amino Acid Score (DIAAS parameter) recommended by FAO (2013) is the most appropriate measure to characterize food as a "source", "high in protein", or "good", as it uses the real digestibility content of essential amino acids in the diet.

Lipids are another important component of cow's milk. Predominantly composed of tri-acylglycerols and saturated fats such as palmitic and stearic acids (27%,9% e 12,2%, respectively), as well as complex fatty acids and some fat-soluble vitamins (Gómez-Cortés et al., 2018). Milk fats are considered natural and almost exclusive sources of fatty acids, essential as nutrients and energy sources (Cimmino et al., 2023). In contrast, plant-based beverages exhibit diverse lipid profiles and, unlike cow's milk, do not contain cholesterol, which makes them attractive to consumers seeking to avoid their consumption (Matos et al., 2024). Although plant-based beverages are often formulated to meet specific nutritional requirements, their lipid composition cannot be overlooked. Lipids play a crucial role in the sensory and technological properties of these products. From a sensory perspective, lipids contribute to texture, creaminess, and mouthfeel, enhancing the overall consumer experience. Technologically, they influence product stability, affecting phase separation, emulsification, and shelf life. Therefore, even though the primary focus of these beverages may be on protein content and other nutrients, the presence and quality of lipids must be carefully considered to ensure a well-balanced and high-quality final product (Chalupa-Krebzdak et al., 2018; Silva et al., 2024).

Dietary fibers are crucial to the composition of plant-based beverages, influencing their nutritional value and technological properties. Plant-based beverages often contain significant fiber derived from raw materials such as cereals, legumes, and oilseeds (0.4–5.5 g/200 mL portion) (Frühauf et al., 2023). From a nutritional perspective, fibers support digestive health, modulate the microbiota, and reduce the glycemic index, making these beverages a functional alternative to traditional dairy products. Technologically, fibers impact viscosity, colloidal stability, and mouthfeel, helping to prevent solid sedimentation and improve overall texture. Incorporating and adjusting fiber type and quantity are essential strategies for developing customized plant-based beverages, ensuring well-balanced and consumer-attractive products (Fructuoso et al., 2021; Hidalgo-Fuentes et al., 2024; Xie et al., 2023).

The analyzed beverages, derived from different matrices such as soy, nuts, seeds, grains, and vegetables, showed significant variation in their nutritional profiles. The energy value ranged from 6 to 183 Kcal/100 mL, while the macronutrient and micronutrient contents also showed significant discrepancies, such as protein from 0 to 12.43 g/100 mL and calcium from 0 to 1252.94 mg/100 mL. More than half of the beverages were fortified with calcium, reaching levels equal to or higher than cow's milk, although fortification with vitamins D and B12 was considered insufficient. These beverages generally had low sodium, saturated fat, and calories. However, their nutritional characteristics vary significantly across types, reinforcing the importance of paying attention when replacing cow's milk with these alternatives and informing consumers about their benefits and limitations (Craig & Fresán, 2021; Fructuoso et al., 2021).

Bioactive compounds in plant-based beverages are often analyzed due to their potential health benefits. These compounds, including phytosterols, polyphenols, flavonoids, and others, exhibit antioxidant, anti-inflammatory, and cardioprotective activities and can reduce oxidative stress and modulate the gut microbiota. The composition and concentration of these bioactive compounds vary depending on the source of raw materials used, making their monitoring essential to ensure the functionality and added value of these beverages (Criste et al., 2023; Jiang et al., 2020; Xie et al., 2023).

A full consideration of the components present in plant-based beverages is indispensable for defining practical processing approaches, minimizing undesirable degradation, and ensuring the final product's quality. The beverage's composition—including proteins, lipids, carbohydrates, fibers, and bioactive compounds—directly influences its stability, rheological properties, and sensory acceptability, and an also the best type of processing step for that product (Silva et al., 2024; Xie et al., 2023).

5.2.2 Sensory aspects of plant-based beverages

The application of technological treatments (whether basic processes, such as pasteurization, or more elaborate processes, such as ohmic heating) directly affects the sensory aspects of milk and its derived beverages (Liu et al., 2025). (Table 5.2) presents a sensory comparison of cow's milk and dairy products.

Table 5.2 Sensory comparison of milk and dairy products ↑ indicates an increase and ↓ a decrease in the value of the hedonic scale.

Beverage	Methods		References
	No. treatment	Treatment	
Fermented dairy beverage made from goat's milk	↑ color (7%) and texture (5,57%); ↓ aroma (5,71%)	Thermal: ↑ aroma (5,86%); ↓ color (6,57%) and texture (5,29%)	Mishra, Machireddy, and Vuppu (2024)
Whey and grape juice beverage processed by supercritical carbon dioxide technology	↓ viscosity (2,9%), texture (6,35%), aroma and flavor (6,15% each)	Thermal-chemical: ↑ viscosity (3,0%), texture (6,78%), and aroma and flavor (6,33% each)	Amaral et al. (2018)
Vanilla flavored protein milk drink	↑ color intensity (4,5%); ↓ aroma intensity (3,5%)	Thermal: ↑ aroma intensity (4,1%) and viscosity (5,53%) ↓ color intensity (2,9%);	Liu et al. (2025)
Yogurt fortified with microencapsulated iron	↑ texture (7,40%) and color (7,33%)	Chemical: ↓Texture (7,2%) and color (6,5%)	Nole-Jaramillo et al. (2024)
Smoothie made with milk and cereals	↑ color (7,93%) and flavor (7,79)	Thermal: ↓ color (7,79%), flavor (7,61%), and Sweetness(7,57%)	Rekha et al. (2024)

Sensory attributes (color, texture, aroma, flavor, and sweetness) are fundamental to consumer acceptance, as they directly influence the product quality (Amaral et al., 2018). Fermented dairy beverage made from goat's milk showed improvement in color, but loss of texture and aroma after fermentation, while Yogurt fortified with microencapsulated iron showed slight loss of texture, compensated by stability of color and aroma (Ranadheera et al., 2016). Meanwhile, the increase in color intensity and the reduction in texture and aroma stand out, suggesting that, although the treatment improved the visual aspect of the Whey and grape juice beverage processed by supercritical carbon dioxide technology, there was an interference in the freshness and creaminess of the beverages (Amaral et al., 2018). Thus, although it is not surprising, it seems that different technological treatments directly affect sensory attributes (Nole-Jaramillo et al., 2024); it is always necessary to evaluate the balance between gains and losses to ensure a good final product.

Sensory attributes are crucial in determining consumer acceptance and preference for a given product. Among these attributes, color is one of the most decisive factors in initial perception, as it shapes expectations for flavor, freshness, and overall quality. A visually appealing product is more likely to attract consumers and influence their purchasing decisions. Beyond color, other sensory aspects such as aroma, texture, and taste also contribute significantly to the overall acceptability of plant-based beverages, reinforcing the importance of a well-balanced formulation to meet consumer expectations (Spence, 2015; Egea, Dantas, et al., 2023).

Color is a crucial sensory attribute for consumer acceptance. Natural pigments, derived from fruits, vegetables, and some microorganisms, can add nutritional value to beverages and act as an alternative to synthetic pigments (Martins et al., 2024).

Plant pigments can be classified into four main categories: chlorophyll, carotenoids, flavonoids, and betalains (Pailliè-Jiménez et al., 2020). Many fruits contain small levels of these pigments and other macronutrients such as proteins, fibers, and lipids (Kamalesh et al., 2025). These pigments have structures called chromophores, which are responsible for their characteristic properties and colors. Chromophores capture light energy and promote the excitation of electrons to higher-energy orbitals. The unabsorbed energy is reflected as visible light, conferring coloration that is perceptible to the human eye (Rodríguez-Mena et al., 2023).

Natural pigments such as carotenoids and anthocyanins are important in plant-based beverages, providing color and significant functional properties including antioxidant, antimicrobial, and anti-inflammatory activities (Brauch, 2016). These compounds have been associated with reduced cardiovascular disease risk, neuroprotective effects, and a stronger immune system. Unlike synthetic pigments, which are cost-effective but pose potential health risks, natural pigments stand out as a healthier option, offering functional benefits while avoiding adverse side effects (Dey & Nagababu, 2022).

In the study by Frühauf et al. (2023), the soy drink presented the highest color saturation value ($C^* = 12.64$), associated with a yellowish hue ($h° = 87.86$ degrees). It was considered to have an "adequate" or "above ideal" color by 81% of the evaluators, contributing to its high acceptability index. The oat drink, with values of $C^* = 6.95$ and $h° = 94.21$ degrees, was also visually well evaluated by 69% of the participants, reinforcing the preference for warmer and more saturated hues. On the other hand, the cashew drink presented the lowest saturation value ($C^* = 4.69$) and the smallest hue angle ($h° = 80.21$ degrees), being perceived as less visually attractive, which may have contributed to its low acceptance (33.61%). These data show that more intense colors, especially those closer to yellowish tones, tend to be associated with greater freshness, flavor, and quality, and are decisive in consumers' choice of plant-based beverages.

Furthermore, beverages with flocculation or suspended particles — such as those made from spelt and cashew nuts — were perceived as less attractive, regardless of flavor. These data show that a clean, stable visual appearance with attractive color is crucial for consumer acceptance and is a determining factor in purchasing plant-based beverages (Frühauf et al., 2023).

With the advancement of microbiological technologies, the production of natural pigments by microorganisms has become a viable alternative, offering high stability, low cost, and greater resistance to adverse environmental conditions (Pintos et al., 2022; Ramesh et al., 2019). Applying techniques such as encapsulation has proven effective in protecting these pigments against degradation by light, oxygen, and heat, thereby preserving their properties and enhancing the beverage's visual appeal. In this way, natural pigments not only contribute to the appearance of beverages but also enhance their nutritional benefits, reinforcing the importance of their inclusion in plant-based formulations (Martins et al., 2024; Mkhari et al., 2023).

Although the plant-based beverage market has grown, concerns about flavor and unfamiliarity with taste are still determining factors in replacing conventional milk with plant-based beverages (Giacalone et al., 2022). Unlike other sensory characteristics, flavor remains one of the main challenges in processing plant-based beverages.

Ultra High Temperature (UHT) treatment is widely used in the processing of plant-based beverages, from the pre-processing of raw materials (such as pulps and purees) to the final product (such as juices). This technique primarily aims to eliminate pathogenic and spoilage microorganisms present food (Matos et al., 2024). However, the applied heat can change the conformation of proteins, carbohydrates, and lipids, directly affecting the product's stability, flavor, and nutritional value (Linhares et al., 2020). Therefore, authors such as (Alves Filho et al., 2018; de Castro et al., 2020; Oliveira et al., 2018) advocate the use of non-thermal technologies, which can result in an increase in the content of bioactive compounds, greater inactivation of enzymes and harmful microorganisms, in addition to minimizing the adverse effects on the food structural matrix.

Some acids found naturally in foods, such as citric acid, malic acid, tartaric acid, and oxalic acid, can be used as preservatives. These acids play crucial roles, such as reducing pH, inhibiting microbiological growth, and preventing oxidative reactions (Fernandes et al., 2025). However, technologies such as exposure to heat or adding chemical preservatives can cause sensory and/or nutritional losses to foods (de Castro et al., 2020) due to the acids' degradation. Alternatives such as controlling excessive temperatures, protecting against the action of oxygen, maintaining pH, and adequate storage can be effective in preserving the functionality of natural acids, ensuring the quality and safety of beverages (Badejo et al., 2020).

Nutritional imbalance is another factor that impacts the acceptance of new plant-based beverage formulations. Although high protein levels can be a differentiator for many plant-based beverages (Fernandes et al., 2025), an imbalance in protein quality and quantity can result in a bitter, earthy, bean-like flavor, which reduces the products's sensory acceptanc (Ramesh et al., 2022, pp. 91–106). These effects can be mitigated through technological processes such as fermentation (Agarbati et al., 2024) and hydrolysis (Islam et al., 2023), which help to reduce anti-nutritional compounds and improve aftertaste.

Texture and viscosity are essential to consumer acceptance of plant-based beverages, as they directly impact the sensory experience. To increase viscosity and improve the body of the beverage while also reducing the perception of the presence of particles, many of these beverages use stabilizers and thickeners, such as guar gum and xanthan gum, or natural pulps to adjust the density and improve homogeneity (Frühauf et al., 2023; Silva et al., 2021). However, increasing viscosity must be balanced, as an excessively thick beverage can be unpleasant to the palate, especially when consumed cold.

Frühauf et al. (2023) related that the texture, assessed mainly by viscosity, is one of the main determinants of sensory quality in plant-based beverages. Instrumental viscosity, measured in mPa s, varied significantly between samples, directly reflecting consumer perceptions. The oat beverage had the highest viscosity (16.8 mPa s^{-1}), was perceived as creamier, and received a positive sensory evaluation from 65% of participants in the "just-about-right" (JAR) test, who classified it as having an adequate or better-than-ideal texture. The soy beverage, with a viscosity of 11.3 mPa s^{-1}, was also well evaluated, with 81% of consumers considering its texture satisfactory, contributing to its high acceptability index (71.75%). Rice beverage presented the lowest viscosity (5.0 mPa s-1) and was perceived as excessively fluid, which may have impaired its acceptance, despite its physical-chemical stability.

On the other hand (Santos et al., 2019), demonstrated that when the soy beverage was fermented, and the pH decreased, there was a tendency for sensory acceptability to decrease, especially related to appearance, due to phase separation in the beverage. As reported for fermented soymilk, the cashew nut drink, with intermediate viscosity (7.5 mPa s^{-1}), was poorly evaluated sensorially, probably due to the presence of sediments and a feeling of instability (Frühauf et al., 2023).

In addition to influencing viscosity perception, texture also affects flavor. Thicker beverages tend to linger in the mouth, creating a more characteristic sensation, while more fluid beverages have a lighter and faster sensation. Controlling viscosity, combined with techniques such as homogenization, allows you to adjust the sensory properties without compromising the stability or nutritional benefits of the beverages (Egea, Santos, et al., 2023).

Developing the ideal texture for plant-based beverages requires considering the interaction between viscosity, flavor, and other sensory components. Innovation remains key to generating products that meet consumers' expectations while preserving nutritional quality. Appropriate technologies and additives are essential to ensure a product's attractiveness while maintaining the quality of plant-based beverages (Moss et al., 2022; Chalupa-Krebzdak et al., 2018).

5.2.3 Influence of interactions between ingredients in plant-based beverages

The stability and quality of plant-based beverages made from soy, oats, and almonds are influenced by several factors related to the ingredients' physical and chemical properties and the technological processes used. The interactions between their chemical components can directly affect the texture, nutritional value, and shelf life of the products. Combining these materials in beverage formulations requires an in-depth understanding of their interactions. Unconventional technologies, such as ultrasound and high-pressure homogenization, have effectively improved the physical and sensory stability of these products. The addition of additives such as sweeteners and stabilizers can positively influence sensory characteristics as long as they do not compromise nutritional value (Esposito et al., 2024; Fructuoso et al., 2021; Sharma et al., 2024).

Soybeans are widely used for their high protein content (35%–40%) (Qin et al., 2022). Still, the presence of anti-nutritional compounds such as lipoxygenases, phytates, and saponins can interfere with the availability of essential minerals. In addition, compounds such as lecithin can affect glucose absorption and vitamins. Technologies such as ultrasound, pulsed electric field, and high-pressure homogenization can reduce the particle size of soybean extract, promoting greater physical and sensory stability. Oats are valued for their soluble fiber content (8%–40%) (Leszczyńska et al., 2023), especially beta-glucans, which are essential for beverage stability. Still, their high water-binding capacity can influence aerobic stability and the fermentation pattern. Almonds are appreciated for their healthy lipid profile (50% of the kernel weight) (Lacivita et al., 2024). Bioactive compounds such as dietary fibers, hydroxycinnamic, hydroxybenzoic, and phenolic acids, triterpenoids, flavanones, flavonols, and flavanols, depending on the part or variety evaluated (Lacivita et al., 2024). Still, they have a low protein content (2.1%–8.8%) (Lacivita et al., 2024), and contamination with aflatoxins can compromise the quality of beverages, requiring adequate processing to ensure safety and preserve final quality (Butovskaya et al., 2025; Maree et al., 2024).

Based on this, the correct selection and dosage of each raw material used in the formulation of plant-based beverages are essential. This approach helps prevent undesirable reactions between components that could negatively impact the product's sensory and technological properties. At the same time, controlled reactions can be strategically induced to enhance the mixture's color, flavor, and overall stability. The proper formulation ensures not only consumer acceptance but also the physicochemical integrity of the beverage, contributing to a more appealing and high-quality final product (Silva et al., 2024).

5.3 Microbiological characteristics of plant-based beverages

The microbiological characteristics of plant-based beverages are crucial in determining their quality, safety, and overall shelf life. The native microbiota, which includes naturally occurring microorganisms such as bacteria, yeasts, and molds, plays a significant role in fermentation and spoilage processes. These microorganisms can have beneficial effects, contributing to developing desirable flavors, textures, and potential health benefits, particularly through probiotic activity. However, plant-based beverages' microbiological quality and safety must be carefully managed to prevent contamination by pathogenic organisms, resulting in significant health risks. Effective monitoring techniques are essential to ensure that plant-based beverages remain environmentally safe, meet regulatory standards, and deliver high-quality products to consumers.

5.3.1 Native microbiota of plant-based beverages

The native microbiota present in plant-based beverages plays a very important role in ensuring microbiological stability, sensory quality, and shelf life. Recent studies have shown that these microorganisms can have beneficial or harmful effects, depending on processing conditions and product composition (Canaviri-Paz et al., 2021). During fermentation, the native microbiota contributes positively, highlighting sensory attributes such as flavor and texture. In this context, *Lactobacillus* species are particularly important for their ability to produce lactic acid, which reduces pH and inhibits spoilage organisms (Leeuwendaal et al., 2022). In addition to preserving, certain microbial strains act as probiotics, supporting intestinal health and promoting the formation of bioactive compounds, such as peptides and short-chain fatty acids. These compounds are associated with anti-inflammatory properties and improved nutrient absorption (Afzaal et al., 2022).

However, not all native microorganisms are beneficial. Some can be pathogenic and pose health risks. Pathogenic microorganisms have been identified in commercial juices, highlighting the importance of rigorous microbiological monitoring during processing (Lin et al., 2023; da Cunha Júnior et al., 2021). In addition, spoilage-related bacteria, such as *Alicyclobacillus*, can produce undesirable off-flavors and odors in fruit-based beverages (Nesterova et al., 2024). To maximize the positive impact of beneficial microbiota while minimizing contamination risks, approaches such as the use of well-characterized starter cultures and biopreservation techniques have been proposed. These techniques improve product stability while preserving its sensorial qualities (Udayakumar et al., 2022). Furthermore, metagenomic tools have enabled a more comprehensive understanding of microbial communities, thereby improving fermentation and product safety (Villarreal-Morales et al., 2018). Thus, understanding the native microbiota is essential for developing safe and high-quality plant-based beverages (Aleman et al., 2024).

5.3.2 Microbiological quality and safety of plant-based beverages

The microbiological quality of plant-based beverages is essential for product safety and commercial viability. Contamination by bacteria, yeasts, and fungi can negatively impact product stability, pose public health risks, and affect consumer confidence in products (Bartula et al., 2023; Hernández et al., 2018). Among foodborne pathogens, for example, *Listeria monocytogenes* can cause serious disease, particularly in vulnerable populations, reinforcing the importance of continuous monitoring (de Abreu Costa et al., 2022).

Microbiological control is based on a combination of classical and modern techniques. Traditional methods include cultivation in selective media and biochemical tests. Selective culture media allow quantification and identification of viable microorganisms, while biochemical assays assist in the differentiation of species based on metabolic activities (Arbefeville et al., 2024; Mishra, Aravind, et al., 2024).

Molecular techniques such as the polymerase chain reaction (PCR) are widely used for their specificity and sensitivity, allowing the detection of pathogens even at low concentrations (LCDL, 1991). Other approaches, such as flow cytometry and real-time monitoring systems, have been increasingly incorporated into quality control programs, allowing for faster detection and intervention (Gombas et al., 2017; He et al., 2020).

Broadly speaking, rigorous microbiological control strategies are essential to ensure that plant-based beverages meet safety standards and maintain product quality during storage and distribution.

(Table 5.3)

However, microbiological control of plant-based beverages faces considerable challenges. The diversity of raw materials, such as soybeans, oats, and almonds, can introduce a variety of microorganisms, making their detection and control difficult (Gützkow et al., 2024). In addition, post-processing contamination, resulting from inadequate equipment cleaning practices or the survival of bacterial spores, is a constant risk. Environmental factors like high humidity and temperature also favor microbial growth. An integrated approach combines physical methods, such as pasteurization, to address these challenges, and natural and artificial preservatives (Aadil et al., 2019, pp. 1–38). Continuous monitoring and using advanced technologies will ensure the production of safe plant-based beverages, comply with regulatory standards, and meet consumer expectations (Manju and

Table 5.3 Methods for monitoring microbiological quality in plant-based beverages.

Method	Description	References
Culture in culture media	Used to identify and quantify microorganisms, essential in fermented plant-based and dairy products to ensure quality and safety.	Mishra, Machireddy, and Vuppu (2024)
Biochemical tests	They detect microorganisms based on their metabolic activities, allowing differentiation of bacterial species and ensuring accurate identification in fermented products.	Arbefeville et al. (2024)
PCR (polymerase chain reaction)	Molecular technique that allows rapid and accurate detection of pathogens, even in tiny quantities. It is frequently used in diagnostics due to its high sensitivity and specificity, facilitating the identification of pathogens in food.	LCDL (1991)
Flow cytometry and real-time monitoring	Advanced technologies that allow real-time detection and quantification of microorganisms in food products, such as plant-based and fermented beverages, ensure their quality and safety. Techniques like nano-flow cytometry facilitate rapid bacterial analysis and continuous contamination monitoring.	Gombas et al. (2017), He et al. (2020)

Mishra, 2021). Technological evolution will be essential to overcome emerging challenges in microbiological management, ensuring high-quality products with a longer shelf life.

5.4 Preservation strategies for plant-based beverages

Among the techniques used in preserving plant-based beverages are thermal and non-thermal (Fig. 5.2). Using heat to produce plant-based beverages can cause the transformation of proteins, carbohydrates, and lipids, and significant changes in characteristics, such as viscosity, separation stability, flavor, and nutritional value (Matos et al., 2024). While non-thermal options are promising for producing enzymatically safe beverages with reduced quality loss, thermal options cause damage to various nutritional and sensorial properties (Krishnan Kesavan et al., 2023).

Table 5.4. presents beverage preservation techniques with their strategic conservation action and application examples.

5.4.1 Thermal techniques

5.4.1.1 Pasteurization

Pasteurization aims to extend the shelf life of products by reducing microorganisms and inactivating enzymes such as polyphenol oxidase and peroxidase, which can cause sensory and nutritional changes (Alim et al., 2023; Zou et al., 2024). The temperature can vary from 71 to 100°C for a period of 30–460 s, depending on the type of beverage (Bonilla et al., 2024; Krishnan Kesavan et al., 2023; Negri Rodríguez et al., 2021; Zou et al., 2024).

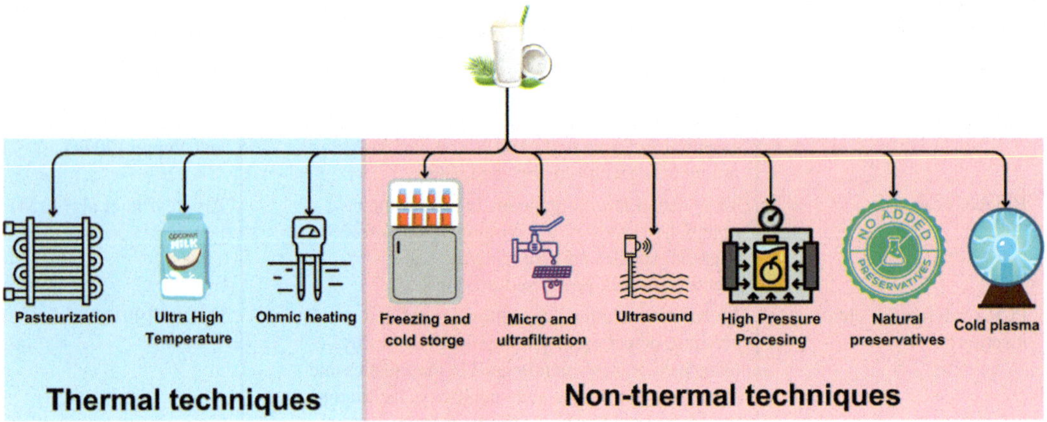

FIGURE 5.2

Thermal and non-thermal techniques used in the preservation of plant-based beverages.

This is one of the most widely techniques (de Paiva et al., 2024). developed a concentrated "Detox" beverage using pineapple, kale, mint, spinach, lemon, psyllium, and spirulina. The authors evaluated the influence of the pasteurization process on the beverage, considering the physicochemical, bioactive, and antioxidant characteristics, stability, and bioaccessibility of the minerals present. Despite the heat treatment, the developed beverage maintained a high antioxidant capacity without changing the color and pH (Bonilla et al., 2024). found that pasteurization (71.1°C for 3 s) allowed greater retention of bioactive compounds and had a more minor impact on the physicochemical properties of a blackberry-soybean-linseed beverage compared to the commercial sterilization process (heating to 87°C followed by immediate hot filling).

Disadvantages such as possible changes in flavor and aroma, loss of nutrients, and changes in texture and color mean that pasteurization must be replaced or associated with another conservation technique. The use of microwave-assisted thermal pasteurization has been studied as a strategy with a lower impact on bioactive compounds (Amaro & Tadini, 2021; Oishi et al., 2022; Kaiky Cesar Amaro & Tadini, 2024; Amaro & Tadini, 2021). Inhibition of pectin methylesterase activity and improved retention of ascorbic acid content is achieved using microwave heating. Furthermore, microwave-assisted pasteurization conditions at 90 and 100°C and holding times between 2 and 10 s in orange juice provide >98% inactivation of pectin methylesterase with minimal impact on vitamin C retention (Kaiky Cesar Amaro & Tadini, 2024).

5.4.1.2 Ultra High Temperature (UHT)

The relatively low temperature of pasteurization does not eliminate all microorganisms present in beverages, so the search for strategies using higher temperatures is being investigated. However, higher temperatures (135–150°C) for short periods (1–10 s) can cause damage, such as loss of nutrients and flavors, protein denaturation, and changes in texture (Matos et al., 2024; Zhang et al., 2024).

Although some adverse effects may occur, Ultra High Temperature (UHT) is a fast and efficient method for producing plant-based beverages, offering numerous benefits to both the food industry and

Table 5.4 Beverage preservation techniques.

Techniques		Definition	Example	Main results	References
Thermal	Pasteurization	Heat the beverage to moderate temperatures to eliminate pathogenic microorganisms	Blackberry-soy-flaxseed beverage	↑retention of bioactive compounds; and ↓ impact on physicochemical properties	Bonilla et al. (2024)
			Orange juice	↓ ascorbic acid, carotenoid and phenolic; and ↓ *E. coli*	Ambreen et al. (2023)
	Ultra high temperature (UHT)	Heating at very high temperatures for just a few seconds, ensuring greater conservation	Lettuce juice	↓ color, chlorophyll, total soluble solids, and vitamins	Zhang et al. (2024)
			Faba bean drink	↑ creaming index and levels of acetic acid; and ↓ volatile profiling	Nawaz et al. (2021)
	Ohmic heating	Using electric current to heat the beverage, reducing thermal damage evenly	Mandarin juice	↓ luminosity and microbial counts; and ↑ enzyme inactivation and loss in total phenolics	(Basak et al., 2025)
			Aguamiel	↓ darkening due to caramelization of sugars	Rascón et al. (2020)
Non-thermal	Freezing and cold storage	Storing beverages at low temperatures, reducing or inhibiting the growth of microorganisms	Apple, orange and pineapple fruit juice	Consumption <2 weeks, as after this period it loses its stability to retain bioactive and antioxidant compounds	Alim et al. (2023)
			Coconut water	↑ total phenolic content, antioxidant activity, total dissolved solids, and potassium	(Pandey et al., 2024)
	Microfiltration and ultrafiltration	Removes microorganisms and other components without altering the	Kombucha	↓ flow over time at each pressure; and ultrafiltration membrane was more stable	Daneluz et al. (2023)

Continued

Table 5.4 Beverage preservation techniques.—cont'd

Techniques		Definition	Example	Main results	References
		characteristics of the product	Cashew apple juice	↓ turbidity, microorganisms and suspended solids; and ↑ sensory and nutritional perfil	Abdullah et al. (2023)
	Ultrasound	Using sound waves to inactivate microorganisms	Kutkura juices	↓ microbial counts; and ↑ retention of ascorbic acid, flavonoid, phenolic and antioxidant activity	Krishnan Kesavan et al. (2023)
			Kiwi juice	↑ reductions in *L. innocua*, soluble solids, total phenolics and chlorophylls	Bhutkar et al. (2024)
	High pressure processing	Application of high pressure to inactivate microorganisms, preserving flavor and nutrients	Lettuce juice	↑ color, chlorophyll, total soluble solids, and vitamins	Zhang et al. (2024)
			Jabuticaba juice	↑ antioxidant capacities, total phenolic, flavonoid, and monomeric anthocyanin content; and ↓ browning degrees	Hu et al. (2020)
	Natural preservatives	Addition of natural antimicrobial compounds, which help prevent the growth of microorganisms without the use of synthetic preservatives	Apple juice	↓ number *E. coli*, *S. aureus* and *C. albicans* using the essential oils of *Mentha virdis*, *Mentha longifolia* and *limonene*	El-Kased and El-Kersh (2022)
			Sugarcane juice	↑ polyphenoloxidase inactivation and sensory perfil with lemongrass essential oil	Bag et al. (2022)

Table 5.4 Beverage preservation techniques.—cont'd

Techniques		Definition	Example	Main results	References
	Cold plasma	Use of low-temperature ionized gas to eliminate microorganisms and prolong conservation, without affecting the chemical composition	Tomato-based beverage	↑ color, retention of ascorbic acid and phenolic content; and ↓ microbial counts	Mehta et al. (2019)
			Tomato juice	↓ lactic acid bacteria, coliform bacteria, and yeast below the limit of quantification	Starek et al. (2020)
	UV-radiation	Use of electromagnetic radiation to damage the genetic material of bacteria, viruses and yeasts, without significantly heating the product	Cold brew coffee	↑ in 7 days in useful life, total polyphenols, and concentration of non-volatile compounds	Orjuela et al. (2025)
			Coconut water	↑ in 12 days in useful life and b* chroma; and ↓ luminosity	Ceballos et al. (2025)

consumers. The combination of high temperature and low time, followed by rapid cooling, must be controlled to ensure efficient sterilization (Matos et al., 2024; Zhang et al., 2024) compared UHT (115°C/5 s) and pasteurization (95°C/60 s) of lettuce juice and found that the parameters of color, total soluble solids content, pH, total aerobic bacteria, yeasts, and fungi did not present significant differences between the two treatments. However, the content of chlorophyll *a* and some vitamins (E, K, and B3) was higher in the UHT treatment.

The plant-based beverage matrix influences the effects caused by UHT treatment (Deng et al., 2024). found that UHT can maintain coconut milk's original aroma and nutritional value. However (Tao et al., 2025), verified the loss of aroma of green tea beverages, with the presence of malty (e.g., 3-methyl butanal), floral (e.g., linalool), sweet (e.g., methional), and smoky (2-methoxy-4-vinylphenol) compounds, contributing to the development of a cooked aftertaste.

5.4.1.3 Ohmic heating

Ohmic heating is an advanced thermal processing technology that has gained attention for its potential application in plant-based beverage treatment. Compared to conventional heating techniques, ohmic heating minimizes thermal degradation, preserving bioactive compounds, vitamins, and sensory attributes such as color and flavor (Ramaswamy et al., 2014, pp. 1–495; Sain et al., 2024; Shimoyamada et al., 2015).

This method uses electrical resistance to generate heat within the product, ensuring rapid and uniform temperature distribution. Additionally, it can improve microbial safety while maintaining the physicochemical stability of the beverage. Due to its efficiency and ability to enhance product quality, ohmic heating represents a promising alternative for the sustainable processing of plant-based beverages (dos Santos et al., 2024; Rascón et al., 2020; Shimoyamada et al., 2015).

This treatment allows microbiologically stable beverages for 60 days, in addition to increasing the total antioxidant capacity, a high level of acceptance among consumers, with a greater preference for color, compared to pasteurization (Rodríguez-Mena et al., 2023).

Key parameters in the application of ohmic heating for plant-based beverages include electrical conductivity —ensuring uniform heating and requiring adjustments—, and processing temperature and time. The time x temperature binomial here has the same importance as it does in other processes in the food industry: ensuring microbial inactivation with the preservation of quality attributes. Optimizing process characteristics such as voltage and frequency and beverage characteristics such as viscosity and particle size distribution are essential to achieve uniform heating, product safety, and sensory appeal. Proper control of these factors ensures the effectiveness and quality of the process (dos Santos et al., 2024; Kamonpatana et al., 2022).

5.4.2 Non-thermal techniques

5.4.2.1 Freezing and cold storage

The storage method in the refrigerator at 4°C or frozen at −10 to −20°C is the most widely used by consumers. However, low temperatures and storage conditions can cause significant changes in the physical-chemical appearance and decrease the total phytochemical content, consequently affecting antioxidant activities (Mohamad Salin et al., 2022).

Alim et al. (2023) found that fruit juices should not be stored for more than 14 days at 4°C in refrigerated conditions and that after 7 days, they already showed a significant loss of bioactivity. Furthermore, the authors found a reduction in the content of total phenolic compounds, which was attributed to the loss of fluid from fruit juices during storage in the refrigerator, causing dehydration and loss of nutrients.

Mohamad Salin et al. (2022) studied the storage of watermelon juice at room temperature (25°C), refrigerator cold (4°C), refrigerator freeze (−8°C), and freeze at −80°C. The authors found that the best storage was frozen in the refrigerator, followed by cold in the refrigerator, and at room temperature. Freezing provided less darkening of the juices, less degradation of total phenolic compounds, and greater antioxidant capacity during storage for 7 days.

Some authors suggest combining cold storage with other treatments, such as a magnetic field (Zhao et al., 2024) and ultraviolet radiation (Ceballos et al., 2025). This strategy offers advantages regarding food safety, nutritional, and sensory quality. Each of these technologies has a specific impact on the preservation process, and when combined, they can enhance the beneficial effects of beverage preservation.

5.4.2.2 Microfiltration and ultrafiltration

Membrane filtration allows clarification and microbial stabilization in a single step. Based on the membrane porosity, there are microfiltration (0.1–10 μm) and ultrafiltration (1–100 nm). Microfiltration is widely used to sterilize beverages, clarify wines and beers, and concentrate some components. Ultrafiltration is used for protein fractionation and concentration, clarification of beverages, filtration of juices, and oil recovery (Daneluz et al., 2023). What often ends up makes membrane filtration unfeasible are the relatively high investment costs and the phenomenon of concentration polarization (Sarbatly et al., 2023; Urošević et al., 2017).

These techniques effectively remove suspended solids, microorganisms, and undesirable macromolecules, improving clarity, extending shelf life, and preserving nutritional and sensory attributes. For instance, a study on lemon juice functional beverages demonstrated that microfiltration and ultrafiltration significantly influenced parameters such as vitamin C content, antioxidant activity, pH, viscosity, and color, with microfiltration yielding higher retention of these qualities than reverse osmosis (Ikrawan et al., 2024). Additionally, research on apple juice processing revealed that ultrafiltration, especially when combined with high-pressure processing, effectively reduced the microbial load while maintaining the juice's sensory and nutritional properties (Zhao et al., 2014). These findings underscore the importance of selecting appropriate membrane filtration methods to achieve desired quality characteristics in plant-based beverages.

5.4.2.3 Ultrasound

Ultrasound technology is based on physical phenomena that are distinct from those of conventional pasteurization. Food stabilization is achieved through the acoustic cavitation mechanism induced by low-frequency ultrasound. Using ultrasound to preserve plant-based beverages has emerged as an alternative to pasteurization, as it enhances their physical, chemical, and technological characteristics. However, from a sensorial perspective, lighter color, lower fluidity, and the perception of granule formation can negatively affect acceptance (da Silveira Maia et al., 2025).

Ultrasonication can be used in conjunction with other treatments, such as high-temperature (thermosonication), to increase its action against deteriorating agents, where ultrasound alone may not be able to achieve the desired result (Krishnan Kesavan et al., 2023). Krishnan Kesavan et al. (2023) found no significant changes in the physicochemical properties of kutkura juices treated by pasteurization and thermosonication. However, the total phenolic and flavonoid contents were higher in the thermosonicated samples, indicating that increasing the sonication temperature (30, 40, and 50°C) positively affects the bioactive properties.

5.4.2.4 High pressure processing (HPP)

Among non-thermal technologies, high-pressure processing (HPP) is gaining wide industrial acceptance among food processors. This is due to the preservation of functional compounds, such as vitamins, polyphenols, flavonoids, and micronutrients in foods (Ravichandran et al., 2023; Zhang et al., 2024). The pressure varies from 100 to 800 MPa, with water as the transmission medium (Zou et al., 2024).

Plant-based beverages are particularly vulnerable to color degradation caused by microbial fermentation, enzymatic discoloration, and other biochemical changes. HPP has the potential to delay these factors, proving effective in minimizing undesirable color changes and preserving product quality, depending on the characteristics and processing parameters used (Ravichandran et al., 2023; Zhang et al., 2024) confirmed that HPP treatment, compared to pasteurization and UHT, promoted a brighter color; prevented the degradation of vitamins E, B1, B2, B12, and niacin; preserved the chlorophyll concentration; and maintained sensory acceptance in lettuce juices.

Furthermore, HPP can promote the release of volatile compounds, improving the volatile profile of the beverage (Zou et al., 2024). The presence of sugars is vital because they sweeten beverages and release aromas. Optimized sugar levels and pressure during processing help maintain the same aroma release and sweet taste (Ravichandran et al., 2023). However, regarding macronutrients, some disadvantages have been reported for proteins. High pressure can alter protein structure through unfolding, aggregation, gelation, and denaturation. Pressures below 300 MPa cause induced denaturation, and above 300 MPa irreversible denaturation (Ravichandran et al., 2023).

5.4.2.5 Use of natural preservatives

Synthetic preservatives, such as potassium metabisulfite, sodium benzoate, or sodium bicarbonate, are often added to prevent microbial spoilage or retain beverages' optimal sensorial properties. However, these components are expensive and can pose potential health risks if ingestion exceeds a specific concentration or time (Javed et al., 2024; Zahan et al., 2024). Because of this, natural preservatives through extracts or essential oils have been standing out for their bioactivities as antioxidants and antimicrobials (Maleš et al., 2022).

Various extracts and essential oils can be used as additives for preserving plant-based beverages. Some examples of studies found are peppermint essential oil in apple juice (Karaman and Sagdic, 2019); orange and pomegranate peel extracts in a functional beverage (Selahvarzi et al., 2021); thyme extracts (*Thymus vulgaris*), *Mentha virdis*, *Mentha longifolia*, rosemary (*Rosmarinus officinalis*), lavender (*Lavandula dentata*), oregano (*Origanum majorana*), lemongrass (*Cymbopogon citratus*), and *Eucalyptus globulus* in apple juice (El-Kased & El-Kersh, 2022); moringa extract in beverage *Ficus carica* L. (Javed et al., 2024); sappan heartwood extracts in beetroot beverages (Muangrat & Thipsuwan, 2024); and extracts of ginger, hops, tea, and mint in isotonic grape beverage (Bendaali et al., 2024).

The use of natural preservatives in plant-based beverages must consider several factors, including their effectiveness against target microorganisms, compatibility with the beverage matrix, impact on sensory attributes (taste, color, and aroma), stability under processing and storage conditions, regulatory limitations, and consumer acceptance (Novais et al., 2022; Vara et al., 2019).

5.4.2.6 Cold plasma

Cold plasma is an emerging technology for treating fruit and vegetable beverages, which do not need to be pasteurized or thermally sanitized. In addition to improving shelf life, it can also enhance nutritional properties and bioactivity, being advantageous over other preservation methods (Pohl et al., 2022).

Another advantage of using cold plasma is the increase in sensory attributes. (Xu et al., 2024) observed the attributes of coconut water, butter, and popcorn flavors in cold plasma-treated coconut water. Furthermore, cold plasma showed good retention of essential aroma actives (2-acetyl-1-pyrroline and nonanal).

Mehta et al. (2019) developed a tomato-based beverage and investigated the effects of pasteurization, ultrasonication, ultraviolet, and cold plasma. The beverage processed with cold plasma retained the highest ascorbic acid content. Tomato beverages treated with cold plasma for 10 min and ultrasonication for 15 min were equivalent to thermal processing in microbial reduction. In addition, cold plasma for 10 min was equivalent to pasteurization in reducing yeast and mold counts.

5.5 Conclusions and future perspectives

Plant-based beverages have gained significant popularity due to their nutritional benefits and the growing demand for dairy alternatives. Ensuring their stability and quality requires a deep understanding of ingredient interactions and microbiota, and carefully selecting preservation methods. Various preservation methods are suited to different raw materials and the properties that must be maintained during processing and storage. The choice of technique should balance efficiency, product stability, and sustainability. While some methods may require higher energy consumption or additives, growing consumer preference for natural and minimally processed products drives the search for alternative, more sustainable solutions. Research continues to focus on optimizing preservation strategies to reduce environmental impact while ensuring these beverages' sensory and nutritional quality.

Emerging trends indicate a growing interest in more natural and sustainable preservation methods. Research into new techniques that involve less energy consumption and fewer chemical additives aims to meet consumer preferences for more natural alternatives and reduce product (and environmental) impacts. Technologies such as biopreservation, beneficial microbial cultures, and new, more environmentally friendly preservation processes have great potential to shape the future of plant-based beverages. The continued development of these innovations can lead to more efficient and sustainable production, in line with the expectations of conscious consumers and the global market's needs.

Acknowledgments

The authors thank CAPES, CNPq, FAPEG, FAPERJ, FAPERGS, and IF Goiano for their financial support.

References

Aadil, R. M., Madni, G. M., Roobab, U., Ur Rahman, U., & Zeng, X. A. (2019). *Quality control in beverage production: An overview quality control in the beverage industry: Volume 17: The science of beverages*. Pakistan: Elsevier. https://doi.org/10.1016/B978-0-12-816681-9.00001-1

Abdullah, S., Karmakar, S., Mishra, S., & Pradhan, R. C. (2023). Ultrafiltration of cashew Apple juice using hollow fibers for shelf life extension: Process optimization, flux modelling and storage study. *Journal of Food Measurement and Characterization, 17*(3), 2182–2192. https://doi.org/10.1007/s11694-022-01790-8

Acquah, J. B., Amissah, J. G. N., Affrifah, N. S., Wooster, T. J., & Danquah, A. O. (2023). Consumer perceptions of plant based beverages: The Ghanaian consumer's perspective. *Future Foods, 7*. https://doi.org/10.1016/j.fufo.2023.100229

Afzaal, M., Saeed, F., Shah, Y. A., Hussain, M., Rabail, R., Socol, C. T., Hassoun, A., Pateiro, M., Lorenzo, J. M., Rusu, A. V., & Aadil, R. M. (2022). Human gut microbiota in health and disease: Unveiling the relationship. *Frontiers in Microbiology, 13*. https://doi.org/10.3389/fmicb.2022.999001

Agarbati, A., Canonico, L., Ciani, M., Morresi, C., Damiani, E., Bacchetti, T., & Comitini, F. (2024). Functional potential of a new plant-based fermented beverage: Benefits through non-conventional probiotic yeasts and antioxidant properties. *International Journal of Food Microbiology, 424*, Article 110857. https://doi.org/10.1016/j.ijfoodmicro.2024.110857

Aleman, R. S., Montero-Fernández, I., Marcía, J. A., Saravia Maldonado, S. A., & Martín-Vertedor, D. (2024). Application of fermentation as a strategy for the transformation and valorization of vegetable matrices. *Fermentation, 10*(3). https://doi.org/10.3390/fermentation10030124

Alim, M. A., Karim, A., Shohan, M. A. R., Sarker, S. C., Khan, T., Mondal, S., Esrafil, M., Linkon, K. M. M. R., Rahman, M. N., Akther, F., & Begum, R. (2023). Study on stability of antioxidant activity of fresh, pasteurized, and commercial fruit juice during refrigerated storage. *Food and Humanity, 1*, 1117–1124. https://doi.org/10.1016/j.foohum.2023.09.008

Alves Filho, E. G., Silva, L. M. A., de Brito, E. S., Wurlitzer, N. J., Fernandes, F. A. N., Rabelo, M. C., Fonteles, T. V., & Rodrigues, S. (2018). Evaluation of thermal and non-thermal processing effect on non-prebiotic and prebiotic acerola juices using 1H qNMR and GC–MS coupled to chemometrics. *Food Chemistry, 265*, 23–31. https://doi.org/10.1016/j.foodchem.2018.05.038

Amaral, G. V., Silva, E. K., Cavalcanti, R. N., Martins, C. P. C., Andrade, L. G. Z. S., Moraes, J., Alvarenga, V. O., Guimarães, J. T., Esmerino, E. A., Freitas, M. Q., Silva, M. C., Raices, R. S. L., Sant' Ana, A. S., Meireles, M. A. A., & Cruz, A. G. (2018). Whey-grape juice drink processed by supercritical carbon dioxide technology: Physicochemical characteristics, bioactive compounds and volatile profile. *Food Chemistry, 239*, 697–703. https://doi.org/10.1016/j.foodchem.2017.07.003

Amaro, K. C., & Tadini, C. C. (2021). The optimal time-temperature conditions for orange juice microwave–assisted pasteurization. *LWT, 150*, Article 111907. https://doi.org/10.1016/j.lwt.2021.111907

Ambreen, S., Arshad, M. U., Imran, A., Afzaal, M., & Madilo, F. K. (2023). A comparative study of high-pressure processing and thermal processing techniques on characteristics and microbial evaluation of orange juice. *International Journal of Food Properties, 26*(2), 3214–3225. https://doi.org/10.1080/10942912.2023.2271678

Arbefeville, S. S., Timbrook, T. T., & Garner, C. D. (2024). Evolving strategies in microbe identification - A comprehensive review of biochemical, MALDI-TOF MS and molecular testing methods. *Journal of Antimicrobial Chemotherapy, 79*, i2. https://doi.org/10.1093/jac/dkae275

Badejo, A. A., Duyilemi, T. I., Falarunu, A. J., & Akande, O. A. (2020). Inclusion of baobab (Adansonia digitata l.) fruit powder enhances the mineral composition and antioxidative potential of processed tigernut (Cyperus esculentus) beverages. *Preventive Nutrition and Food Science, 25*(4), 400–407. https://doi.org/10.3746/PNF.2020.25.4.400

Bag, B. B., Panigrahi, C., Gupta, S., & Mishra, H. N. (2022). Efficacy of plant-based natural preservatives in extending shelf life of sugarcane juice: Formulation optimization by MOGA and correlation study by principal component analysis. *Applied Food Research, 2*(2). https://doi.org/10.1016/j.afres.2022.100164

Bartula, K., Begley, M., Latour, N., & Callanan, M. (2023). Growth of food-borne pathogens Listeria and Salmonella and spore-forming Paenibacillus and Bacillus in commercial plant-based milk alternatives. *Food Microbiology, 109*, Article 104143. https://doi.org/10.1016/j.fm.2022.104143

Basak, S., Thakur, P., & Chakraborty, S. (2025). Pasteurization of mandarin juice by ohmic heating and evaluation of its shelf-life under refrigerated and ambient conditions. *Sustainable Food Technology, 3*(1), 239–252. https://doi.org/10.1039/d4fb00267a

Bendaali, Y., Escott, C., Vaquero, C., González, C., & Morata, A. (2024). Physicochemical, antioxidant activity, and sensory properties of grape juice-herbs extract based isotonic beverages. *International Journal of Gastronomy and Food Science, 37*, Article 100986. https://doi.org/10.1016/j.ijgfs.2024.100986

Berardy, A. J., Rubín-García, M., & Sabaté, J. (2022). A scoping review of the environmental impacts and nutrient composition of plant-based milks. *Advances in Nutrition, 13*(6), 2559–2572. https://doi.org/10.1093/advances/nmac098

Bhutkar, S., Brandão, T. R. S., Silva, C. L. M., & Miller, F. A. (2024). Application of ultrasound treatments in the processing and production of high-quality and safe-to-drink kiwi juice. *Foods, 13*(2). https://doi.org/10.3390/foods13020328

Bonilla, A. I., Usaga, J., Cortés, C., & Pérez, A. M. (2024). Effect of thermal treatment on selected bioactive compounds and physicochemical properties of a blackberry-soy-flaxseed beverage. *NFS Journal, 35*. https://doi.org/10.1016/j.nfs.2024.100177

Brauch, J. (2016). Underutilized fruits and vegetables as potential novel pigment sources. In *Handbook on natural pigments in food and beverages* (pp. 305–335). Elsevier.

Butovskaya, E., Caprai, E., Peloso, M., Gasparini, M., Borgia, M., Ehtesham Abdul, M., Candotti, P., & Menotta, S. (2025). Plant-based milk alternatives: Assessing the occurrence of chemical and microbiological contaminants in soy, oat, rice and almond beverages from Italian market. *Food Control, 169*, Article 111005. https://doi.org/10.1016/j.foodcont.2024.111005

Canaviri-Paz, P., Oscarsson, E., Kjellström, A., Olsson, H., Jois, C., & Håkansson, Å. (2021). Effects on microbiota composition after consumption of quinoa beverage fermented by a novel xylose-metabolizing L. *Plantarum Strain . Nutrients, 13*(10), 3318. https://doi.org/10.3390/nu13103318

Ceballos, M. W., Jafari, S., Fikry, M., Shiekh, K. A., Kijpatanasilp, I., & Assatarakul, K. (2025). Changes in quality attributes of coconut water treated with UV-radiation and nisin during cold storage: Kinetics modelling and shelf-life prediction. *Food Control, 167*. https://doi.org/10.1016/j.foodcont.2024.110801

Chalupa-Krebzdak, S., Long, C. J., & Bohrer, B. M. (2018). Nutrient density and nutritional value of milk and plant-based milk alternatives. *International Dairy Journal, 87*, 84–92. https://doi.org/10.1016/j.idairyj.2018.07.018

Cimmino, F., Catapano, A., Villano, I., Di Maio, G., Petrella, L., Traina, G., Pizzella, A., Tudisco, R., & Cavaliere, G. (2023). Invited review: Human, cow, and donkey milk comparison: Focus on metabolic effects. *Journal of Dairy Science, 106*(5), 3072–3085. https://doi.org/10.3168/jds.2022-22465

Craig, W. J., & Fresán, U. (2021). International analysis of the nutritional content and a review of health benefits of non-dairy plant-based beverages. *Nutrients, 13*(3), 1–14. https://doi.org/10.3390/nu13030842

Criste, A. D., Urcan, A. C., Coroian, C. O., Copolovici, L., Copolovici, D. M., Burtescu, R. F., & Oláh, N. K. (2023). Plant-based beverages from germinated and ungerminated seeds, as a source of probiotics, and bioactive compounds with health benefits—part 1: Legumes. *Agriculture, 13*(6). https://doi.org/10.3390/agriculture13061185

Daneluz, J., Ferreira da Silva, G., Duarte, J., Circe Turossi, T., dos Santos, V., Baldasso, C., & Daneluz, A. C. (2023). Characterization of microfiltration and ultrafiltration membranes for application in kombucha filtration. *Journal of Industrial and Engineering Chemistry, 126*, 264–269. https://doi.org/10.1016/j.jiec.2023.06.015

de Abreu Costa, J., Teixeira de Oliveira Santos, J., Gomes Abreu Bacelar, R., Martins Carneiro, R., Darlisson Slag Neri Silva, Maria Marlúcia Gomes Pereira Nóbrega, & Maria Christina Sanches Muratori. (2022). Dairy drink fermented with chia seed and acerola syrup: Physicochemical, microbiological, and sensory characterization. *Ciencia Animal Brasileira, 23*. https://doi.org/10.1590/1809-6891v23e-72395e

de Castro, D. R. G., Mar, J. M., da Silva, L. S., da Silva, K. A., Sanches, E. A., de Araújo Bezerra, J., Rodrigues, S., Fernandes, F. A. N., & Campelo, P. H. (2020). Dielectric barrier atmospheric cold plasma applied on camu-camu juice processing: Effect of the excitation frequency. *Food Research International, 131*. https://doi.org/10.1016/j.foodres.2020.109044

da Cunha Júnior, P. C., de Sá de Oliveira, L., Paiva Gouvêa, L.de, de Alcantara, M., Rosenthal, A., & Ferreira, E. H.d. R. (2021). Symbiotic drink based on Brazil nuts (Bertholletia excelsa H.B.K): Production, characterization, probiotic viability and sensory acceptance. *Ciência Rural, 51*(2). https://doi.org/10.1590/0103-8478cr20200361

de Oliveira, B. R., Egea, M. B., Lemes, S. A.d. F., Hernandes, T., & Takeuchi, K. P. (2024). Beverage of Brazil nut and Bocaiuva almond enriched with minerals: Technological quality and nutritional effect in Male Wistar rats. *Foods, 13*(16). https://doi.org/10.3390/foods13162533

de Paiva, K. F., Sousa, L. L., Cavalcante, M. P., Barros, S. L., Santos, N. C., Santos, F. A. O., de Menezes, F. L., Sitonio Eça, K., & Vasconcelos, L. B. (2024). Investigating the impact of pasteurization on the bioactive-rich potential of psyllium and spirulina in a concentrated beverage. *Measurement: Food, 13*. https://doi.org/10.1016/j.meafoo.2023.100129

da Silveira Maia, I. C., Macedo, E. B. C., dos Santos, L. P., de Oliveira Bordin, E., de Oliveira Lima, L., Feihrmann, A. C., Marcolino, V. A., Barão, C. E., & Pimentel, T. C. (2025). Ultrasound as an alternative for pasteurization of cashew nut milks: Improvements in the rheological and technological properties, fatty acid profile and acceptance. *Food Bioscience, 63*, Article 105649.

Deng, B., Yang, L., Yang, Y., & Xie, W. (2024). Advantages of UHT in retaining coconut milk aroma and insights into thermal changes of aroma compounds. *Food Research International, 194*, Article 114937. https://doi.org/10.1016/j.foodres.2024.114937

Dey, S., & Nagababu, B. H. (2022). Applications of food color and bio-preservatives in the food and its effect on the human health. *Food Chemistry Advances, 1*, Article 100019. https://doi.org/10.1016/j.focha.2022.100019

dos Santos, I. F., Pimentel, T. C., da Cruz, A. G., Stringheta, P. C., Martins, E., & Campelo, P. H. (2024). Ohmic heating in food processing: An overview of plant-based protein modification. *Processes, 12*(9). https://doi.org/10.3390/pr12091800

Egea, M. B., Dantas, L. A., Sousa, T. L.d., Lima, A. G., & Lemes, A. C. (2023). The potential, strategies, and challenges of Monascus pigment for food application. *Frontiers in Sustainable Food Systems, 7*. https://doi.org/10.3389/fsufs.2023.1141644

Egea, M. B., Santos, D. C. D., Neves, J. F., Lamas, I. B., Filho, J. G.d. O., & Takeuchi, K. P. (2023). Physicochemical characteristics and rheological properties of soymilk fermented with kefir. *Biointerface Research in Applied Chemistry, 13*(2). https://doi.org/10.33263/BRIAC132.127

El-Kased, R. F., & El-Kersh, D. M. (2022). GC–MS profiling of naturally extracted essential oils: Antimicrobial and beverage preservative actions. *Life, 12*(10). https://doi.org/10.3390/life12101587

Esposito, M., Battacchi, D., Castigliego, T., Lovatti, E., Re, M., Nava, C., Rizzo, M., Rondena, M., Papini, A., Pettinaroli, C., Pignatelli, D., Salvi, S., Tomasi, M., Scarafoni, A., & Scaglia, B. (2024). Insoluble residues from soybean, rice, oat and almond -based beverage: Landscape of the product category, chemical characterisation and valorization in the food industry. *Trends in Food Science and Technology, 152*, Article 104669. https://doi.org/10.1016/j.tifs.2024.104669

Fact.MR. (2024). *Plant-based Beverage market is estimated to reach $56.73 billion with a 11.9% CAGR by 2034 in (Vol. 2025)*. https://www.globenewswire.com/news-release/2024/11/20/2984360/0/en/Plant-based-Beverage-Market-is-Estimated-to-Reach-56-73-Billion-with-a-11-9-CAGR-By-2034-Fact-MR-Reports.html: GlobeNewswire. . 2025.

FAO. (2013). *Dietary protein quality evaluation in human nutrition: Report of an FAO expert consultation* (Vol 92). Rome: FAO.

Fernandes, F. A., Roriz, C., Calhelha, R. C., Rodrigues, P., Pires, T. C., Prieto, M. A., Ferreira, I. C., Barros, L., & Heleno, S. A. (2025). Valorization of natural resources-development of a functional plant-based beverage. *Food Chemistry, 472*, Article 142813.

Frühauf, V., Egea, M., Hernandes, T., & Takeuchi, K. (2023). Relationship between physicochemical and sensory characteristics of commercial plant-based beverages. *Journal of Culinary Science & Technology, 21*(6), 886–902. https://doi.org/10.1080/15428052.2021.2024470

Fructuoso, I., Romão, B., Han, H., Raposo, A., Ariza-Montes, A., Araya-Castillo, L., & Zandonadi, R. P. (2021). An overview on nutritional aspects of plant-based beverages used as substitutes for cow's milk. *Nutrients, 13*(8). https://doi.org/10.3390/nu13082650

Gómez-Cortés, P., Juárez, M., & de la Fuente, M. A. (2018). Milk fatty acids and potential health benefits: An updated vision. *Trends in Food Science and Technology, 81*, 1–9. https://doi.org/10.1016/j.tifs.2018.08.014

Gützkow, K. L., Lencioni, A., Schwake-Anduschus, C., Müller, A., Kabisch, J., Grundmann, V. L., Stöckl, M., & Maul, R. (2024). Comprehensive investigation of undesired substances and microbial contamination in plant-based drinks. *Food Control, 166*, Article 110599. https://doi.org/10.1016/j.foodcont.2024.110599

Giacalone, D., Clausen, M. P., & Jaeger, S. R. (2022). Understanding barriers to consumption of plant-based foods and beverages: Insights from sensory and consumer science. *Current Opinion in Food Science, 48*. https://doi.org/10.1016/j.cofs.2022.100919

Gombas, D., Luo, Y., Brennan, J., Shergill, G., Petran, R., Walsh, R., Hau, H., Khurana, K., Zomorodi, B., Rosen, J., Varley, R., & Deng, K. (2017). Guidelines to validate control of cross-contamination during washing of fresh-cut leafy vegetables. *Journal of Food Protection, 80*(2), 312–330. https://doi.org/10.4315/0362-028x.jfp-16-258

Grau-Fuentes, E., Rodrigo, D., Garzón, R., & Rosell, C. M. (2023). Understanding the marketed plant-based beverages: From ingredients technological function to their nutritional value. *Journal of Functional Foods, 106*, Article 105609. https://doi.org/10.1016/j.jff.2023.105609

He, S., Hong, X., Zhang, M., Wu, L., & Yan, X. (2020). Label-free detection of bacteria in fruit juice by nano-flow cytometry. *Analytical Chemistry, 92*(3), 2393–2400. https://doi.org/10.1021/acs.analchem.9b01869

Hernández, A., Pérez-Nevado, F., Ruiz-Moyano, S., Serradilla, M. J., Villalobos, M. C., Martín, A., & Córdoba, M. G. (2018). Spoilage yeasts: What are the sources of contamination of foods and beverages? *International Journal of Food Microbiology, 286*, 98–110. https://doi.org/10.1016/j.ijfoodmicro.2018.07.031

Hidalgo-Fuentes, B., Jesús-José, E. de, Cabrera-Hidalgo, A.d. J., Sandoval-Castilla, O., Espinosa-Solares, T., González-Reza, R. M., Zambrano-Zaragoza, M. L., Liceaga, A. M., & Aguilar-Toalá, J. E. (2024). Plant-based fermented beverages: Nutritional composition, sensory properties, and health benefits. *Foods, 13*(6). https://doi.org/10.3390/foods13060844

Hu, Y. H., Wang, C. Y., & Chen, B. Y. (2020). Effects of high-pressure processing and thermal pasteurization on quality and microbiological safety of jabuticaba (Myrciaria cauliflora) juice during cold storage. *Journal of Food Science and Technology, 57*(9), 3334–3344. https://doi.org/10.1007/s13197-020-04366-w

Ikrawan, Y., Rukmana, J., Gozaly, T., & Triani, R. (2024). Wildan qoharisma salam, Hari Hariadi, comparison of filtration processes using microfiltration, ultrafiltration, nanofiltration and reverse osmosis methods on the characteristics of lemon juice functional beverages at pilot Scale. *Jurnal Penelitian Pertanian Terapan, 24*(4), 517–531. https://doi.org/10.25181/jppt.v24i4.3759

Islam, M., Huang, Y., Jain, P., Fan, B., Tong, L., & Wang, F. (2023). Enzymatic hydrolysis of soy protein to high moisture textured meat analogue with emphasis on antioxidant effects: As a tool to improve techno-functional property. *Biocatalysis and Agricultural Biotechnology, 50*, Article 102700. https://doi.org/10.1016/j.bcab.2023.102700

Javed, F., Tehseen, S., Ashfaq, F., Sameen, A., Khalid, W., Batool, R., Bilal, A., Zubair Khalid, M., Alsulami, T., Mugabi, R., & Ahmad Nayik, G. (2024). Stabilization of Ficus carica L. Drink by utilizing varying levels of ultrasound-assisted moringa extract as a natural preservative. *Ultrasonics Sonochemistry, 111*. https://doi.org/10.1016/j.ultsonch.2024.107133

Jiang, L. L., Gong, X., Ji, M. Y., Wang, C. C., Wang, J. H., & Li, M. H. (2020). Bioactive compounds from plant-based functional foods: A promising choice for the prevention and management of hyperuricemia. *Foods, 9*(8). https://doi.org/10.3390/foods9080973

Kamalesh, R., Saravanan, A., Yaashikaa, P. R., & Vijayasri, K. (2025). Innovative approaches to harnessing natural pigments from food waste and by-products for eco-friendly food coloring. *Food Chemistry, 463*(Pt 4), Article 141519. https://doi.org/10.1016/j.foodchem.2024.141519

Kamonpatana, P., Gavahian, M., & Sastry, S. K. (2022). Ohmic heating for food processing: Methods and procedures related to process parameters. In *Emerging food processing technologies* (pp. 181–193). Springer.

Karaman, K., & Sagdic, O. (2019). Zygosaccharomyces bailii and Z. rouxii induced ethanol formation in apple juice supplemented with different natural preservatives: A response surface methodology approach. *Journal of Microbiological Methods, 163*, Article 105659. https://doi.org/10.1016/j.mimet.2019.105659

krishnan Kesavan, R., Gogoi, S., & Nayak, P. K. (2023). Influence of thermosonication and pasteurization on the quality attributes of kutkura (Meyna spinosa) juice. *Applied Food Research, 3*(1), Article 100268. https://doi.org/10.1016/j.afres.2023.100268

Lacivita, V., Derossi, A., Caporizzi, R., Lamacchia, C., Speranza, B., Guerrieri, A., Racioppo, A., Corbo, M. R., Sinigaglia, M., & Severini, C. (2024). Discover hidden value of almond by-products: Nutritional, sensory, technological and microbiological aspects. *Future Foods, 10*, Article 100398. https://doi.org/10.1016/j.fufo.2024.100398

LCDL. (1991). National laboratory of enteric pathogens, Bureau of Microbiology, Laboratory Centre for Disease Control. The polymerase chain reaction: An overview and development of diagnostic PCR protocols at the LCDC. *Canadian Journal of Infectious Diseases and Medical Microbiology, 2*, 89–91.

Leeuwendaal, N. K., Stanton, C., O'toole, P. W., & Beresford, T. P. (2022). Fermented foods, health and the gut microbiome. *Nutrients, 14*(7). https://doi.org/10.3390/nu14071527

Leszczyńska, D., Wirkijowska, A., Gasiński, A., Średnicka-Tober, D., Trafiałek, J., & Kazimierczak, R. (2023). Oat and oat processed Products—Technology, composition, nutritional value, and health. *Applied Sciences, 13* (20), Article 11267. https://doi.org/10.3390/app132011267

Lin, X., Duan, N., Wu, J., Lv, Z., Wang, Z., & Wu, S. (2023). Potential food safety risk factors in plant-based foods: Source, occurrence, and detection methods. *Trends in Food Science and Technology, 138*, 511–522. https://doi.org/10.1016/j.tifs.2023.06.032

Linhares, M.d. F. D., Alves Filho, E. G., Silva, L. M. A., Fonteles, T. V., Wurlitzer, N. J., de Brito, E. S., Fernandes, F. A. N., & Rodrigues, S. (2020). Thermal and non-thermal processing effect on açai juice composition. *Food Research International, 136*. https://doi.org/10.1016/j.foodres.2020.109506

Liu, J., Klebach, M., Visser, M., & Hofman, Z. (2019). Amino acid availability of a dairy and vegetable protein blend compared to single casein, whey, soy, and pea proteins: A Double-Blind, cross-over trial. *Nutrients, 11* (11), 2613. https://doi.org/10.3390/nu11112613

Liu, Y., Sunkesula, V., Barbano, D. M., & Drake, M. A. (2025). Comparison of vanilla-flavored milk protein beverages thermally processed by direct steam injection, retort, and autoclave. *Journal of Dairy Science, 108* (8), 7996–8011. https://doi.org/10.3168/jds.2025-26660

Mańkiewicz-Żurawska, I., Lutogniewska, W., Skała-Zamorowska, E., & Jarosz-Chobot, P. (2023). Nutrition analysis – With particular focus on carbohydrate content in kefirs and natural yoghurts in the Polish consumer market. *Pediatric Endocrinology, Diabetes and Metabolism, 29*(3), 166–174. https://doi.org/10.5114/pedm.2023.132026

Maleš, I., Pedisić, S., Zorić, Z., Elez-Garofulić, I., Repajić, M., You, L., Vladimir-Knežević, S., Butorac, D., & Dragović-Uzelac, V. (2022). The medicinal and aromatic plants as ingredients in functional beverage production. *Journal of Functional Foods, 96*, Article 105210. https://doi.org/10.1016/j.jff.2022.105210

Manju, G., & Mishra, S. (2021). Microbiological environmental monitoring in food processing. *Indian Food Industry Mag, 3*, 46–56.

Maree, E., Blignaut, J., Du Toit, C., Meissner, H., & Ederer, P. (2024). The need for holistic, sector-tailored sustainability assessments for milk and plant-based beverages. *Animal*, Article 101348.

Martins, I. R., Martins, L. H.d. S., Chisté, R. C., Picone, C. S. F., & Joele, M. R. S. P. (2024). Betalains from vegetable peels: Extraction methods, stability, and applications as natural food colorants. *Food Research International, 195*. https://doi.org/10.1016/j.foodres.2024.114956

Matos, J.d. S., Azevedo, P. Z., Costa, J. E. G., Justino, H.d. F. M., Lamarão, C. V., Sanches, E. A., Bezerra, J.d. A., Stringheta, P. C., Martins, E., & Campelo, P. H. (2024). UHT processing in the context of plant-based beverages: A scientific review on product characteristics and the functional role of plant proteins. *Food Chemistry Advances, 5*. https://doi.org/10.1016/j.focha.2024.100848

Mehta, D., Sharma, N., Bansal, V., Sangwan, R. S., & Yadav, S. K. (2019). Impact of ultrasonication, ultraviolet and atmospheric cold plasma processing on quality parameters of tomato-based beverage in comparison with thermal processing. *Innovative Food Science and Emerging Technologies, 52*, 343–349. https://doi.org/10.1016/j.ifset.2019.01.015

Mishra, S., Aravind, S. M., Ajlouni, S., Ranadheera, C. S., Singh, B. P., & Chakkaravarthi, S. (2024). Optimization of fermentation process and characterization of non-alcoholic functional beverage from pigmented rice varieties. *Biocatalysis and Agricultural Biotechnology, 58*. https://doi.org/10.1016/j.bcab.2024.103213

Mishra, T., Machireddy, J., & Vuppu, S. (2024). Comprehensive Study on hygiene and quality assessment practices in the production of drinkable dairy-based and plant-based fermented products. *Fermentation, 10*(9), 489. https://doi.org/10.3390/fermentation10090489

Mkhari, T., Kaseke, T., & Fawole, O. A. (2023). Encapsulation of betalain-rich extract from beetroot postharvest waste using a binary blend of gum Arabic and maltodextrin to promote a food circular bioeconomy. *Frontiers in Nutrition, 10*. https://doi.org/10.3389/fnut.2023.1235372

Mohamad Salin, N. S., Md Saad, W. M., Abdul Razak, H. R., & Salim, F. (2022). Effect of storage temperatures on Physico-Chemicals, phytochemicals and antioxidant properties of watermelon juice (Citrullus lanatus). *Metabolites, 12*(1). https://doi.org/10.3390/metabo12010075

Moss, R., Barker, S., Falkeisen, A., Gorman, M., Knowles, S., & McSweeney, M. B. (2022). An investigation into consumer perception and attitudes towards plant-based alternatives to milk. *Food Research International, 159*, Article 111648. https://doi.org/10.1016/j.foodres.2022.111648

Muangrat, R., & Thipsuwan, Y. (2024). Enhancing bacterial inhibition in beetroot beverages: The potent combination of sappan heartwood extracts via accelerated solvent extraction and pulsed electric field methods. *Journal of Agriculture and Food Research, 18*, Article 101268. https://doi.org/10.1016/j.jafr.2024.101268

Munekata, P. E. S., Domínguez, R., Budaraju, S., Roselló-Soto, E., Barba, F. J., Mallikarjunan, K., Roohinejad, S., & Lorenzo, J. M. (2020). Effect of innovative food processing technologies on the physicochemical and nutritional properties and quality of non-dairy plant-based beverages. *Foods, 9*(3). https://doi.org/10.3390/foods9030288

Nawaz, M. A., Singh, T. K., Stockmann, R., Jegasothy, H., & Buckow, R. (2021). Quality attributes of ultra-high temperature-treated model beverages prepared with faba bean protein concentrates. *Foods, 10*(6). https://doi.org/10.3390/foods10061244

Negri Rodríguez, L. M., Arias, R., Soteras, T., Sancho, A., Pesquero, N., Rossetti, L., Tacca, H., Aimaretti, N., Rojas Cervantes, M. L., & Szerman, N. (2021). Comparison of the quality attributes of carrot juice pasteurized by ohmic heating and conventional heat treatment. *LWT, 145*. https://doi.org/10.1016/j.lwt.2021.111255

Nesterova, E., Morozova, P., Gladkikh, M., Kazemzadeh, S., & Syromyatnikov, M. (2024). Molecular methods for detecting microorganisms in beverages. *Beverages, 10*(2), 46. https://doi.org/10.3390/beverages10020046

Nole-Jaramillo, J. M., Muñoz-More, H. D., Ruiz-Flores, L. A., Gutiérrez-Valverde, K. S., Nolazco-Cama, D. M., Espinoza-Silva, C. R., & Espinoza-Espinoza, L. A. (2024). Evaluation of the physicochemical, bioactive, and sensory properties of yogurt fortified with microencapsulated iron. *Applied Food Research, 4*(2). https://doi.org/10.1016/j.afres.2024.100525

Novais, C., Molina, A. K., Abreu, R. M. V., Santo-Buelga, C., Ferreira, I. C. F. R., Pereira, C., & Barros, L. (2022). Natural food colorants and preservatives: A review, a demand, and a challenge. *Journal of Agricultural and Food Chemistry, 70*(9), 2789–2805. https://doi.org/10.1021/acs.jafc.1c07533

Oishi, T. K., Pouzada, E. V. S., & Gut, J. A. W. (2022). Experimental validation of a multiphysics model for the microwave-assisted pasteurization of apple juice. *Digital Chemical Engineering, 5*, Article 100053. https://doi.org/10.1016/j.dche.2022.100053

Oliveira, A. F. A., Mar, J. M., Santos, S. F., da Silva Júnior, J. L., Kluczkovski, A. M., Bakry, A. M., Bezerra, J. d. A., Nunomura, R.d. C. S., Sanches, E. A., & Campelo, P. H. (2018). Non-thermal combined treatments in the processing of açai (Euterpe oleracea) juice. *Food Chemistry, 265*, 57–63. https://doi.org/10.1016/j.foodchem.2018.05.081

Orjuela, M. A., Moreno, F. L., Córdoba, N., Osorio, C., & Ruiz-Pardo, R. Y. (2025). Effect of ultraviolet irradiation on the shelf life and chemical composition of cold brew coffee. *Food and Bioproducts Processing, 149*, 58–69. https://doi.org/10.1016/j.fbp.2024.11.007

Pailliè-Jiménez, M. E., Stincone, P., & Brandelli, A. (2020). Natural pigments of microbial origin. *Frontiers in Sustainable Food Systems, 4*. https://doi.org/10.3389/fsufs.2020.590439

Pandey, A., Gaikwad, K. K., & Maiti, A. (2024). Improvement of coconut water shelf-life through low-temperature concentration process: Understanding impact of non-thermal process on shelf-life. *Journal of Food Process Engineering, 47*(6). https://doi.org/10.1111/jfpe.14673

Pintos, F. M., Lemoine, M. L., Gergoff Grozeff, G. E., Hasperué, H. J., Vicente, A. R., & Rodoni, L. M. (2022). Use of riboflavin to reduce decay and extend the shelf-life of fresh-cut sweet pepper. *Postharvest Biology and Technology, 188*. https://doi.org/10.1016/j.postharvbio.2022.111882

Pohl, P., Dzimitrowicz, A., Cyganowski, P., & Jamroz, P. (2022). Do we need cold plasma treated fruit and vegetable juices? A case study of positive and negative changes occurred in these daily beverages. *Food Chemistry, 375*, Article 131831. https://doi.org/10.1016/j.foodchem.2021.131831

Popova, A., Mihaylova, D., & Lante, A. (2023). Insights and perspectives on plant-based beverages. *Plants, 12* (19), 3345. https://doi.org/10.3390/plants12193345

Qin, P., Wang, T., & Luo, Y. (2022). A review on plant-based proteins from soybean: Health benefits and soy product development. *Journal of Agriculture and Food Research, 7*, Article 100265. https://doi.org/10.1016/j.jafr.2021.100265

Ramaswamy, H. S., Marcotte, M., Sastry, S., & Abdelrahim, K. (2014). *Ohmic heating in food processing ohmic Heating in Food Processing*. Canada: CRC Press. https://doi.org/10.1201/b16605

Ramesh, S. V., Shameena Beegum, P. P., Pandiselvam, R., Manikantan, M. R., & Hebbar, K. B. (2022). *Plant-Based milk alternatives: Nutritional potential and challenges conceptualizing plant-based nutrition: Bio-resources, nutrients repertoire and bioavailability.* India: Springer Nature. https://doi.org/10.1007/978-981-19-4590-8_5

Ramesh, C., Vinithkumar, N. V., Kirubagaran, R., Venil, C. K., & Dufossé, L. (2019). Multifaceted applications of microbial pigments: Current knowledge, challenges and future directions for public health implications. *Microorganisms, 7*(7). https://doi.org/10.3390/microorganisms7070186

Ranadheera, C. S., Evans, C. A., Adams, M., & Baines, S. K. (2016). Co-culturing of probiotics influences the microbial and physico-chemical properties but not sensory quality of fermented dairy drink made from goats' milk. *Small Ruminant Research, 136*, 104–108. https://doi.org/10.1016/j.smallrumres.2016.01.016

Rascón, L., Cruz, M., Rodríguez-Jasso, R. M., Neira-Vielma, A. A., Ramírez-Barrón, S. N., & Belmares, R. (2020). Effect of ohmic heating on sensory, physicochemical, and microbiological properties of "aguamiel" of agave salmiana. *Foods, 9*(12). https://doi.org/10.3390/foods9121834

Ravichandran, C., Jayachandran, L. E., Kothakota, A., Pandiselvam, R., & Balasubramaniam, V. M. (2023). Influence of high pressure pasteurization on nutritional, functional and rheological characteristics of fruit and vegetable juices and purees-an updated review. *Food Control, 146*, Article 109516. https://doi.org/10.1016/j.foodcont.2022.109516

Rekha, R., Sabikhi, L., & Sathish Kumar, M. H. (2024). Storage stability, nutritional profiling and consumer acceptability of a milk-sorghum-based breakfast smoothie. *Sustainable Food Technology, 2*(3), 729–740. https://doi.org/10.1039/d4fb00038b

Roberts, S. B., & Flaherman, V. (2022). Dietary energy. *Advances in Nutrition, 13*(6), 2681–2685. https://doi.org/10.1093/advances/nmac092

Rodríguez-Mena, A., Ochoa-Martínez, L. A., González-Herrera, S. M., Rutiaga-Quiñones, O. M., González-Laredo, R. F., & Olmedilla-Alonso, B. (2023). Natural pigments of plant origin: Classification, extraction and application in foods. *Food Chemistry, 398*. https://doi.org/10.1016/j.foodchem.2022.133908

Sain, M., Minz, P. S., John, H., Singh, A., & Pandiselvam, R. (2024). Effect of ohmic heating on food products: An In-Depth review approach associated with quality attributes. *Journal of Food Processing and Preservation, 2024*, 1–17. https://doi.org/10.1155/2024/2025937

Silva, J. C. D. M., Santana, R. V., Almeida, A. B.de, Pereira Takeuchi, K., & Egea, M. B. (2021). Changes in the chemical, technological, and microbiological properties of kefir-fermented soymilk after supplementation with Inulin and Acrocomia aculeata pulp. *Applied Sciences, 11*(12), 5575. https://doi.org/10.3390/app11125575

Santana, R. V., Santos, D. C.d., Santana, A. C. A., Oliveira Filho, J. G.d., Almeida, A. B.d., Lima, T. M.d., Silva, F. G., & Egea, M. B. (2020). Quality parameters and sensorial profile of clarified "Cerrado" cashew juice supplemented with Sacharomyces boulardii and different sweeteners. *LWT, 128*. https://doi.org/10.1016/j.lwt.2020.109319

Santos, D. C.d., Oliveira Filho, J. G.d., Santana, A. C. A., Freitas, B. S. M.d., Silva, F. G., Takeuchi, K. P., & Egea, M. B. (2019). Optimization of soymilk fermentation with kefir and the addition of inulin:

Physicochemical, sensory and technological characteristics. *LWT, 104*, 30–37. https://doi.org/10.1016/j.lwt.2019.01.030

Sarbatly, R., Sariau, J., & Krishnaiah, D. (2023). Recent developments of membrane technology in the clarification and concentration of fruit juices. *Food Engineering Reviews, 15*(3), 420–437. https://doi.org/10.1007/s12393-023-09346-2

Selahvarzi, A., Ramezan, Y., Sanjabi, M. R., Mirsaeedghazi, H., Azarikia, F., & Abedinia, A. (2021). Investigation of antimicrobial activity of orange and pomegranate peels extracts and their use as a natural preservative in a functional beverage. *Journal of Food Measurement and Characterization, 15*(6), 5683–5694. https://doi.org/10.1007/s11694-021-01141-z

Sethi, S., Tyagi, S. K., & Anurag, R. K. (2016). Plant-based milk alternatives an emerging segment of functional beverages: A review. *Journal of Food Science and Technology, 53*(9), 3408–3423. https://doi.org/10.1007/s13197-016-2328-3

Sharma, N., Yeasmen, N., Dubé, L., & Orsat, V. (2024). A review on current scenario and key challenges of plant-based functional beverages. *Food Bioscience, 60*, Article 104320. https://doi.org/10.1016/j.fbio.2024.104320

Shimoyamada, M., Itabashi, Y., Sugimoto, I., Kanauchi, M., Ishida, M., Tsuzuki, K., Egusa, S., & Honda, Y. (2015). Characterization of soymilk prepared by ohmic heating and the effects of voltage applied. *Food Science and Technology Research, 21*(3), 439–444. https://doi.org/10.3136/fstr.21.439

Shkembi, B., & Huppertz, T. (2023). Glycemic responses of milk and plant-based drinks: Food matrix effects. *Foods, 12*(3), 453. https://doi.org/10.3390/foods12030453

Silva, A. R. A.d., Santelli, R. E., Braz, B. F., Silva, M. M. N., Melo, L., Lemes, A. C., & Ribeiro, B. D. (2024). A comparative Study of dairy and non-dairy milk types: Development and characterization of customized plant-based milk options. *Foods, 13*(14). https://doi.org/10.3390/foods13142169

Silva, A. R. A., Silva, M. M. N., & Ribeiro, B. D. (2020). Health issues and technological aspects of plant-based alternative milk. *Food Research International, 131*, Article 108972. https://doi.org/10.1016/j.foodres.2019.108972

Spence, C. (2015). On the psychological impact of food colour. *Flavour, 4*, 1–16.

Starek, A., Sagan, A., Andrejko, D., Chudzik, B., Kobus, Z., Kwiatkowski, M., Terebun, P., & Pawłat, J. (2020). Possibility to extend the shelf life of NFC tomato juice using cold atmospheric pressure plasma. *Scientific Reports, 10*(1). https://doi.org/10.1038/s41598-020-77977-0

Tan, M., Nawaz, M. A., & Buckow, R. (2023). Functional and food application of plant proteins–a review. *Food Reviews International, 39*(5), 2428–2456. https://doi.org/10.1080/87559129.2021.1955918

Tao, M., Guo, W., Jin, L., & Liu, Z. (2025). Unraveling the key cooked off-flavor compounds in thermally sterilized green tea beverages, and masking effect of tea raw material baking. *Food Chemistry, 464*(Pt 1), Article 141671. https://doi.org/10.1016/j.foodchem.2024.141671

Udayakumar, S., Rasika, D. M. D., Priyashantha, H., & Vidanarachchi, J. K. (2022). Chaminda senaka ranadheera, probiotics and beneficial microorganisms in biopreservation of plant-based foods and beverages. *Applied Sciences, 12*(22), Article 11737. https://doi.org/10.3390/app122211737

Urošević, T., Povrenović, D., Vukosavljević, P., Urošević, I., & Stevanović, S. (2017). Recent developments in microfiltration and ultrafiltration of fruit juices. *Food and Bioproducts Processing, 106*, 147–161. https://doi.org/10.1016/j.fbp.2017.09.009

Vara, S., Karnena, M. K., & Dwarapureddi, B. K. (2019). Natural preservatives for nonalcoholic beverages. In *Preservatives and preservation approaches in beverages* (pp. 179–201). Elsevier.

Villarreal-Morales, S. L., Montañez-Saenz, J. C., Aguilar-González, C. N., & Rodriguez-Herrera, R. (2018). Metagenomics of traditional beverages. *Advances in Biotechnology for Food Industry, 14*, 301–326. https://doi.org/10.1016/B978-0-12-811443-8.00011-6

Walther, B., Guggisberg, D., Badertscher, R., Egger, L., Portmann, R., Dubois, S., Haldimann, M., Kopf-Bolanz, K., Rhyn, P., Zoller, O., Veraguth, R., & Rezzi, S. (2022). Comparison of nutritional composition between plant-based drinks and cow's milk. *Frontiers in Nutrition, 9.* https://doi.org/10.3389/fnut.2022.988707

Wang, S., Fang, Y., Xu, Y., Zhu, B., Piao, J., Zhu, L., Yao, L., Liu, K., Wang, S., Zhang, Q., Qin, L., & Wu, J. (2022). The effects of different extraction methods on physicochemical, functional and physiological properties of soluble and insoluble dietary fiber from Rubus chingiiHu. fruits. *Journal of Functional Foods, 93*, Article 105081. https://doi.org/10.1016/j.jff.2022.105081

Xie, A., Dong, Y., Liu, Z., Li, Z., Shao, J., Mohan, L., & Yue, X. (2023). A review of plant-based drinks addressing nutrients, flavor, and processing technologies. *Foods, 12*(21), 3952. https://doi.org/10.3390/foods12213952

Xie, A., Shen, X., Hong, R., Xie, Y., Zhang, Y., Chen, J., Li, Z., Li, M., Yue, X., & Young Quek, S. (2025). Unlocking the potential of donkey milk: Nutritional composition, bioactive properties and future prospects. *Food Research International, 209*, Article 116307. https://doi.org/10.1016/j.foodres.2025.116307

Xu, L., Li, Z., Yang, S., Jiang, H., Deng, J., Zhang, W., Wang, J., Xie, M., & Yun, Y.-H. (2024). Cold plasma–A new technology for maintaining key aroma compounds and flavor in coconut water. *Innovative Food Science & Emerging Technologies, 96*, Article 103752.

Zahan, I., Khan, M. M., Rana, M. S., Sahabuddin, M., Rasik, M. R., & Uddin, M. B. (2024). Effect of selective preservatives on shelf-life of guava juice extracted using pectinase enzyme. *Heliyon, 10*(18). https://doi.org/10.1016/j.heliyon.2024.e37596

Zhang, J., Cheng, J., Li, Z., Weng, M., Zhang, X., Tang, X., & Pan, Y. (2024). Effects of ultra-high pressure, thermal pasteurization, and ultra-high temperature sterilization on color and nutritional components of freshly-squeezed lettuce juice. *Food Chemistry, 435*, Article 137524. https://doi.org/10.1016/j.foodchem.2023.137524

Zhao, L., Wang, Y., Qiu, D., & Liao, X. (2014). Effect of ultrafiltration combined with high-pressure processing on safety and quality features of fresh Apple juice. *Food and Bioprocess Technology, 7*(11), 3246–3258. https://doi.org/10.1007/s11947-014-1307-9

Zhao, S., Wu, J., Guo, Z., Wang, D., Chen, J., Liu, Q., Ding, C., Guo, L., & Tao, T. (2024). Magnetic field technology in improving the quality of food refrigeration and freezing: Mechanisms, applications, and challenges. *Journal of Stored Products Research, 106*, Article 102254. https://doi.org/10.1016/j.jspr.2024.102254

Zou, W., Niu, H., Yi, J., & Zhou, L. (2024). Passion fruit juicing with or without seeds treated by high-pressure processing and thermal pasteurization: Effects on the storage stability of enzymes and quality properties. *Innovative Food Science & Emerging Technologies, 91*, Article 103554. https://doi.org/10.1016/j.ifset.2023.103554

CHAPTER

6 Advancements in ensuring safety standards for alcoholic beverages: A scientific perspective

Akriti Verma[1], Himanshu Chandelkar[1], Roji Waghmare[1] and Manoj Kumar[2]

[1]*Department of Food Engineering and Technology, Institute of Chemical Technology, Mumbai, Maharashtra, India;* [2]*Chemical and Biochemical Processing Division, ICAR-Central Institute for Research on Cotton Technology, Mumbai, Maharashtra, India*

6.1 Introduction

Alcoholic beverages have been a significant part of culture and diet for centuries. They offer a variety of flavors and effects due to differences in ingredients and production methods. People enjoy these drinks for their taste, and they play a key role in social and cultural traditions around the world. Understanding the definition, types, and global consumption trends of alcoholic beverages gives important insights into their effects on health, society, and the economy. Alcoholic drinks contain ethanol, which is produced when yeast ferments sugars (Lin et al., 2023). They are categorized according to their production methods, components, and alcohol levels (Trius-Soler et al., 2023). The use of alcohol around the world is very different from one region to another. This variation is influenced by cultural, economic, and legal factors (Kilian et al., 2023). In high-income countries, more people are seeking low-alcohol and alcohol-free options. This trend indicates that consumers are choosing healthier lifestyles (De-Loyde et al., 2024). Laws like minimum unit pricing and taxes have helped people drink less by making alcoholic drinks more expensive, especially for those who have less money. Also, rules that limit when alcohol can be sold, such as shorter sales hours, have been effective in lowering the total amount of alcohol people consume (Kilian et al., 2023). Nonetheless, enforcing safety regulations in the production of alcohol faces difficulties stemming from trade conflicts and opposition from the industry (Milsom et al., 2021). The alcohol industry contributes to the economy by creating jobs and generating revenue (Verma et al., 2024). At the same time, alcohol-related issues, including healthcare expenses and lost productivity, impose substantial economic burdens (Herdiana, 2025).

Throughout history, alcoholic drinks have had a significant impact on food security, public health, and economic systems, influencing both beneficial and detrimental outcomes (Anderson, Meloni, & Swinnen, 2019). Although alcohol has provided energy and medicinal advantages, its overconsumption has resulted in numerous health issues. Throughout history, global trends in alcohol consumption have experienced notable changes, especially during times of globalization. These changes have prompted improvements in production methods and shifts in the structure of alcohol

The Science and Safety of Beverages. https://doi.org/10.1016/B978-0-443-36536-2.00005-3

companies. Policies such as taxes and government regulations have both affected and been shaped by these changing patterns, influencing the ways alcohol is made, distributed, and consumed around the globe (Anderson, Meloni, & Swinnen, 2019). The early stages of alcohol production were mostly without regulation, and there is evidence of brewing methods that go back over 8000 years (McGovern et al., 2017). In ancient Greece and Rome, wine was the preferred alcoholic beverage, whereas beer was often viewed with disdain (Rabin & Forget, 2014). Distilled spirits emerged around the eighth century BCE, initially for medicinal purposes. As commerce expanded, alcohol consumption patterns evolved in response to local production capacities and cultural preferences (Anderson, Meloni, & Swinnen, 2019). Despite its widespread acceptance, alcohol was also recognized as a potential source of harm. Ancient societies implemented various regulations to control alcohol consumption. In China, during the Shang Dynasty (1750–1100 BCE), excessive drinking among rulers was blamed for the dynasty's decline, prompting stricter drinking laws in later periods. Egyptian texts warned against drunkenness, with wall paintings depicting intoxicated individuals in negative contexts. The Code of Hammurabi (1770 BCE) regulated beer prices and penalized dishonest tavern owners in Babylon. While many cultures acknowledged the social and health benefits of moderate drinking, excessive alcohol consumption was seen as a threat to social order, leading to restrictions and societal pressures for moderation (Rabin & Forget, 2014). The Industrial Revolution in the mid-19th century marked a turning point in alcohol production. Technological advancements led to increased availability of cheaper alcohol, which, in turn, resulted in widespread social issues related to excessive consumption and alcoholism. Temperance movements emerged, advocating for reduced alcohol consumption and stricter regulations. Governments introduced excise taxes and quality controls to manage production and consumption levels. This period established more formal safety standards as public health concerns gained prominence (Anderson, Meloni, & Swinnen, 2019). Post-WWII, alcohol safety standards evolved with stricter regulations, including age restrictions, warning labels, advertising limitations, and taxation to control consumption. Globalization and the growth of craft producers added complexity. This made it necessary to update safety measures (Rabin & Forget, 2014). Historically, regulations focused on taxes and purity while medieval monasteries improved brewing methods. The distillation boom in the 18th century raised concerns about adulteration. This led to laws like England's Gin Acts. Industrialization brought risks such as methanol poisoning, resulting in the Pure Food and Drug Act in 1906. Prohibition from 1920 to 1933 showed the dangers of unregulated alcohol. This led to stricter quality controls after it was repealed. Today, modern standards, including the Codex Alimentarius, address contaminants using better analytical tools and bioactive compounds. As scientific understanding grows, regulations must balance public health and industry interests to ensure alcohol safety worldwide (Rabin & Forget, 2014). This chapter examines recent innovations in alcoholic beverage safety. It discusses improvements in production methods, contamination control, analytical testing, and regulatory standards. The chapter provides a scientific perspective on how these developments enhance product safety, help meet regulations, and protect public health.

6.2 Alcoholic beverages processing

A significant part of everyday life, alcoholic beverages are made by fermenting carbohydrates to produce ethyl alcohol and other by-products. Although there are many different kinds of alcohol found in nature, ethyl alcohol is the main ingredient in all alcoholic drinks. It is a thin, transparent liquid with an intense burning taste and significant volatility used for its exhilarating and calming effects.

Alcoholic beverages are defined as those that contain more than 0.5% ethyl alcohol (ethanol) by volume (Safety & Act, 2023). The ethanol needed to make them must come from agriculture. There are two categories for alcoholic beverages: un-distilled and distilled, as shown in Fig. 6.1. Beer, wine, cider, and toddy are un-distilled beverages made only by fermentation. Spirits, tequila, vodka, gin, and rum are distilled beverages (Lopes et al., 2019). However, ethanol produced by fermenting grains, fruits, vegetables, molasses, or other carbohydrate sources is then distilled to create distilled alcoholic beverages, sometimes called spirits or liquors. While other fruits can be used, grapes are the main ingredient in wine; barley, hops, yeast, and water are the ingredients of beer; and cereals, cane sugar, potatoes, beets, or molasses are usually used to make spirits (Scoccianti, 2015). Water is frequently added to spirits to dilute them and change the amount of alcohol present (Mudgil & Barak, 2018).

Alcohol consumption has increased recently in both developed and developing nations. Moderate consumption of alcoholic beverages, especially wine, may have some health benefits. However, excessive consumption has been associated with several health hazards, such as gastrointestinal problems, cancer, liver disease, pancreatitis, and psychological disorders like anxiety, depression, and suicidal thoughts. In addition, excessive alcohol use during pregnancy can cause damage to the fetus, neurological system difficulties, and cardiovascular issues. In light of these dangers, laws, rules, and public education campaigns are becoming more and more necessary to limit alcohol use and inform people of its possible adverse health effects (Mudgil & Barak, 2018).

6.2.1 Undistilled beverage

Fermented alcoholic beverages that are not distilled are known as undistilled beverages. Examples of beverages that preserve the natural flavors and qualities of their unprocessed constituents include wine, beer, cider, perry, toddy, and mead. These drinks usually contain between 3% and 15% alcohol by

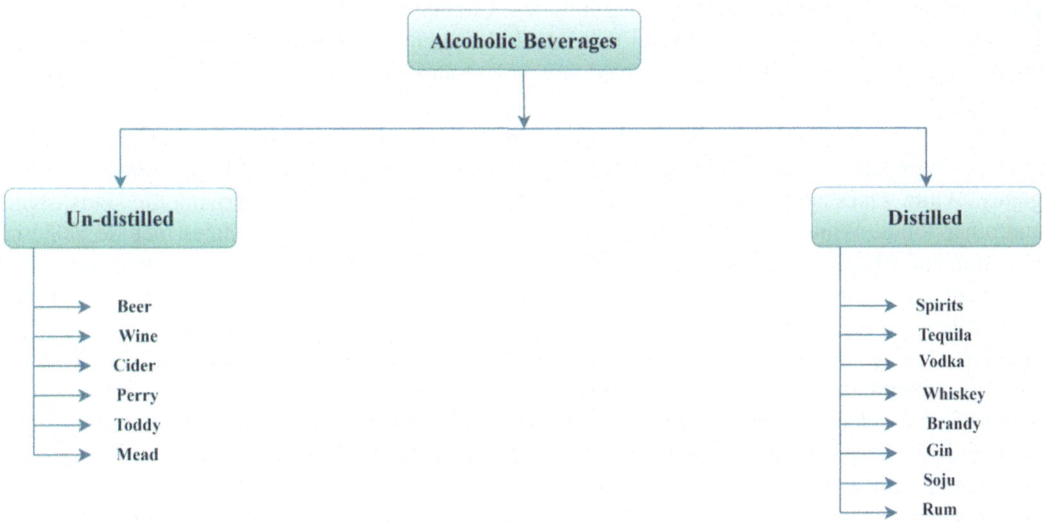

FIGURE 6.1

Classification of alcoholic beverages.

volume (ABV) (Besse & Dechaine, 2014), which is less than the amount found in distilled spirits. During the fermentation process, yeast converts sugars into carbon dioxide and alcohol, which affects the final product's flavor, texture, and aroma. Product safety depends on quality control and safety procedures such as appropriate fermentation conditions, microbiological monitoring, and contamination avoidance. Undistilled beverages are popular in many cultures and geographical areas because they come in various flavors and styles.

6.2.1.1 Wine

Wine is one of the world's oldest and most popular alcoholic beverages. The International Organisation of Vine and Wine (IOV) reported that global wine consumption reached between 227 million hectoliters (mhl) and 235 mhl in 2024 (Mishra, 2024). The United States, France, Italy, Germany, and China are the world's largest wine consumers, consuming an average of 120 mhl annually. The appeal of wine tasting, combined with rich cultural traditions in specific locations, leads to its popularity over other alcoholic beverages (Gutiérrez-Escobar et al., 2021).

The classification of wine can be complicated because innumerable varietals differ in many aspects (Jackson, 2023). However, a more general method enables wines to be grouped according to their general makeup without exploring the more specific differences highlighted by experts. Four basic features can be used to categorize wine (Jackson, 2008).

Wine can be classified into still or sparkling, red or white, dry or sweet, and fortified or unfortified. Still wines, commonly known as table or dinner wines, are fully fermented before bottling. As a result, they contain only the quantity of carbon dioxide naturally dissolved in the liquid, which maintains equilibrium with the air under typical handling conditions. In contrast, sparkling wines are bottled before fermentation, trapping carbon dioxide gas in the liquid at a pressure greater than atmospheric pressure. This causes the wine to effervesce when served. Carbon dioxide pressure usually ranges between 4 and 6 atm. Sparkling wines can range from dry to sweet and light to robust, with well-known examples including sparkling Burgundy and Champagne.

Wines are also classed according to their alcohol content: those with 7%–9% alcohol are called "light" wines, those with 9%–16% are "medium" wines, and those with 16%–21% are called "strong" wines (Bisht & Singh, 2025).

Red wines are prepared by fermenting juice with grape skins, stems, and other pieces, which removes pigments and gives the wine its distinctive color. Examples include Port, Chianti, and Burgundy. White wines are prepared by fermenting only the grape juice and removing the skins, stems, and other solids. White wine colors range from mild straw to rich gold. Examples include Sauterne, Riesling, and Champagne (Joshi et al., 2017). Dry wines are those in which fermentation has turned nearly all sugar into alcohol. Their alcohol concentration is usually between 8% and 12%, and they have little to no sugar. Burgundy, Hock, and Moselle are a few examples. Sweet wines contain higher amounts of sugar, which can be determined by taste. These wines possess some unfermented sugar and have an alcohol concentration ranging from 13%–15% by weight, entirely due to fermentation. Sauterne and Tokay are among the examples (Reboredo-Rodríguez et al., 2015). Fortified wines contain distilled spirits, such as grape brandy, to boost the alcohol content above what fermentation alone can produce. These wines typically contain between 18% and 22% alcohol. Sherry, port, and champagne are some examples. Unfortified wines have an alcohol concentration solely derived from fermentation and contain no additional spirits. Unfortified wines include the dry and sweet wines listed above dry or sweet wines.

Winemakers use various methods to make wine, although the process is natural. The oldest system is the division of still table wines (the most popular type) into red, white, and rosé, which reflects variations in flavor, use, and production techniques (Jackson, 2008). Grape sugar metabolism through yeast-driven alcoholic fermentation produces a long shelf life for wine. Proteins, polysaccharides, phenolic compounds, organic acids, glucose, fructose, glycerol, ethanol, volatile chemicals, and vital minerals like potassium are some of its main constituents (Chaudhary et al., 2014).

6.2.1.2 Wine processing

The process for producing wine generally consists of five main steps: harvesting, crushing and pressing, fermentation, clarifying, aging, and bottling (Jackson, 2020) (Fig. 6.2).

Harvesting is the first phase in the winemaking process and is critical to producing high-quality wine. Grapes are the only fruit that naturally contains the acids, esters, and tannins needed for consistent wine production. Tannins contribute to the wine's bitterness and astringency while giving it a dry mouthfeel. The grape variety used to make the wine influences its acidity, sweetness, and flavor. Harvesting can be done both manually and mechanically. Grapes are picked and then sorted to remove any rotting or under-ripe fruit. After harvesting, the next steps are crushing and pressing. The grapes are de-stemmed and crushed after sorting. Grapes were traditionally stomped with feet, but mechanical presses are now employed to smash the grapes and extract fresh juice, known as "must," which comprises skins, seeds, and solids. Mechanical pressing has improved the durability and quality of the wine while also delivering considerable sanitary benefits. White wine is made by rapidly crushing and pressing the grapes to extract the juice from the solids, seeds, and skins (Ribereau-Gayon et al., 2006).

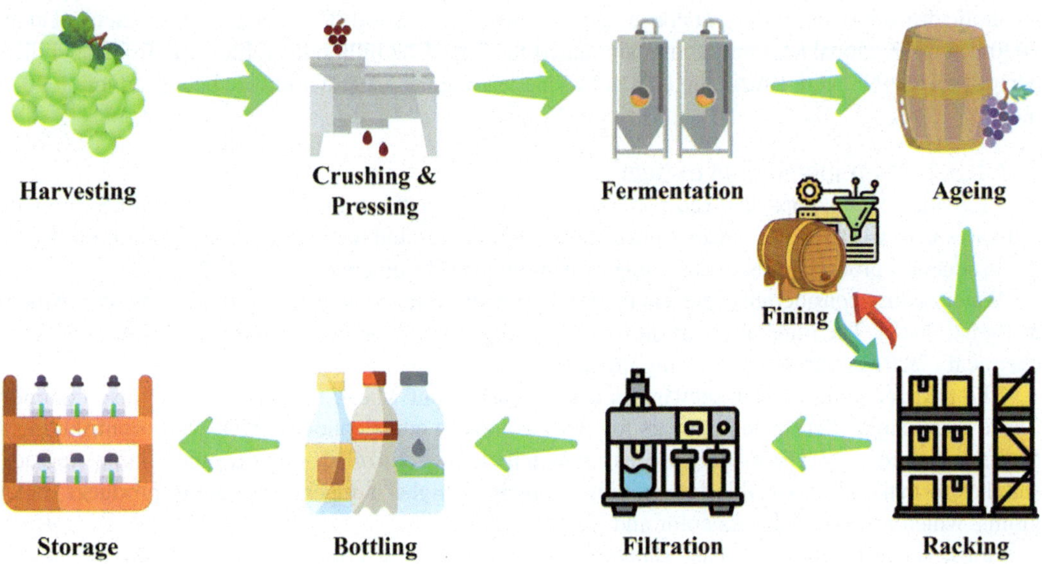

FIGURE 6.2

Basic steps of the making process.

The icons illustrated in this figure were obtained from Flaticon.com.

This keeps tannins and undesirable colors from leaking into the finished product. In contrast, red wine's juice can touch the skin to absorb additional tannins, color, and flavor, which are crucial to the wine's qualities. The must (or juice) undergoes fermentation in 6–12 h following crushing and pressing. Dry wine is the result of continuing until all of the sugar has been transformed into alcohol. The fermentation process is halted before the sugar is converted to sweet wine.

Temperature affects the duration of fermentation, which can range from 10 days to more than a month. The rate at which sugar is converted increases with temperature. For instance, fermentation occurs more quickly at 30°C than at 25°C, while fermentation occurs more rapidly at 25°C than at 20°C. The process of clarity begins once fermentation is complete. The wine's proteins, tannins, and dead yeast cells are eliminated in this process. The wine is moved into stainless steel containers or oak barrels during racking. Filtration or fining is then used to obtain clarification. While filtration eliminates bigger particles from the wine, fining adds particular compounds to the wine to help clean it (Buglass, 2010). After that, the clarified wine is moved to a different container to be bottled or allowed to age further. Then aging and bottling, these two steps constitute the latter phase of the winemaking process. You can age wine in oak barrels, stainless steel tanks, or bottles. Because it exposes the wine to more oxygen, aging in oak barrels produces a smoother, rounder wine with a vanilla flavor. This procedure improves the fruitiness of the wine and lowers the tannin concentration. Typically, zesty white wines are aged in stainless steel containers. The wine is bottled with a screw cap or a cork after it has finished maturing (Okafor, 2007).

6.2.1.3 Beer

Beer is a fermented, carbonated alcoholic beverage that dates back to the Sumerians and the beginning of civilization, making it one of the first beverages produced by humans. It is the most popular alcoholic drink and the sixth most consumed beverage in the world (Paiva et al., 2021; Rachwał et al., 2020). In 2023, global beer production amounted to about 1.88 billion hectoliters, up from 1.3 billion hectoliters in 1998, with Brazil, the US, and China leading the way (Worldwide beer production 2023, n.d.).

6.2.1.3.1 Main ingredients of beer

Water, malted cereal, hops, and yeast are the four main ingredients used in conventional beer brewing (Olivares-Galván et al., 2022). Combining these components and the various brewing methods used in the production process leads to the range of beer styles (Pferdmenges et al., 2022).

Water quality considerably impacts the final product, as it accounts for up to 97% of beer (Mudgil & Barak, 2018). The mineral composition of brewing water is crucial because it influences different chemical reactions during the brewing process.

The primary grain used in brewing is malted barley, but wheat, rye, and oats are also common. These grains supply fermentable sugars for yeast to convert into alcohol and CO_2 while contributing to beer's color and body. The malting process, which includes controlled sprouting and kilning, degrades starches to make them suitable for brewing. Longer or higher temperature kilning produces darker grains, which affects the beer's color and flavor.

Hops, scientifically known as *Humulus lupulus*, thrive in cold climates and require specific cultivation conditions (Almeida et al., 2020). It offers bitterness to balance malt sweetness while also providing a variety of flavors and smells ranging from citrusy and piney to earthy and spicy. Hops are the conical blooms of a fast-growing cannabis vine. The bitterness stems from alpha acids found in the flower's lupulin glands, which must be chemically changed through boiling to be effective (Féchir et al., 2023; Kimura et al., 2021).

Yeast, a single-celled eukaryotic organism from the fungi kingdom (Sahaya Glingston et al., 2021). Yeast plays a critical part in beer production by fermenting sugars from grains to produce CO_2, alcohol, and numerous by-products, such as esters and phenols, which contribute to the beer's flavor, fragrance, and overall character (Mudgil & Barak, 2018). Brewing yeast is divided into two types: ale yeast (*Saccharomyces cerevisiae*), a top-fermenting strain that thrives at warmer temperatures (18–24°C) and produces fruity or spicy flavors due to higher phenol and ester production, and lager yeast (*Saccharomyces pastorianus*), a bottom fermenting strain that ferments at cooler temperatures (7–13°C), minimizing by-products and resulting in a cleaner yeast profile (Wunderlich & Back, 2009).

6.2.1.4 Beer processing

There are some basic steps in the brewing process Fig. 6.3 milling, mashing, filtering, boiling, treatment, fermentation, maturation, filtration, and pasteurization (Carvalho et al., 2023). Although some stages are unnecessary for beer production, major industrial breweries usually incorporate them to improve the end product and meet consumer preferences.

Three main goals are achieved during the milling stage, which is intended to break down malt grains uniformly: exposing the endosperm (the inner part of the grain) by lengthwise peeling the husk; enhancing enzymatic activity on starches and proteins by entirely disintegrating the endosperm; and reducing the amount of excessively fine flour particles (Mosher & Trantham, 2021). Mashing combines milled malt with water at a specified temperature according to a predefined program. This process dissolves water-soluble malt components and facilitates enzymatic hydrolysis, converting starch and proteins into fermentable sugars and amino acids. Following mashing, wort is filtered in a receptacle called a lauter tun. The wort is filtered using malt husks as a natural filtering layer, yielding a clear liquid free of husks, seedlings, and other insoluble substances (Blšáková et al., 2022). The filtering layer is washed with water to increase sugar extraction and process yield (Hennemann et al., 2021). Wort boiling is the next step in the brewing process, and it stabilizes the wort composition, sterilizes germs, extracts and changes hop chemicals for bitterness and fragrance, and eliminates undesired volatiles (Carvalho et al., 2023). After boiling, wort treatment eliminates precipitated hops and proteins, cools the wort, and aerates it in preparation for fermentation. Oxygen is then supplied to help the yeast grow. Beer's sensory profile is defined by the ethanol, CO_2, and taste chemicals that yeast produces during fermentation. However, unwanted byproducts may emerge, necessitating maturation, which involves cooling the beer (0–10°C) to allow yeast to metabolize these chemicals and improve clarity, stability, and flavor (Mosher & Trantham, 2017). For further clarification, industrial breweries eliminate yeast and haze-forming particles before bottling using filtration techniques like dead-end, crossflow, or dynamic microfiltration (Rögener, 2021). Finally, by inactivating yeast and spoilage bacteria, pasteurization, a gentle heat treatment that ranges from 60 to 90°C, extends the shelf life of beer, albeit it may marginally change its taste qualities (Milani & Silva, 2022; Nunes Filho et al., 2021).

6.2.1.5 Cider

Cider, also known as hard cider, is an alcoholic beverage produced through the fermentation of apple juice and undergoes three key stages. In autumn, ripe apples are crushed, followed by juice extraction through pressing. Fermentation lasts for weeks or months, with the cider typically bottled by late

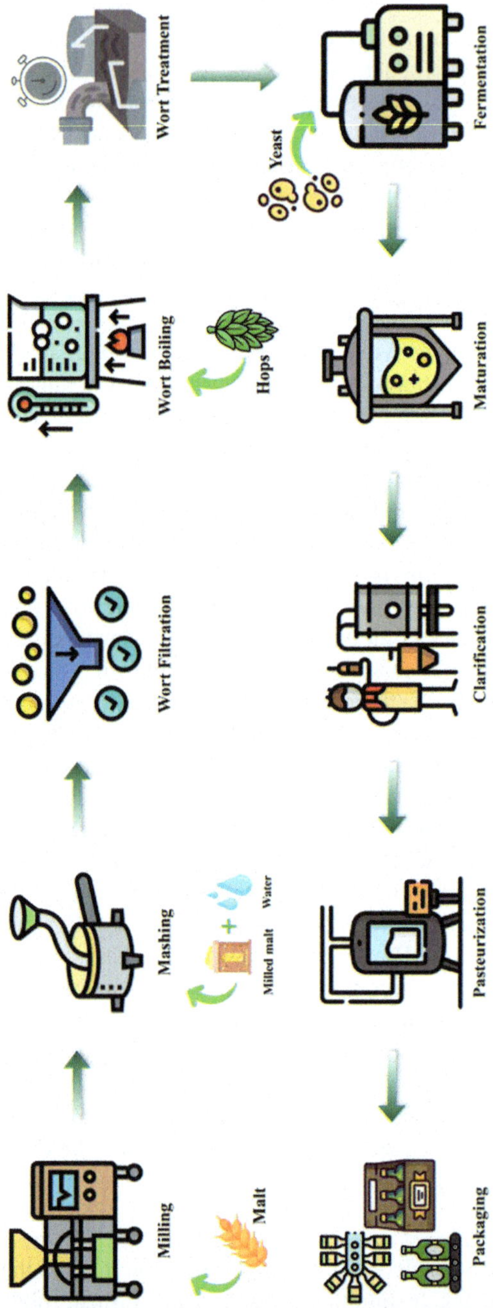

FIGURE 6.3

Basic steps of the beer-making process.

The icons illustrated in this figure were obtained from Flaticon.com.

winter. The UK is the leading cider producer, with the most popular variety being a clear, carbonated, and mildly flavored beverage. Typically sold in bottles or cans, this cider contains an alcohol content ranging from 1.2% to 8.5% ABV (Lea et al., 2013).

6.2.2 Steps involved in cider making

The choice of apples is a crucial phase in producing hard cider. Harvesting, sweating, washing, crushing, pressing, blending, testing, the process of fermentation, racking off, filtration or fining, bottling, and storing are some of the 12 steps Fig. 6.4 involved in making cider (Proulx & Nichols, 2003).

The quality of apple juice starts with proper harvesting techniques. Apples should be picked at peak maturity, which is determined by factors such as starch conversion, sugar levels (Brix), and firmness. Harvesting is finished manually or mechanically, depending on the orchard size and apple variety (Ibrahim et al., 2017). Proper timing ensures a balance of acidity and sweetness, which is essential for producing high-quality juice. Overripe apples may ferment prematurely, while under-ripe ones can result in excessive tartness. Research suggests that apples harvested at 13%–16% Brix produce the best juice quality (Janick et al., 2008). After harvesting, apples may undergo a process known as sweating, where they are stored for 1–2 weeks in a cool, dry area. This step enhances sugar concentration and aroma through enzymatic activity, improving juice yield and flavor complexity (Beech, 1972). Following sweating, the apples are washed to eliminate dirt and microbial contaminants, a step essential for maintaining the microbiological safety of the fermentation process. Then, apples are crushed into a fine pulp using mechanical mills. This process ruptures the cells to release the juice and allows for better polyphenol extraction (Beech, 1972).

The crushed apple pulp is then pressed to extract the juice. The method of pressing, whether traditional rack and cloth or modern hydraulic, can influence the tannin and phenolic content of the resulting juice, impacting the cider's flavor and astringency (Beech, 1972). After pressing, juice from different varieties of apple is often blended to balance sugar, acid, and tannin levels. Blending is a common practice in European and North American cider production to achieve stylistic consistency (Janick et al., 2008). Before fermentation begins, the juice is tested for pH, °Brix (sugar content), titratable acidity, and tannin levels. These parameters help cider makers determine potential alcohol content and ensure ideal fermentation conditions (Wang et al., 2024). Based on the results, adjustments may be made to achieve the desired flavor or yeast performance.

Fermentation is then initiated using wild/native yeasts or cultured strains such as *Saccharomyces cerevisiae*. Fermentation typically lasts 1–3 weeks at controlled temperatures (13–21°C), during which sugars are converted into C_2H_5OH and CO_2 (Wang et al., 2024). Secondary fermentation may follow to soften the cider and allow malolactic fermentation, which converts malic acid to lactic acid, reducing acidity and creating a smoother mouthfeel (Cousin et al., 2017). After fermentation, the cider is transferred from the fermentation vessel to separate it from the sediment or lees at the bottom. This step improves clarity and prevents off-flavors caused by yeast autolysis (Cousin et al., 2017). The cider can be further clarified and stabilized by fining or filtering. While fining agents like bentonite can bond with tannins or proteins to improve visual clarity and sensory quality, filtration eliminates suspended particles and yeasts (Cousin et al., 2017).

The finished cider is then bottled under hygienic conditions. It can be bottled still (noncarbonated) or sparkling, with carbonation introduced naturally (via bottle conditioning) or mechanically (force-

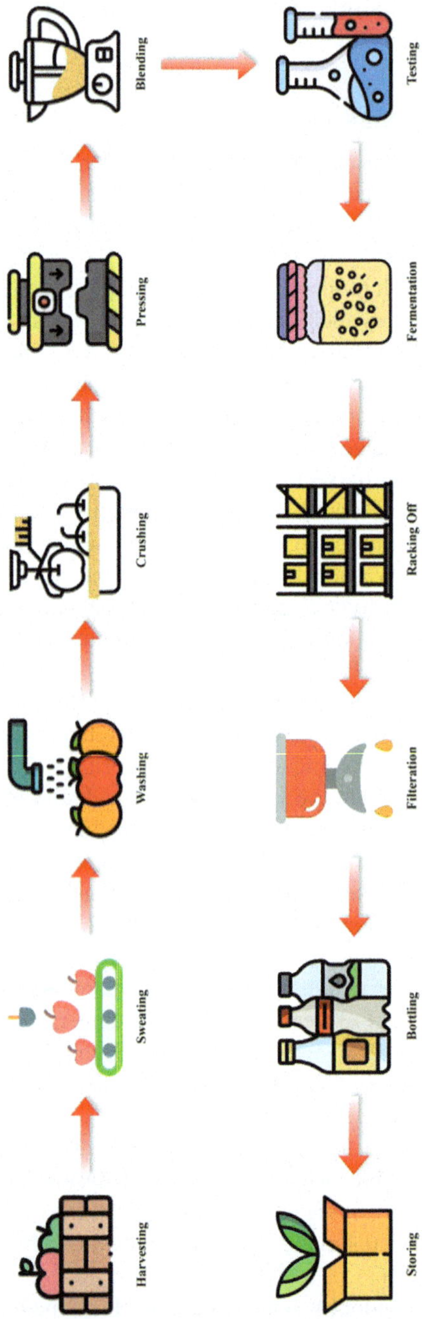

FIGURE 6.4

Basic steps of the cider-making process.

The icons illustrated in this figure were obtained from Flaticon.com.

carbonated). Lastly, the cider is stored in a cool, dark place. Short-term storage (1–3 months) is sufficient for young, fruity ciders, while more complex, tannic ciders benefit from longer aging (up to 6–12 months) to develop depth and complexity (Janick et al., 2008).

6.2.2.1 Perry

Perry is a fermented beverage made from pears, similar to cider. The pear varieties used in perry production typically have high tannin content and natural sugars ranging from 10%–15% Brix. Fermentation uses *Saccharomyces cerevisiae* strains at temperatures between 12–18°C, with an alcohol content usually ranging from 4%–8%. Traditional perry-making methods date back to the Middle Ages, particularly in England and France (cherry ripe, 2009).

6.2.2.2 Perry processing

The process begins with selecting, washing, and crushing ripe perry pears. The crushed fruit is then pressed to extract juice, which may undergo enzymatic treatment to improve clarity and enhance flavor release. Fermentation is carried out using either native wild yeasts or inoculated strains such as Saccharomyces cerevisiae. In some cases, a secondary malolactic fermentation is encouraged to reduce acidity and enrich the mouthfeel (Aparnna et al., 2024).

Following fermentation, the perry is clarified through racking and filtration, and then matured in stainless steel vessels or oak barrels to allow flavor development and stabilization. Depending on the desired final product, Perry may be bottled as a still beverage or undergo carbonation through natural secondary fermentation or forced carbonation. The finished perry is a well-balanced, aromatic beverage characterized by its soft effervescence, floral and fruity notes, and a refreshing acidity that reflects the unique chemical profile of the pears used (Aparnna et al., 2024).

6.2.2.3 Toddy

Toddy is the colloquial term for a fermented palm beverage in India. It is made by fermenting fresh sap from various palm tree species, including the palmyra, silver date, and coconut palms, all of which belong to the Arecaceae family. In India, toddy is a popular refreshing beverage and has sociocultural significance, particularly among ethnic groups (Das & Tamang, 2023a). The sap contains 10%–17% sugar and naturally ferments within 12–24 h due to wild yeasts, reaching alcohol levels of 4%–6% (Steinkraus, 2018). The fermentation process can be controlled or spontaneous, with temperature crucial to the final product quality.

6.2.2.4 Toddy processing

The production of toddy, a naturally fermented alcoholic beverage derived from palm sap, begins with the skilled activity of tapping the palm tree. A trained toddy tapper ascends the palm, typically a coconut or palm tree, and makes a small, well-placed incision near the upper portion of the trunk or at the base of the inflorescence, depending on regional practice and tree species (Das & Tamang, 2021). A hollow bamboo tube is inserted into this incision to serve as a conduit for the sap. The opposite end of the bamboo is positioned to drain into a clean, round-shaped earthen pot that is securely fastened to the tree. Over the course of several hours, fresh palm sap, locally referred to as *neera*, is collected drop by drop as it naturally exudes from the wound site (Das & Tamang, 2023b). Once sufficient sap has been gathered, the pot is brought down, and the raw sap is filtered through a fine-mesh strainer or muslin cloth to remove visible impurities such as plant particles, dust, or insects. The clarified sap is then transferred into a clean, preferably sterilized, container and left undisturbed at ambient room temperature to undergo spontaneous fermentation. This natural fermentation process typically lasts for 2–3 days and is initiated by indigenous microflora, primarily wild yeasts and lactic acid bacteria present in the environment and on the collection vessels (Prathiviraj et al., 2022). As fermentation progresses, these microorganisms metabolize the sugars in the sap, producing ethanol, carbon dioxide, and organic acids. The final product toddy is a mildly alcoholic beverage characterized by its slightly sweet, tangy flavor and gentle effervescence. It is traditionally consumed fresh due to its tendency to sour rapidly if left unrefrigerated or exposed to air for extended periods (Karamoko et al., 2019).

6.2.2.5 Mead

Mead is a traditional alcoholic beverage made when yeasts ferment diluted honey to produce alcohol with a volumetric alcoholic strength of 8% and 18%. In addition to being widely consumed in England, Germany, and the Baltic states, it is also a popular beverage in eastern Europe (Poland, Slovenia), particularly in African nations like South Africa and Ethiopia. Mead is still created by hand in Portugal using traditional and empirical methods. This alcoholic beverage is said to be the earliest that people have ever consumed, possibly even older than wine, and it was most likely the precursor of beer (Pereira et al., 2017). *Saccharomyces cerevisiae* is commonly used to ferment the honey sugars, typically around 80% fructose and glucose. Modern mead production has seen yeast selection and fermentation control innovations to enhance flavor complexity and stability (Sousa-Dias et al., 2021).

6.2.3 Mead processing

The production of mead involves three primary stages: preparation of the honey must, fermentation, and maturation. Each of these stages can be carried out using various techniques and modifications Fig. 6.5, all of which significantly impact the final product.

These variations can alter the physicochemical properties, the composition of volatile and phenolic compounds, and ultimately influence the sensory and organoleptic characteristics of the mead. The process begins with preparing the honey must, which involves diluting honey with water to achieve a suitable sugar concentration for fermentation. The type of honey selected is critical, as it contributes a unique set of aromatic and phenolic compounds depending on its floral source. For instance, linden and chestnut honeys have been shown to impart different flavors, with chestnut honey providing a fuller body but also greater bitterness due to higher levels of insoluble solids (Kuś et al., 2022; Vidrih & Hribar, 2007). The honey-to-water ratio, commonly ranging between 1:4 and 1:0.5, not only determines the potential alcohol content but also affects fermentation efficiency. A higher honey concentration often leads to sweeter, more alcoholic meads but can inhibit yeast activity if not properly balanced (Sroka & Tuszyński, 2007). Since honey is naturally low in nitrogen and other micronutrients essential for yeast metabolism, nutrient supplementation particularly with diammonium phosphate (DAP) is a common practice to enhance fermentation performance and prevent off-flavors or stalled fermentations (Pereira et al., 2015). Flavoring agents, such as fruits, grains, and certain spices, are sometimes added during this stage, which not only contribute to the sensory characteristics but may also serve as supplementary nutrient sources (Araújo et al., 2022). Another important but optional step is pasteurization or boiling of the must, which can eliminate wild microbes but also risk the loss of volatile aroma compounds and reduction in honey character due to heat-induced changes (Bednarek & Szwengiel, 2020; Kuś et al., 2022).

The next stage, fermentation, is where yeast converts the sugars in the must into ethanol and other metabolites. The choice of yeast species and strain has a significant impact on the mead's fermentation

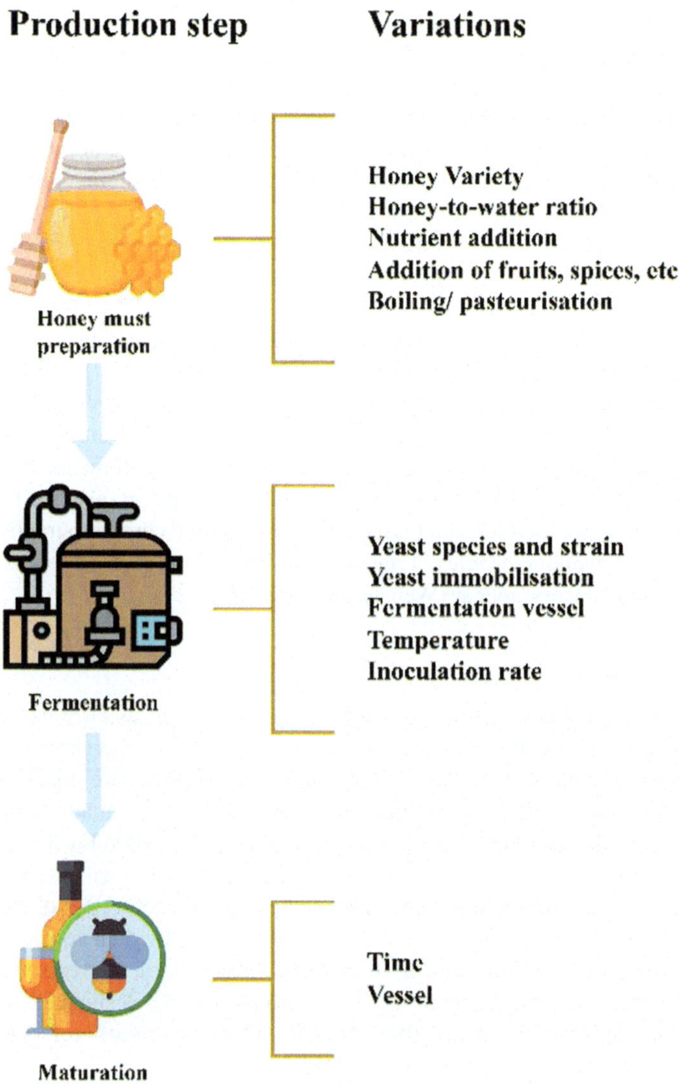

FIGURE 6.5

Mead production process, with examples of possible variations at each stage.

The icons illustrated in this figure were obtained from Flaticon.com.

kinetics and sensory profile. The yeast *Saccharomyces cerevisiae* is most commonly used due to its high C_2H_5OH and SO_2 tolerance, and ability to thrive in acidic conditions typical of mead (Lopes et al., 2020). Other yeast strains, including *S. bayanus* and probiotic yeasts like *S. boulardii*, are also explored for specific flavor profiles or health-related properties (de Souza et al., 2024). Yeast may be used in free form or immobilized, and inoculation rates can be varied to influence fermentation speed and aroma compound production (Pereira et al., 2013, 2014). Fermentation conditions such as temperature, vessel type, and oxygen exposure are also critical. Warmer temperatures speed up fermentation but can also increase unwanted by-products like volatile acidity (Gomes et al., 2013). The process can be terminated early through filtration, sulfite addition, or chilling to retain residual sugars and produce sweeter meads (Ramalhosa et al., 2011).

Once fermentation is done, mead undergoes maturation and stabilization. It is usually racked to separate it from spent yeast (lees), and then aged to develop flavor complexity and reduce harshness. Aging can last from a few months to over a year, and may occur in stainless steel vessels, bottles, or oak barrels. Oak aging, especially with chips or staves, has been shown to enhance phenolic content and antioxidant activity (Fortes et al., 2023). Pasteurization or chemical stabilization methods like sulfur dioxide addition are employed to ensure microbial stability, especially if back-sweetening with honey is applied post-fermentation (Pascoal et al., 2019). In some cases, a secondary fermentation is induced to create sparkling mead.

Quality control throughout production is essential to prevent faults and ensure product consistency. Common issues include microbial spoilage, nutrient deficiency-induced off-flavors, and excessive formation of 5-hydroxymethylfurfural (HMF), a heat-induced compound with possible carcinogenic properties (Chen et al., 2013; Kahoun et al., 2017). Though rare, methanol formation (if fruit is used) and the presence of *Clostridium botulinum* spores in raw honey are also concerns, although the alcohol and acidic conditions in mead generally prevent botulism risk in adults (Harder et al., 2021). Analytical techniques such as gas chromatography (GC) and high-performance liquid chromatography (HPLC) are used to assess the volatile and phenolic profiles of meads, which are closely tied to aroma, flavor, antioxidant properties, and overall sensory appeal (Webster et al., 2025).

6.2.4 Distilled alcoholic beverage

Distillation is the process of extracting greater alcohol from fermented beverages using heat to evaporate and then condense it, raising the alcohol content. In essence, distillation increases the alcohol concentration of a liquid. Spirits, including vodka, brandy, rum, and whiskey, are aqueous ethanol solutions produced by this technique. While these alcoholic beverages can be made from various source materials, they all use a similar manufacturing process to obtain a high ABV. Each type of liquor is made in three stages: enzymes are used to break down basic materials, fermentation transforms carbohydrates into ethanol, and distillation isolates and purifies the alcohol. After distillation, the finishing procedure varies based on the spirit type and the distiller's individual formula. Each liquor category is subject to stringent rules, and failing to achieve these criteria prevents the product from being marketed under that specific designation. For example, to be designated as "vodka," the ethanol must be distilled to at least 190 proofs (95% ethanol). The term "proof" refers to the alcoholic strength of the finished product (Besse & Dechaine, 2014).

6.2.4.1 Spirits

Distilled spirits are alcoholic beverages made by fermenting and distilling carbohydrate-rich raw materials like grains, fruits, or sugary components. Fermentation is the first step in the production process, during which yeast turns sugars into ethanol and other byproducts that contribute to the scent and flavor of the spirit. This fermented liquid normally has 8%–12% alcohol before being distilled, which concentrates and refines the alcohol's taste. Distillation is done with either pot stills or column stills. Pot stills work in batches and retain more congeners flavor compounds that contribute to the complexity of the spirit while column stills allow for continuous distillation and higher purity, producing a cleaner, more neutral spirit (Black & Walker, 2023). The production of spirits distilled alcoholic beverages relies on a precise combination of fermentation and distillation to concentrate ethanol and develop complex flavors. Unlike beer or wine, spirits have a higher alcohol content and distinct sensory profiles, shaped by both traditional techniques and modern innovations. The process begins with selecting raw materials such as grains (barley, rye, corn), fruits, potatoes, or sugarcane, each contributing unique flavor traits. Rye, for example, is valued for its robustness and spicy character, especially in traditional Polish distillates (Black & Walker, 2023). Preparation involves converting starches into fermentable sugars through malting and mashing for grains, or pressing for fruits. The sugary solution wort or must is then fermented with yeast, transforming sugars into ethanol and influencing aroma based on factors like temperature, pH, and yeast strain (Douady et al., 2019).

After fermentation, distillation separates and concentrates ethanol. Pot stills are often used for spirits like whiskey and brandy, while column stills suit high-efficiency vodka production. Advanced systems like pervaporation membranes offer cleaner separation and energy savings (Douady et al., 2019). During fractional distillation, only the "hearts" are retained for quality, while the "heads" and "tails," containing unwanted compounds, are discarded.

Flavor refinement continues during distillation, carefully managing volatile compounds like esters and aldehydes. Cognac distillation research, for instance, highlights how heat control preserves these aroma compounds (Douady et al., 2019). Aging in oak barrels further matures the spirit, contributing flavors like vanillin and tannins. Factors like barrel age and size affect this evolution (Alcarde et al., 2014).

Post-aging steps include filtration to improve clarity and blending to ensure consistency. Master blenders combine batches of different ages or origins to meet flavor standards. The final spirit is diluted to 35%–50% ABV and bottled, with packaging playing a key role in branding. Throughout, rigorous testing ensures safety, quality, and compliance (Black & Walker, 2023).

6.2.4.2 Tequila

Tequila is a Mexican distilled alcoholic beverage made exclusively from the blue agave plant (*Agave tequilana* Weber var. azul) (Hobbs, 2023). The procedure starts with collecting mature agave plants, usually 5–7 years old. Skilled jimadores remove the leaves to obtain the heart, or piña. Piñas are roasted in stone ovens or autoclaves, converting inulin into fermentable sugars. The cooked agave is crushed to remove the sweet fluid, called mosto, which is then fermented with yeast, most often *Saccharomyces cerevisiae*. The choice of yeast has a major impact on the synthesis of volatile taste components such as esters and higher alcohols, as demonstrated in studies on yeast strain selection in agave fermentation (Arellano et al., 2008; Lachance, 1995). After fermentation, ethanol and other necessary flavoring ingredients are purified and concentrated by repeated distillation of the liquid. Tequila is divided into four categories based on how long it is kept in oak barrels: Blanco (unaged), Reposado (2–11 months), Añejo (1–3 years), and Extra Añejo (beyond 3 years). Tequila's elemental composition, particularly the amounts of metals like calcium, magnesium, copper, and zinc, has been utilized as a quality and authenticity indicator in addition to fermentation and aging, as shown by analytical studies employing inductively coupled plasma optical emission spectrometry. The unique profile and regulatory integrity of genuine tequila are influenced by a combination of these chemical processes (Ceballos-Magaña et al., 2009).

6.2.4.3 Vodka

Vodka is a clear, high-purity distilled alcoholic beverage that typically contains approximately 40% ABV. It is originally prepared from grains, potatoes, or sugar beets, which are fermented before distillation. Although vodka is frequently described as neutral in taste, it can include trace amounts of natural chemicals that influence its flavor and scent. The raw ingredients utilized, as well as the distillation and filtration procedures, account for these slight variances. Activated carbon is widely used to filter vodka and eliminate impurities, making it smoother. Even if they contain the same amount of alcohol, different vodka brands may have slightly different flavors. The number of distillations often determines the vodka's smoothness and purity. Ingredients like fruit, herbs, or spices are used to flavor some vodkas. Vodka has a lengthy history and cultural significance in Russia and Eastern Europe, where it is most popular. Vodka's quality and character are dependent on careful production choices, despite its straightforward look (Wiśniewska et al., 2015).

6.2.4.4 Gin

Gin is a distilled alcoholic beverage that originated in Europe. It is typically flavored with juniper berries and has evolved into numerous kinds and brands over time. To achieve its characteristic flavor profile, modern gin is made by redistilling neutral grain alcohol with a blend of botanicals such as herbs, spices, and fruits. Chemical investigations have revealed important components in gin, including monoterpenes and terpenoids, that contribute to its aroma and flavor. Recent research utilizing ultrahigh-resolution mass spectrometry has discovered that each gin has distinct chemical fingerprints, which aid in quality control and authenticity verification (Dou et al., 2023). Gin became popular in England during the "Gin Craze" of the 18th century, resulting in social concerns and subsequent regulatory measures such as the Gin Act of 1751 (Gately, 2008). In modern times, the worldwide gin market is expanding, driven by customer interest in premium and flavored gins, particularly among younger generations. Gin production innovations include using sustainable ingredients like peas to lessen environmental impact. When drunk in moderation, Gin's possible health advantages are ascribed to the antioxidants found in juniper berries. Overall, gin remains a flexible and dynamic spirit reflecting its rich history and contemporary innovations (Dou et al., 2023).

6.2.4.5 Whiskey

Whiskey (or whisky, depending on the country of origin) is a distilled spirit derived from fermented grains and matured in wooden barrels. The aging process imparts diverse tastes like vanilla, caramel, spice, and smoke. Whiskey is classified according to its components, distillation methods, and geographical origins. Scotch whisky, created mostly from malted barley, is recognized for its smoky and peaty flavors, whilst Irish whiskey is usually triple-distilled for a smoother profile. Bourbon (made from at least 51% maize and matured in new charred oak barrels) and rye whiskey (produced from at least 51% rye and has a spicier flavor) are two types of American whiskey. Japanese whisky, influenced by Scotch, is renowned worldwide for its accuracy and workmanship (Narula, 2019; Russell & Stewar, 2003).

6.2.4.6 Brandy

Brandy is a distilled alcoholic beverage manufactured mostly from fermented grape juice, but other fruits such as apples and pears can also be used. It typically contains between 35% and 60% ABV. Brandy is frequently aged in oak barrels, giving it a deep amber color and smooth, subtle flavors. The term "brandy" is derived from the Dutch term brandewijn, which means "burnt wine," and refers to the distillation process. Cognac and Armagnac are well-known brands of brandy from various regions of France. The aging process is critical to the development of brandy's scent and flavor, with older brandies typically being smoother. Brandy is typically consumed neat, in cocktails, or as a digestif. Its flavor is usually warm, fruity, and slightly sweet. The production method, which includes the type of fruit, fermentation, distillation, and barrel aging, has a significant impact on final quality. Brandy plays an important role in traditional and artisanal spirits worldwide (Dhiman & Attri, 2011).

6.2.4.7 Rum

Rum is a sugarcane-based alcohol created by fermenting and distilling sugarcane juice or molasses. It originated in the Caribbean, and it is still the dominant spirit. Rum's flavor varies widely depending on production methods and aging. White rums are light and crisp, and are commonly used in cocktails such as mojitos and daiquiris, but dark rums are aged longer, creating deep tastes of caramel, spice, and wood. Tropical climates favor overproof rums, which frequently approach 50% ABV. Some high-end rums use a solera aging procedure, like sherry, to blend younger and older spirits for consistency (Qian et al., 2019).

6.2.4.8 Soju

Soju is the most well-known and popular Korean spirit. In Korea, "soju" refers to both distilled and diluted liquor. The process of producing diluted soju was created during the Japanese colonial period in response to liquor taxation restrictions (Kwon et al., 2023). According to a market strategy analysis on alcoholic beverages in Korea, diluted soju controls the local liquor market. In 2021, it accounted for USD 3096 million, or 40.1% of the overall market, trailing only beer at 41.0%. In comparison, traditional liquors accounted for only 1.1% of the market. Its market share grew from KRW 40.0 billion to KRW 94.2 billion (0.43%–1.07%) between 2017 and 2021. Notably, distilled soju accounted for 11.4% of traditional liquor sales, and its value increased from KRW 33.2 billion to KRW 64.6 billion (Hwang et al., 2024). This expansion has been aided by an increase in the number of distilled soju manufacturing licenses from 64 to 152 enterprises over the same time period (Hwang et al., 2024).

6.3 Chemical composition and potential contaminants

6.3.1 Common ingredients in alcoholic beverages

Alcoholic beverages are made with various raw components, contributing to their flavor, aroma, and overall personality. Fermentable sugars or starches are the fundamental constituents, and they ferment to make ethanol. Grains, including barley, corn, rye, wheat, rice, and sorghum, are often used in beer, whiskey, and vodka, and their starches must be broken down into fermentable sugars through enzymatic conversion (Bamforth, 2009; Russell & Stewart, 2014). Grapes, apples, plums, cherries, and pears are natural sugar sources for fermentation and are used to make wine, brandy, cider, and fruit-based liqueurs (Soni et al., 2021, pp. 67–98; Waterhouse et al., 2024). Rum and cachaça are made from sugarcane and molasses, whereas mead and certain liqueurs use honey to provide floral and nuanced flavors (Bogdanov et al., 2008). Furthermore, agave plants are the primary ingredient in tequila and mezcal, providing a particular character derived from their natural sugars (López-Alvarez et al., 2012).

Water is essential to all alcoholic beverages, acting as the principal solvent during fermentation and distillation. Water's mineral composition can considerably impact flavor, especially in beer and spirits (De Keukeleire, 2000). Another key component is yeast, which is in charge of turning carbohydrates into alcohol and carbon dioxide. Saccharomyces cerevisiae, the most prevalent strain, is commonly utilized in beer, winemaking, and spirit distillation (Fleet, 2003). Still, wild yeasts and bacteria contribute to spontaneous fermentations in lambic beers, sour ales, and traditional spirits like baijiu. Enzymes and microbial starters are used in addition to yeast to help with fermentation (Kitagaki & Kitamoto, 2013).

Beyond the main components, various additives improve the flavor profile of alcoholic beverages. Hops are utilized in beer to offer bitterness, aroma, and preservation, whereas botanicals like juniper berries, coriander, wormwood, and anise define spirits like gin and absinth (Neve, 1991). Spices such as cinnamon, clove, nutmeg, and vanilla enhance the flavor of spiced rums, flavored whiskeys, and herbal liqueurs. Aging in oak barrels is also important, adding aromas of vanilla, caramel, and smoke to spirits such as whiskey, brandy, and aged rum (Russell & Stewar, 2003). Sweeteners such as sugar, maple syrup, and caramel are also used in liqueurs and flavored spirits to balance and enhance their flavor. These components and techniques, combined, define the vast spectrum of alcoholic beverages consumed around the world (Guth, 1997).

6.3.2 Types of contaminants

The problem of chemical contaminants that are either present where they shouldn't be or found at quantities above permissible limits must be addressed in order to ensure food safety, as it is with all items intended for human consumption. Any food safety violation might have detrimental effects on one's health, both now and in the future. Consequently, it is crucial to recognize and reduce these matters (Rather et al., 2017).

The International Agency for Research on Cancer (IARC) monographs describe alcohol contaminants as small components that are "not necessary to the flavors or properties of a product" but admit that some may offer toxicological or carcinogenic hazards (IARC Working Group on the Evaluation of Carcinogenic Risks to Humans & International Agency for Research on Cancer, 2010). Unlike most foods, alcoholic beverages pose a low risk of microbial contamination. Their high acidity, polyphenol content, and alcohol levels naturally hinder pathogen growth by providing limited nutrients for microbial survival (Azevedo et al., 2016). As a result, the main issue with alcohol contamination is chemical risks, which can occur during any phase of manufacture, storage, or as unintended by-products of chemical or microbiological activities. Even though a lot of research has been done on identifying and quantifying these contaminants, it is still difficult to determine the precise stage at which they enter. Table 6.1 represents a condensed list of the contaminants that have been found, along with their potential sources.

The majority of samples in a 1980 moonshine study in Georgia had toxic levels of heavy metals; several samples had arsenic, with one sample having a dangerously high concentration of 415 μg/L (safe limit: 10 μg/L); most samples had copper levels that were up to 14 times higher than the safe limit (1000 μg/L); more than half of the samples had lead, some with extremely high levels; two samples had elevated zinc, one exceeding the 5000 μg/L safety threshold; and the alcohol content was the same in all samples (Gerhardt et al., 1980). In contrast to the contamination found in Georgia moonshine, commercial Rakı showed much safer chemical profiles. Ethyl carbamate was absent, and furfural levels ranged from undetectable to 3.97 mg/L (well below the 50 mg/L limit). Ethanol and methanol levels met legal standards, except in a few counterfeit samples. Arsenic was found only in two samples at negligible levels (0.018 and 0.022 mg/L). Copper ranged from 0.046 to 0.414 mg/L (limit: 5 mg/L), lead was at ppb levels, and zinc ranged from 0.01 to 0.39 mg/L (limit: 5 mg/L) (Menevseoglu & Cabaroglu, 2021). Acetaldehyde (AA) levels ranged from 0.033 mg/L (soft drinks) to 55.6 mg/L

Table 6.1 List of different contaminants detected in alcohol products.

Contaminants	Contaminants concentrations	Products	References
Zinc (Zn)	>5000 μg/L	Moonshine	Gerhardt et al. (1980)
Copper (Cu)	2100–14,000 μg/L		
Arsenic (As)	415 μg/L.x		
Arsenic (As)	0.02 mg/L	Turkish Rakı	Menevseoglu and Cabaroglu (2021)
Copper (Cu)	0.05–0.41 mg/L		
Lead (Pb)	0.03 mg/L		
Zinc (Zn)	0.01–0.39 mg/L		
Acetaldehyde (AA)	29.4 mg/L	Grappa	Ioannidou et al. (2016)
	17.1 mg/L	Tsipouro	
	6.8 mg/L	Beer	
	3.7 mg/L	Red wine	
	7.2 mg/L	Retsina	
DEHP(Di(2-Ethylhexyl) phthalate)	10–300 ng/mL	Vodka, rum, whiskey, whisky, gin, and brandy	He et al. (2024)
DEHA(Di(2ethylhexyl) adipate)	0.7–95 ng/mL		
BBZP(Butyl benzyl phthalate)	11–14 ng/mL	Randy	
Aflatoxin	1.8–6.8 μg/L	Maize beers	Okaru et al. (2017)
Copper (Cu)	0.936 mg/L	Local dry gin	Okafor et al. (2022)
Iron (Fe)	0.075 mg/L	Imported red wine	
Lead (Pb)	0.078 mg/L	Local dry gin	

(tsipouro). High levels were found in grappa (37 mg/L), tsipouro (22 mg/L), and red wine (9 mg/L), while soft drinks (0.056 mg/L) and mineral water (0.06 mg/L) had the lowest. Beers with higher alcohol had more AA—6.8 mg/L at 9% versus 2.9 mg/L at 4.9%. Storing retsina in plastic raised AA from 7.2 to 66.8 mg/L (Ioannidou et al., 2016). Seven plasticizers were detected, with DEHP and DEHA most common (in 16/37 samples). DEHP ranged from 10 to 300 ng/mL; DEHA, 13–95 ng/mL. BBzP was only in Brandy; DEP in eight samples (He et al., 2024). Heavy metal analysis of alcoholic beverages showed Cd (>0.01 mg/L) and Cr (>0.05 mg/L) exceeded limits in IDG (Imported Dry Gin), LDG (Local Dry Gin), and Wine. Cu (0.936 mg/L) and Fe (0.075 mg/L) were highest in LDG and IRW (Imported Red Wine). Pareto analysis highlighted Cu and Zn as dominant metals (80%–92%, 82%–90%). Cd and Cr were major contaminants; others were minimal. Pollution Load Index (PLI <1) indicated no pollution, though HI > 1 for H (1.48) and PW (1.89) suggests potential health risks (Okafor et al., 2022). Aflatoxin levels ranged 1.8–6.8 mg/L (mean 3.5), with 500 mL exposure at 0.015–0.057 mg/kg bw (mean 0.030), MOE 15–58 (Okaru et al., 2017). The validated method showed high accuracy (95.1%–105.3%), precision (%RSD 0.80–4.56), and sensitivity (LODs 0.01–0.16 ppb, LOQs 0.10–1.6 ppb). In 32 homemade samples, metals were detected in ppb ranges: Al (7.05–253.30), Cr (22.78–52.10), Mn (3.44–69.58), Co (0.11–2.38), Cu (3.92–82.50), Zn (30.88–350.06), Pb (0.26–52.29). One sample (SKK) exceeded the aluminum limit (253.60 ppb), five exceeded lead limits. Commercial samples contained only Cu (9.02–15.3) and Zn (3.21–10.2) (Tsenang et al., 2023). Mycotoxins were found in all beer and 88% of wine samples. AOH was most frequent in beer (90%, 19.39 μg/L) and wine (52%), while PAT and β-ZAL had the highest concentrations (up to 43.18 μg/L in beer, 25.86 μg/L in wine). OTA dominated in cava (80%, 1.36 μg/L); cider showed high β-ZAL (61.48 μg/L). Co-occurrence appeared in 45% of beer, 38% of wine, and 60% of cava (Carballo et al., 2021).

6.4 Microbiological safety: Managing contamination risks

Alcoholic beverage microbiological safety is essential for both product quality and customer health. The sourcing of raw materials, fermentation, and storage are only a few of the industrial processes where microbial contamination can occur. While some microorganisms are helpful for fermentation, undesired molds, bacteria, and wild yeasts can cause spoiling, change sensory qualities, and compromise safety. Recent improvements in microorganism detection and control remedies have raised the standard for alcoholic beverage safety.

6.4.1 Types of microbial contaminants in alcoholic beverages

Microbial contamination in alcoholic beverages can occur from a variety of sources, such as raw materials, fermentation vessels, and post-fermentation storage conditions. The most popular contaminants are:

Bacteria: The production of alcoholic beverages may be affected by certain bacteria, including *Lactobacillus*, *Acetobacter*, *Pediococcus* and *Gluconobacter.* At the same time, some lactic acid bacteria genera like *Pediococcus* and *Lactobacillus* may endure in the alcoholic and acidic environments of beverages. The quality of the beverage may be compromised by their growth, which could lead to haze formation, unpleasant tastes, and increased acidity. Because they can outcompete desired yeast strains under less-than-ideal conditions, these bacteria can be particularly problematic in the production of wine and beer.

Acetic acid bacteria species such as *Acetobacter* and *Gluconobacter* oxidize ethanol to acetic acid, causing the beverage to sour. They are notorious for contaminating wine and beer, particularly when exposed to oxygen during production or storage (Torres-Guardado et al., 2022).

Molds can contaminate alcoholic beverages through ingredients like fruits and grains or inappropriate storage conditions, posing health risks. Mycotoxin-producing molds such as *Aspergillus*, *Penicillium*, and *Fusarium* species create harmful secondary metabolites, especially ochratoxin A, which can be nephrotoxic to humans (O'Brien & Dietrich, 2005). Mycotoxin contamination of raw materials has been reported in wine and beer production, notably in poorly preserved grains and grapes (Mateo et al., 2007; Pietri et al., 2001).

Wild yeast strains (*Saccharomyces cerevisiae*) are required for controlled fermentation; wild yeasts like *Brettanomyces* can induce unwanted sensory alterations in wine and beer, such as excessive phenolic and barnyard-like odors (Agnolucci et al., 2017). Wild yeast contamination can be difficult to handle, necessitating stringent sanitation and yeast management techniques.

6.4.2 The importance of controlling fermentation and storage conditions

The biochemical process of making alcoholic beverages is extremely complex and requires exact control over a wide range of factors to ensure that the final product satisfies requirements for safety, quality, and sensory appeal. The two most important phases in this process are fermentation and storage, both of which are crucial in establishing the beverage's chemical makeup, organoleptic properties, and general stability. In order to preserve product consistency, reduce spoilage, and enhance the unique characteristics that set apart various beverage categories, including wine, cider, spirits, and beer, these steps must be carefully managed.

The metabolic process known as fermentation, which is mostly carried out by *Saccharomyces cerevisiae* and related species are essential for the production of alcohol as well as a variety of flavor-active substances. Temperature, pH, nutrient concentration, oxygen availability, and the type of yeast used all have a substantial impact on the rate and completeness of sugar conversion as well as the makeup of secondary metabolites that are produced during fermentation (Pires et al., 2014). For example, high fermentation temperatures can speed up the metabolism of yeast, which increases the production of esters and fusel alcohols, which can give the beverage a solvent-like or too fruity flavor (Ribereau-Gayon et al., 2006). Overly low temperatures, on the other hand, may cause slow or incomplete fermentation, leaving residual sugars in the finished product. This could cause instability and inadvertent refermentation in packaged goods. Because different strains of yeast have varying capacities for producing higher alcohols, esters, organic acids, and sulfur-containing compounds, the choice of strain further influences the beverage's flavor and aroma (Mendes Ferreira & Mendes-Faia, 2020).

The significance of storage conditions increases after fermentation. Alcoholic beverages are especially vulnerable to environmental factors that might hasten unwanted chemical changes, including temperature, light, and oxygen exposure. For instance, oxidation can cause color browning, aldehyde formation, and the breakdown of fragrance components, all of which can result in stale or "cardboard" flavors (Mendes Ferreira & Mendes-Faia, 2020). The notorious "skunky" off-flavor in beer is caused by 3-methyl-2-butene-1-thiol, which is formed when hopderived chemicals undergo a photochemical reaction in beer exposed to light, particularly ultraviolet light (Bamforth, 2023). In addition to being bad for flavor, these reactions can diminish shelf life and lower consumer approval. Long-term development is influenced by storage conditions during the prolonged maturing process that some beverage types most notably wines and spirits go through. In barrel-aged spirits, the contact with wood introduces a range of taste components such as vanillin, tannins, and lactones, while in wines, slow oxidation and esterification processes during aging contribute to complexity and mouthfeel (Jackson, 2008). Temperature, barrel type, humidity, and even airflow must all be carefully regulated during this aging process in order to produce the ideal product profile. Over-oaked, imbalanced, or oxidized items that don't satisfy sensory requirements can be the result of improper conditions.

From a production perspective, strict regulation of fermentation and storage conditions improves operational effectiveness as well as product quality. It decreases waste, lowers batch variability, and facilitates adherence to legal requirements for food safety and labeling. Furthermore, the necessity for processing precision increases as customers expect beverages with natural components, consistent flavor, and few additives (Pretorius, 2000).

6.5 Analytical techniques for quality assurance

Alcohol, specifically ethyl alcohol or ethanol, is a colorless and flammable liquid primarily used in alcoholic beverages, which are produced through the fermentation of sugars from grains, fruits, and other starches (Wardencki, 2018). Its substantial socio-cultural relevance in many countries is highlighted by the fact that the worldwide alcoholic beverage business was valued at over $1 trillion in 2018 and is expected to rise by 3% over the next 5 years (Tabago et al., 2021). The three primary categories of alcoholic beverages are wines, spirits, and beers. The alcohol concentration of these beverages varies and is commonly expressed as ABV (Wardencki, 2018). The alcohol content in these beverages can range from 1% to 76% ABV, with beverages above 76% classified as medicines (Wardencki, 2018). The determination of alcohol content is crucial for quality assurance and regulatory compliance in the production of alcoholic beverages, employing various analytical methods for accuracy (Spedding, 2016). The quality assurance of alcohol products is a critical aspect of the beverage industry, ensuring that alcoholic beverages meet both consumer expectations and regulatory standards. Analytical techniques such as distillation, gas chromatography, and machine learning regression models play pivotal roles in assessing alcohol content and detecting contaminants (Manual_Alcoholic_Beverages, 2019; Wardencki, 2018). Moreover, rigorous quality assurance programs are essential for maintaining the integrity of alcohol testing, particularly in breath-alcohol analysis (Anghel, 2025). The use of standardized methods, as outlined by organizations like the International Organisation of Vine and Wine (OIV), further ensures uniformity in testing procedures across different regions (Methods of analysis for spirituous beverages and alcohols | OIV, 2025). By leveraging these techniques and standards, producers can optimize production processes and enhance product quality, ultimately contributing to consumer satisfaction and compliance with regulatory requirements (Methods of analysis for spirituous beverages and alcohols | OIV, 2025).

6.5.1 Chromatographic techniques

The schematic illustrates the diverse analytical methods employed for both the qualitative and quantitative assessment of significant compounds found in beer and its primary ingredients. Key analytes, including proteins, carbohydrates, polyphenols, bitter acids, and both volatile and nonvolatile compounds, are systematically organized in Fig. 6.6, along with the relevant analytical techniques used for their identification and quantification. Some of these methods include mass spectrometry (MS), gas chromatography (GC), high-performance liquid chromatography (HPLC), and spectrophotometry (Anderson, Santos *et al.*, 2019). Gas chromatography is an important technique for analyzing volatile substances in alcoholic drinks. The headspace solid-phase microextraction-gas chromatography-barrier discharge ionization detector (HS-SPME-GC-BID) method is commonly used for beverages like cachaça and whisky. This technique improves measurement accuracy by eliminating solvent interference. It also achieves low detection limits, with limits of detection (LOD) ranging from 0.26 to 0.51 mg/L and limits of quantification (LOQ) from 0.78 to 1.55 mg/L. The recovery rates fall between 81.24% and 106.94% (Oliveira do Nascimento et al., 2022). Gas chromatography-olfactometry (GC-O) is a method that combines sensory analysis to assess both good and bad odor compounds. It aids in quality control when choosing raw materials and during fermentation and aging processes. This process includes techniques like solvent extraction, headspace analysis, and SPME isolation (Plutowska & Wardencki, 2008).

GC-BID and GC-MS techniques are used for precise analysis of volatile compounds. They help HPLC-DAD identify aging indicators like acetaldehyde and furfural (Nascimento, 2023). Sophisticated gas chromatography techniques, such as GC $\times$ GC-HRTOF-MS and enantioselective GC $\times$ GC-MS/FID, improve the classification and authentication of alcoholic drinks. This is especially true when used alongside chemometric methods like Principal Component Analysis (PCA) and Hierarchical Cluster Analysis (HCA) (Koljančić et al., 2024).

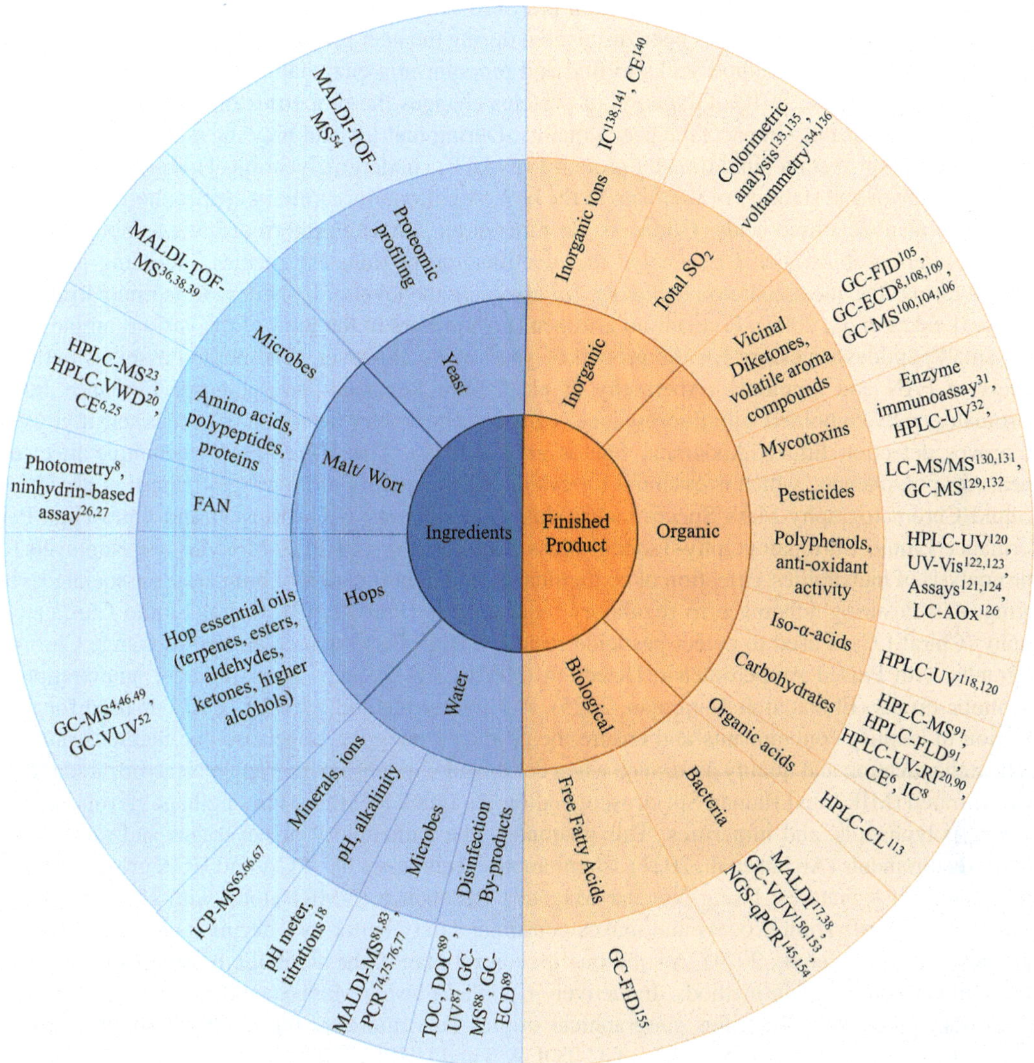

FIGURE 6.6

Overview of analytical methods for identifying key compounds in beer and its ingredients.

Figure reproduced from the work by Anderson, H. E., Santos, I. C., Hildenbrand, Z. L., Schug, K. A., (2019). A review of the analytical methods used for beer ingredient and finished product analysis and quality control. Analytica Chimica Acta. 18734324. 1085, 1–20. https://doi.org/10.1016/j.aca.2019.07.061 with the permission of Elsevier.

High-Performance Liquid Chromatography (HPLC) and its newer versions are important for analyzing non-volatile compounds in alcoholic drinks. HPLC is often used to measure polyphenols, organic acids, and carbohydrates. Reducing matrix interference helps with precise quantification, especially when using refractive index (RI) and ultraviolet (UV) detectors. Researchers can analyze proteins, polypeptides, and amino acids found in beer using HPLC. In HPLC analyses at a wavelength of 265 nm, acid hydrolysis and derivatization prepared samples from various Indian rice brews (Das et al., 2014). Protein glycation has been discovered during the beer brewing process through "shotgun" analysis of HPLC. This method seeks to find and pinpoint non-enzymatic glycations in barley malt (Petry-Podgórska et al., 2010). Glycation of proteins changes the properties of malt and the foam in beer, which significantly impacts the beer's quality. During malting and brewing, key proteins such as Protein Z and non-specific lipid transfer protein 1 (ns-LTP1) undergo glycation. This process improves the overall flavor and stability of the foam in the beer. Additionally, capillary electrophoresis (CE) can be used to analyze amino acids (Cortacero-Ramirez et al., 2003). Furthermore, it was noted that the rapid separation abilities of CE enabled the identification of transient species, including particular protein forms. The most common technique for assessing the level of FAN in wort is ninhydrin-based assays (Lekkas et al., 2007). Free amino nitrogen (FAN) refers to the total of the various amino acids and small peptides necessary for the growth of yeast cells. However, this method assesses both the levels of FAN and ammonia (Abernathy et al., 2009). Reversed-phase high-performance liquid chromatography combined with fluorescence or mass spectrometry detection enhances sensitivity and improves detection limits (Anderson, Santos *et al.*, 2019). The HPLC-DAD technique precisely measures polyphenols, which is essential for evaluating the quality of beverages (Bharti et al., 2024). Liquid Chromatography-Mass Spectrometry/Mass Spectrometry (LC-MS/MS) and Ultra-High-Performance Liquid Chromatography-Tandem Mass Spectrometry (UHPLC-MS/MS) are employed for the analysis of metabolites, detection of contaminants, and identification of biomarkers associated with aging, thus ensuring adherence to regulatory requirements (Preti, 2019). Chiral Liquid Chromatography (Chiral LC) is used to detect pesticide residues. High-Performance Anion-Exchange Chromatography with Pulsed Amperometric Detection (HPAEC-PAD) helps identify sugar adulteration in alcoholic drinks (Elumalai & Natarajan, 2025). A different method, UHPLC-CAD, is used for verification to identify contaminants and ensure the product's integrity. Spectroscopic methods improve both authentication and quality assurance when combined with chromatography. Near-Infrared (NIR), Mid-Infrared (MIR), and Raman Spectroscopy allow for quick identification of ethanol levels, acidity, sugars, polyphenols, and impurities. This guarantees the authenticity of beverages and meets regulatory requirements (Arslan et al., 2021). Chemometric techniques like PCA and HCA group drinks by their chemical signatures. Using Nuclear Magnetic Resonance (NMR) along with chromatography improves the verification process and makes consumer safety better by offering a clearer analysis of composition (Bharti et al., 2024). A solid quality control plan in the alcoholic beverage industry uses different chromatographic methods. Inductively Coupled Plasma Mass Spectrometry (ICP-MS) analyzes trace elements and verifies geographical origin. This improves the quality assurance process (Preti, 2019). The combination of GC $\times$ GC-TOF-MS and UHPLC-HRMS enables a detailed analysis of volatile compounds. It distinguishes between different types of beverages and assists in metabolomic research. This enhances the detection of fraud and the evaluation of product quality (Preti, 2019). Gas chromatography-mass spectrometry (GC-MS) has proven effective for the detailed chemical analysis of alcoholic beverages. This method enabled the detection of key aging markers such as vanillin, syringaldehyde, and methyl octadecane in wines aged in oak barrels. It made it easier to verify aging methods and assess wood interaction. It also helped identify artificial flavoring agents like methyl anthranilate, dimethyl acrylate, and triacetin in lower quality and fruit wines. Additionally, it detected higher levels of preservatives such as sorbic and benzoic acids. These results highlight the importance of GC-MS for evaluating authenticity, identifying fraud, and ensuring safety and regulatory compliance in the analysis of alcoholic beverages (Savchuk et al., 2020). The use of specialized chromatographic and spectroscopic methods greatly improves quality assurance for alcoholic drinks. These methods verify authenticity, identify fraud, and assess contaminants. Combining gas and liquid chromatography with chemometric tools boosts product safety, helps meet regulations, and builds consumer trust. As technology progresses, these techniques will play a larger role in maintaining the integrity of alcoholic beverages. This ensures that both producers and consumers can trust the quality of the products available in the marketplace.

6.5.2 Spectroscopy techniques

The study of alcoholic beverages uses spectroscopic methods for quality control, authenticity, and composition assessment. Different spectroscopic techniques offer information on ethanol levels, product quality, and the identification of adulterants. Methods like Near-Infrared (NIR) spectroscopy play an important role in measuring ethanol, evaluating quality, and confirming authenticity. These methods are often combined with chemometric approaches to improve accuracy (Arslan et al., 2021; Fulgêncio et al., 2023). Mid-Infrared (MIR) and Fourier Transform Infrared (FTIR) spectroscopy are key techniques for studying ethanol, sugar compounds, and acids. They help identify fraud and determine where something comes from Arslan et al. (2021) and Lachenmeier (2007). MIR spectroscopy provides a molecular fingerprint analysis of polysaccharides, organic acids, and phenolic compounds in alcoholic drinks (Koljančić et al., 2024). Raman spectroscopy is an effective method for monitoring fermentation processes and identifying brands in whiskey production. Nuclear Magnetic Resonance (NMR) spectroscopy plays a key role in verifying authenticity and detecting fraud. Using fluorescence spectroscopy along with Electronic Nose and Electronic Tongue sensor technologies, as well as Colorimetric Sensor Arrays, is crucial for detecting adulterants like methanol and assessing aroma and volatile compounds. This aids in ensuring compliance with regulations (Arslan et al., 2021). UV-visible (UV-Vis) spectroscopy checks color consistency and oxidation states. This method helps keep the sensory and visual quality of wines and spirits (Bharti et al., 2024). Thermal Infrared Enthalpimetry (TIE) provides a cost-effective and efficient way to measure alcohol content in distilled drinks. It also lowers energy use and the need for solvents (Santos et al., 2019). Combining infrared (NIR, MIR) spectroscopy with UV-visible spectroscopy and sensor technologies allows for quick, non-destructive evaluations. These evaluations assist with quality control, meet regulations, and help prevent fraud (Heyman & Ebeler, 2017). The progress in spectroscopy significantly enhances the safety, authenticity, and overall quality of alcoholic beverages. Near-infrared spectroscopy (NIR), along with tools like iSPA-PLS and DD-SIMCA, provides a quick, solvent-free, and non-destructive option compared to traditional analytical methods. This approach greatly cuts down on the need for reagents and reduces waste while ensuring high accuracy in measuring alcohol content and density. It also classifies cachaça accurately based on its geographic origin. Using multivariate analysis boosts the reliability and strength of the models, making this method ideal for regular quality control and compliance with regulations in the alcoholic beverage industry. This case study illustrates how vibrational spectroscopy, combined with data analysis, guarantees product authenticity and enhances the traceability of regional spirits (Oliveira et al., 2023).

6.5.3 Physical and sensory analysis

Maintaining the quality of alcoholic drinks requires a combination of physical, chemical, and sensory evaluations. Different analytical methods, such as spectroscopy, chromatography, and chemometrics, are essential for assessing composition, confirming authenticity, and measuring consumer acceptance. Traditional techniques like distillation and pycnometry have been widely used for measuring density. However, Flow Thermal Infrared Enthalpimetry (TIE-F) offers a quicker alternative (Santos et al., 2019). In combination with spectroscopy, both densitometry and refractometry are important for analyzing, controlling quality, and verifying ethanol (Arslan et al., 2021). The physical examination measures different factors. These include alcohol concentration, which is determined using densitometry and refractometry. It also checks pH and acidity through titration and pH meters. For soluble solids, hydrometers and refractometers are used. Finally, color and clarity are evaluated with spectrophotometers and turbidimeters (Heyman & Ebeler, 2017). The quality of alcoholic beverages is assessed using descriptive sensory analysis. This method examines the visual aspects, aroma, flavor, and texture (Wardencki, 2018). Sophisticated tools that assist with sensory evaluation include Gas Chromatography (GC-O), Fourier Transform Infrared Spectroscopy (FTIR), and the Electronic Nose (e-nose). To analyze volatile and non-volatile compounds, methods such as Gas Chromatography (GC), High-Performance Liquid Chromatography (HPLC), and Mass Spectrometry (MS) are often used. Chemometric techniques improve the accuracy and reliability of these analyses (Heyman & Ebeler, 2017). Recent innovations use machine learning to improve quality evaluation. Support Vector Machines (SVM) have shown high accuracy in predicting beer quality based on its chemical and sensory characteristics (Dong et al., 2014). Accelerated storage evaluations predict sensory stability by simulating aging effects. This allows manufacturers to keep consumer approval over time (O'Sullivan, 2012, pp. 42–65). Research on fermented drinks, especially those made from pineapple byproducts, shows how the composition of the raw materials affects key sensory traits. These traits include mouthfeel, sweetness, and tartness (Sabino et al., 2023). Physical and sensory analysis methods are essential for evaluating alcoholic beverages. They offer valuable insights into quality and consumer appeal. For rum, sensory profiling was done using Quantitative Descriptive Analysis (QDA). Trained judges described the product based on its sensory traits, including aroma, taste, and mouthfeel. The analysis identified unique aromas like brown sugar, caramel, maple, vanilla, and smoky notes. It also showed a smooth, warming mouthfeel and a bitter flavor. These measurable sensations were important for spotting differences between samples and maintaining consistent product quality (Ickes & Cadwallader, 2017). The joint use of physical mapping and sensory analysis was demonstrated through Napping with Ultra-Flash Profiling (UFP) in assessing brandy. Evaluators arranged samples in a spatial format based on perceived similarities. They noted sensory characteristics such as color (e.g., dark gold, copper-tinged), aroma (e.g., chocolate, tobacco, herbaceous), and mouthfeel (e.g., oily, watery). This mix of visual mapping and descriptive profiling helped clearly distinguish between high-alcohol beverage samples. It illustrated how physical arrangement and sensory traits work together to improve product evaluation (Louw et al., 2013). Merging chemometric techniques with sensory and instrumental analyses can really improve the assessment of the quality of alcoholic beverages. Using analytical methods and machine learning models also improves quality control and increases consumer satisfaction.

6.5.4 Microbiological & toxicological assessments

Alcoholic beverages must undergo rigorous microbiological testing to maintain quality, ensure safety, and prevent spoilage. Studies indicate that raw materials and processing techniques influence microbial diversity in fermented alcoholic beverages (FABs). Among commercial FABs, including beer, fruit wine, refined rice wine, and yakju, micro brewed beer exhibited the highest microbial counts. *Bacillus cereus* was detected in 54.8% of samples, with aerobic plate counts reaching 3.5 log CFU/mL (Jeon et al., 2015). Similarly, Ethiopian Tella contained high levels of yeast (6.13–8.43 log CFU/mL) and lactic acid bacteria (LAB) (6.09–8.13 log CFU/mL). However, the presence of Enterobacteriaceae in early fermentation stages suggested contamination concerns (Nemo & Bacha, 2020). Traditional beverages such as Caxiri, a Brazilian cassava-based drink, were dominated by Saccharomyces cerevisiae, while Bacillus species and *Pediococcus acidilactici* were the predominant bacteria. Microbial activity in fermentation was evident through a pH drop from 4.76 to 3.15 and an ethanol increase to 83.9 g/L (Santos et al., 2019). Beyond fermentation, enteric bacteria, including *Enterococcus faecium* and *Pantoea conspicua*, were introduced via contaminated ice cubes. However, alcoholic and carbonated beverages significantly reduced microbial survival (Gaglio et al., 2017). Alcoholic beverages may also contain hazardous chemicals. Studies found high acetaldehyde concentrations in fruit-based liqueurs and grappa, reaching 499 mg/L (Jeon et al., 2015). Additionally, Chinese rice wines contained notable levels of ethyl carbamate, a toxic compound raising concerns over nutritional safety (Jeon et al., 2015). Detected in beer and wine, mycotoxins, such as aflatoxins and ochratoxin A, further contribute to toxicological risks (He & Bayen, 2020). Contaminants from plastic packaging and processing equipment also pose safety concerns. Phthalates were identified in alcoholic beverages, underscoring the need for stricter regulatory oversight (Nemo & Bacha, 2020). Heavy metals, including lead, cadmium, and arsenic, were detected in spirits, with cadmium levels ranging from 6 to 40 μg/L (Pflaum et al., 2016). Furthermore, ethyl carbamate concentrations in fruit spirits reached up to 22,000 μg/kg, presenting significant health risks (He & Bayen, 2020). While traditional beverages like Ethiopian Tella and Brazilian Caxiri contain beneficial microorganisms such as *Saccharomyces cerevisiae* and LAB, they may also harbor harmful enteric bacteria, particularly when contaminated ice is used (He & Bayen, 2020; Mulaw et al., 2025). Additionally, pectinase-producing bacteria during fermentation have been linked to methanol contamination, a severe microbiological hazard associated with poisoning incidents worldwide (Ohimain, 2016). To mitigate microbiological and toxicological risks, stringent quality control measures, improved fermentation methods, and stricter safety regulations are essential. Implementing enhanced microbiological testing, monitoring packaging materials, and refining production processes will help ensure the safety and quality of alcoholic beverages worldwide.

6.6 Regulatory frameworks and compliance

6.6.1 Standards of WHO for alcoholic beverages

The World Health Organization (WHO) classifies blood alcohol concentration (BAC) limits based on driver type, enforcing stricter rules for young and novice drivers. BAC limits vary across countries, ranging from ≤0.01 g/dL (zero tolerance) to ≤0.08 g/dL, with India setting the threshold at ≤0.03 g/dL for all drivers (Blood Alcohol Concentration (BAC) limit for drivers, 2025). Excise taxes on alcohol are implemented in 148 countries, though 22 exempt wines. Beer and wine are typically taxed by volume, while spirits are taxed based on alcohol content. The median excise tax share is 13.4% for beer and 24.8% for spirits. However, only 23.1% of countries adjust alcohol taxes for inflation, and 21 nations earmark tax revenues for health initiatives. Despite its effectiveness in reducing alcohol-related harm, taxation remains an underutilized tool (Global report on the use of alcohol taxes. (2023)).

Public alcohol consumption is regulated in many countries through restrictions such as bans on drinking in streets, parks, and beaches unless within designated areas. Open container laws are strictly enforced in countries like the U.S. but are more relaxed in Germany. Drinking is often prohibited on public transport, and strict drunk driving laws are upheld. Legal drinking ages also vary, with India setting it at 18 and the U.S. at 21. Some exceptions permit public drinking during festivals or in licensed zones (Restrictions on alcohol use in public places, 2018).

As of 2016, 80 countries (46%) had a written national alcohol policy, with higher adoption rates in high-income nations (67%) and Europe, while low-income countries (15%) and Africa lagged behind. These policies were categorized as alcohol-specific (40%) or integrated into broader frameworks such as substance abuse (25%), noncommunicable diseases (23%), or public health policies (20%). The approval process varied, with 59% of policies adopted by national governments, 28% by parliaments, and 11% by health ministries. High-income nations demonstrated stronger policy enforcement, whereas low-income countries faced challenges in both adoption and implementation (Adopted written national policy on alcohol, 2016).

Several countries, particularly in the Eastern Mediterranean and African regions, enforce a total ban on alcohol. Nations such as Afghanistan, Iran, Kuwait, Libya, Mauritania, Saudi Arabia, Somalia, Sudan, and Yemen prohibit the sale, production, and consumption of alcohol, impose strict penalties, and ban alcohol advertising. Others, like Pakistan, Bangladesh, and Brunei, enforce partial bans, restricting alcohol access to non-Muslim populations or designated areas. To prevent illegal alcohol sales, governments employ taxation, licensing, strict penalties, monitoring systems, and public awareness campaigns, with 144 nations using police investigations and surveillance to track illicit alcohol (National legislation to prevent illegal alcohol sales, 2025).

Advertising regulations vary, with 26% of countries enforcing a total ban on alcohol advertising on national television, while others impose partial restrictions. However, 35 countries still lack any regulations on alcohol advertising (Advertising Restrictions on National Television, 2016). Additionally, 55% of countries with a licensing system regulate alcohol at all market levels, including export, while 30% (50 nations) maintain a government monopoly over one or more aspects of the alcohol market, including export control (Licensing required for exports of alcoholic beverages, 2025).

Warning labels on alcohol products and advertisements are mandatory in several countries, with messages varying by nation. Examples include the USA ("may cause health effects"), Gabon ("alcohol is dangerous for health"), Ethiopia ("don't drink if you drive"), Kenya ("excessive alcohol consumption impairs your judgment; do not drive or operate machinery"), and Sweden ("alcohol may cause cerebral hemorrhage and cancer"). Some countries, such as South Africa and Panama, also include warnings on alcohol-related violence and crime (Health warning labels on alcohol advertising, 2025).

In summary, global alcohol regulations encompass diverse policies on BAC limits, taxation, public consumption, national policies, advertising restrictions, and warning labels. While high-income nations demonstrate stronger implementation, low-income countries face challenges in enforcement. Strengthening international cooperation and policy enforcement remains essential to reducing alcohol-related harm.

6.6.2 Standards of the WTO for alcoholic beverages

The World Trade Organisation (WTO) does not establish specific safety standards for alcoholic beverages but plays a crucial role in regulating international trade laws that impact alcohol policies

(Baumberg, 2010). Several key WTO agreements govern alcohol trade, including the Technical Barriers to Trade (TBT) Agreement, which prohibits unnecessary obstacles created by domestic technical regulations and standards (Barlow et al., 2022). Other relevant agreements include the Sanitary and Phytosanitary (SPS) Agreement, which addresses health-related standards, the General Agreement on Tariffs and Trade (GATT) for fair trade and tariffs, and the Agreement on Trade-Related Aspects of Intellectual Property Rights (TRIPS) concerning geographical indications.

While the WTO permits health-based regulations, these must be scientifically justified to prevent trade disputes. Some critics argue that its rules may hinder strong alcohol control policies, though exceptions exist for public health measures (Baumberg, 2010). The proposed Framework Convention on Alcohol Control (FCAC) seeks to reinforce regulatory frameworks but faces political resistance (Baumberg, 2010). WTO laws influence alcohol policies by limiting protectionist measures while allowing health-based regulations. However, strict trade rules and the "necessity test" may discourage countries from implementing stringent alcohol control measures, potentially exacerbating alcohol-related harm (Baumberg & Anderson, 2008).

A notable example of WTO-driven policy shifts is Taiwan's 2002 accession, which led to deregulation, increased foreign competition, and tax reforms. While this altered consumer preferences, overall alcohol consumption remained stable (Chen et al., 2021). Given these dynamics, there is a growing call for binding regulations to prevent industry influence on policy decisions, ensuring that health warnings and other measures are effectively enforced (Monteiro & Sanchez, 2022). Thus, WTO agreements significantly impact global alcohol policies, with the TBT Agreement providing a framework to balance trade and health objectives. However, the influence of the alcohol industry presents challenges in implementing effective public health measures. Future efforts should increase transparency and strengthen international cooperation to prioritize public health over commercial interests.

6.6.3 Standards of Codex Alimentarius for alcoholic beverages

Due to limited risk assessment capacity, WTO members, particularly developing countries, often rely on Codex food safety standards. As a result, many national regulations either defer to or closely align with Codex standards (Schwegel, 2018). The Codex Committee on Food Labeling (CCFL) addressed alcohol labeling during its 48th session in 2024, with discussions focusing on mandatory alcohol content labeling, health warnings, and nutrition claims. However, the European Union opposed the creation of a separate Codex standard. At the same time, the Organisation Internationale de la Vigne et du Vin (OIV) updated wine labeling regulations (Related Standards | CODEXALIMENTARIUS FAO-WHO, 2024).

The International Enological Codex 2024 establishes stringent regulations for alcohol, particularly rectified alcohol of viticultural and agricultural origins. It mandates a minimum ethanol content of 96% at 20°C to ensure purity and quality (INTERNATIONAL ŒNOLOGICAL CODEX, 2024). Additionally, strict contaminant limits are set to prevent health risks, including lead (<0.5 mg/L), mercury (<0.2 mg/L), and arsenic (<0.5 mg/kg). The concentration of methanol must not go beyond 50 g/hL of ethanol because of its possible harmful effects (INTERNATIONAL ŒNOLOGICAL CODEX, 2024).

To guarantee safety and adherence to regulations, alcoholic beverages need to be kept in non-reactive containers that avoid contamination, and labels should display batch numbers and product details for tracking purposes. To confirm purity and identify impurities, advanced methodologies such as gas chromatography, isotopic analysis, and physicochemical assessments are necessary for analytical standards (INTERNATIONAL ŒNOLOGICAL CODEX, 2024). The Codex is also consistent with international food safety regulations, such as directives from the European Union, guidelines from the U.S. FDA, and standards established by the OIV, thereby ensuring uniformity in global alcohol quality standards (INTERNATIONAL ŒNOLOGICAL CODEX, 2024).

6.6.4 Standards of FSSAI for alcoholic beverages

Food Safety and Standards Authority of India (FSSAI) has formulated (Food Safety and Standards (Alcoholic Beverages) Regulations,. (2018)) which outline specific standards and requirements to ensure the safety and quality of alcoholic beverages. These regulations classify alcoholic beverages into categories such as distilled spirits, wines, fermented drinks and beer, each having clearly defined ethanol levels, allowable contaminants, and labeling standards. Distilled beverages like whisky, brandy, rum, vodka, and gin must contain an ethanol content ranging from 36%–50% ABV and must adhere to maximum contaminant limits, including lead (0.2 mg/L), copper (5 mg/L), and methanol (100–300 mg/100L absolute alcohol). Wines and other fermented beverages, such as fortified wines (15%–24% ABV) and fruit wines (0.5%–9% ABV), must be free from coliforms and pathogens, while methanol levels should not exceed 250–400 mg/L. Beer, classified into regular (0.5%–5.0% ABV) and strong (5.0%–8.0% ABV), must be pasteurized or filter-sterilized, except for draught beer, which may be unpasteurized. Additionally, low-alcoholic beverages (0.5%–8% ABV) must declare expiry dates and avoid misleading claims like "non-intoxicating." Labeling requirements prohibit nutritional and health claims, except for optional energy content (kcal) from March 2024, and mandate a statutory warning stating, "Consumption of Alcohol is Injurious to Health." The regulations ensure that water used for dilution meets IS:10,500 drinking water standards, and alcoholic beverages adhere to FSSAI's food additive and processing regulations. The Food Safety and Standards (Contaminants, Toxins, and Residues) Regulations, 2018 (Food Safety and Standards (Alcoholic Beverages) Regulations,. (2018)) Table 6.2, sets specific limits for contaminants in alcoholic beverages to ensure consumer safety. Naturally occurring toxic substances such as agaric acid (100 ppm), hydrocyanic acid (5 ppm), hypericine (1 ppm), and saffrole (10 ppm) are regulated to prevent potential health risks. Additionally, metal contaminants like lead and arsenic are restricted to a maximum of 0.2 mg/kg, reducing the risk of heavy metal exposure. For canned alcoholic beverages, the permissible limit for tin is 150 mg/kg to prevent contamination from packaging materials. These standards help maintain the quality and safety of alcoholic beverages available in the market.

6.7 Conclusion

Alcoholic beverage safety has improved immensely due to innovation in science and regulation reforms. As this chapter elucidates, safety of the alcoholic beverages matters for credibility within the industry and adherence to stringent safety measures, in addition to consumers' health. Application of sophisticated analytical methods, microbiological precautions for safety, and regulatory systems has enabled remarkable identification and prevention of possible hazards during manufacturing of alcoholic beverages. Scientific progress has been the key to creating quality control methods. The creation of advanced analytical tools such as GC, LC, and MS has enabled the detection of toxic chemicals such

Table 6.2 Standards of FSSAI for alcoholic beverages.

Category	Ethanol content (% ABV)	Key requirements	Contaminant limits	Labeling & processing standards
General standards	–	No chloral hydrate, paraldehyde, narcotics, or psychotropic substances. Only ethanol of agricultural origin.	Methanol: 10–300 mg/100L alcohol depending on beverage. Heavy metals (Pb: 0.2 mg/L, As: 0.25 mg/L, Cd: 0.01 mg/L). No pathogenic microorganisms.	Alcohol tolerance: ±0.3% (up to 20% ABV), ±1.0% (above 20% ABV). Water quality: IS:10,500 standards. Additives per FSSAI regulations.
Distilled beverages	36%–50%	Includes brandy, Whisky, vodka, Rum, gin, Feni. If "matured," must be aged ≥1 year in oak barrels.	Lead: 0.2 mg/L, Copper: 5.0 mg/L methyl alcohol: Max 100–300 mg/100L alcohol	Label alcohol %, 'standard drinks' info, and GI tags (if applicable). No health claims are allowed.
Wine & fermented beverages	7.0%–15.5% (table Wine), 15%–24% (Fortified Wine), 0.59% (cider, Perry, fruit Wine)	Made from grapes, fruits, or plant sap. Fortified wine must contain ≥7% alcohol from fermentation.	Methanol: 250,400 mg/L wine. Must be free from coliforms & pathogens.	Must declare grape variety, sugar content, and vintage year. Wine containing >10 mg/L sulfur dioxide must be labeled with 'contains sulfites'.
Beer	0.5%–5.0% (Regular), 5.0%–8.0% (Strong), 0.0% (Alcoholfree)	Made from malted grains & hops. Can be lager, ale, wheat, stout, or porter. Draught beer may be unpasteurized.	Methanol: Max 50 mg/L, Total plate count: <10 cfu/mL, No coliforms	Must be pasteurized or filter-sterilized (except draught beer). 'AlcoholFree' must have 0.0% ABV.
Low alcoholic beverages	0.5%–8.0%	Includes ready-todrink flavored beverages. Residue on evaporation max 25%.	Methanol: Max 25 mg/100L alcohol, pH: 2.0–5.0, sugar max 20%.	Must declare expiry date. No 'nonintoxicating' claims investment in R&D will be needed to ensure responses to developing issues in alcoholic drink safety. Climate change, shifting consumer preferences, and increased international trade

Continued

Table 6.2 Standards of FSSAI for alcoholic beverages.—cont'd

Category	Ethanol content (% ABV)	Key requirements	Contaminant limits	Labeling & processing standards
				require ongoing adaptation of safety and regulatory guidelines. Cooperation between researchers, industry, and regulators will be critical to speeding up advances while upholding high levels of safety. Lastly, the safety of alcoholic drinks calls for a multi-faceted strategy involving scientific inquiry and regulatory rules. Through leveraging these developments, the industry can maintain consumer confidence, safeguard public health, and usher in a more open and sustainable era of alcohol beverage manufacturing. If alcohol >0.5%.
Packaging & labeling	–	No nutrition claims, except optional energy content (kcal) (from March 2024). No health claims.	–	Mandatory health warning: 'Consumption of alcohol is Injurious to health.' must follow FSSAI packaging & Labeling rules, 2011.

Food Safety and Standards Authority of India. (2021, March 4). Compendium: Food Safety and Standards (Alcoholic Beverages) Regulations, 2018. https://www.fssai.gov.in/upload/uploadfiles/files/Compendium_Alcoholic_Beverages_Regulations_04_03_2021.pdf.

as methanol, heavy metals, and pesticide residues with accuracy. Spectroscopic methods, including IR and NMR spectroscopy, have assisted in guaranteeing the quality of alcoholic beverages. This has enhanced the capacity of the industry to supply high-quality products while safeguarding public health. Microbiological safety is essential since fermentation processes depend on microbial activity, which needs to be adequately controlled. Microbiological screening technology has enabled rapid and precise identification of spoilage organisms and pathogens. In addition, compliance with good manufacturing procedures has enhanced safety practices, reduced the risk of contamination, and improved overall beverage quality. International regulatory bodies like the WHO, WTO and food safety authorities in various countries have been instrumental in driving compliance with safety standards. For compliance within the industry, these regulatory systems establish tolerable ingredient limits, enforce labeling requirements, and conduct safety audits. The continuous refinement of such policies, as more scientific data becomes available, has strengthened consumer protection from unsafe products and deception.

Looking ahead, continued investment in research and development will be necessary to address emerging issues in alcoholic drink safety. Climate change, shifting consumer preferences, and increased international trade require ongoing adaptation of safety and regulatory guidelines. Cooperation among researchers, industry, and regulators will be crucial to accelerating advances while maintaining high levels of safety. Lastly, the safety of alcoholic drinks calls for a multi-faceted strategy involving scientific inquiry and regulatory rules. Through leveraging these developments, the industry can maintain consumer confidence, safeguard public health, and usher in a more open and sustainable era of alcohol beverage manufacturing.

References

Abernathy, D. G., Spedding, G., & Starcher, B. (2009). Analysis of protein and total usable nitrogen in beer and wine using a microwell ninhydrin assay. *Journal of the Institute of Brewing, 115*(2), 122–127. https://doi.org/10.1002/j.2050-0416.2009.tb00356.x, 00469750.

Adopted written national policy on alcohol. (2016). https://www.who.int/data/gho/data/indicators/indicator-details/GHO/adopted-written-national-policy-on-alcohol.

Agnolucci, M., Tirelli, A., Cocolin, L., & Toffanin, A. (2017). Brettanomyces bruxellensis yeasts: Impact on wine and winemaking. *World Journal of Microbiology and Biotechnology, 33*(10). https://doi.org/10.1007/s11274-017-2345-z

Alcarde, A. R., Souza, L. M., & Bortoletto, A. M. (2014). Formation of volatile and maturation-related congeners during the aging of sugarcane spirit in oak barrels. *Journal of the Institute of Brewing, 120*(4), 529–536. https://doi.org/10.1002/jib.165

Almeida, A.d. R., Maciel, M. V.d. O. B., Machado, M. H., Bazzo, G. C., de Armas, R. D., Vitorino, V. B., Vitali, L., Block, J. M., & Barreto, P. L. M. (2020). Bioactive compounds and antioxidant activities of Brazilian hop (Humulus lupulus L.) extracts. *International Journal of Food Science and Technology, 55*(1), 340–347. https://doi.org/10.1111/ijfs.14311

Anderson, H. E., Santos, I. C., Hildenbrand, Z. L., & Schug, K. A. (2019). A review of the analytical methods used for beer ingredient and finished product analysis and quality control. *Analytica Chimica Acta, 1085*, 1–20. https://doi.org/10.1016/j.aca.2019.07.061

Anderson, K., Meloni, G., & Swinnen, J. (2019). *Global alcohol markets: Evolving consumption patterns, regulations, and industrial organizations, 73* (pp. 671–712). World Scientific Pub Co Pte Lt. https://doi.org/10.1142/9789811202094_0026

Anghel, M. A. (2025). *Quality assurance in breath-alcohol analysis.*

Aparnna, V. P., Chauhan, A. K., & Singh, S. (2024). Palm-based beverages around the world: A review. *Current Nutrition & Food Science, 20*(1), 16–27. https://doi.org/10.2174/1573401319666230417083106

Araújo, G. S., Ribeiro, G. O., de Souza, S. M. A., da Silva, G. P., de Carvalho, G. B. M., Bispo, J. A. C., & Martínez, E. A. (2022). Rice (Oryza sativa) bran and soybean (Glycine max) meal: Unconventional supplements in the mead production. *Food Technology and Biotechnology, 60*(1), 89–98. https://doi.org/10.17113/ftb.60.01.22.7183

Arellano, M., Pelayo, C., Ramírez, J., & Rodriguez, I. (2008). Characterization of kinetic parameters and the formation of volatile compounds during the tequila fermentation by wild yeasts isolated from agave juice. *Journal of Industrial Microbiology & Biotechnology, 35*(8), 835–841. https://doi.org/10.1007/s10295-008-0355-4

Arslan, M., Tahir, H. E., Zareef, M., Shi, J., Rakha, A., Bilal, M., Xiaowei, H., Zhihua, L., & Xiaobo, Z. (2021). Recent trends in quality control, discrimination and authentication of alcoholic beverages using nondestructive instrumental techniques. *Trends in Food Science and Technology, 107*, 80–113. https://doi.org/10.1016/j.tifs.2020.11.021

Azevedo, S., Battaglene, T., Hodson, G., & Aurand, J.-M. (2016). Microbiologically, wine is a low food safety risk consumer product. *BIO Web of Conferences, 7*, Article 04003. https://doi.org/10.1051/bioconf/20160704003

Bamforth, C. (2009). *Beer tap into the art and science of brewing.* Oxford University Press.

Bamforth, C. W. (2023). *Beer: Tap into the art and science of brewing.* New York: Oxford University Press. https://doi.org/10.1093/oso/9780199996742.001.0001

Barlow, P., Gleeson, D., O'Brien, P., & Labonte, R. (2022). Industry influence over global alcohol policies via the world trade organization: A qualitative analysis of discussions on alcohol health warning labelling, 2010–19. *The Lancet Global Health, 10*(3), Article e429. https://doi.org/10.1016/S2214-109X(21)00570-2

Baumberg, B., & Anderson, P. (2008). Trade and health: How world trade organization (WTO) law affects alcohol and public health. *Addiction, 103*(12), 1952–1958. https://doi.org/10.1111/j.1360-0443.2008.02322.x

Baumberg, B. (2010). World trade law and a framework convention on alcohol control. *Journal of Epidemiology and Community Health, 64*(6), 473–474. https://doi.org/10.1136/jech.2008.084855

Bednarek, M., & Szwengiel, A. (2020). Distinguishing between saturated and unsaturated meads based on their chemical characteristics. *LWT, 133*, Article 109962. https://doi.org/10.1016/j.lwt.2020.109962

Beech, F. W. (1972). Cider making and cider research: A review. *Journal of the Institute of Brewing, 78*(6), 477–491. https://doi.org/10.1002/j.2050-0416.1972.tb03485.x

Besse, J., & Dechaine, D. (2014). *Distillery design: Producing vodka and other spirits.*

Bharti, A., Jain, U., & Chauhan, N. (2024). Progressive analytical techniques utilized for the detection of contaminants attributed to food safety and security. *Talanta Open, 10*, Article 100368. https://doi.org/10.1016/j.talo.2024.100368

Bisht, A., & Singh, S. P. (2025). A comprehensive review on the study of wines and their clinical effect on human health to cite this version: HAL id: Hal-04946850. *Archives of Ecotoxicology.*

Black, K., & Walker, G. (2023). Yeast fermentation for production of neutral distilled spirits. *Applied Sciences, 13*(8), 4927. https://doi.org/10.3390/app13084927

Blood Alcohol Concentration (BAC) limit for drivers. (2025). https://www.who.int/data/gho/data/indicators/indicator-details/GHO/blood-alcohol-concentration-(bac)-limit-for-drivers.

Blšáková, L., Gregor, T., Mešťánek, M., Hřivna, L., & Kumbár, V. (2022). The use of unconventional malts in beer production and their effect on the wort viscosity. *Foods, 11*(1), 31. https://doi.org/10.3390/foods11010031

Bogdanov, S., Jurendic, T., Sieber, R., & Gallmann, P. (2008). Honey for nutrition and health: A review. *Journal of the American College of Nutrition, 27*(6), 677–689. https://doi.org/10.1080/07315724.2008.10719745

Buglass, A. J. (2010). Handbook of alcoholic beverages: Technical, analytical and nutritional aspects. In *Handbook of alcoholic beverages: Technical, analytical and nutritional aspects, 1–2*South Korea: John Wiley and Sons. https://doi.org/10.1002/9780470976524

Carballo, D., Fernández-Franzón, M., Ferrer, E., Pallarés, N., & Berrada, H. (2021). Dietary exposure to mycotoxins through alcoholic and non-alcoholic beverages in Valencia, Spain. *Toxins, 13*(7), 438. https://doi.org/10.3390/toxins13070438

Carvalho, G., Leite, A. C., Leal, R., & Pereira, R. (2023). The role of emergent processing technologies in beer production. *Beverages, 9*(1). https://doi.org/10.3390/beverages9010007

Ceballos-Magaña, S. G., Jurado, J. M., Martín, M. J., & Pablos, F. (2009). Quantitation of twelve metals in tequila and mezcal spirits as authenticity parameters. *Journal of Agricultural and Food Chemistry, 57*(4), 1372–1376. https://doi.org/10.1021/jf803626kSpain

Chaudhary, C., Yadav, B. S., & Grewal, R. (2014). Preparation of red wine by blending of grape (Vitis vinifera L.) and jamun (Syzygiumcuminii L. Skeels) juices before fermentation. *International Journal of Agriculture and Food Science Technology, 5*, 239–348.

Chen, C. H., Wu, Y. L., Lo, D., & Wu, M. C. (2013). Physicochemical property changes during the fermentation of longan (Dimocarpus longan) mead and its aroma composition using multiple yeast inoculations. *Journal of the Institute of Brewing, 119*(4), 303–308. https://doi.org/10.1002/jib.95

Chen, C.-C., Cheng, K.-W., Chang, H.-Y., & Chang, S.-S. (2021). Changes in alcoholic beverage preference and consumption in Taiwan following accession to the world trade organization. *Addiction, 116*(3), 497–505. https://doi.org/10.1111/add.15184

cherry ripe, Perry. (2009). *Gastronomica, 9*(4), 58–61. https://doi.org/10.1525/gfc.2009.9.4.58

Cortacero-Ramirez, S., Hernáinz-Bermúdez de Castro, M., Segura-Carretero, A., Cruces-Blanco, C., & Fernández-Gutiérrez, A. (2003). Analysis of beer components by capillary electrophoretic methods. *TrAC Trends in Analytical Chemistry, 22*(7), 440–455. https://doi.org/10.1016/s0165-9936(03)00704-0

Cousin, F., Le Guellec, R., Schlusselhuber, M., Dalmasso, M., Laplace, J.-M., & Cretenet, M. (2017). Microorganisms in fermented apple beverages: Current knowledge and future directions. *Microorganisms, 5*(3), 39. https://doi.org/10.3390/microorganisms5030039

Das, S., & Tamang, J. P. (2021). Changes in microbial communities and their predictive functionalities during fermentation of toddy, an alcoholic beverage of India. *Microbiological Research, 248*. https://doi.org/10.1016/j.micres.2021.126769

Das, S., & Tamang, J. P. (2023a). Fermentation dynamics of naturally fermented palm beverages of West Bengal and Jharkhand in India. *Fermentation, 9*(3), 301. https://doi.org/10.3390/fermentation9030301

Das, S., & Tamang, J. P. (2023b). Metagenomics and metabolomics of Toddy, an Indian fermented date palm beverage. *Food Research International, 172*. https://doi.org/10.1016/j.foodres.2023.113205

Das, A. J., Khawas, P., Miyaji, T., & Deka, S. C. (2014). HPLC and GC-MS analyses of organic acids, carbohydrates, amino acids and volatile aromatic compounds in some varieties of rice beer from northeast India. *Journal of the Institute of Brewing, 120*(3), 244–252. https://doi.org/10.1002/jib.134

De Keukeleire, D. (2000). Fundamentals of beer and hop chemistry. *Química Nova, 23*(1), 108–112. https://doi.org/10.1590/S0100-40422000000100019

de Souza, H. F., Monteiro, G. F., Di Próspero Gonçalves, V. D., dos Santos, J. V., de Oliveira, A. C. D., Pereira, K. N., Carosia, M. F., de Carvalho, M. V., Brandi, I. V., & Kamimura, E. S. (2024). Evaluation of sensory acceptance, purchase intention and color parameters of potentially probiotic mead with saccharomyces boulardii. *Food Science and Biotechnology, 33*(7), 1651–1659. https://doi.org/10.1007/s10068-023-01459-y

De-Loyde, K., Ferrar, J., Pilling, M. A., Hollands, G. J., Clarke, N., Matthews, J. A., Maynard, O. M., Wood, T., Heath, C., Munafò, M. R., & Attwood, A. S. (2024). The impact of introducing alcohol-free beer options in bars and public houses on alcohol sales and revenue: A randomised crossover field trial. *Addiction, 119*(6), 1071–1079. https://doi.org/10.1111/add.16449

Dhiman, A., & Attri, S. (2011). Production of brandy. In *Handbook of enology: Principles, practices and recent innovations, 3* (p. 60).

Dong, J. J., Li, Q. L., Yin, H., Zhong, C., Hao, J. G., Yang, P. F., Tian, Y. H., & Jia, S. R. (2014). Predictive analysis of beer quality by correlating sensory evaluation with higher alcohol and ester production using multivariate statistics methods. *Food Chemistry, 161*, 376–382. https://doi.org/10.1016/j.foodchem.2014.04.006

Dou, Y., Mäkinen, M., & Jänis, J. (2023). Analysis of volatile and nonvolatile constituents in gin by direct-infusion ultrahigh-resolution ESI/APPI FT-ICR mass spectrometry. *Journal of Agricultural and Food Chemistry, 71* (18), 7082–7089. https://doi.org/10.1021/acs.jafc.3c00707

Douady, A., Puentes, C., Awad, P., & Esteban-Decloux, M. (2019). Batch distillation of spirits: Experimental study and simulation of the behaviour of volatile aroma compounds. *Journal of the Institute of Brewing, 125* (2), 268–283. https://doi.org/10.1002/jib.560

Elumalai, A., & Natarajan, V. (2025). Advancements in analytical technologies for ensuring food quality and authentication: A comprehensive review. *Journal of Food Composition and Analysis, 139*, Article 107075. https://doi.org/10.1016/j.jfca.2024.107075

Féchir, M., Weaver, G., Roy, C., & Shellhammer, T. H. (2023). Exploring the regional identity of Cascade and mosaic® hops grown at different locations in Oregon and Washington. *Journal of the American Society of Brewing Chemists, 81*(3), 480–492. https://doi.org/10.1080/03610470.2022.2089010

Fleet, G. (2003). Yeast interactions and wine flavour. *International Journal of Food Microbiology, 86*(1–2), 11–22. https://doi.org/10.1016/s0168-1605(03)00245-9

Food Safety and Standards (Alcoholic Beverages) Regulations. (2018). *Fssai*. https://fssai.gov.in/upload/uploadfiles/files/Comp_Alcoholic_Beverages(III)_28_08_2023.pdf.

Fortes, J. P., Franco, F. W., Baranzelli, J., Ugalde, G. A., Ballus, C. A., Rodrigues, E., Mazutti, M. A., Somacal, S., & Sautter, C. K. (2023). Enhancement of the functional properties of mead aged with oak (Quercus) chips at different toasting levels. *Molecules, 28*(1). https://doi.org/10.3390/molecules28010056

Fulgêncio, A. C.d. C., Resende, G. A. P., Teixeira, M. C. F., Botelho, B. G., & Sena, M. M. (2023). Combining portable NIR spectroscopy and multivariate calibration for the determination of ethanol in fermented alcoholic beverages by a multi-product model. *Talanta Open, 7*. https://doi.org/10.1016/j.talo.2023.100180

Gaglio, R., Francesca, N., Di Gerlando, R., Mahony, J., De Martino, S., Stucchi, C., Moschetti, G., & Settanni, L. (2017). Enteric bacteria of food ice and their survival in alcoholic beverages and soft drinks. *Food Microbiology, 67*, 17–22. https://doi.org/10.1016/j.fm.2017.04.020

Gately, I. (2008). *Drink: A cultural history of alcohol*. Penguin.

Gerhardt, R. E., Crecelius, E. A., & Hudson, J. B. (1980). Trace element content of moonshine. *Archives of Environmental Health, 35*(6), 332–334. https://doi.org/10.1080/00039896.1980.10667515

Global report on the use of alcohol taxes. (2023). https://www.who.int/publications/i/item/9789240086104.

Gomes, T., Barradas, C., Dias, T., Verdial, J., Morais, J. S., Ramalhosa, E., & Estevinho, L. M. (2013). Optimization of mead production using response surface methodology. *Food and Chemical Toxicology, 59*, 680–686. https://doi.org/10.1016/j.fct.2013.06.034

Guth, H. (1997). Quantitation and sensory studies of character impact odorants of different white wine varieties. *Journal of Agricultural and Food Chemistry, 45*(8), 3027–3032. https://doi.org/10.1021/jf970280a

Gutiérrez-Escobar, R., Aliaño-González, M. J., & Cantos-Villar, E. (2021). Wine polyphenol content and its influence on wine quality and properties: A review. *Molecules, 26*(3). https://doi.org/10.3390/molecules26030718. Available from: http://www.mdpi.com/journal/molecules.

Harder, M. N. C., Martins Benetole, B., Gomes, W. P. C., Paiva Generoso, E., Verde de Campos, S., Costa Harder, L. N., & Arthur, V. (2021). Mead of natural fermentation. *Journal of Microbiology, Biotechnology and Food Sciences, 11*(1), Article e3628. https://doi.org/10.15414/jmbfs.3628

He, N. X., & Bayen, S. (2020). An overview of chemical contaminants and other undesirable chemicals in alcoholic beverages and strategies for analysis. *Comprehensive Reviews in Food Science and Food Safety, 19* (6), 3916–3950. https://doi.org/10.1111/1541-4337.12649

He, N., Yargeau, V., Liu, L., & Bayen, S. (2024). Development of a targeted and non-targeted direct-injection analysis of plastic-related contaminants in liquor products. *Food Control, 162*, Article 110424. https://doi.org/10.1016/j.foodcont.2024.110424

Health warning labels on alcohol advertising. (2025). https://www.who.int/data/gho/data/indicators/indicator-details/GHO/health-warning-labels-on-alcohol-advertising.

Hennemann, M., Gastl, M., & Becker, T. (2021). Influence of particle size uniformity on the filter cake resistance of physically and chemically modified fine particles. *Separation and Purification Technology, 272*, Article 118966. https://doi.org/10.1016/j.seppur.2021.118966

Herdiana, Y. (2025). Alcohol in daily products: Health risks, cultural considerations, and economic impacts. *Risk Management and Healthcare Policy, 18*, 217–237. https://doi.org/10.2147/rmhp.s495493

5—Rapid methods to analyze alcoholic beverages. Heymann, H., & Ebeler, S. E. (Eds.), *Sensory and instrumental evaluation of alcoholic beverages*, (pp. 84–104). (2017). Academic Press. https://doi.org/10.1016/B978-0-12-802727-1.00005-3

Hobbs, C. E. (2023). The chemistry of Tequila. In *Chemistry of alcoholic beverages* (pp. 37–61). ACS Publications.

Hwang, I. S., Kim, C. W., Kim, B. R., Lim, B. R., & Choi, J. H. (2024). A comparative analysis of aroma profiles of Soju and other distilled spirits from Northeastern Asia. *Foods, 13*(21). https://doi.org/10.3390/foods13213368

Ibrahim, M., Agarwal, M., Giles, H., Muslim, A., & Ren, Y. (2017). Optimization of environmental factors to measure physiological parameters of two rose varieties. *Open Journal of Applied Sciences, 07*(10), 585–595. https://doi.org/10.4236/ojapps.2017.710042

Ickes, C. M., & Cadwallader, K. R. (2017). Characterization of sensory differences in mixing and premium rums through the use of descriptive sensory analysis. *Journal of Food Science, 82*(11), 2679–2689. https://doi.org/10.1111/1750-3841.13936

INTERNATIONAL ŒNOLOGICAL CODEX. (2024). https://www.oiv.int/sites/default/files/publication/2024-03/CODEX%20oenologique%20EN%202024.pdf.

Ioannidou, M. D., Samouris, G., & Achilias, D. S. (2016). Acetaldehyde contamination of water, alcoholic, and non-alcoholic beverages stored in glass or plastic bottles. *Toxicological and Environmental Chemistry, 98*(10), 1183–1190. https://doi.org/10.1080/02772248.2015.1115505

Jackson, R. S. (2008). *Wine science: Principles and applications* (3rd ed.). Amsterdam; Boston: Elsevier/Academic Press.

Jackson, R. S. (2020). *Wine science: Principles and applications*. Academic press.

Jackson, R. S. (2023). Styles and types of wine. In *Wine tasting* (pp. 333–379). Elsevier. https://doi.org/10.1016/B978-0-323-85263-0.00012-0

Janick, J., Valois, S., & Padilla-Zakour, O. I. (2008). Cider apples and cider-making techniques in Europe and North America. *Horticultural Reviews, 34*, 365–415. https://doi.org/10.1002/9780470380147.ch6

Jeon, S. H., Kim, N. H., Shim, M. B., Jeon, Y. W., Ahn, J. H., Lee, S. H., Hwang, I. G., & Rhee, M. S. (2015). Microbiological diversity and prevalence of spoilage and pathogenic bacteria in commercial fermented alcoholic beverages (beer, fruit wine, refined rice wine, and yakju). *Journal of Food Protection, 78*(4), 812–818. https://doi.org/10.4315/0362-028X.JFP-14-431

Joshi, V. K., Sharma, S., & Thakur, A. D. (2017). Wines. In *Current developments in biotechnology and bioengineering* (pp. 353–406). Elsevier. https://doi.org/10.1016/B978-0-444-63666-9.00013-3

Kahoun, D., Řezková, S., & Královský, J. (2017). Effect of heat treatment and storage conditions on mead composition. *Food Chemistry, 219*, 357–363. https://doi.org/10.1016/j.foodchem.2016.09.161

Karamoko, D., Bouatenin, J., Yoro, D., Djeni, N., & Djè, M. (2019). Dynamics of lactic acid bacteria isolated from palm wine during the exploitation of two varieties of oil palm for the production of new beverages. *Journal of Global Bioscience, 8*(3), 5990–6002.

Kilian, C., Lemp, J. M., Llamosas-Falcón, L., Carr, T., Ye, Y., Kerr, W. C., Mulia, N., Puka, K., Lasserre, A. M., Bright, S., Rehm, J., & Probst, C. (2023). Reducing alcohol use through alcohol control policies in the general population and population subgroups: A systematic review and meta-analysis. *eClinicalMedicine, 59*. https://doi.org/10.1016/j.eclinm.2023.101996

Kimura, M., Ito, T., Sato, H., & Higashi, M. (2021). Theoretical study on isomerization of α-acids: A DFT calculation. *Food Chemistry, 364*, Article 130418. https://doi.org/10.1016/j.foodchem.2021.130418

Kitagaki, H., & Kitamoto, K. (2013). Breeding research on sake yeasts in Japan: History, recent technological advances, and future perspectives. *Annual Review of Food Science and Technology, 4*(1), 215–235. https://doi.org/10.1146/annurev-food-030212-182545

Koljančić, N., Furdíková, K., Gomes, A.de A., & Špánik, I. (2024). Wine authentication: Current progress and state of the art. *Trends in Food Science & Technology, 150*, Article 104598. https://doi.org/10.1016/j.tifs.2024.104598

Kuś, P. M., Czabaj, S., & Jerković, I. (2022). Comparison of volatile profiles of meads and related unifloral honeys: Traceability markers. *Molecules, 27*(14), 4558. https://doi.org/10.3390/molecules27144558

Kwon, Y. S., Lee, J., Kim, M. S., Han, S., & Choi, H. S. (2023). Potential production strategy for distilled soju by fermenting nonsteamed rice using commercial enzyme products. *Korean Journal of Food Preservation, 30*(4), 669–682. https://doi.org/10.11002/kjfp.2023.30.4.669

Lachance, M. A. (1995). Yeast communities in a natural tequila fermentation. *Antonie Van Leeuwenhoek, 68*(2), 151–160. https://doi.org/10.1007/BF00873100

Lachenmeier, D. W. (2007). Rapid quality control of spirit drinks and beer using multivariate data analysis of Fourier transform infrared spectra. *Food Chemistry, 101*(2), 825–832. https://doi.org/10.1016/j.foodchem.2005.12.032

Lea, A. G. H., Lea, A. G. H., & Piggott, J. R. (2003). *Fermented beverage production*. Springer Science & Business Media.

Lekkas, C., Stewart, G. G., Hill, A. E., Taidi, B., & Hodgson, J. (2007). Elucidation of the role of nitrogenous wort components in yeast fermentation. *Journal of the Institute of Brewing, 113*(1), 3–8. https://doi.org/10.1002/j.2050-0416.2007.tb00249.x

Licensing required for exports of alcoholic beverages. (2025). https://www.who.int/data/gho/data/indicators/indicator-details/GHO/licensing-required-for-exports-of-alcoholic-beverages.

Lin, M., Yang, B., Dai, M., Xu, Y., Li, X., & Sun, B. (2023). East meets west in alcoholic beverages: Flavor comparison, microbial metabolism and health effects. *Food Bioscience, 56*, Article 103385. https://doi.org/10.1016/j.fbio.2023.103385

Lopes, A. C. A., Eda, S. H., Andrade, R. P., Amorim, J. C., & Duarte, W. F. (2019). New alcoholic fermented beverages-potentials and challenges fermented beverages: Volume 5. In *The science of beverages* (pp. 577–603). Brazil: Elsevier. https://doi.org/10.1016/B978-0-12-815271-3.00014-2

Lopes, A. C. A., Costa, R., Andrade, R. P., Lima, L. M. Z., Santiago, W. D., das Graças Cardoso, M., & Duarte, W. F. (2020). Impact of Saccharomyces cerevisiae single inoculum and mixed inoculum with Meyerozyma caribbica on the quality of mead. *European Food Research and Technology, 246*(11), 2175–2185.

López-Alvarez, A., Díaz-Pérez, A. L., Sosa-Aguirre, C., Macías-Rodríguez, L., & Campos-García, J. (2012). Ethanol yield and volatile compound content in fermentation of agave must by Kluyveromyces marxianus UMPe-1 comparing with Saccharomyces cerevisiae baker's yeast used in tequila production. *Journal of Bioscience and Bioengineering, 113*(5), 614–618. https://doi.org/10.1016/j.jbiosc.2011.12.015

Louw, L., Malherbe, S., Naes, T., Lambrechts, M., van Rensburg, P., & Nieuwoudt, H. (2013). Validation of two napping® techniques as rapid sensory screening tools for high alcohol products. *Food Quality and Preference, 30*(2), 192–201. https://doi.org/10.1016/j.foodqual.2013.05.016

Manual_Alcoholic_Beverages. (2019). https://fssai.gov.in/upload/uploadfiles/files/Manual_Alcoholic_Beverages_04_07_2019.pdf.

Mateo, R., Medina, A., Mateo, E. M., Mateo, F., & Jiménez, M. (2007). An overview of ochratoxin A in beer and wine. *International Journal of Food Microbiology, 119*(1–2), 79–83. https://doi.org/10.1016/j.ijfoodmicro.2007.07.029

McGovern, P., Jalabadze, M., Batiuk, S., Callahan, M. P., Smith, K. E., Hall, G. R., Kvavadze, E., Maghradze, D., Rusishvili, N., Laurent, B., Failla, O., Cola, G., Mariani, L., Boaretto, E., Bacilieri, R., This, P., Wales, N., & Lordkipanidze, D. (2017). Early Neolithic wine of Georgia in the South Caucasus. *Proceedings of the National Academy of Sciences, 114*(48). https://doi.org/10.1073/pnas.1714728114

Mendes Ferreira, A., & Mendes-Faia, A. (2020). The role of yeasts and lactic acid bacteria on the metabolism of organic acids during winemaking. *Foods, 9*(9), 1231. https://doi.org/10.3390/foods9091231

Menevseoglu, A., & Cabaroglu, T. (2021). Evaluating the chemical and metal contamination of commercial Rakı, a grape-based alcoholic beverage from Turkey. *OENO One, 55*(3), 261–271. https://doi.org/10.20870/oeno-one.2021.55.3.4669

Methods of analysis for spirituous beverages and alcohols | OIV. (2025). https://www.oiv.int/standards/compendium-of-international-methods-of-analysis-for-spirituous-beverages-and-alcohols/spirituous-beverages-and-alcohols/methods-of-analysis-for-spiri.

Milani, E. A., & Silva, F. V. M. (2022). Pasteurization of beer by non-thermal technologies. *Frontiers in Food Science and Technology, 1.* https://doi.org/10.3389/frfst.2021.798676

Milsom, P., Smith, R., Modisenyane, S. M., & Walls, H. (2021). Do international trade and investment agreements generate regulatory chill in public health policymaking? A case study of nutrition and alcohol policy in South Africa. *Globalization and Health, 17*(1), Article 17448603. https://doi.org/10.1186/s12992-021-00757-6

Mishra, S. (December 3, 2024). *Wine production in 2024 projected to reach lowest level since 1961.* Just Drinks. https://www.just-drinks.com/news/global-wine-production-in-2024/.

Monteiro, M. G., & Sanchez, Z. M. (2022). How can we get sober from the influence of the alcohol industry? *The Lancet Global Health, 10*(3), Article e315. https://doi.org/10.1016/S2214-109X(22)00024-9

Mosher, M., & Trantham, K. (2017). Brewing science: A multidisciplinary approach. In *Brewing science: A multidisciplinary approach.* https://doi.org/10.1007/978-3-319-46394-0

Mosher, M., & Trantham, K. (2021). Brewing science: A multidisciplinary approach. In *Brewing science: A multidisciplinary approach.* https://doi.org/10.1007/978-3-030-73419-0

Mudgil, D., & Barak, S. (2018). *Beverages: Processing and technology.* Scientific Publishers. https://books.google.co.in/books?id=3Q2NDwAAQBAJ.

Mulaw, G., Gebregziabher, T., & Tesfay, T. (2025). A review on the microbiology of Ethiopian traditional fermented beverage products. *Frontiers in Nutrition, 12.* https://doi.org/10.3389/fnut.2025.1519547

Narula, A. P. S. (2019). Fragrance and attractionB. Guthrie, J. D. Beauchamp, A. Buettner, S. Toth, & M. C. Qian (Eds.). *ACS Symposium Series, 1321*, 1–16. https://doi.org/10.1021/bk-2019-1321.ch001

Nascimento, H. O. D. (2023). *Federal university of ceara science center postgraduate program in chemistry department of analytical and physical chemistry.*

National legislation to prevent illegal alcohol sales. (2025). https://www.who.int/data/gho/data/indicators/indicator-details/GHO/national-legislation-to-prevent-illegal-alcohol-sales.

Nemo, R., & Bacha, K. (2020). Microbial, physicochemical and proximate analysis of selected Ethiopian traditional fermented beverages. *LWT, 131*, Article 109713. https://doi.org/10.1016/j.lwt.2020.109713

Neve, R. A. (1991). *Hops.* Netherlands: Springer.

Nunes Filho, R. C., Galvan, D., Effting, L., Terhaag, M. M., Yamashita, F., Benassi, M.d. T., & Spinosa, W. A. (2021). Effects of adding spices with antioxidants compounds in red ale style craft beer: A simplex-centroid mixture design approach. *Food Chemistry*, 365. https://doi.org/10.1016/j.foodchem.2021.130478

O'Sullivan, M. G. (2012). *Principles of sensory shelf-life evaluation and its application to alcoholic beverages.* Elsevier BV. https://doi.org/10.1533/9780857095176.1.42

O'Brien, E., & Dietrich, D. R. (2005). Ochratoxin A: The continuing enigma. *Critical Reviews in Toxicology, 35* (1), 33–60. https://doi.org/10.1080/10408440590905948

Ohimain, E. I. (2016). *Methanol contamination in traditionally fermented alcoholic beverages: The microbial dimension*. Nigeria: SpringerOpen, Article 21931801. https://doi.org/10.1186/s40064-016-3303-1

Okafor, V. N., Omokpariola, D. O., Okabekwa, C. V., & Umezinwa, E. C. (2022). Heavy metals in alcoholic beverages consumed in awka, South-East Nigeria: Carcinogenic and non-carcinogenic health risk assessments. *Chemistry Africa, 5*(6), 2227–2239. https://doi.org/10.1007/s42250-022-00477-3

Okafor, N. (2007). *Modern industrial microbiology and biotechnology*. Science Publishers.

Okaru, A. O., Abuga, K. O., Kibwage, I. O., Hausler, T., Luy, B., Kuballa, T., Rehm, J., & Lachenmeier, D. W. (2017). Aflatoxin contamination in unrecorded beers from Kenya – A health risk beyond ethanol. *Food Control, 79*, 344–348. https://doi.org/10.1016/j.foodcont.2017.04.006

Olivares-Galván, S., Marina, M. L., & García, M. C. (2022). Extraction of valuable compounds from brewing residues: Malt rootlets, spent hops, and spent yeast. *Trends in Food Science & Technology, 127*, 181–197. https://doi.org/10.1016/j.tifs.2022.06.002

Oliveira do Nascimento, H., da Silva, M. Z. F., Alexandre, J. B., Vidal, C. B., Carvalho, T. V., & Ferreira do Nascimento, R. (2022). New HS-SPME-GC-BID method for the determination of volatile constituents in distilled beverages. *Microchemical Journal, 181*, Article 107669. https://doi.org/10.1016/j.microc.2022.107669

Oliveira, S., Duarte, E., Gomes, M., Nagata, N., Fernandes, D. D.d. S., & Veras, G. (2023). A green method for the authentication of sugarcane spirit and prediction of density and alcohol content based on near infrared spectroscopy and chemometric tools. *Food Research International, 170*. https://doi.org/10.1016/j.foodres.2023.112830

Paiva, R. A. M., Mutz, Y. S., & Conte-Junior, C. A. (2021). A review on the obtaining of functional beers by addition of non-cereal adjuncts rich in antioxidant compounds. *Antioxidants, 10*(9). https://doi.org/10.3390/antiox10091332. Available from: https://www.mdpi.com/2076-3921/10/9/1332/pdf.

Pascoal, A., Anjos, O., Feás, X., Oliveira, J. M., & Estevinho, L. M. (2019). Impact of fining agents on the volatile composition of sparkling mead. *Journal of the Institute of Brewing, 125*(1), 125–133. https://doi.org/10.1002/jib.549

Pereira, A. P., Mendes-Ferreira, A., Oliveira, J. M., Estevinho, L. M., & Mendes-Faia, A. (2013). High-cell-density fermentation of Saccharomyces cerevisiae for the optimisation of mead production. *Food Microbiology, 33*(1), 114–123. https://doi.org/10.1016/j.fm.2012.09.006

Pereira, A. P., Mendes-Ferreira, A., Oliveira, J. M., Estevinho, L. M., & Mendes-Faia, A. (2014). Effect of Saccharomyces cerevisiae cells immobilisation on mead production. *LWT - Food Science and Technology, 56*(1), 21–30. https://doi.org/10.1016/j.lwt.2013.11.005

Pereira, A. P., Mendes-Ferreira, A., Oliveira, J. M., Estevinho, L. M., & Mendes-Faia, A. (2015). Mead production: Effect of nitrogen supplementation on growth, fermentation profile and aroma formation by yeasts in mead fermentation. *Journal of the Institute of Brewing, 121*(1), 122–128. https://doi.org/10.1002/jib.184

Pereira, A. P., Oliveira, J. M., Mendes-Ferreira, A., Estevinho, L. M., & Mendes-Faia, A. (2017). *Mead and other fermented beverages current developments in biotechnology and bioengineering: Food and beverages industry* (pp. 407–434). Portugal: Elsevier Inc.. https://doi.org/10.1016/B978-0-444-63666-9.00014-5. Available from: http://www.sciencedirect.com/science/book/9780444636669.

Petry-Podgórska, I., Žídková, J., Flodrová, D., & Bobálová, J. (2010). 2D-HPLC and MALDI-TOF/TOF analysis of barley proteins glycated during brewing. *Journal of Chromatography B, 878*(30), 3143–3148. https://doi.org/10.1016/j.jchromb.2010.09.023

Pferdmenges, L. E., Schröter, A., Lohmayer, R., Striegel, L., Rychlik, M., Müller, A., Meinhardt, A. K., Trierweiler, B., Hartmann, B. M., & Frommherz, L. (2022). Characterization of the nutrient composition of German beer styles for the German nutrient database. *Journal of Food Composition and Analysis, 105*. https://doi.org/10.1016/j.jfca.2021.104181. Available from: http://www.elsevier.com/inca/publications/store/6/2/2/8/7/8/index.htt.

Pflaum, T., Hausler, T., Baumung, C., Ackermann, S., Kuballa, T., Rehm, J., & Lachenmeier, D. W. (2016). Carcinogenic compounds in alcoholic beverages: An update. *Archives of Toxicology, 90*(10), 2349–2367. https://doi.org/10.1007/s00204-016-1770-3

Pietri, A., Bertuzzi, T., Pallaroni, L., & Piva, G. (2001). Occurrence of ochratoxin A in Italian wines. *Food Additives and Contaminants, 18*(7), 647–654. https://doi.org/10.1080/02652030119480

Pires, E. J., Teixeira, J. A., Brányik, T., & Vicente, A. A. (2014). Yeast: The soul of beer's aroma - A review of flavour-active esters and higher alcohols produced by the brewing yeast. *Applied Microbiology and Biotechnology, 98*(5), 1937–1949. https://doi.org/10.1007/s00253-013-5470-0

Plutowska, B., & Wardencki, W. (2008). Application of gas chromatography–olfactometry (GC–O) in analysis and quality assessment of alcoholic beverages – A review. *Food Chemistry, 107*(1), 449–463. https://doi.org/10.1016/j.foodchem.2007.08.058

Prathiviraj, R., Rajeev, R., Jose, C. M., Begum, A., Selvin, J., & Kiran, G. S. (2022). Fermentation microbiome and metabolic profiles of Indian palm wine. *Gene Reports, 27*. https://doi.org/10.1016/j.genrep.2022.101543. Available from: http://www.journals.elsevier.com/gene-reports.

Preti, R. (2019). Progress in beverages authentication by the application of analytical techniques and chemometrics. In *Quality control in the beverage industry: Volume 17: The science of beverages* (pp. 85–121). Italy: Elsevier. https://doi.org/10.1016/B978-0-12-816681-9.00003-5. Available from: http://www.sciencedirect.com/science/book/9780128166819.

Pretorius, I. S. (2000). Tailoring wine yeast for the new millennium: Novel approaches to the ancient art of winemaking. *Yeast, 16*(8), 675–729. https://doi.org/10.1002/1097-0061(20000615)16:8<675::AID-YEA585>3.0.CO;2-B

Proulx, A., & Nichols, L. (2003). *Cider: Making, using & enjoying sweet & hard cider*. Storey Publishing.

Qian, M. C., Hughes, P., & Cadwallader, K. (2019). Overview of distilled spirits. In *Sex, smoke, and spirits: The role of chemistry* (pp. 125–144). ACS Publications.

Rabin, D., & Forget, C. (2014). *Dictionary of beer and brewing* (2nd ed.). Taylor and Francis.

Rachwał, K., Waśko, A., Gustaw, K., & Polak-Berecka, M. (2020). Utilization of brewery wastes in food industry. *PeerJ, 8*, Article e9427. https://doi.org/10.7717/peerj.9427

Ramalhosa, E., Gomes, T., Pereira, A. P., Dias, T., & Estevinho, L. M. (2011). Mead production: Tradition versus modernity. *Advances in Food and Nutrition Research, 63*, 101–118. https://doi.org/10.1016/B978-0-12-384927-4.00004-X

Rather, I. A., Koh, W. Y., Paek, W. K., & Lim, J. (2017). The sources of chemical contaminants in food and their health implications. *Frontiers in Pharmacology, 8*. https://doi.org/10.3389/fphar.2017.00830. Available from: http://www.frontiersin.org/Pharmacology.

Reboredo-Rodríguez, P., González-Barreiro, C., Rial-Otero, R., Cancho-Grande, B., & Simal-Gándara, J. (2015). Effects of sugar concentration processes in grapes and wine aging on aroma compounds of sweet Wines—A review. *Critical Reviews in Food Science and Nutrition, 55*(8), 1053–1073. https://doi.org/10.1080/10408398.2012.680524

Related standards | CODEXALIMENTARIUS FAO-WHO. (2024). https://www.fao.org/fao-who-codexalimentarius/committees/committee/related-standards/en/?committee=CCFL.

Restrictions on alcohol use in public places. (2018). https://www.who.int/data/gho/data/indicators/indicator-details/GHO/restrictions-on-alcohol-use-in-public-places.

Ribereau-Gayon, P., Dubourdieu, D., Doneche, B., & Lonvaud, A. (2006). Handbook of enology: The microbiology of wine and vinifications. In (2nd ed.,, *1. Handbook of Enology: The Microbiology of Wine and Vinifications* (pp. 1–497). wiley. https://doi.org/10.1002/0470010363

Rögener, F. (2021). Filtration technology for beer and beer yeast treatment. *IOP Conference Series: Earth and Environmental Science, 941*(1), Article 012016. https://doi.org/10.1088/1755-1315/941/1/012016

Russell, I., & Stewar, G. (2003). *Whisky: Technology, production and marketing whisky: Technology, production and marketing* (pp. 1–366). United Kingdom: Elsevier Ltd.. https://doi.org/10.1016/B978-0-12-669202-0.X5014-3. Available from: http://www.sciencedirect.com/science/book/9780126692020.

Russell, I., & Stewart, G. (2014). Whisky: Technology, production and marketing. In *Technology, production and marketing* (2nd ed., pp. 1–417). United States: Elsevier. https://doi.org/10.1016/C2012-0-00481-4

Sabino, L. L., de Oliveira Silva, M. F., & de Castilhos, M. B. M. (2023). Production of fermented beverage using pineapple residue as an alcoholic fermentation substrate: A physicochemical and sensory approach. *Food Research and Technology, 249*(2), 387–396. https://doi.org/10.1007/s00217-022-04124-6

Sahaya Glingston, R., Yadav, J., Rajpoot, J., Joshi, N., & Nagotu, S. (2021). Contribution of yeast models to virus research. *Applied Microbiology and Biotechnology, 105*(12), 4855–4878. https://doi.org/10.1007/s00253-021-11331-w

Santos, R. B.d., Filoda, P. F., Teixeira, I. D., Helfer, G. A., Santos, R. O., Oliveira, A. S., Barin, J. S., Tischer, B., & Costa, A. B.d. (2019). Flow thermal infrared enthalpimetry: Rapid and inexpensive determination of the alcohol content of distilled beverages. *Talanta, 200*, 67–71. https://doi.org/10.1016/j.talanta.2019.03.044

Savchuk, S. A., Palacio, C., Gil, A., Tagliaro, F., Kuznetsov, R. M., Brito, A., & Appolonova, S. A. (2020). Determination of the chemical composition of alcoholic beverages by gas chromatography-mass spectrometry. *Journal of Food Processing and Preservation, 44*(9), Article 17454549. https://doi.org/10.1111/jfpp.14676

Schwegel, J. (2018). Super unleaded malbec? A case Study in flawed international standard setting at the codex alimentarius. *Journal of Food Law & Policy, 14*(2). https://doi.org/10.54119/jflp.pctd3508

Scoccianti, C. (2015). *Carcinogens: Identification of carcinogens encyclopedia of food and health* (pp. 658–662). France: Elsevier Inc.. https://doi.org/10.1016/B978-0-12-384947-2.00118-5

Soni, S. K., Swami, U., Trivedi, N., & Soni, R. (2021). *Wine as a complete functional beverage: A perspective.* Informa UK Limited. https://doi.org/10.1201/9781351034265-4

Sousa-Dias, M. L., Paula, V. B., Dias, L. G., & Estevinho, L. M. (2021). Mead production using immobilized cells of saccharomyces cerevisiae: Reuse of sodium alginate beads. *Processes, 9*(4). https://doi.org/10.3390/pr9040724

Spedding, G. (2016). Alcohol and its measurement. In *Brewing materials and processes* (pp. 123–149). Elsevier. https://doi.org/10.1016/B978-0-12-799954-8.00007-1

Sroka, P., & Tuszyński, T. (2007). Changes in organic acid contents during mead wort fermentation. *Food Chemistry, 104*(3), 1250–1257. https://doi.org/10.1016/j.foodchem.2007.01.046

Steinkraus, K. (2018). In K. H. Steinkraus (Ed.), *Handbook of indigenous fermented foods* (2nd ed.). CRC Press.

Tabago, M. K. A. G., Calingacion, M. N., & Garcia, J. (2021). Recent advances in NMR-based metabolomics of alcoholic beverages. *Food Chemistry: Molecular Sciences, 2*. https://doi.org/10.1016/j.fochms.2020.100009. Available from: www.journals.elsevier.com/food-chemistry-molecular-sciences.

Torres-Guardado, R., Esteve-Zarzoso, B., Reguant, C., & Bordons, A. (2022). Microbial interactions in alcoholic beverages. *International Microbiology, 25*(1), 1–15. https://doi.org/10.1007/s10123-021-00200-1

Trius-Soler, M., Praticò, G., Gürdeniz, G., Garcia-Aloy, M., Canali, R., Fausta, N., Brouwer-Brolsma, E. M., Andrés-Lacueva, C., & Dragsted, L. O. (2023). Biomarkers of moderate alcohol intake and alcoholic beverages: A systematic literature review. *Genes and Nutrition, 18*(1). https://doi.org/10.1186/s12263-023-00726-1

Tsenang, M., Pheko-ofitlhile, T., Mokgadi, J., Masamba, W., & Phokedi, G. N. (2023). A validated ICP-MS method for the screening and quantitative analysis of heavy metal contaminants in home-brewed alcoholic beverages of Botswana. *Food and Humanity, 1*, 1125–1133. https://doi.org/10.1016/j.foohum.2023.09.013

Verma, G., Singh, V. P., Rajpurohit, G. S., Singh, S., Shah, S. N., Kumari, R., Bala, M., Gupta, L., Rani, R., Neha, & Yadav, R. K. (2024). Crafting responsibility: Strategies for balancing economic growth with public health and environmental sustainability in India's liquor sector. *Journal of Drug and Alcohol Research, 13*(7). https://doi.org/10.4303/JDAR/236307

Vidrih, R., & Hribar, J. (2007). Studies on the sensory properties of mead and the formation of aroma compounds related to the type of honey. *Acta Alimentaria, 36*(2), 151–162. https://doi.org/10.1556/aalim.36.2007.2.2

Wang, Z., Svyantek, A., Miller, Z., & Watrelot, A. A. (2024). Fermentation process effects on fermented McIntosh apple ciders. *Fermentation, 10*(3), 115. https://doi.org/10.3390/fermentation10030115

Wardencki, W. (2018). Alcoholic beverages. In *Reference module in chemistry, molecular sciences and chemical engineering*. Elsevier. https://doi.org/10.1016/B978-0-12-409547-2.14330-6

Waterhouse, A. L., Sacks, G. L., & Jeffery, D. W. (2024). *Understanding wine chemistry.* John Wiley & Sons.

Webster, C. E., Barker, D., Deed, R. C., & Pilkington, L. I. (2025). Mead production and quality: A review of chemical and sensory mead quality evaluation with a focus on analytical methods. *Food Research International, 202*, Article 18737145. https://doi.org/10.1016/j.foodres.2024.115655

Wiśniewska, P., Śliwińska, M., Dymerski, T., Wardencki, W., & Namieśnik, J. (2015). The analysis of vodka: A review paper. *Food Analytical Methods, 8*(8), 2000–2010. https://doi.org/10.1007/s12161-015-0089-7

Worldwide beer production 2023. (n.d.). Statista. https://www.statista.com/statistics/270275/worldwide-beer-production/.

Wunderlich, S., & Back, W. (2009). 1—Overview of manufacturing beer: Ingredients, processes, and quality criteria. In V. R. Preedy (Ed.), *Beer in health and disease prevention* (pp. 3–16). Academic Press. https://doi.org/10.1016/B978-0-12-373891-2.00001-8

Further reading

Food Safety and Standards Authority of India. (2018). *Compendium: Food safety and standards (alcoholic beverages) regulations.* https://www.fssai.gov.in/upload/uploadfiles/files/Compendium_Alcoholic_Beverages_Regulations_04_03_2021.pdf.

Kurt, M. D. (1994). Quality assurance in breath-alcohol analysis. *Journal of Analytical Toxicology, 18*(6), 306–311. https://doi.org/10.1093/jat/18.6.306

CHAPTER

7 Microbiological composition, fermentation methods and quality attributes of non-alcoholic fermented beverages

Mariana Buranelo Egea[1], Larissa Graziele Rauber Duarte[2] and Ailton Cesar Lemes[3]

[1]*Goiano Federal Institute of Education, Science and Technology, Campus Rio Verde, Rio Verde, GO, Brazil;* [2]*Instituto Federal do Sul de Minas, IFSULdeMINAS, Machado, MG, Brazil;* [3]*School of Chemistry, Federal University of Rio de Janeiro, Rio de Janeiro, RJ, Brazil*

7.1 Introduction

The growing consumer awareness of the relationship between diet and overall well-being has significantly fueled demand for food and beverages beyond mere hunger satisfaction or basic nutrition. Modern consumers actively seek products that offer additional health benefits, such as enhancing gut health, strengthening the immune system, and reducing the risk of chronic diseases. This shift in dietary preferences has been driven by scientific advancements highlighting the role of foods and beverages in disease prevention, as well as a growing interest in personalized nutrition and wellness. Consequently, the food industry has responded by developing innovative products incorporating bioactive compounds, probiotics, prebiotics, and other nutritionally enhanced ingredients, catering to an increasingly health-conscious market. In this context, non-alcoholic fermented beverages have gained prominence due to their potential to modulate the gut microbiota, strengthen the immune system, and provide bioactive compounds with various potentially beneficial properties. These beverages, associated with more balanced dietary practices, meet the demands of increasingly health-conscious consumers who prioritize the quality of life and well-being (Altay et al., 2013; Santos et al., 2024).

Historically, non-alcoholic fermented beverages have played a significant role in various cultures worldwide. These products have been valued for their nutritional and sensory properties, from traditional fermented dairy beverages to cereal-based beverages. Today, the, associated with more balanced dietary practices, interest in these beverages aligns with scientific advancements highlighting their potential health benefits, providing their adaptation for current consumers (Marsh et al., 2014).

Non-alcoholic fermented beverages are obtained through the controlled action of microorganisms, such as lactic acid bacteria and yeasts, which convert fermentable substrates into bioactive metabolites, organic acids, and other compounds of interest (Table 7.1). Unlike alcoholic beverages, this fermentation process is designed to minimize ethanol production, prioritizing the formation of

The Science and Safety of Beverages. https://doi.org/10.1016/B978-0-443-36536-2.00008-9

Table 7.1 Types of fermentation, microorganisms, final metabolites and possible applications.

Fermentation type	Microorganisms	Final metabolites	Examples/ Applications	References
Alcoholic	Yeasts (Saccharomyces)	Ethanol + CO_2	Beer, wine, bread	Saranraj et al. (2024)
Lactic	Lactic acid bacteria (*Lactobacillus, Streptococcus*)	Lactic acid	Yogurt, cheeses, kefir	Praveen and Brogi (2025)
Acetic	Acetic bacteria (Acetobacter)	Acetic acid	Vinegar	Hao et al. (2025)
Butyric	*Clostridium butyricum*	Butyric acid + gas H_2/CO_2	Fermentation of organic waste	Kumar et al. (2025)
Propionic	*Propionibacterium*	Propionic acid + CO_2	Swiss cheese	Ağagündüz et al. (2025)
Mixed fermentation	Enterobacteria	Various (acids, gases, ethanol)	Intestinal fermentations	Kocsis et al. (2025)

compounds that influence functionality, nutritional, and sensory profiles, as well as product (Agarbati et al., 2024; Altay et al., 2013; Ignat et al., 2020). The production and standardization of these beverages require strict control of microbiological and technological parameters to ensure food safety, the viability of beneficial microorganisms, and the maintenance of desirable characteristics throughout storage (Chong et al., 2023; Ignat et al., 2020).

The global market for non-alcoholic fermented beverages has followed this growing consumer demand, generating revenue of $3.6 billion in 2023, with projections indicating growth to approximately $4.9 billion by 2031 (Global, 2024). Within this market, these beverages can be produced from various raw materials, each imparting distinct nutritional, sensory, and bioactive properties. Traditionally, cereals, legumes, fruits, and vegetables are used individually or in blends (Basinskiene et al., 2016; Cichońska & Ziarno, 2022; Jooyandeh, 2013). From the selected raw material or properly treated blend, fermentation enhances nutrient digestibility, increases the bioavailability of bioactive compounds, and generates new metabolites with functional properties, such as organic acids, exopolysaccharides, and bioactive peptides. Additionally, fermentation modifies key sensory attributes, including flavor, aroma, and texture, improving consumer acceptance of the final product (Brugnoli et al., 2023; Shahbazi et al., 2018).

Despite the numerous benefits of these beverages, their production processes must be carefully designed to enable industrial-scale production without compromising their nutritional, technological, and sensory properties. Standardizing fermentation conditions, including microbial strain selection, temperature control, fermentation time, and medium composition, is essential to ensure product stability and the reproducibility of its beneficial effects (Ignat et al., 2020; Nedyalkov et al., 2019). Additionally, processing strategies should be implemented to preserve the viability of beneficial microorganisms, the integrity of bioactive compounds, and sensory quality throughout storage, ensuring that the final product meets market demands and regulatory requirements (Cunha et al., 2022; Tamang & Thapa, 2022, pp. 130–148; Valero-Cases et al., 2020).

Furthermore, producing non-alcoholic fermented beverages aligns with sustainability goals by utilizing agricultural by-products, reducing food waste, and promoting resource-efficient fermentation methods. This approach supports environmental responsibility and contributes to the development of more accessible and cost-effective functional beverages (Alexandre et al., 2023; Salas-Millán & Aguayo, 2024).

In this context, understanding fermentation processes, microbial interactions, and the factors affecting the viability and functionality of microorganisms is essential for optimizing formulation and standardizing these products. Thus, this chapter explores the associated microbiota, fermentation processes, and key quality parameters required for the safe and standardized production of non-alcoholic fermented beverages.

7.2 Fermentation methods in non-alcoholic beverages

Throughout history, the human ability to understand and control natural processes has been essential for technological advancements and the development of products that meet evolving consumer demands. The need for differentiated food and beverage options with enhanced sensory, nutritional, and functional properties has driven the observation and refinement of biological processes. Once used empirically, fermentation has been increasingly understood and optimized to transform raw materials into a wide range of products, from preserved foods to functional beverages. With scientific and technological progress, it has become possible to enhance fermentation efficiency and modulate it for the production of non-alcoholic fermented beverages, which offer a combination of desirable sensory attributes, stability, and potential health benefits (Cuvas-Limon et al., 2021; Kitessa, 2024).

Fermentation is a complex biochemical process driven by the metabolic activity of microorganisms, including bacteria and yeasts, which convert organic substrates into valuable compounds. This transformation occurs through enzymatic reactions that break down carbohydrates, proteins, and lipids, producing metabolites such as organic acids, alcohols, and gases. The specific metabolic pathways involved depend on the type of microorganism and fermentation conditions, which can be carefully controlled to obtain targeted products with distinct sensory, nutritional, and functional properties. Fermentation has been widely used in food and beverage production for centuries, contributing to the preservation and enhancement of raw materials and the development of unique flavors, textures, and bioactive compounds (Kaur et al., 2019; Verardo et al., 2020). In non-alcoholic fermented beverages, the fermentation process is carefully controlled to minimize ethanol production while enhancing the formation of beneficial metabolites, contributing to the development of functional and health-promoting beverages (Behera et al., 2019). Lactic fermentation stands out among the main fermentation methods for these beverages (Baschali et al., 2017).

The main requirements involve the selection of viable strains of beneficial microorganisms (such as *Lactobacillus* and yeasts that do not produce excessive ethanol), rigorous temperature control (generally 20–40°C to avoid alcoholic production), pH (4.0–5.5 to inhibit pathogens), fermentation time (24–120 h depending on the product), and medium composition (fermentable sugars $<5–10\%$ to minimize ethanol). These factors ensure desired metabolites such as organic acids, prebiotics, and bioactive compounds, while meeting food safety regulations (e.g., $<0.5\%$ ethanol for non-alcoholic classification) and sensory/nutritional standards (Behera et al., 2019).

Lactic fermentation occurs through the action of bacteria of the *Lactobacillus*, *Streptococcus*, and *Bifidobacterium* genera, which convert lactose and other sugars into lactic acid (Behera et al., 2019). This process is widely used in producing beverages such as kefir, kombucha, kvass (a Slavic beverage made from fermented rye bread), among others (Chong et al., 2023).

The association of more than one fermentation method is widespread. It is carried out to create unique sensory profiles and increase the possibility of health benefits due to the numerous metabolites produced by the beverage's microbiota (Baschali et al., 2017). For example, propionic fermentation, carried out by bacteria of the *Propionibacterium* genus, can contribute to the complexity of fermented beverages by producing propionic acid and carbon dioxide (Behera et al., 2019). Table 7.2 summarizes the key microbiological and process parameters for non-alcoholic fermented beverages.

Consuming these beverages offers health benefits associated with the substrates and microorganisms used in the fermentation process, as well as the metabolites produced (Marsh et al., 2014). Fermented beverages offer various health benefits by supporting digestion, promoting beneficial gut microbiota, and aiding in the breakdown of complex food components. They also modulate the immune system by producing antimicrobial peptides and other bioactive compounds. Additionally, fermentation enhances sensory attributes by developing richer flavors and refining texture. This process also improves nutrient bioavailability, facilitating the absorption of essential vitamins and minerals, such as B vitamins, iron, and calcium, thereby contributing to overall well-being (Baschali et al., 2017).

Fermenting non-alcoholic beverages is an ancient practice with deep cultural roots that continues to evolve through scientific and technological advancements. Over time, this process has been refined to preserve and enhance beverage sensory qualities, develop innovative flavors, and deliver functional health benefits. Whether through traditional artisanal techniques or modern biotechnological approaches, non-alcoholic fermented beverages are gaining increasing relevance in contemporary diets,

Table 7.2 Key microbiological and process parameters for non-alcoholic fermented beverages.

Parameter	Description/Typical range	Importance
Microbial strains	*Lactobacillus*, *Streptococcus*, *Bifidobacterium*, yeasts (e.g., non-ethanol producing *Saccharomyces*)	Produce beneficial metabolites and minimize ethanol (Behera et al., 2019)
Substrate	Cereals, fruits, plant-based milk, teas (sugars 5%–15%)	Source of fermentable nutrients for lactic acids and bioactives
Temperature	20–40°C (optimum 30–37°C for lactic)	Controls metabolic rate and prevents contamination (Behera et al., 2019)
Initial/final pH	4.5–6.5 initial; 3.5–4.5 final	Inhibits pathogens and stabilizes product
Fermentation time	24–120 h	Optimizes metabolite formation without excess ethanol
Ethanol concentration	<0.5% v/v	Legal classification as non-alcoholic
Aeration/Agitation	Anaerobic or microaerophilic	Influences metabolic pathways (e.g., lactic vs. acetic)
Storage	4–10°C post-fermentation	Maintains microbial viability and sensory quality (Chong et al., 2023)

offering health-conscious consumers natural, microbiota-supporting alternatives that align with current trends in nutrition, wellness, and sustainable food production (Baschali et al., 2017; Cuvas-Limon et al., 2021; Marsh et al., 2014).

7.3 Microbiological composition of non-alcoholic fermented beverages

Non-alcoholic fermented beverages represent a microbial transformation process deeply rooted in diverse cultural traditions worldwide. In particular, African countries possess a rich and longstanding heritage of cereal-based fermentations, which have led to the development of a wide variety of non-alcoholic beverages. These traditional products are often produced through spontaneous fermentation processes and are characterized by complex microbial ecosystems, including diverse species of lactic acid bacteria, yeasts, and other functional microorganisms. Such beverages not only reflect local customs and knowledge but also contribute to nutritional security and dietary diversity in many regions (Madilo et al., 2024; Pswarayi & Gänzle, 2022).

The microbial composition of these beverages follows a structured succession rather than occurring randomly, with different groups of microorganisms replacing each other throughout the fermentation process. Various factors influence this dynamic shift, including substrate composition, fermentation conditions, and microbial interactions. In the initial stages, fast-growing microorganisms dominate the process by rapidly consuming available sugars and producing metabolites like organic acids and antimicrobial compounds. As fermentation progresses, changes in pH, oxygen levels, and nutrient availability create a selective environment that favors the growth of more specialized or stress-tolerant microbial populations. This sequential microbial succession not only influences the final sensory attributes of the beverage but also affects its nutritional profile and functional properties, ensuring the development of a stable and beneficial end product (Shen et al., 2021; Wang et al., 2023; Zheng et al., 2018). More precisely, initially, plant-associated Enterobacteriaceae are present in the raw materials. As fermentation progresses, these early microorganisms are replaced by specialized fermentative species. At intermediate stages, lactic acid bacteria (LAB), such as Enterococci, Lactococci, Leuconostoc, and Weissella, dominate, shaping the beverage's sensory profile (Hao et al., 2021). In the final stages, acid-tolerant bacteria, including *Pediococci, Lactiplantibacillus plantarum*, and *Limosilactobacillus fermentum*, take over, contributing to acidity and further refining sensory attributes (Pswarayi & Gänzle, 2022).

Several factors play a crucial role in shaping the microbiological composition of non-alcoholic fermented beverages. The selection of raw materials, such as corn, sorghum, wheat, or other cereal and plant-based substrates, significantly influences the specific microbial communities that dominate the fermentation process (Gautam et al., 2024). Each substrate provides distinct nutrients, including carbohydrates, proteins, and micronutrients, which selectively promote the growth of particular bacterial and yeast strains. Additionally, environmental conditions, such as temperature, pH, oxygen availability, and the presence of indigenous microbiota, contribute to microbial succession, thereby affecting fermentation kinetics and metabolite production (Louw et al., 2023). The interplay between these factors ultimately determines the final beverage's sensory attributes, nutritional profile, and functional properties.

A comprehensive understanding of microbial interactions in these beverages is essential for optimizing and standardizing production while ensuring consistent quality and functionality.

Investigating the dynamic relationships between native microbiota and controlled inoculation strategies allows researchers to identify key microbial species and metabolic pathways that contribute to desirable sensory attributes, enhanced microbiological stability, and potential health benefits. Comparative studies help determine how spontaneous fermentations differ from those guided by selected starter cultures, offering insights into methods that can improve flavor complexity, probiotic potential, and bioactive compound formation. These findings deepen our understanding of traditional food fermentation practices and pave the way for the development of novel functional beverages with tailored nutritional and therapeutic properties.

7.3.1 Lactic acid bacteria (*Lactobacillus, Lactococcus,* and *Streptococcus*)

Lactic acid bacteria (LAB) play a key role in producing non-alcoholic fermented beverages, shaping their nutritional, sensory, and functional properties. By converting sugars into lactic acid, LAB helps preserve the product, inhibits spoilage microorganisms, and enhances flavor complexity by producing organic acids and aromatic compounds. Additionally, they produce bioactive compounds, such as bacteriocins and peptides, that support gut health and exert antimicrobial effects. Their presence ensures product stability, safety, and additional health benefits, making them essential for developing high-quality functional beverages (Mandha et al., 2021, pp. 127–158; Pswarayi & Gänzle, 2022). These bacteria are generally facultative anaerobes and acid-tolerant, with an optimal growth range of pH 5.5-6.0. Regarding temperature, many mesophilic species grow between 20°C and 45°C, while thermotolerant strains can grow at temperatures above 50°C (Liu et al., 2024; Sionek et al., 2024; Souza et al., 2017).

In traditional African and Latin American fermentation practices, dominant LAB species include *Lactobacillus plantarum*, *L. brevis*, *L. fermentum*, and *Lactococcus lactis*. These bacteria metabolize cereal substrates, producing 0.5%–2.0% lactic acid, reducing pH from 6.0–7.0 to 3.5–4.5, and generating exopolysaccharides (up to 10–50 mg/L) and bacteriocins (1–100 AU/mL) that enhance both sensory quality and nutritional value (Carboni et al., 2023; Mashau et al., 2021).

Beyond their role in fermentation, LAB possess significant functional potential, particularly through their probiotic properties. These microorganisms contribute to gut health by enhancing intestinal microbiota balance (increasing beneficial *Bifidobacterium* counts by 10–100 fold), inhibiting pathogenic bacteria through competitive exclusion and bacteriocin production (reducing pathogens like *E. coli* by 2–4 log CFU/mL), and strengthening the immune system (elevating IgA levels by 20%–50%). Additionally, LAB improves digestibility by breaking down complex macromolecules—degrading 30%–70% of proteins and 20%–50% of phytates—into more bioavailable forms, facilitating nutrient absorption. Their enzymatic activity also aids in reducing anti-nutritional factors, such as phytic acid (by 40%–90%), further enhancing the nutritional quality of fermented beverages. As a result, LAB plays a crucial role in preserving and enhancing non-alcoholic fermented beverages' health benefits (Aburjaile et al., 2022, pp. 207–219; Anumudu et al., 2024; Ilango & Antony, 2021). Some LAB strains stimulate mucin production in the intestinal lining by 1.5–3 fold, strengthening its protective barrier while inhibiting pathogenic microorganisms. Additionally, they enhance the nutritional profile of non-alcoholic beverages by increasing B-vitamin content (e.g., B12 up to 5–20 μg/100 mL) (Anumudu et al., 2024).

Studies in Europe and Africa highlight the potential of plant-based probiotic beverages fermented with LAB (Mandha et al., 2021, pp. 127–158). Ingredients like rice, wheat, and corn are optimal substrates, each favoring specific microbial communities (Ziarno & Cichońska, 2021). Fermentation improves the bioavailability of essential nutrients, vitamins, and minerals, making these beverages highly nutritious (Moiseenko et al., 2024).

Technological advancements have enabled more precise control of LAB fermentation, optimizing microbial growth conditions, enhancing metabolite production, and improving sensory and functional properties in fermented beverages. Selecting specific strains like *Lactobacillus helveticus* allows for tailored sensory and functional characteristics (Jemima & John, 2024, pp. 159–190; Zhao et al., 2024). These developments support the production of customized non-alcoholic beverages that align with consumer preferences and health needs, offering enhanced probiotic potential, extended shelf life, and improved overall product quality.

Ultimately, LAB bridges traditional fermentation practices with modern scientific approaches, expanding their applications in the functional beverage industry. By controlling fermentation conditions, manufacturers can enhance product safety, quality, and nutritional value, transforming these beverages into functional foods with significant health benefits (Mbaye et al., 2023).

7.3.2 Yeasts (*Saccharomyces, Candida,* and *Brettanomyces*)

Yeasts are fundamental in producing non-alcoholic fermented beverages, contributing to traditional and modern biotechnological applications. Their significance goes beyond conventional fermentation, as they facilitate the development of beverages with distinctive sensory attributes (e.g., esters at 10–50 mg/L contributing to fruity aromas), improved nutritional properties (e.g., B-vitamins increased by 20%–100%), and controlled alcohol content (<0.5% v/v ethanol). Producers can carefully select and optimize yeast strains to enhance flavor complexity, texture, and functional benefits while maintaining minimal or negligible ethanol levels, catering to consumer demand for healthier and innovative beverage options (Jemima & John, 2024, pp. 159–190). Most yeasts exhibit optimal growth at a pH range of 4.0–6.0 and temperatures between 25°C and 35°C (growth rates 0.1–0.3 h^{-1}), although thermotolerant species can grow above 40°C. Additionally, many yeasts display osmotic resistance (tolerating up to 30%–50% sugars) and the ability to adapt to environments with high sugar concentrations or low oxygen availability (DO < 1 mg/L), making them versatile for food, biotechnological, and industrial applications (Liu et al., 2015; Yalcin & Ozbas, 2008).

Recent studies highlight the potential of non-*Saccharomyces* yeasts as promising alternatives in non-alcoholic beverage production (Vaštík et al., 2022). Certain yeast strains can be strategically selected to minimize ethanol production (e.g., <0.2% after 72h fermentation) while preserving desirable sensory attributes. Some ferment simple sugars without generating significant alcohol (ethanol yields <1 g/L glucose consumed), making them ideal for producing low-alcohol beverages (Nyhan et al., 2023).

The metabolic versatility of yeasts, particularly *Brettanomyces* and *Saccharomyces,* allows for innovative fermentations. These yeasts contribute to the valorization of dairy by-products (e.g., lactose utilization 70%–90%) and facilitate the fermentation of complex sugars, expanding the development of functional beverages (Lawton et al., 2021; Rivera Flores et al., 2021). Their ability to transform underutilized substrates into nutritious and flavorful beverages (e.g., phenolic content increased 2–5 fold) further underscores their biotechnological value.

Kombucha and other symbiotic fermentations illustrate the intricate microbial interactions between yeasts and bacteria. These relationships create unique flavor profiles (acetic acid 0.5–3 g/L) and enhance probiotic and nutritional benefits (live cells $>10^6$ CFU/mL). This complex microbial ecosystem is a fascinating frontier in beverage production, merging traditional techniques with modern scientific perspectives (Harrison et al., 2023).

Fruit-based fermented beverages represent another key application of yeast-driven fermentation (Kesa et al., 2021). Careful yeast strain selection allows for beverages with enhanced functionality (antioxidant capacity up 30%–50%), extended shelf life (TTC >90 days at 4°C), and distinct sensory experiences. This process transforms simple fruit-derived substrates, yielding complex beverages with unique flavors, beneficial bioactive compounds, and potential health-promoting effects, further expanding the scope of functional fermented drinks (Bueno et al., 2021).

Research on yeast-based fermentation suggests a promising future for the non-alcoholic beverage industry. The metabolic diversity of yeasts enables the creation of customized beverages that cater to nutritional and sensory consumer demands. Continuous innovation in yeast applications reinforces their pivotal role in developing healthy and appealing fermented beverages.

7.3.3 Acetic bacteria (*Acetobacter, Gluconobacter*)

Acetic acid bacteria (AAB) such as *Acetobacter* and *Gluconobacter* are crucial in producing non-alcoholic fermented beverages, transforming simple substrates into complex, functional products. These Gram-negative aerobic microorganisms excel in converting ethanol (yields up to 90%–98% acetic acid from ethanol), sugars (glucose oxidation 50%–80%), and other compounds into organic acids through oxidative fermentation, achieving acetic acid concentrations of 3–10 g/L (Hata et al., 2023; Jemima & John, 2024, pp. 159–190). They exhibit optimal growth at a pH of 4.0–6.5 (tolerating down to pH 2.5–3.0), demonstrating high tolerance to acidic environments with growth rates of 0.05–0.15 h^{-1}. The optimal temperature range for their development is between 25°C and 30°C (doubling time 4–8 h), although some species can grow at higher temperatures up to 38–40°C (Gomes et al., 2018; Puerari et al., 2012).

The metabolic versatility of AAB, particularly *Acetobacter* and *Gluconobacter*, supports the development of innovative non-alcoholic beverages with distinct sensory and nutritional attributes (e.g., gluconic acid 5–20 g/L, enhancing antioxidant capacity by 20%–40%) (Brugnoli et al., 2023). Studies have shown their potential in converting agricultural waste and unconventional fruits into functional beverages (substrate utilization 70%–95%), broadening the scope of sustainable beverage production (Calderón-Martínez et al., 2024, pp. 157–216).

Kombucha and similar fermented beverages showcase the integral role of AAB in creating complex microbial ecosystems (AAB populations 10^6–10^8 CFU/mL). These bacteria produce beneficial compounds, including glucuronic acid (0.5–2.5 g/L), exopolysaccharides (10–100 mg/L), and organic acids (total 5–15 g/L), enhancing these beverages' nutritional and functional properties (Bueno et al., 2021).

Beyond traditional fermentation, research explores AAB applications in developing health-promoting beverages from various substrates, such as dates and agricultural by-products (bioconversion efficiency 60%–85%). Their ability to produce bioactive metabolites (e.g., phenolic content increased 1.5–3 fold) and transform simple ingredients into valuable nutritional components makes them essential for innovation in functional beverages (Cantadori et al., 2022).

Microbial ecology studies have highlighted the intricate interactions between AAB and other microorganisms (synergistic growth boosting metabolite yields by 30%–50%), demonstrating their profound impact on sensory characteristics (acetic acid contributing 40%–70% of total acidity) and potential health benefits (De Roos & De Vuyst, 2018; Lavefve et al., 2019). These dynamic microbial relationships represent a cutting-edge area in beverage science, bridging traditional fermentation practices with modern advancements.

7.3.4 Microbial interactions: Synergy between yeasts and bacteria in fermentation

Microbial interactions during fermentation form a complex network of cooperation, in which yeasts and bacteria engage in metabolic exchanges that transform simple substrates into functional beverages (Ignat et al., 2020; Maicas, 2020). The interaction between lactic acid bacteria (LAB) and yeasts is well documented in indigenous fermentation practices, especially in African food systems (Adesulu-Dahunsi et al., 2020). These interactions extend beyond coexistence, involving cross-feeding mechanisms in which microorganisms mutually benefit from each other's metabolic by-products (Ferreira et al., 2022). For instance, yeasts degrade complex carbohydrates into simpler sugars, facilitating LAB metabolism, while LAB produces organic acids that modulate pH, creating favorable conditions for yeast activity (Table 7.3). Additionally, producing aromatic compounds, exopolysaccharides, and

Table 7.3 Microbiological composition of non-alcoholic fermented beverages.

Microbial group	Main genera	Role in fermentation	Associated beverages	Optimal growth conditions	References
Lactic acid bacteria (LAB)	*Lactobacillus, Lactococcus, Streptococcus, Leuconostoc, Weissella, Pediococcus*	Produce lactic acid, reduce pH, and improve flavor and microbiological stability.	Plant-based probiotic beverages (e.g., cereal and fruit-based), Kefir (LAB + yeasts)	pH 5.5–6.0; Temperature 20°C–45°C	(Mandha et al., 2021, pp. 127–158; Pswarayi & Gänzle, 2022)
Yeasts	*Saccharomyces, Candida, Brettanomyces, Starmerella*	Ferment sugars contribute to flavor and aroma and aid in texture.	Non-alcoholic beers (with *Saccharomycodes ludwigii*), Kvass	pH 4.0–6.0; Temperature 25°C–35°C	(Vaštík et al., 2022; Nyhan et al. 2023)
Acetic acid bacteria (AAB)	*Acetobacter, Gluconobacter*	Oxidize ethanol to acetic acid and produce bioactive compounds.	Kombucha, Fermented fruit beverages (e.g., agave-based)	pH 4.0–6.5; Temperature 25°C–30°C	(Hata et al., 2023; Brugnoli et al., 2023)
Microbial interactions	Combinations of LAB, yeasts, and AAB	Metabolic synergy: production of complex flavors and increased nutrient bioavailability.	Kefir (LAB + yeasts), Kombucha (yeasts + AAB), Fermented fruit beverages	Variable depending on substrate and environmental conditions	(Bueno et al., 2021; Kesa et al., 2021)

bioactive metabolites through microbial synergy enhances fermented beverages' sensory profile, texture, and functional properties. These cooperative interactions also contribute to microbiological stability and safety, preventing the proliferation of spoilage organisms and pathogens. Understanding and harnessing these microbial dynamics allows for developing more consistent, high-quality, and health-promoting non-alcoholic fermented beverages (El Youssef et al., 2020; Ferreira et al., 2022; Zanirati et al., 2015).

Co-fermentation of non-conventional probiotic yeasts with LAB has shown notable potential in enhancing the functional properties (e.g., probiotic viability $>10^7$ CFU/mL, 20%–50% increase in metabolite diversity), sensory characteristics (acceptance index 65%–85%, volatile compounds up 1.5–3 fold), and nutritional value (polyphenols 0.5–2.0 mg GAE/mL, exopolysaccharides 10–50 mg/L) of beverages (Agarbati et al., 2024; Freire et al., 2017). Studies on traditional Nigerian beverages like Kunu highlight how strategic microbial combinations can improve probiotic potential (LAB counts log 9.0–9.6 CFU/mL after 24–48h, pH reduction to 3.8–4.2) (Ndukwe et al., 2023).

Recent research suggests that these interactions can be deliberately manipulated to optimize fermentation, particularly in functional non-alcoholic beverages derived from substrates like rice and millet (Banwo et al., 2024; Mishra et al., 2024). Careful selection and pairing of specific yeast and bacterial strains can significantly influence the final product's sensory and functional attributes.

These microbial relationships extend beyond basic fermentation, constituting a highly developed biochemical network where microorganisms engage in competitive and cooperative interactions. This dynamic interplay influences the fermentation efficiency and the development of unique metabolites that enhance the final product's sensory, nutritional, and functional attributes. As scientific understanding of these microbial interactions advances, researchers uncover novel strategies to engineer beverages with precisely tailored characteristics, seamlessly integrating traditional fermentation wisdom with cutting-edge biotechnological innovations.

7.3.5 Native microbiota versus controlled inoculation: Impact on final product quality

The comparison between native microbiota and controlled inoculation highlights the complexity of microbial dynamics in fermented beverage production (Ojeda-Linares et al., 2022). Spontaneous fermentation, driven by indigenous microorganisms, often results in diverse and rich microbial communities that significantly influence the beverage's characteristics.

Studies have shown native microbiota exhibit greater bacterial diversity than controlled inoculation methods (Jemima & John, 2024, pp. 159–190). For instance, traditional fermented beverages often develop more complex microbial communities, with clay fermentation vessels acting as natural reservoirs contributing to unique flavor profiles and functional properties (Han et al., 2024).

While controlled inoculation offers greater predictability, it typically results in a more limited microbial consortium. This approach allows for the targeted selection of bacterial and yeast strains to enhance specific traits such as flavor, nutritional value, and long-term stability (Peña González et al., 2023). The deliberate introduction of selected microorganisms enables consistent and reproducible fermentation processes.

Beyond microbial composition, inoculation strategies also influence the metabolomic profile of fermented beverages. Significant differences in metabolite concentrations and profiles have been observed between native and controlled fermentation approaches (de Mello Sampaio et al., 2025).

These changes can dramatically affect the final product's sensory attributes, nutritional value, and functional properties.

Traditional fermentation practices balance microbial diversity with controlled selection. While native microbiota provide complexity and unique regional characteristics, controlled inoculation ensures consistency and the ability to achieve specific desirable traits (Altay et al., 2013). The future of non-alcoholic fermented beverages lies in understanding and integrating the strengths of both approaches. By studying microbial interactions and metabolic processes, researchers can develop innovative strategies that preserve the richness of traditional fermentation while meeting modern quality and consistency standards.

7.4 Types of non-alcoholic fermented beverages

Non-alcoholic fermented beverages result from microbial activity, primarily involving bacteria and yeast, which metabolize sugars into diverse bioactive compounds while minimizing ethanol production. These beverages stand out for their distinctive flavor profiles, probiotic potential, and associated health benefits. Among the most well-known examples are kombucha, water kefir, and rejuvelac—each offering unique sensory experiences and functional properties. Their rising popularity reflects a broader consumer shift toward natural, health-enhancing alternatives in the beverage industry. This is driven by an increasing awareness of gut health and the demand for minimally processed functional foods.

7.4.1 Kefir

Kefir is a fermented beverage originating in the Caucasus Mountains in Russia, resulting from the action of the natural microbiota present in the so-called "grains" or kefir lumps, with microbial populations reaching 10^8–10^{10} CFU/g in mature grains. Also known as tibicos or Tibetan mushrooms, when cultivated in milk, the beverage is called "yogurt plant" or "yogurt mushroom", characterized as fermented milk produced from kefir biomass (Van Wyk, 2019, pp. 473–527). The kefir biomass consists of a symbiotic consortium of lactic acid bacteria (LAB: 65%–90% of total microbiota, 10^7–10^9 CFU/g), acetic acid bacteria (10^5–10^7 CFU/g), yeasts (10^6–10^8 CFU/g), and fungi, all encased within a polysaccharide matrix known as kefiran (1%–5% w/w of grain mass). This unique microbial composition includes LAB such as *Lactobacillus* (30%–50%), *Lactococcus* (20%–30%), *Leuconostoc* (5%–15%), *Pediococcus* (2%–10%), and *Streptococcus* (5%–10%), alongside yeasts from genera such as *Saccharomyces* (20%–40%) and *Kluyveromyces* (15%–30%), which collectively contribute to kefir's characteristic taste (lactic acid 0.8%–1.5%), texture, and health benefits (Egea et al., 2020).

Due to its diverse microbial composition (bacteria:yeasts ratio 10:1 to 80:1) and the health benefits of its consumption, kefir biomass is a valuable source of probiotic microorganisms (viability $>10^7$ CFU/mL post-digestion). These microbes exhibit remarkable resilience, demonstrating resistance to bile salts (survival >70% at 0.3%–0.5% bile) and acidic pH conditions (viability >80% at pH 2.0–3.0 for 3h) essential for survival in the gastrointestinal tract. Also, kefir-associated probiotics can adhere to the intestinal epithelium (adhesion rates 10%–50% to Caco-2 cells), promoting gut colonization (increasing beneficial taxa by 1–2 log) and microbiota balance. Moreover, they are crucial in inhibiting pathogenic bacteria (reductions of 3–5 log CFU/mL against *E. coli* and *Salmonella*), enhancing gut health, and potentially supporting the immune system (elevated IgA by 20%–50%) (Diosma et al., 2014). *Lactococcus lactis* is an essential probiotic microorganism (populations 10^8–10^9 CFU/g) and is frequently present in kefir culture (Wang et al., 2015), as is *Lactobacillus kefiranofaciens* (dominant at 10^7–10^8 CFU/g) (Georgalaki et al., 2021; Zanirati et al., 2015), *Lactococcus lactis* ssp. *cremoris* (Vieira et al., 2017; Xing et al., 2017), *Lactobacillus diolivorans* and *Lactobacillus casei* (Zanirati et al., 2015), among others.

Kefir grains can have different sizes, ranging from 0.5 to 3.5 cm in diameter (average 1.5–2.5 cm) and presenting volumes between 0.5 and 20.0 mL per unit (typical 5–15 mL). Their shape is irregular, and the color can vary between whitish and yellowish tones, depending on the culture medium (Egea et al., 2020). When cultivated in milk, they acquire a light yellow hue (water content 85%–90%); in brown sugar, they take on an ochre or brown coloration; and when fermented in grape juice, they present a purple hue (Witthuhn et al., 2005; Wszolek et al., 2001) (Fig. 7.1).

The microbial composition of kefir biomass may vary according to the region of origin (LAB 60%–90%, yeasts 10%–40%), time of use, handling techniques, and culture medium (de Oliveira Filho et al., 2023). One of the key advantages of kefir production is the ability to recover and reuse the biomass for successive fermentation cycles (up to 10–20 cycles with 20%–50% biomass growth per cycle). After the fermentation process (24–48h at 25–30°C), the kefir culture can be separated from the liquid substrate (recovery yield 80%–95%), allowing for the production of the fermented beverage while simultaneously promoting biomass growth (grain multiplication rate 5%–15% daily). This feature ensures a continuous supply of active cultures (viability $>10^8$ CFU/g) and contributes to the sustainability and economic feasibility of kefir production (Satir & Guzel-Seydim, 2016). However, scaling up kefir production to an industrial level presents significant challenges, particularly in maintaining the nutritional and sensory consistency of the final product (probiotic counts variation ± 2 log CFU/mL). The natural kefir biomass is highly complex and irregular due to its diverse microbial composition, which can fluctuate based on environmental conditions, handling practices, and the substrate used in fermentation (pH 3.8–4.5, titratable acidity 0.8%–1.5%). These variations may lead to flavor, texture, and probiotic content inconsistencies, posing difficulties for large-scale manufacturing. To address this issue and ensure product standardization (viability stability $<10\%$

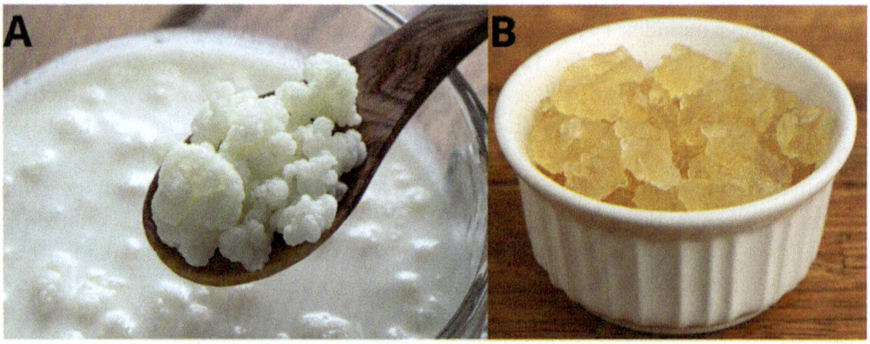

FIGURE 7.1

Kefir grains grown in milk (A) and brown sugar (B).

variation), researchers have explored the use of defined starter cultures, which consist of carefully selected microbial strains (LAB:yeast ratio 10:1) that replicate the key characteristics of traditional kefir fermentation while offering greater control over the process (Egea et al., 2020).

Furthermore, beverages fermented with kefir biomass may contain kefiran, an exopolysaccharide isolated from kefir grains (yield 50–200 mg/L). Kefiran is a water-soluble glucogalactan produced mainly by *Lactobacillus kefiranofaciens* in the center of the grains, under anaerobic conditions and is recognized for its immune system modulator (increasing IgA 20%–40%), antioxidant (DPPH scavenging 30%–60%), anti-inflammatory (TNF-α reduction 25%–50%), wound healing (contraction rate 40%–70% faster), and antimicrobial properties (inhibition zones 15–25 mm against *E. coli*), among others (de Oliveira Filho et al., 2023; Medrano et al., 2011; Vinderola et al., 2006).

In developing non-alcoholic fermented beverages, kefir has been widely used because it has good resistance to food conditions such as pH (stability at 3.5–4.5) and temperature (viability $>10^7$ CFU/mL at 4–10°C for 28 days) during storage. Several types of substrates can be used for the production of beverages, including fruits and vegetables (fermentation efficiency 70%–90%), cereals and oilseeds (sugar utilization 60%–85%), among others (de Melo Silva et al., 2021; Mendes et al., 2021; Ozcelik et al., 2021).

The raw material used in producing fermented juice impacts not only the flavor and aroma of the beverage but also the viability of the probiotic microorganisms (survival rates 70%–95% after 28 days) (dos Santos et al., 2023). The specific composition of the juice, including the type and concentration of sugars (5–12°Brix), organic acids (0.2%–1.0%), and other bioactive compounds, directly affects microbial growth (doubling time 2–4h), fermentation kinetics (rate 0.1–0.3 g/L/h lactic acid), and metabolite production. Maintaining an optimal balance between sugar content and acidity is crucial for creating favorable conditions that enhance fermentation efficiency (yield 80%–95%), ensuring the survival and metabolic activity of kefir microorganisms throughout the process (Ozcelik et al., 2021).

Another important aspect to consider is the dynamic interaction between microbial metabolism and the physicochemical properties of the fermentation medium. As microorganisms in kefir consume available carbohydrates (utilization 70%–95%) and produce lactic acid (0.8%–1.5%), the pH of the beverage gradually decreases (from 6.0–6.5 to 3.8–4.5). This acidification plays a dual role: while it helps inhibit the growth of pathogenic microorganisms (3–5 log reduction), contributing to the product's microbiological safety, it can also impact the texture and stability of the final beverage (viscosity 50–200 cP). This effect is particularly noticeable in water-soluble extracts of oilseeds, such as soy-based substrates. Since the isoelectric point of soy proteins is close to the final pH of fermented beverages (pI 4.5), the reduction in solubility can lead to protein aggregation (20%–50% precipitation), precipitation, and eventual phase separation. This phenomenon may compromise the sensory attributes and uniformity of the product and need formulation adjustments, such as pH control or stabilizing agents (0.1%–0.5% w/v), to enhance plant-based fermented beverages' overall texture and stability (Gamba et al., 2020; Rui et al., 2019; Santos et al., 2019). Therefore, it is expected that there will be a need to add some additive that can contribute to the body of fermented drinks of this type (Silva et al., 2021).

The microorganisms in the kefir culture and their complex symbiotic interaction give the beverages therapeutic properties, including antioxidant properties (ORAC values 5–15 μmol TE/mL), healing (wound closure 50%–80% faster), anti-inflammatory (IL-6 reduction 30%–60%), lipid metabolism modulators (cholesterol reduction 10%–25%), among others (Fahmy & Ismail, 2015; Fathi et al., 2016; Fiorda et al., 2016).

7.4.2 Kombucha

Kombucha is a sweet drink of Asian origin produced by fermenting tea from *Camellia sinensis* var. *sinensis* (green tea, 2–5 g/L leaves) or *Camellia sinensis* var. *assamica* (black tea, polyphenols 20%–30% oxidized) with added sugar (50–100 g/L sucrose or glucose) (Yang et al., 2010). Fermentation occurs by a symbiotic association of bacteria and yeast called SCOBY (Symbiotic Culture of Bacteria and Yeast), with microbial populations of 10^7–10^9 CFU/mL (LAB 40%–60%, AAB 20%–30%, yeasts 10%–20%), housed in a cellulose matrix (pellicle thickness 2–10 mm, 1%–5% w/w dry weight) synthesized by acetic bacteria (*Komagataeibacter* spp., 10^6–10^8 CFU/mL) formed during each fermentation process (7–30 days at 20–30°C, pH drop from 4.5–5.5 to 2.5–3.5, acetic acid 3–15 g/L) that is passed from one person to another (Fig. 7.2A-C) (Wang et al., 2022).

SCOBY may contain acetic bacteria such as *Acetobacter xylinum* (10^6–10^8 CFU/mL), *Acetobacter xylinoides, Bacterium gluconicum, Acetobacter aceti, Acetobacter pasteurianus* (20%–40% of AAB population), and yeasts such as *Schizosaccharomyces pombe, Saccharomycodes ludwigii, Kloeckera apiculata, Saccharomyces cerevisiae* (10^7–10^9 CFU/mL), *Zygosaccharomyces bailii, Brettanomyces bruxellensis, Brettanomyces lambicus, Brettanomyces custersii, Candida*, and *Pichia* species (Laavanya et al., 2021).

During the fermentation process, the catechins (50–150 mg/L) and xanthines (20–60 mg/L) present in tea stimulate the synthesis of cellulose (1–5 g/L) by bacteria, especially by *Komagataeibacter xylinus* (previously known as *Acetobacter xylinum*), which has this ability (productivity 0.5–2 g/L/day), contributing to the formation of the SCOBY structure (pellicle yield 2–10 mm thick) (Laureys et al., 2020). The yeasts convert the previously added sucrose (50–100 g/L) into fructose (20–40 g/L), glucose (30–50 g/L), and ethanol (0.5–3 g/L). Glucose and fructose are metabolized by acetic bacteria,

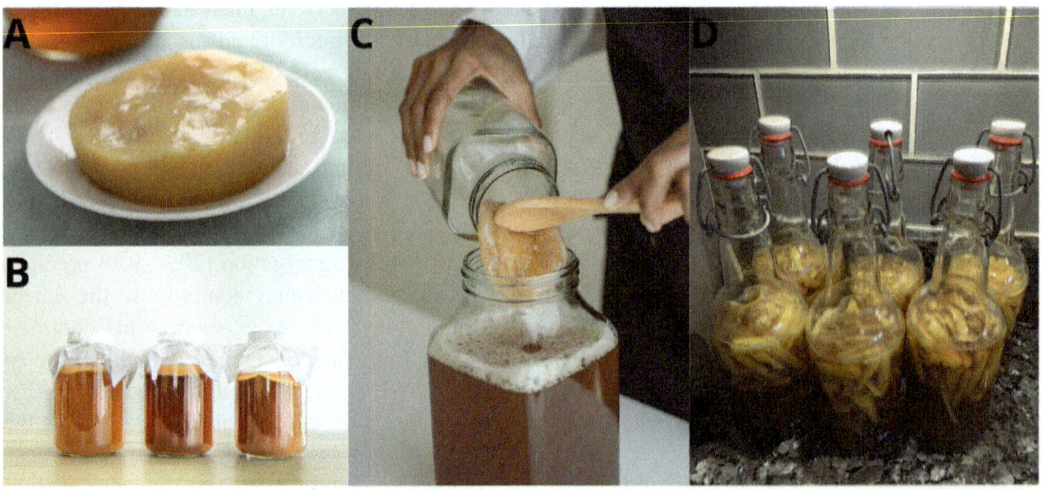

FIGURE 7.2

Symbiotic culture of bacteria and yeast (SCOBY) separated (A), fermentation process forming new SCOBY (B) and transferring to new fermentation process (C) and second fermentation for production of flavored kombucha (D).

producing glucuronic acid (0.5–2 g/L), acetic acid (3–15 g/L), gluconic acid (2–10 g/L), glucosamines (0.1–0.5 g/L), lactic acid (0.5–2 g/L), vitamins (B-vitamins 0.1–1 mg/L), amino acids (50–200 mg/L), and substances with natural antimicrobial properties (Alamgir & Alamgir, 2018, pp. 25–164).

The presence of acetic acid (3–15 g/L) stimulates yeast to produce ethanol (conversion efficiency 80%–95%), which in turn is used by acetic bacteria to produce additional acetic acid (yield 90%–98%). In addition, the presence of characteristic concentrations of ethanol (0.5–3 g/L) and acetic acid (3–15 g/L) can act as an antimicrobial agent, inhibiting undesirable microorganisms' growth (3–5 log CFU/mL reduction) and maintaining the fermentation system's symbiotic balance (Raspor & Goranovič, 2008). In addition, glucuronic acid (0.5–2 g/L) has been linked to the modulation of lipid metabolism in this beverage by binding to fat-soluble molecules (affinity 70%–90%) and facilitating their elimination (Adriani et al., 2011).

Regarding the product's characteristics, the flavor of kombucha changes throughout the fermentation process (7–30 days), changing from a slightly sparkling acidic fruit flavor (pH 3.5–4.5, volatiles 50–200 mg/L) to a milder vinegar flavor (pH 2.5–3.5, acetic acid >10 g/L) when incubation is prolonged (Sanwal et al., 2023). In addition, the color varies depending on the type of tea used in the fermentation process and/or the addition of fruit in the second fermentation stage (Fig. 7.2D) (da Silva et al., 2024).

Regarding the beneficial effects of kombucha beverage intake, there is antimicrobial activity against several pathogenic microorganisms (inhibition zones 10–25 mm), modulation of lipid and glucose metabolism (cholesterol reduction 15%–30%, glucose 10%–25%), and anticancer activity (cell viability reduction 20%–60% in vitro), among others. However, all these biological activities were evaluated in vitro or in vivo in animal models and must be confirmed in human experiments (Adriani et al., 2011; Sreeramulu et al., 2000; Srihari et al., 2013).

7.4.3 Fermented beverages using probiotic starter cultures

Probiotics are live microorganisms that, when administered in appropriate amounts ($\geq 10^6$–10^7 CFU/day), confer significant health benefits to the host (Hill et al., 2014). These microorganisms must remain viable (>10^7 CFU/g at production, >10^6 CFU/g at end of shelf life), metabolically active (acid tolerance >80% survival at pH 2.0–3.0 for 3h), and present in sufficient concentrations throughout the product's shelf life (28–90 days at 4–10°C) to be considered adequate. Specifically, probiotic-containing beverages should maintain a minimum count of 10^7 CFU/g of total lactic acid bacteria (viability retention 70%–95%) and 10^4–10^6 CFU/g of specific yeasts (survival >60% post-storage) to ensure their functional properties and health-promoting effects (dos Santos et al., 2023). Factors such as storage conditions (4–8°C optimal), pH (3.8–4.5 stability range), and interactions with other microbial communities (competitive exclusion reducing pathogens 2–4 log CFU/mL) can influence the survival and stability of probiotics in the final product.

Probiotic microorganism strains must be safe for humans (GRAS status, no antibiotic resistance genes) and resistant to low pH (survival 70%–90% at pH 2.5), gastric (90 min exposure) and pancreatic juices (120 min exposure), and bile salts (>60% tolerance at 0.3%–0.5% bile for 2h) (Fijan, 2014). In addition, these microorganisms must adhere to the intestinal epithelium and mucus (adhesion rates 10%–50% to Caco-2/HT-29 cells), antagonize pathogenic microorganisms (bacteriocin production 100–1000 AU/mL), and exhibit antimicrobial activity (inhibition zones 10–25 mm) and systemic effects on the intestinal barrier system (TEER increase 20%–50%) (Servin, 2004). The main bacteria used as supplements in probiotic functional foods belong to the genera *Lactobacillus* (populations 10^8–10^9 CFU/g) and *Bifidobacterium* spp. (10^7–10^8 CFU/g) (Cizeikiene & Jagelaviciute, 2021).

The development of probiotic foods, which contain beneficial microbial cultures (>10^7 CFU/g initial load), has become a niche market for the food industry but still faces significant challenges (Fig. 7.3) (dos Santos et al. 2023). The addition of probiotics can impact sensory characteristics, such as odor (volatile compounds increase 20%–50%), flavor (acidity 0.6%–1.2%), and texture (viscosity 50–300 cP), throughout the product's shelf life (viability decline 0.5–1.5 log CFU/month). This occurs due to the continuous metabolism of glucose (60%–90% utilization) by microorganisms, resulting in the production of metabolites (lactic acid, 0.5–2.0 g/L) and biomass (0.1%–1% w/v). These changes vary depending on the substrate (sugar content 5–15°Brix), the microorganism used (growth rates 0.1–0.3 h^{-1}), and the food processing conditions (fermentation 24–72h at 30–37°C) (Mohammadi et al., 2011; Prajapati et al., 2023).

Studies indicate that the addition of probiotic microorganisms can generate competitiveness between microorganisms (pathogen reduction 2–5 log CFU/mL), increase metabolite production (lactic acid 0.5–2.0 g/L, bacteriocins 100–1000 AU/mL), and extend shelf life (viability retention 70%–95% over 28–90 days at 4–10°C) due to their antimicrobial action (Aladeboyeje et al., 2022; Kadyan et al., 2021).

In addition to the microbiological aspects, fermented beverages with probiotics can improve their sensory and nutritional profile. Studies show that these beverages increase phenolic compounds

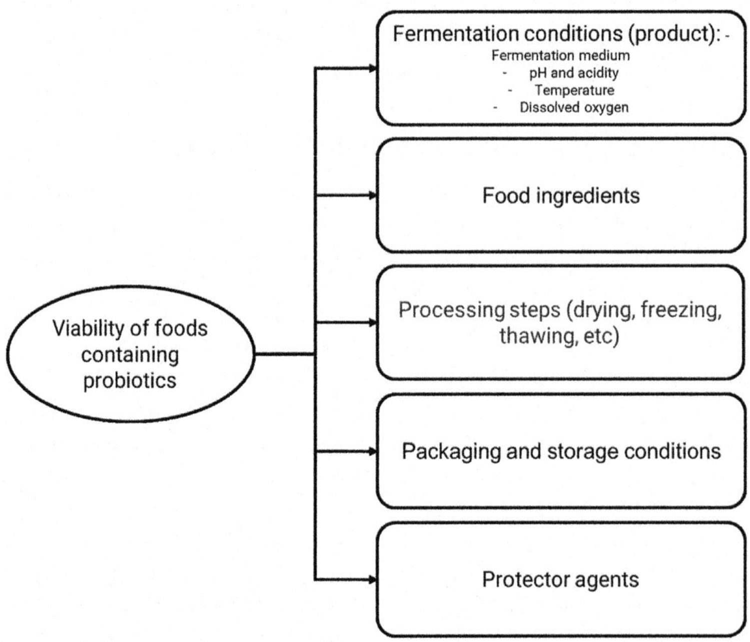

FIGURE 7.3

Scheme of introducing probiotics into food products to maintain their functionality during their shelf life.

Source: The authors.

(20%–150% or 0.5–3.0 mg GAE/mL) and antioxidants (DPPH scavenging 30%–70%), providing additional health benefits (Capece et al., 2018; Santana et al., 2020). Including probiotic beverages improved sensory perception (acceptance scores 6.5–8.5/9, CO_2 1.5–3.5 g/L for natural carbonation) (Kadyan et al., 2021; Santana et al., 2020).

Another major challenge is the aseptic introduction of probiotic strains into food (post-pasteurization contamination $<10^2$ CFU/g). For a product to be considered probiotic, microorganisms must remain viable ($>10^6$ CFU/g at end of shelf life). Therefore, cultures must be added after thermal (72°C/15s) or non-thermal processes (HPP 400–600 MPa) reducing natural microbiota (>5 log reduction), creating critical control points to avoid risks (Fenster et al., 2019).

The concentration of added probiotics must ensure sufficient viable cells throughout shelf life despite pH (3.5–4.5), temperature (4–10°C), and chemical conditions. Frozen cultures require ~10^{10} CFU/g (recovery >80%), lyophilized powders 10^{11} CFU/g (viability 70%–90% post-rehydration), depending on species (Saxelin et al., 2005).

One strategy to improve viability is adding cell protectants (10%–20% w/v): skimmed milk powder (survival 85%–95%), whey protein (80%–90%), glycerol (75%–85%), betaine (70%–80%), lactose (65%–75%), polymers like dextran/PEG (80%–92%) before drying (Hubálek, 2003).

Encapsulation immobilizes probiotics in matrices (particle size 10 nm-5 mm), achieving survival rates 80%–98% under adverse conditions (pH 2.5, 0.3% bile). Controlled release occurs at target sites (gastrointestinal pH 6.5–7.5) (Chávarri et al., 2012; Manojlović et al., 2010, pp. 269–302).

Emulsification with hydrocolloids (alginate 1%–3%, carrageenan 0.5%–2%, pectin 1%–2%) yields high survival (85%–95%), small capsules (20–200 μm), but lacks size standardization (variation 20%–50%), affecting release control (Camelo-Silva et al., 2022).

Extrusion with hydrocolloids produces uniform capsules (500 μm^{-2} mm), protecting viability (90%–98% retention, GIT survival 70%–90%) during storage (6–12 months at 4°C) and gastrointestinal transit (How et al., 2022; Rodrigues et al., 2020).

The choice of encapsulation technique depends on food characteristics, microorganism (growth rate 0.1–0.3 h^{-1}), and processing (temperature <40°C). Combined strategies enhance efficacy (viability +30–50%) and acceptance (sensory scores +15–25%) (Rodrigues et al., 2020).

Therefore, advancing technologies to protect and enable probiotics represents a significant step forward for the food industry. The search for efficient methods to ensure the survival and functionality of these cultures in the final product continues to be a fundamental field of research, enabling the development of innovative foods with scientifically proven health benefits.

7.5 Conclusions and future perspectives

Non-alcoholic fermented beverages are experiencing significant market growth, driven by increasing consumer demand for products that promote health and well-being. This sector has gained attention from individuals seeking natural alternatives rich in bioactive compounds and beneficial for gut microbiota, establishing itself as a rapidly expanding global trend.

However, developing these beverages requires carefully balancing quality parameters, microbial selection, and sensory attributes. Many fermentation processes remain artisanal or lack standardization, leading to variations in the final product profile. Ensuring stability and consumer acceptance necessitates a thorough understanding and control of the factors influencing fermentation, from microbial culture selection to final formulation. Additionally, aspects such as raw material sourcing, fermentation time, and storage conditions must be optimized to preserve the final product's functional properties and sensory appeal.

Within the non-alcoholic fermented beverage sector, there is a growing need for advancements in culture standardization, ensuring the presence of viable and beneficial microorganisms throughout shelf life. Innovations in biotechnology, including strain selection and fermentation optimization, can enhance probiotic viability and bioactive compound production. Moreover, diversifying flavors and blends represents a key competitive advantage, offering new sensory experiences to consumers while meeting dietary preferences and restrictions.

Developing stable, scalable, and safe fermentation processes is essential for consolidating this category in the food industry. Investment in research and technological advancements will play a fundamental role in overcoming current challenges, facilitating market expansion, and positioning non-alcoholic fermented beverages as reliable, accessible, and scientifically validated health-promoting alternatives. The future of this sector will depend not only on microbial innovation but also on consumer education and regulatory frameworks that support the growth of functional and natural beverage options worldwide.

Acknowledgments

The authors thank CAPES, CNPq, FAPEG, FAPERJ, UFRJ, and IF Goiano for their financial support.

References

Ağagündüz, D., Ertas Öztürk, Y., Ayhan, B., Bulmus-Tüccar, T., Özenir, Ç., Erdoğan Gövez, N., Ozogul, Y., Esatbeyoglu, T., & Ozogul, F. (2025). Certain fermented dairy foods as a source of multibiotics and multi-metabolites: A comprehensive review. *Frontiers in Nutrition, 12*. https://doi.org/10.3389/fnut.2025.1678150

Aburjaile, F. F., de Jesus, L. C. L., da Silva, T. F., Drumond, M. M., de Oliveira Carvalho, R. D., Azevedo, V., & Mancha-Agresti, P. D. C. (2022). *Lactic acid bacteria in gut microbiota, probiotics and disease prevention lactic acid bacteria in food biotechnology: Innovations and functional aspects*. Brazil: Elsevier Science Ltd.. https://doi.org/10.1016/B978-0-323-89875-1.00001-8

Adesulu-Dahunsi, A. T., Dahunsi, S. O., & Olayanju, A. (2020). Synergistic microbial interactions between lactic acid bacteria and yeasts during production of Nigerian Indigenous fermented foods and beverages. *Food Control, 110*. https://doi.org/10.1016/j.foodcont.2019.106963

Adriani, L., Mayasari, N., Angga, A., & Kartasudjana, R. (2011). The effect of feeding fermented kombucha tea on HLD, LDL and total cholesterol levels in the duck bloods. *Biotehnologija u stocarstvu, 27*(4), 1749–1755. https://doi.org/10.2298/bah1104749a

Agarbati, A., Canonico, L., Ciani, M., Morresi, C., Damiani, E., Bacchetti, T., & Comitini, F. (2024). Functional potential of a new plant-based fermented beverage: Benefits through non-conventional probiotic yeasts and antioxidant properties. *International Journal of Food Microbiology, 424*, Article 110857. https://doi.org/10.1016/j.ijfoodmicro.2024.110857

Aladeboyeje, O. T., Sanli, N. O., & Buyuk, U. (2022). Evaluation of the antimicrobial efficacy of some fermented traditional Turkish beverages with probiotic potentials: The first study to evaluate antimicrobial properties of isolates from five beverages against a broad spectrum of human microbial pathogens. *Johnson Matthey Technology Review, 66*(3), 337–350. https://doi.org/10.1595/205651322X16388083409013

Alamgir, A., & Alamgir, A. (2018). Phytoconstituents—Active and inert constituents, metabolic pathways, chemistry and application of phytoconstituents, primary metabolic products, and bioactive compounds of primary metabolic origin. In *Therapeutic use of medicinal plants and their extracts: Volume 2: Phytochemistry and bioactive compounds*.

Alexandre, E. M. C., Aguiar, N. F. B., Voss, G. B., & Pintado, M. E. (2023). Properties of fermented beverages from food Wastes/by-products. *Beverages, 9*(2). https://doi.org/10.3390/beverages9020045

Altay, F., Karbancıoglu-Güler, F., Daskaya-Dikmen, C., & Heperkan, D. (2013). A review on traditional Turkish fermented non-alcoholic beverages: Microbiota, fermentation process and quality characteristics. *International Journal of Food Microbiology, 167*(1), 44–56. https://doi.org/10.1016/j.ijfoodmicro.2013.06.016

Anumudu, C. K., Miri, T., & Onyeaka, H. (2024). Multifunctional applications of lactic acid bacteria: Enhancing safety, quality, and nutritional value in foods and fermented beverages. *Foods, 13*(23). https://doi.org/10.3390/foods13233714

Banwo, K., Jimoh, O., Olojede, A., & Ogundiran, T. (2024). Functional properties and antioxidant potentials of Kunun-zaki (A non-alcoholic millet beverage) produced using Pediococcus pentosaceus and Pichia kudriavzevii. *Food Biotechnology, 38*(2), 159–179. https://doi.org/10.1080/08905436.2024.2345775

Baschali, A., Tsakalidou, E., Kyriacou, A., Karavasiloglou, N., & Matalas, A. L. (2017). Traditional low-alcoholic and non-alcoholic fermented beverages consumed in European countries: A neglected food group. *Nutrition Research Reviews, 30*(1), 1–24. https://doi.org/10.1017/S0954422416000202

Basinskiene, L., Juodeikiene, G., Vidmantiene, D., Tenkanen, M., Makaravicius, T., & Bartkiene, E. (2016). Non-alcoholic beverages from fermented cereals with increased oligosaccharide content. *Food Technology and Biotechnology, 54*(1), 36–44. https://doi.org/10.17113/ftb.54.01.16.4106

Behera, S. S., Ray, R. C., Das, U., Panda, S. K., & Saranraj, P. (2019). Microorganisms in fermentation. In *Essentials in Fermentation Technology* (pp. 1–39).

Brugnoli, M., Cantadori, E., Arena, M. P., De Vero, L., Colonello, A., & Gullo, M. (2023). Zero-and low-alcohol fermented beverages: A perspective for non-conventional healthy and sustainable production from red fruits. *Fermentation, 9*, 457.

Bueno, R. S., Ressutte, J. B., Hata, N. N. Y., Henrique-Bana, F. C., Guergoletto, K. B., de Oliveira, A. G., & Spinosa, W. A. (2021). Quality and shelf life assessment of a new beverage produced from water kefir grains and red pitaya. *LWT, 140*. https://doi.org/10.1016/j.lwt.2020.110770

Calderón-Martínez, F. E., González-Laredo, R. F., González-Escobar, J. L., Nicolás-García, M., Muñiz-Márque, D. B., & Veana, F. (2024). *Fermented beverages from agro-industrial wastes and non-conventional sources biosystems engineering applications for quality food production: Waste valorization and new product development*. Mexico: Apple Academic Press. Available from: https://www.appleacademicpress.com/biosystems-engineering-applications-for-quality-food-production-waste-valorization-and-new-product-development/9781774916681.

Camelo-Silva, C., Verruck, S., Ambrosi, A., & Di Luccio, M. (2022). Innovation and trends in probiotic microencapsulation by emulsification techniques. *Food Engineering Reviews, 14*(3), 462–490. https://doi.org/10.1007/s12393-022-09315-1

Cantadori, E., Brugnoli, M., Centola, M., Uffredi, E., Colonello, A., & Gullo, M. (2022). Date fruits as raw material for vinegar and non-alcoholic fermented beverages. *Foods, 11*(13), 1972. https://doi.org/10.3390/foods11131972

Capece, A., Romaniello, R., Pietrafesa, A., Siesto, G., Pietrafesa, R., Zambuto, M., & Romano, P. (2018). Use of *Saccharomyces cerevisiae* var. boulardii in co-fermentations with *S. cerevisiae* for the production of craft beers with potential healthy value-added. *International Journal of Food Microbiology, 284*, 22–30. https://doi.org/10.1016/j.ijfoodmicro.2018.06.028

Carboni, A. D., Martins, G. N., Gómez-Zavaglia, A., & Castilho, P. C. (2023). Lactic acid bacteria in the production of traditional fermented foods and beverages of Latin America. *Fermentation, 9*(4). https://doi.org/10.3390/fermentation9040315

Chávarri, M., Marañón, I., & Villarán, M. C. (2012). Encapsulation technology to protect probiotic bacteria. In *Probiotics*. IntechOpen.

Chong, A. Q., Lau, S. W., Chin, N. L., Talib, R. A., & Basha, R. K. (2023). Fermented beverage benefits: A comprehensive review and comparison of Kombucha and Kefir microbiome. *Microorganisms, 11*(5). https://doi.org/10.3390/microorganisms11051344

Cichońska, P., & Ziarno, M. (2022). Legumes and legume-based beverages fermented with lactic acid bacteria as a potential carrier of probiotics and prebiotics. *Microorganisms, 10*(1), 91. https://doi.org/10.3390/microorganisms10010091

Cizeikiene, D., & Jagelaviciute, J. (2021). Investigation of antibacterial activity and probiotic properties of strains belonging to lactobacillus and bifidobacterium genera for their potential application in functional food and feed products. *Probiotics and Antimicrobial Proteins, 13*(5), 1387–1403. https://doi.org/10.1007/s12602-021-09777-5

Cunha, P. C.d., Oliveira, L.d. S.d., Blanco, J. C., Silva, M. T.d. C., Gálvez, S. G. L., Rosenthal, A., & Ferreira, E. H. d. R. (2022). Elaboration, characterization, and probiotic viability of synbiotic non-dairy drink based on coconut. *Ciência Rural, 53*, Article e20210723.

Cuvas-Limon, R. B., Nobre, C., Cruz, M., Rodriguez-Jasso, R. M., Ruíz, H. A., Loredo-Treviño, A., Texeira, J. A., & Belmares, R. (2021). Spontaneously fermented traditional beverages as a source of bioactive compounds: An overview. *Critical Reviews in Food Science and Nutrition, 61*(18), 2984–3006. https://doi.org/10.1080/10408398.2020.1791050

da Silva, S. F., Cavalcante, M. P., Sensheng, Y., Silva, S.d. S., & Frota Gaban, S. V. (2024). Physicochemical properties, antioxidant activity, and sensory profiles of Kombucha and Kombucha-like beverages prepared using passion fruit (Passiflora edulis) and apple (Malus pumila). *ACS Agricultural Science and Technology, 4*(9), 938–946. https://doi.org/10.1021/acsagscitech.4c00372

de Mello Sampaio, V., Wiele, N., da Silva Vale, A., Woiciechowski, A. L., Karp, S. G., Soccol, C. R., & de Melo Pereira, G. V. (2025). Modulation of aroma and chemical composition of coffee beans through simultaneous and sequential inoculation of Pichia fermentans and Pediococcus pentosaceus during wet fermentation. *Systems Microbiology and Biomanufacturing, 5*(1), 335–346. https://doi.org/10.1007/s43393-024-00253-z

de Melo Silva, J. C., Santana, R. V., Almeida, A. B.de, Pereira Takeuchi, K., & Egea, M. B. (2021). Changes in the chemical, technological, and microbiological properties of kefir-fermented soymilk after supplementation with inulin and acrocomia aculeata pulp. *Applied Sciences, 11*(12), 5575. https://doi.org/10.3390/app11125575

de Oliveira Filho, J. G., de Oliveira Silva, C., Egea, M. B., de Azeredo, H. M. C., & Mattoso, L. H. C. (2023). Employing alternative culture media in kefiran exopolysaccharide production: Impact on microbial diversity, physicochemical properties, and bioactivities. *International Journal of Biological Macromolecules, 246*, Article 125648.

De Roos, J., & De Vuyst, L. (2018). Acetic acid bacteria in fermented foods and beverages. *Current Opinion in Biotechnology, 49*, 115–119. https://doi.org/10.1016/j.copbio.2017.08.007

Diosma, G., Romanin, D. E., Rey-Burusco, M. F., Londero, A., & Garrote, G. L. (2014). Yeasts from kefir grains: Isolation, identification, and probiotic characterization. *World Journal of Microbiology and Biotechnology, 30*(1), 43–53. https://doi.org/10.1007/s11274-013-1419-9

Dong, H., Bao, X., Wang, Y., Liao, X., Wang, K., Chen, J., Li, X., Yang, Z., & Wang, Y. (2024). The impact of lactic acid bacteria inoculation on the fermentation and metabolomic dynamics of Indigenous beijing douzhi microbial communities. *Frontiers in Microbiology, 15*. https://doi.org/10.3389/fmicb.2024.1435834

dos Santos, D. C., da Oliveira Filho, J. G., Andretta, J. R., Silva, F. G., & Egea, M. B. (2023). Challenges in maintaining the probiotic potential in alcoholic beverage development. *Food Bioscience*, Article 102485.

Egea, M., Santos, D.d., Oliveira Filho, J.d., Ores, J.d. C., Takeuchi, K., & Lemes, A. (2020). A review of nondairy kefir products: Their characteristics and potential human health benefits. *Critical Reviews in Food Science and Nutrition*, 1–17.

El Youssef, C., Bonnarme, P., Fraud, S., Péron, A.-C., Helinck, S., & Landaud, S. (2020). Sensory improvement of a pea protein-based product using microbial co-cultures of lactic acid bacteria and yeasts. *Foods, 9*(3), 349. https://doi.org/10.3390/foods9030349

Fahmy, H. A., & Ismail, A. F. M. (2015). Gastroprotective effect of kefir on ulcer induced in irradiated rats. *Journal of Photochemistry and Photobiology B: Biology, 144*, 85–93. https://doi.org/10.1016/j.jphotobiol.2015.02.009

Fathi, Y., Faghih, S., Zibaeenezhad, M. J., & Tabatabaei, S. H. R. (2016). Kefir drink leads to a similar weight loss, compared with milk, in a dairy-rich non-energy-restricted diet in overweight or Obese premenopausal women: A randomized controlled trial. *European Journal of Nutrition, 55*(1), 295–304. https://doi.org/10.1007/s00394-015-0846-9

Fenster, K., Freeburg, B., Hollard, C., Wong, C., Laursen, R. R., & Ouwehand, A. C. (2019). The production and delivery of probiotics: A review of a practical approach. *Microorganisms, 7*(3), 83. https://doi.org/10.3390/microorganisms7030083

Ferreira, I., de Sousa Melo, D., Menezes, A. G. T., Fonseca, H. C., de Assis, B. B. T., Ramos, C. L., Magnani, M., Dias, D. R., & Schwan, R. F. (2022). Evaluation of potentially probiotic yeasts and lactiplantibacillus plantarum in co-culture for the elaboration of a functional plant-based fermented beverage. *Food Research International, 160*. https://doi.org/10.1016/j.foodres.2022.111697

Fijan, S. (2014). Microorganisms with claimed probiotic properties: An overview of recent literature. *International Journal of Environmental Research and Public Health, 11*(5), 4745–4767. https://doi.org/10.3390/ijerph110504745

Fiorda, F. A., de Melo Pereira, G. V., Thomaz-Soccol, V., Medeiros, A. P., Kumar Rakshit, S., & Soccol, C. R. (2016). Development of kefir-based probiotic beverages with DNA protection and antioxidant activities using soybean hydrolyzed extract, colostrum and honey. *LWT - Food Science and Technology, 68*, 690–697. https://doi.org/10.1016/j.lwt.2016.01.003

Freire, A. L., Ramos, C. L., da Costa Souza, P. N., Cardoso, M. G. B., & Schwan, R. F. (2017). Nondairy beverage produced by controlled fermentation with potential probiotic starter cultures of lactic acid bacteria and yeast. *International Journal of Food Microbiology, 248*, 39–46. https://doi.org/10.1016/j.ijfoodmicro.2017.02.011

Gamba, R. R., Yamamoto, S., Abdel-Hamid, M., Sasaki, T., Michihata, T., Koyanagi, T., & Enomoto, T. (2020). Chemical, microbiological, and functional characterization of kefir produced from cow's milk and soy milk. *International Journal of Microbiology, 2020*. https://doi.org/10.1155/2020/7019286

Gautam, A., Poopalarajah, R., Ahmed, A. R., Rana, B. N., Denekew, T. W., Ahn, N., Utenova, L., Kunwar, Y. S., Bhandari, N. N., & Jha, A. R. (2024). *Ecological factors that drive microbial communities in culturally diverse fermented foods*. Nepal: bioRxiv. https://doi.org/10.1101/2024.08.20.608727

Georgalaki, M., Zoumpopoulou, G., Anastasiou, R., Kazou, M., & Tsakalidou, E. (2021). Lactobacillus kefiranofaciens: From isolation and taxonomy to probiotic properties and applications. *Microorganisms, 9*(10), 2158. https://doi.org/10.3390/microorganisms9102158

Global. (2024). *Global fermented non-dairy non-alcoholic beverages market – Industry trends and forecast to 2031. In (Vol. 2025)*. https://www.databridgemarketresearch.com/reports/global-fermented-non-dairy-non-alcoholic-beverages-market.

Gomes, R. J., Borges, M.d. F., Rosa, M.d. F., Castro-Gómez, R. J. H., & Spinosa, W. A. (2018). Acetic acid bacteria in the food industry: Systematics, characteristics and applications. *Food Technology and Biotechnology, 56*(2), 139–151. https://doi.org/10.17113/ftb.56.02.18.5593

Hao, Y., Kang, J., Guo, Y., Meng, L., Li, Z., & Qin, X. (2025). Bacterial interactions mediated by acetic acid and their impact on flavor profile during acetic acid fermentation stage of Shanxi aged vinegar. *Food Bioscience, 64*, Article 105996. https://doi.org/10.1016/j.fbio.2025.105996

Hao, F., Tan, Y., Lv, X., Chen, L., Yang, F., Wang, H., Du, H., Wang, L., & Xu, Y. (2021). Microbial community succession and its environment driving factors during initial fermentation of Maotai-flavor baijiu. *Frontiers in Microbiology, 12*. https://doi.org/10.3389/fmicb.2021.669201

Harrison, K., Navarro, R., Jensen, K., Cayler, W., Nielsen, T., & Curtin, C. (2023). Live, probiotic, or neither? Microbial composition of retail-available Kombucha and "hard" Kombucha in the Pacific Northwest of the United States. *Beverages, 9*(3), 59. https://doi.org/10.3390/beverages9030059

Hata, N. N. Y., Surek, M., Sartori, D., Serrato, R. V., & Spinosa, W. A. (2023). Role of acetic acid bacteria in food and beverages. *Food Technology and Biotechnology, 61*(1), 85–103. https://doi.org/10.17113/ftb.61.01.23.7811

Hill, C., Guarner, F., Reid, G., Gibson, G. R., Merenstein, D. J., Pot, B., Morelli, L., Canani, R. B., Flint, H. J., Salminen, S., Calder, P. C., & Sanders, M. E. (2014). The International Scientific Association for Probiotics and Prebiotics consensus statement on the scope and appropriate use of the term probiotic. *Nature Reviews Gastroenterology & Hepatology, 11*(8), 506–514. https://doi.org/10.1038/nrgastro.2014.66

How, Y.-H., Lai, K.-W., Pui, L.-P., & Lian-Aun, L. (2022). In, Co-extrusion and extrusion microencapsulation: Effect on microencapsulation efficiency, survivability through gastrointestinal digestion and storage. *Journal of Food Process Engineering, 45*(3). https://doi.org/10.1111/jfpe.13985

Hubálek, Z. (2003). Protectants used in the cryopreservation of microorganisms. *Cryobiology, 46*(3), 205–229. https://doi.org/10.1016/s0011-2240(03)00046-4

Ignat, M. V., Salantă, L. C., Pop, O. L., Pop, C. R., Tofană, M., Mudura, E., Coldea, T. E., Borsa, A., & Pasqualone, A. (2020). Current functionality and potential improvements of non-alcoholic fermented cereal beverages. *Foods, 9*(8). https://doi.org/10.3390/foods9081031

Ilango, S., & Antony, U. (2021). Probiotic microorganisms from non-dairy traditional fermented foods. *Trends in Food Science & Technology, 118*, 617–638. https://doi.org/10.1016/j.tifs.2021.05.034

Jemima, D., & John, S. (2024). *Microbes in production of non-alcoholic beverages microbial products for health and nutrition*. India: Springer Nature. https://doi.org/10.1007/978-981-97-4235-6_7

Jooyandeh, H. (2013). Production of non-alcoholic fermented plum beverages. *Middle-East Journal of Scientific Research, 13*(6), 836–843. https://doi.org/10.5829/idosi.mejsr.2013.13.6.2623Iran

Kadyan, S., Rashmi, H. M., Pradhan, D., Kumari, A., Chaudhari, A., & Deshwal, G. K. (2021). Effect of lactic acid bacteria and yeast fermentation on antimicrobial, antioxidative and metabolomic profile of naturally carbonated probiotic whey drink. *LWT, 142*, Article 111059. https://doi.org/10.1016/j.lwt.2021.111059

Kaur, P., Ghoshal, G., & Banerjee, U. C. (2019). Traditional bio-preservation in beverages: Fermented beverages. In *Preservatives and preservation approaches in beverages* (pp. 69–113). Elsevier.

Kesa, A. L., Pop, C. R., Mudura, E., Salanță, L. C., Pasqualone, A., Dărab, C., Burja-Udrea, C., Zhao, H., & Coldea, T. E. (2021). Strategies to improve the potential functionality of fruit-based fermented beverages. *Plants, 10*(11). https://doi.org/10.3390/plants10112263

Kitessa, D. A. (2024). Review on effect of fermentation on physicochemical properties, anti-nutritional factors and sensory properties of cereal-based fermented foods and beverages. *Annals of Microbiology, 74*(1). https://doi.org/10.1186/s13213-024-01763-w

Kocsis, B., Szabó, D., & Sipos, L. (2025). Gut microbiome and intestinal colonization with multidrug-resistant strains of enterobacterales: An interplay between microbial communities. *Antibiotics, 14*(9), 890. https://doi.org/10.3390/antibiotics14090890

Kumar, R., Kaur, G., & Brar, S. K. (2025). Tailored production of butyric acid from mixed culture fermentation of food waste. *Food and Bioproducts Processing, 150*, 1–11. https://doi.org/10.1016/j.fbp.2024.12.013

Laavanya, D., Shirkole, S., & Balasubramanian, P. (2021). Current challenges, applications and future perspectives of SCOBY cellulose of Kombucha fermentation. *Journal of Cleaner Production, 295*, Article 126454. https://doi.org/10.1016/j.jclepro.2021.126454

Laureys, D., Britton, S. J., & De Clippeleer, J. (2020). Kombucha tea fermentation: A review. *Journal of the American Society of Brewing Chemists, 78*(3), 165–174. https://doi.org/10.1080/03610470.2020.1734150

Lavefve, L., Marasini, D., & Carbonero, F. (2019). Microbial ecology of fermented vegetables and non-alcoholic drinks and current knowledge on their impact on human health. *Advances in Food and Nutrition Research, 87*, 147–185. https://doi.org/10.1016/bs.afnr.2018.09.001

Lawton, M. R., deRiancho, D. L., & Alcaine, S. D. (2021). Lactose utilization by Brettanomyces claussenii expands potential for valorization of dairy by-products to functional beverages through fermentation. *Current Opinion in Food Science, 42*, 93–101. https://doi.org/10.1016/j.cofs.2021.05.006

Liu, X., Jia, B., Sun, X., Ai, J., Wang, L., Wang, C., Zhao, F., Zhan, J., & Huang, W. (2015). Effect of initial PH on growth characteristics and fermentation properties of *Saccharomyces cerevisiae*. *Journal of Food Science, 80* (4), Article M800. https://doi.org/10.1111/1750-3841.12813China

Liu, J., Zhao, M., Hao, J., Yan, X., Fu, Z., Zhu, N., Jia, Y., Wang, Z., & Ge, G. (2024). Effects of temperature and lactic acid bacteria additives on the quality and microbial community of wilted alfalfa silage. *BMC Plant Biology, 24*(1). https://doi.org/10.1186/s12870-024-05501-x

Louw, N. L., Lele, K., Ye, R., Edwards, C. B., & Wolfe, B. E. (2023). Microbiome assembly in fermented foods. *Annual Review of Microbiology, 77*, 381–402. https://doi.org/10.1146/annurev-micro-032521-041956

Madilo, F. K., Parry-Hanson Kunadu, A., Tano-Debrah, K., Saalia, F. K., & Kolanisi, U. (2024). Diversity of production techniques and microbiology of African cereal-based traditional fermented beverages. *Journal of Food Quality, 2024*. https://doi.org/10.1155/2024/1241614

Maicas, S. (2020). The role of yeasts in fermentation processes. *Microorganisms, 8*(8), 1142. https://doi.org/10.3390/microorganisms8081142

Mandha, J., Shumoy, H., Matemu, A. O., & Raes, K. (2021). *Current trends and opportunities of plant-based non-alcoholic probiotic beverages: A European and African perspective probiotic beverages*. Belgium: Elsevier. https://doi.org/10.1016/B978-0-12-818588-9.00013-9

Manojlović, V., Nedović, V. A., Kailasapathy, K., & Zuidam, N. J. (2010). *Encapsulation of probiotics for use in food products encapsulation technologies for active food ingredients and food processing*. New York, Serbia: Springer. https://doi.org/10.1007/978-1-4419-1008-0_10

Marsh, A. J., Hill, C., Ross, R. P., & Cotter, P. D. (2014). Fermented beverages with health-promoting potential: Past and future perspectives. *Trends in Food Science and Technology, 38*(2), 113–124. https://doi.org/10.1016/j.tifs.2014.05.002

Mashau, M. E., Maliwichi, L. L., & Jideani, A. I. O. (2021). Non-alcoholic fermentation of maize (Zea mays) in Sub-Saharan Africa. *Fermentation, 7*(3). https://doi.org/10.3390/FERMENTATION7030158

Mbaye, B., Wasfy, R. M., Tidjani Alou, M., Borentain, P., Andrieu, C., Caputo, A., Raoult, D., Gerolami, R., Million, M., & fermentum, L. (2023). Lactococcus lactis and Thomasclavelia ramosa are enriched and Methanobrevibacter smithii is depleted in patients with non-alcoholic steatohepatitis. *Microbial Pathogenesis, 180*, Article 106160. https://doi.org/10.1016/j.micpath.2023.106160

Medrano, M., Racedo, S. M., Rolny, I. S., Abraham, A. G., & Pérez, P. F. (2011). Oral administration of Kefiran induces changes in the balance of immune cells in a murine model. *Journal of Agricultural and Food Chemistry, 59*(10), 5299–5304. https://doi.org/10.1021/jf1049968

Mendes, R. M. L., Andrade, R. H. C.d., Marques, M.d. F. F., & Andrade, E. R.d. (2021). Potential use of the passion fruit from caatinga in kefir. *Food Bioscience, 39*. https://doi.org/10.1016/j.fbio.2020.100809

Mishra, S., Aravind, S. M., Ajlouni, S., Ranadheera, C. S., Singh, B. P., & Chakkaravarthi, S. (2024). Optimization of fermentation process and characterization of non-alcoholic functional beverage from pigmented rice varieties. *Biocatalysis and Agricultural Biotechnology, 58*. https://doi.org/10.1016/j.bcab.2024.103213

Mohammadi, R., Mortazavian, A. M., Khosrokhavar, R., & Da Cruz, A. G. (2011). Probiotic ice cream: Viability of probiotic bacteria and sensory properties. *Annals of Microbiology, 61*(3), 411–424. https://doi.org/10.1007/s13213-010-0188-z

Moiseenko, K. V., Glazunova, O. A., & Fedorova, T. V. (2024). Fermentation of rice, oat, and wheat flour by pure cultures of common starter lactic acid bacteria: Growth dynamics, sensory evaluation, and functional properties. *Federation Foods, 13*(15). https://doi.org/10.3390/foods13152414

Ndukwe, J. K., Aduba, C. C., Ughamba, K. T., Chukwu, K. O., Eze, C. N., Nwaiwu, O., & Onyeaka, H. (2023). Diet diversification and priming with Kunu: An indigenous probiotic cereal-based non-alcoholic beverage in Nigeria. *Beverages, 9*(1). https://doi.org/10.3390/beverages9010014

Nedyalkov, P., Denkova, R., Teneva, D., Shopska, V., Goranov, B., Denkova, Z., Kostov, G., & Kaneva, M. (2019). Yeast selection for non-alcoholic and low-alcoholic beverages based on wort. *Food Science and Applied Biotechnology, 2*(2), 140–148. https://doi.org/10.30721/fsab2019.v2.i2.61

Nyhan, L., Sahin, A. W., & Arendt, E. K. (2023). Co-fermentation of non-Saccharomyces yeasts with Lactiplantibacillus plantarum FST 1.7 for the production of non-alcoholic beer. *European Food Research and Technology, 249*(1), 167–181. https://doi.org/10.1007/s00217-022-04142-4

Ojeda-Linares, C. I., Solís-García, I. A., & Casas, A. (2022). Constructing micro-landscapes: Management and selection practices on microbial communities in a traditional fermented beverage. *Frontiers in Ecology and Evolution, 10*. https://doi.org/10.3389/fevo.2022.821268

Ozcelik, F., Akan, E., & Kinik, O. (2021). Use of cornelian cherry, hawthorn, red plum, roseship and pomegranate juices in the production of water kefir beverages. *Food Bioscience, 42*, Article 101219. https://doi.org/10.1016/j.fbio.2021.101219

Peña González, M. A., Jennifer Pamela Ortiz Urgiles, Fernanda Alegría Santander Pérez, Marco Antonio Lazo Vélez, & Rodrigo Sebastián Caroca Cáceres. (2023). Physicochemical changes during controlled laboratory fermentation of cocoa (CCN-51) with the inclusion of fruits and on-farm inoculation. *Brazilian Journal of Food Technology, 26*. https://doi.org/10.1590/1981-6723.01323

Prajapati, N., Patel, J., Singh, S., Yadav, V. K., Joshi, C., Patani, A., Prajapati, D., Sahoo, D. K., & Patel, A. (2023). Postbiotic production: Harnessing the power of microbial metabolites for health applications. *Frontiers in Microbiology, 14*. https://doi.org/10.3389/fmicb.2023.1306192

Praveen, M., & Brogi, S. (2025). Microbial fermentation in food and beverage industries: Innovations, challenges, and opportunities. *Foods, 14*(1), 114. https://doi.org/10.3390/foods14010114

Pswarayi, F., & Gänzle, M. (2022). African cereal fermentations: A review on fermentation processes and microbial composition of non-alcoholic fermented cereal foods and beverages. *International Journal of Food Microbiology, 378*, Article 109815. https://doi.org/10.1016/j.ijfoodmicro.2022.109815

Puerari, C., Magalhães, K. T., & Schwan, R. F. (2012). New cocoa pulp-based kefir beverages: Microbiological, chemical composition and sensory analysis. *Food Research International, 48*(2), 634–640. https://doi.org/10.1016/j.foodres.2012.06.005

Raspor, P., & Goranovič, D. (2008). Biotechnological applications of acetic acid bacteria. *Critical Reviews in Biotechnology, 28*(2), 101–124. https://doi.org/10.1080/07388550802046749

Rivera Flores, V. K., Demarsh, T. A., Gibney, P. A., & Alcaine, S. D. (2021). Fermentation of dairy-relevant sugars by saccharomyces, kluyveromyces, and brettanomyces: An exploratory study with implications for the utilization of acid whey, part I. *Fermentation, 7*(4). https://doi.org/10.3390/fermentation7040266

Rodrigues, F. J., Cedran, M. F., Bicas, J. L., & Sato, H. H. (2020). Encapsulated probiotic cells: Relevant techniques, natural sources as encapsulating materials and food applications – A narrative review. *Food Research International, 137*, Article 109682. https://doi.org/10.1016/j.foodres.2020.109682

Rui, X., Zhang, Q., Huang, J., Li, W., Chen, X., Jiang, M., & Dong, M. (2019). Does lactic fermentation influence soy yogurt protein digestibility: A comparative study between soymilk and soy yogurt at different pH. *Journal of the Science of Food and Agriculture, 99*(2), 861–867. https://doi.org/10.1002/jsfa.9256

Salas-Millán, J.Á., & Aguayo, E. (2024). Fermentation for revalorisation of fruit and vegetable by-products: A sustainable approach towards minimising food loss and waste. *Foods, 13*(22). https://doi.org/10.3390/foods13223680

Santana, R. V., Santos, D. C.d., Santana, A. C. A., Oliveira Filho, J. G.d., Almeida, A. B.d., Lima, T. M.d., Silva, F. G., & Egea, M. B. (2020). Quality parameters and sensorial profile of clarified "cerrado" cashew juice supplemented with Sacharomyces boulardii and different sweeteners. *LWT, 128*. https://doi.org/10.1016/j.lwt.2020.109319

Santos, D. C.d., Oliveira Filho, J. G.d., Santana, A. C. A., Freitas, B. S. M.d., Silva, F. G., Takeuchi, K. P., & Egea, M. B. (2019). Optimization of soymilk fermentation with kefir and the addition of inulin:

Physicochemical, sensory and technological characteristics. *LWT, 104*, 30–37. https://doi.org/10.1016/j.lwt.2019.01.030

Santos, D. C.d., Pimentel, T. C., Sousa, T. L.d., Almeida, A. B.d., Oliveira, M. S., Oliveira Filho, J. G.d., Silva, F. G., & Egea, M. B. (2024). Cerrado cagaita (Eugenia dysenterica) cloudy and clarified beverages: Effect of kefir fermentation and inulin addition. *Food Bioscience, 61*. https://doi.org/10.1016/j.fbio.2024.104767

Sanwal, N., Gupta, A., Bareen, M. A., Sharma, N., & Sahu, J. K. (2023). Kombucha fermentation: Recent trends in process dynamics, functional bioactivities, toxicity management, and potential applications. *Food Chemistry Advances, 3*. https://doi.org/10.1016/j.focha.2023.100421

Saranraj, P., Ray, R. C., Kumar, N. A., Lokeshwari, B., Gayathri, K., & Sivasakthivelan, P. (2024). Microbes in action: Powering sustainable fermentation for food, pharma, and bioeconomy. *Applied Food Biotechnology, 12* (1), 1–24.

Satir, G., & Guzel-Seydim, Z. B. (2016). How kefir fermentation can affect product composition? *Small Ruminant Research, 134*, 1–7. https://doi.org/10.1016/j.smallrumres.2015.10.022

Saxelin, M., Tynkkynen, S., Mattila-Sandholm, T., & de Vos, W. M. (2005). Probiotic and other functional microbes: From markets to mechanisms. *Current Opinion in Biotechnology, 16*(2), 204–211. https://doi.org/10.1016/j.copbio.2005.02.003

Servin, A. L. (2004). Antagonistic activities of lactobacilli and bifidobacteria against microbial pathogens. *FEMS Microbiology Reviews, 28*(4), 405–440. https://doi.org/10.1016/j.femsre.2004.01.003

Shahbazi, H., Hashemi Gahruie, H., Golmakani, M.-Taghi, Eskandari, M. H., & Movahedi, M. (2018). Effect of medicinal plant type and concentration on physicochemical, antioxidant, antimicrobial, and sensorial properties of kombucha. *Food Science and Nutrition, 6*(8), 2568–2577. https://doi.org/10.1002/fsn3.873

Shen, D., Shen, H., Yang, Q., Chen, S., Dun, Y., Liang, Y., Zheng, J., Zhao, S., & Gralnick, J. A. (2021). Deciphering succession and assembly patterns of microbial communities in a two-stage solid-state fermentation system. *Microbiology Spectrum, 9*(2). https://doi.org/10.1128/spectrum.00718-21

Sionek, B., Szydłowska, A., Trząskowska, M., & Kołożyn-Krajewska, D. (2024). The impact of physicochemical conditions on lactic acid bacteria survival in food products. *Fermentation, 10*(6), 298. https://doi.org/10.3390/fermentation10060298

Souza, E. C., Oliveira de Souza de Azevedo, P., Domínguez, J. M., Converti, A., & de Souza Oliveira, R. P. (2017). Influence of temperature and pH on the production of biosurfactant, bacteriocin and lactic acid by Lactococcus lactis CECT-4434. *CyTA - Journal of Food, 15*(4), 525–530. https://doi.org/10.1080/19476337.2017.1306806

Sreeramulu, G., Zhu, Y., & Knol, W. (2000). Kombucha fermentation and its antimicrobial activity. *Journal of Agricultural and Food Chemistry, 48*(6), 2589–2594. https://doi.org/10.1021/jf991333m

Srihari, T., Arunkumar, R., Arunakaran, J., & Satyanarayana, U. (2013). Downregulation of signalling molecules involved in angiogenesis of prostate cancer cell line (PC-3) by kombucha (lyophilized). *Biomedicine & Preventive Nutrition, 3*(1), 53–58. https://doi.org/10.1016/j.bionut.2012.08.001

Tamang, J. P., & Thapa, N. (2022). *Beneficial microbiota in ethnic fermented foods and beverages good microbes in medicine, food production, biotechnology, bioremediation, and agriculture*. India: wiley. https://doi.org/10.1002/9781119762621.ch11

Vaštík, P., Rosenbergová, Z., Furdíková, K., Klempová, T., Šišmiš, M., & Šmogrovičová, D. (2022). Potential of non-saccharomyces yeast to produce non-alcoholic beer. *FEMS Yeast Research, 22*(1). https://doi.org/10.1093/femsyr/foac039

Valero-Cases, E., Cerdá-Bernad, D., Pastor, J. J., & Frutos, M. J. (2020). Non-dairy fermented beverages as potential carriers to ensure probiotics, prebiotics, and bioactive compounds arrival to the gut and their health benefits. *Nutrients, 12*(6). https://doi.org/10.3390/nu12061666

Van Wyk, J. (2019). *Kefir: The champagne of fermented beverages fermented beverages: Volume 5. The Science of beverages*. South Africa: Elsevier. https://doi.org/10.1016/B978-0-12-815271-3.00012-9

Verardo, V., Gómez-Caravaca, A. M., & Tabanelli, G. (2020). Bioactive components in fermented foods and food by-products. *Foods, 9*(2). https://doi.org/10.3390/foods9020153

Vieira, C. P., Cabral, C. C., da Costa Lima, B. R. C., Paschoalin, V. M. F., Leandro, K. C., & Conte-Junior, C. A. (2017). Lactococcus lactis ssp. Cremoris MRS47, a potential probiotic strain isolated from kefir grains, increases cis-9, trans-11-CLA and PUFA contents in fermented milk. *Journal of Functional Foods, 31*, 172–178. https://doi.org/10.1016/j.jff.2017.01.047

Vinderola, G., Perdigón, G., Duarte, J., Farnworth, E., & Matar, C. (2006). Effects of the oral administration of the exopolysaccharide produced by lactobacillus kefiranofaciens on the gut mucosal immunity. *Cytokine, 36*(5–6), 254–260. https://doi.org/10.1016/j.cyto.2007.01.003

Wang, B., Rutherfurd-Markwick, K., Zhang, X. X., & Mutukumira, A. N. (2022). Kombucha: Production and microbiological research. *Foods, 11*(21). https://doi.org/10.3390/foods11213456

Wang, J., Xing, Z., Tang, W., Zheng, Y., & Wang, Y. (2015). Isolation, identification, and potential probiotic characterization of one lactococcus from Kefir grain. *Food Science and Biotechnology, 24*(5), 1775–1780. https://doi.org/10.1007/s10068-015-0231-8

Wang, Y., Zhang, C., Liu, F., Jin, Z., & Xia, X. (2023). Ecological succession and functional characteristics of lactic acid bacteria in traditional fermented foods. *Critical Reviews in Food Science and Nutrition, 63*(22), 5841–5855. https://doi.org/10.1080/10408398.2021.2025035

Witthuhn, R. C., Schoeman, T., & Britz, T. J. (2005). Characterisation of the microbial population at different stages of Kefir production and Kefir grain mass cultivation. *International Dairy Journal, 15*(4), 383–389. https://doi.org/10.1016/j.idairyj.2004.07.016

Wszolek, M., Tamime, A. Y., Muir, D. D., & Barclay, M. N. I. (2001). Properties of kefir made in Scotland and Poland using bovine, caprine and ovine milk with different starter cultures. *LWT - Food Science and Technology, 34*(4), 251–261. https://doi.org/10.1006/fstl.2001.0773

Xing, Z., Tang, W., Geng, W., Zheng, Y., & Wang, Y. (2017). In vitro and in vivo evaluation of the probiotic attributes of Lactobacillus kefiranofaciens XL10 isolated from Tibetan kefir grain. *Applied Microbiology and Biotechnology, 101*(6), 2467–2477. https://doi.org/10.1007/s00253-016-7956-z

Yalcin, S. K., & Ozbas, Z. Y. (2008). Effects of pH and temperature on growth and glycerol production kinetics of two indigenous wine strains of *Saccharomyces cerevisiae* from Turkey. *Brazilian Journal of Microbiology, 39* (2), 325–332. https://doi.org/10.1590/S1517-83822008000200024Turkey

Yang, Z., Zhou, F., Ji, B., Li, B., Luo, Y., Yang, L., & Li, T. (2010). Symbiosis between microorganisms from Kombucha and kefir: Potential significance to the enhancement of Kombucha function. *Applied Biochemistry and Biotechnology, 160*(2), 446–455. https://doi.org/10.1007/s12010-008-8361-6

Zanirati, D. F., Abatemarco, M., Sandes, S. H.d. C., Nicoli, J. R., Nunes, Á. C., & Neumann, E. (2015). Selection of lactic acid bacteria from Brazilian kefir grains for potential use as starter or probiotic cultures. *Anaerobe, 32*, 70–76. https://doi.org/10.1016/j.anaerobe.2014.12.007

Zhao, J., Zeng, X., Xi, Y., & Li, J. (2024). Recent advances in the applications of Lactobacillus helveticus in the fermentation of plant-based beverages: A review. *Trends in Food Science & Technology, 147*, Article 104427. https://doi.org/10.1016/j.tifs.2024.104427

Zheng, Y., Mou, J., Niu, J., Yang, S., Chen, L., Xia, M., & Wang, M. (2018). Succession sequence of lactic acid bacteria driven by environmental factors and substrates throughout the brewing process of Shanxi aged vinegar. *Applied Microbiology and Biotechnology, 102*(6), 2645–2658. https://doi.org/10.1007/s00253-017-8733-3

Ziarno, M., & Cichońska, P. (2021). Lactic acid bacteria-fermentable cereal- and pseudocereal-based beverages. *Microorganisms, 9*(12), 2532. https://doi.org/10.3390/microorganisms9122532

Further reading

Aloulou, A., Hamden, K., Elloumi, D., Ali, M. B., Hargafi, K., Jaouadi, B., Ayadi, F., Elfeki, A., & Ammar, E. (2012). Hypoglycemic and antilipidemic properties of kombucha tea in alloxan-induced diabetic rats. *BMC Complementary and Alternative Medicine, 12*, 1–9.

Baú, T., Garcia, S., & Ida, E. (2015). Changes in soymilk during fermentation with kefir culture: Oligosaccharides hydrolysis and isoflavone aglycone production. *International Journal of Food Sciences & Nutrition, 66*, 845–850.

Fathi, Y., Ghodrati, N., Zibaeenezhad, M.-J., & Faghih, S. (2017). Kefir drink causes a significant yet similar improvement in serum lipid profile, compared with low-fat milk, in a dairy-rich diet in overweight or Obese premenopausal women: A randomized controlled trial. *Journal of Clinical Lipidology, 11*, 136–146.

Jeong, D., Kim, D.-H., Kang, I.-B., Kim, H., Song, K.-Y., Kim, H.-S., & Seo, K.-H. (2017). Characterization and antibacterial activity of a novel exopolysaccharide produced by Lactobacillus kefiranofaciens DN1 isolated from kefir. *Food Control, 78*, 436–442.

Moreira, M. E., Santos, M. H., Pereira, I. O., Ferraz, V., Barbosa, L. C., & Schneedorf, J. M. (2008). Anti-inflammatory activity of carbohydrate produced from aqueous fermentation of kefir. *Química Nova, 31*, 1738–1742.

Moreira, M., Santos, M. D., Zolini, G., Wouters, A., Carvalho, J., & Schneedorf, J. (2008). Anti-inflammatory and cicatrizing activities of a carbohydrate fraction isolated from sugary kefir. *Journal of Medicinal Food, 11*, 356–361.

Rodrigues, K. L., Araújo, T. H., Schneedorf, J. M., de Souza Ferreira, C., Moraes, G.d. O. I., Coimbra, R. S., & Rodrigues, M. R. (2016). A novel beer fermented by kefir enhances anti-inflammatory and anti-ulcerogenic activities found isolated in its constituents. *Journal of Functional Foods, 21*, 58–69.

Rodrigues, K. L., Caputo, L. R. G., Carvalho, J. C. T., Evangelista, J., & Schneedorf, J. M. (2005). Antimicrobial and healing activity of kefir and kefiran extract. *International Journal of Antimicrobial Agents, 25*, 404–408.

Rodrigues, K. L., Carvalho, J. C. T., & Schneedorf, J. M. (2005). Anti-inflammatory properties of kefir and its polysaccharide extract. *Inflammopharmacology, 13*, 485–492.

Santanna, A. F., Filete, P. F., Lima, E. M., Porto, M. L., Meyrelles, S. S., Vasquez, E. C., Endringer, D. C., Lenz, D., Abdalla, D. S. P., Pereira, T. M. C., & Andrade, T. U. (2017). Chronic administration of the soluble, nonbacterial fraction of kefir attenuates lipid deposition in LDLr−/− mice. *Nutrition, 35*, 100–105.

CHAPTER

Processing technologies for safe production of beverages

8

Hirpha Adugna Areti[1], Ayele Assefa Adugna[2], Rabira Lemessa Gudeta[2], Dessalegn Legese Negewo[2] and N. Vamsi Vara Prasad[3]

[1]*Department of Chemical Engineering, Haramaya Institute of Technology, Haramaya University, Dire Dawa, Ethiopia;* [2]*Department of Food Technology and Process Engineering, Haramaya Institute of Technology, Haramaya University, Dire Dawa, Ethiopia;* [3]*Department of Food Engineering and Technology, Institute of Chemical Technology, Mumbai, Maharashtra, India*

8.1 Introduction

The beverage industry is an essential element of global food systems since it provides a variety of products that meet the various consumer preferences. World Health Organization (WHO) has identified this sector as essential as it creates economic value and influence on the population health due to the impact of the consumption of squat/sugar-containing beverages. Research revealed that 50% of the population in the entire globe consumes sugar-sweetened beverages at least one time a week since these beverages augment the possibilities of contracting obesity and noncommunicable diseases (Kraak et al., 2019). The WHO has suggested that an individual is advised to only consume free sugars as up to 10% of total energy intake per day but further health advantages are realized once the level drops to less than 5% (Zhou et al., 2020). Food safety and quality control are essential in the production of beverages since they determine the level of satisfaction and health needs of consumers of the products. According to the World Health Organization, the unsafe food and beverages cause over 200 diseases that cause illness to 600 million people and result into 420,000 deaths annually due to foodborne sicknesses (Zhou et al., 2020). The beverage industry should exercise high standards of safety since these measures will aid in minimizing the current health hazards. The drink industry must adopt Hazard Analysis Critical Control Points (HACCP) due to the research that reveals that the system lowers food safety outbreaks by half in various fields such as the beverages industry (Dosoky & Setzer, 2018). The beverage production process involves four necessary stages that begin with raw material preparation that is followed by extraction, fermentation, and finally packaging. All the production process relies on these stages to provide safe and quality finished products. Washing and sorting procedures of raw materials are the first phase that eliminates 90% of the contaminants on the material (Wiesner et al., 2021). The methods of extraction that involve pressing, brewing are done with the aim of realizing the maximum yield, without damage to the delicate compounds. According to Sivamaruthi et al. (2018), the modern method of high-pressure processing preserves 95% of nutritional qualities of extracted beverages. Fermentation process is one of the crucial stages in the production of drinks since

The Science and Safety of Beverages. https://doi.org/10.1016/B978-0-443-36536-2.00009-0

it produces safe and quality alcoholic and probiotic beverages. The preservatives produced by the fermentation process are two crucial preservatives that are used to improve the quality and safety of beverages by producing alcohol and organic acids. Studies indicate that the control of fermentation brings pathogenic microorganisms to less than 1% (Hetika et al., 2022, pp. 381–386). This is contributed by the inclusion of specific yeast and bacterial strains in the process of production that result in the improvement of beverage sensory properties that increases consumer preference (Vilela et al., 2019). The last phase in the beverage manufacturing process is the packaging that is used as an important factor in ensuring the quality and safety of the products throughout the production process to delivery. It has been discovered that 30% of the spoilage of beverages happens due to ineffective packaging and that proves the necessity of developing better packaging technology (Fentie et al., 2020). The industry is increasingly moving toward the use of smart packaging solutions that can actually monitor and report the quality of the beverage in real-time. Such innovations may reduce food waste by nearly half by making sure that the products are eaten in the optimal time of their freshness (Bahmani et al., 2021). The chapter discusses different technologies used in the processing of beverages to enhance their safety and quality. It is highlighted that the use of superior processing technologies, including nonthermal, fermentation, and filtration systems, is necessary to inactivate or destroy microbial hazards and enhance the sensory quality. As an illustration, selected starter cultures can be used to increase the quality of microbes and nutritional value and reduce safety risks associated with spontaneous fermentation in traditional fermented beverages (Madilo et al., 2024). Also, alternative methods, including the supercritical carbon dioxide processing and ultra-high-pressure homogenization have been discovered as possible substitutes to the traditional thermal processes, which helped in preserving the nutritional and sensory qualities of drinks (Arruda et al., 2023; Codina-Torrella et al., 2023). The role of the filtration technologies to filter impurities and guarantee the microbial stability to retain the quality of the products is also discussed more in-depth in the chapter (Jihill et al., 2025). To sum up, the application of such high-end processing trends is necessary to the beverage industry to address the safety standards and cater to the preferences in the context of which the positive circumstances regarding the health of the population are registered.

8.2 Raw materials and ingredient safety

The source and supply of raw material are very crucial variables in the preparation of the beverages, which carry very important impacts in terms of acceptability, quality, and safety. The raw materials employed in beverage preparation are a wide variety of fruit and vegetable products, crop products, and other derivatives of plants, which introduce unique characteristics to the finished product. The material quality is most vital since it not only affects the sensory property but also defines the nutritional and safety value of beverages. The example is that good quality fruit and vegetable can affect the flavor and nutritional quality, and low-quality ingredients can cause unpleasant tastes and health hazards as Kraak et al. (2019) have noted. To ensure the security of the raw materials, strict quality control should be applied to the raw material. This involves the physical and chemical testing of the ingredients, as well as, contaminants like the pesticides, heavy metals, and pathogens. Maintaining the safety of ingredients contained in drinks is even more of an issue, especially given the increased percentage of contaminants present on agricultural products. Research studies have indicated that pesticides are present in up to 80% of vegetables and fruits, and it is therefore important that the industry should put in place stringent testing and monitoring procedures to ensure quality and safety standards are achieved (Zhou et al., 2020). Moreover, the existence of heavy metals in the raw materials could be accompanied by severe health implications, whereby health-regulating limits of permissible levels of the same in foods and beverages have been set. The identification of the potential hazards regarding the raw materials is centrally determined by the hazard risk assessment and control measures. This is undertaken through the assessment of the risk probability and severity of the contaminants that are known to cause a risk and the installation of controls, which will minimize the effects. The risk of pesticides in vegetables can be significantly lowered by Good Agricultural Practices (GAP). Moreover, application of HACCP principles to beverage manufacturing makes it possible to identify the critical points in the supply chain and identify where the product may be contaminated and control measures implemented (Dosoky & Setzer, 2018). Various international and national organizations, such as the World Health Organization (WHO) and Food and Drug Administration (FDA), come up with quality standards and regulations of raw materials. These regulations provide rules of acceptable amounts of contaminants in addition to labeling and traceable origin of raw inputs. The compliance with these standards is extremely crucial in ensuring the quality and safety of drinks and the maintenance of trust in the industry among the consumers (Wiesner et al., 2021). As an example, the FDA has established regulations to ensure that all drinks and food items do not include poisonous concentrations of contaminants and that their producer should conduct regular tests to ensure the assurance of compliance (Sivamaruthi et al., 2018). In addition to compliance with regulations, the beverage industry is becoming more and more concerned with sustainability and how raw materials are acquired ethically. It includes the sourcing of ingredients from suppliers that comply with ecologically friendly agriculture and promotion of fair terms in which the farm workers will work. Consumers are also demanding beverages which are produced in a sustainable and ethical way. It has made several business operations introduce as transparent as possible measures of procurement and receive receiving certification, including organic or fair trade (Hetika et al., 2022, pp. 381–386). The change will not just lead to improved quality and safety of raw materials but also produce products on the same level as the consumer need for wellness-based products promoting social and environmental values. Technology is being used to enhance the quality and safety of raw materials and ingredients in manufacture of beverages. Emerging technologies, such as nonthermal processing technologies such as high-pressure processing and using pulsed electric fields, can lead to substantial decreases in the number of microbes without impacting the nutrient and sensory properties of raw materials (Vilela et al., 2019). These technologies provide potential replacements to the conventional thermal treatments, which in most cases lead to degradation of sensitive compounds found in vegetables and fruits. By adopting such sophisticated processing technologies, the beverage companies can guarantee the quality and safety of their products, and solve the problem of consumer demands for wellness (Fentie et al., 2020). Moreover, big data and Internet of Things (IoT) have been implemented in the beverage industry, and they transform the process of acquiring raw materials (Areti et al., 2024). Monitoring networks based on IoT can deliver real-time data on the conditions of the environment and, therefore, offer the growers a chance of streamlining the growing and harvesting experience to ensure the risk of contamination is reduced. This kind of data-driven solution makes it possible to control the quality of raw materials in such a way that safe and high-quality beverages are created (Bahmani et al., 2021). Manufacturing of beverages depends on the quality and safety of raw materials. A single system of quality controls, which includes new filtration technologies and molecular detection technologies, plays a leading role in the minimization of contaminants (microorganisms and chemical toxins) (Jihill et al., 2025; Nesterova et al., 2024). The use of new processing technologies, such as high-pressure processing and pulsed electric fields, could ensure the safety of microbes and avoid negative effects on the nutritional qualities of beverages (Vilas-Boas et al., 2022). Moreover, the sustainability of the industry and its ethical procurement is a pointer to a greater shift toward the manufacturing of safe and high-quality drinks that respond to consumer needs (Avîrvarei et al., 2023). According to the previous studies, it is essential to infuse more sanitation measures, new packaging methods, and effective regulations that will ensure high-quality and safety of beverages (Ehtesham et al., 2024; Liao et al., 2023). Continuous studies about the contamination sources, as well as the innovations of the new innovative processes of detection, serve to emphasize the effort of the industry in terms of preserving the community health (Darwish et al., 2024).

8.3 Beverage manufacturing processing technologies

The drinks industry uses a set of processing technologies to guarantee the security of products, increase the level of quality, and increase the shelf life. The key way in which these technologies are divided is into both thermal processing methods and nonthermal technologies. These two levels possess certain approaches to the employment of distinct principles to attain intended results in beverages processing.

8.3.1 Thermal processing technologies

Pasteurization is commonly used in thermal treatment of beverages, to decrease the microbial content of beverages, particularly, juices and dairy beverages. The pasteurization process involves increasing the temperature of the beverage at a certain temperature for a certain duration of time. This helps in effectively inhibiting pathogens while also retaining the quality and food value of the beverage. Batch pasteurization, which heats beverages to 63°C for 30 min, and high-temperature short time pasteurization, where drinks are heated to 72°C for 15 s, are standard pasteurization treatments (Munekata, Dominguez, Budaraju, et al., 2020). Pasteurization enhances the safety of the drinks but also increases its shelf life as the process reduces the organisms responsible for the spoilage of the drink thus ensuring the safety of the final-user (Cosme et al., 2022). Moreover, pasteurization has also been revealed to preserve the nutritious quality of drinks, rendering it a pivotal process in the manufacturing of secure and quality drinks (Aqib et al., 2019).

Pasteurization and sterilization differ in their purpose and the amount of microbes they kill. The primary aim of pasteurization is to get pathogenic microorganisms down to manageable levels, whereas sterilization works to obliterate them entirely, along with the spores. Sterilization has an extended shelf life without refrigeration (Munekata, Domínguez, Budaraju, et al., 2020). This is done through a process called autoclaving in which drinks are treated under steam under a high-pressure regime at temperatures above 121°C for a set period of time (Cosme et al., 2022). In the case of the beverage sector, sterilization is of importance specifically to beverage products like shelf-stable juice and vegetable dairy drinks that have long shelf life as one of the critical factors in the logistics and storage casting (Castro-Muñoz, 2019).

The processes that use sterilization produce products that are safe and microbe-free to their shelf life and consequently develop trust in consumers in the beverage's safety (Aqib et al., 2019). Ultra-high-temperature processing (UHT) is a heat treatment process that involves heating beverages to 135°C or more in a very short period and then cooled down. This is an excellent way of Sterilization of the product and preservation of its flavor and nutritional content (Morata & Guamis, 2020). One of the benefits of UHT processing is that it extends the shelf life of the nonrefrigerated beverages and so it is highly applicable to dairy beverages and fruit juices (Munekata, Domínguez, Budaraj, et al., 2020). Besides ensuring that there is no harmful bacteria, the process also preserves the flavor and the color of the beverage that the consumers adore, without being affected. Other researches have indicated that increase in temperature could introduce some effects in the flavor properties due to the Maillard reaction owing to UHT processing (Morata & Guamis, 2020).

Despite this, some studies indicate that UHT processing may cause subtle effects in terms of flavor profiles by virtue of the Maillard reaction that may occur when temperatures are raised (Morata & Guamis, 2020). Usually, it does not affect flavor at all in most cases. Moreover, the benefits of longer lasting and safer benefits outweigh any disadvantages (Castro-Muñoz, 2019).

When it comes to the safety of beverages, thermal processing has an important role to play. However, it doesn't just stop at that. It also affects the nutritional quality and flavor profiles of beverages. Studies show that some heat-sensitive vitamins, like vitamin C and some of the B vitamins, will get broken down when thermal processing occurs to lower the nutritional quality of the end-product (Lafarga et al., 2018). Maillard reaction as a result of increasing the temperature during the processing may also result in the flavor perception of beverages changing because it may intensify certain flavors and weaken the current ones (Morata & Guamis, 2020).

This is why the use of thermal processing technologies such as pasteurization, sterilization as well as ultra-high-temperature (UHT) processing has some very crucial roles in ensuring safe production of beverages (Table 8.1). Each of the technologies has distinct principles, applications, and effects on the quality of a final beverage. Thermal treatments are invaluable for controlling microbial numbers and shelf-life extensions while having challenges related to retention of nutritional quality and flavor.

Table 8.1 Thermal and nonthermal techniques for beverage processing.

Technique	Type of beverage	Optimized condition	Shelf life/other findings	References
Thermal pasteurization	Bael beverage	95°C for 5 min	30 days at 4°C based on sensory acceptability	Dhar and Chakraborty (2024)
Microwave heating	Ready-to-drink teas	800 W for 30 s	Enhances flavor retention and extends shelf life	Amini et al. (2024)
HPP	Juices, smoothies	300–600 MPa for 1–5 min	Maintains flavor and nutrients	Udayakumar et al. (2022)
Ultrasound processing	Broccoli and carrot by-products beverage	28 days at 4 °C, 6 mg/L Carotenoids, 1.25 g/L glucosinolates	With longer shelf life compared to pasteurized beverage	Pérez et al. (2023)
Cold plasma processing	Juices, alcoholic beverages	-	Reduces microbial load without heat, preserves sensory qualities	Liao et al. (2023)

Innovative processing technologies are doing their best to lower these challenges so that the final products are delivered to the consumers safe, nutritious, and tasty.

8.3.2 Nonthermal processing technologies

The nonthermal processing technologies have also been adopted by the beverages industry in an effort to enhance the quality of end products, shelf life, and nutritional content of end products. This part explains three major nonthermal technologies, namely, HPP, cold plasma technology, and PEF and compares their applicability to thermal conventional technologies.

HPP applies the very high pressure to inactivate microorganisms and enzymes found in the beverage system without a considerable increase in the temperature as a result of application of heat. The principle of operation is to subject a packaged or unpackaged product to 100–600 Mpa of pressure that is applied consistently in the entire product by a medium of transmitting the pressure (Sehrawat et al., 2021). Studies have revealed that cold plasma is able to reduce bacteria and viruses on packaging of beverages. This reduces the risks of cross-contamination in handling and taking of beverages. This method is an efficient method of killing pathogenic and spoilage microorganisms without altering sensory and nutritional properties of beverages and increasing their shelf life (Govaris & Pexara, 2021; Serna-Hernandez et al., 2021). HPP has several advantages. To start with, it severely diminishes the microbial load that constitutes viruses like the norovirus and the hepatitis A virus that are of utmost importance in the beverage safety. Second, HPP does not lose the organoleptic properties of flavor and flavor found in thermal processing (Balakrishna et al., 2020). It has also been found that the HPP-treated products have become more consumer-friendly due to the preservation of fresh-like properties (Pérez-Lamela et al., 2021). Thirdly, HPP has been demonstrated to increase the bioavailability of the selected nutrients thus a desirable technology in health-based drinks formulation. There are a number of applications of HPP in the beverage industry which encompass fruit juice, smoothies, milk-based drinks where HPP has been effectively used to assure safety without necessarily compromising on quality (Pinto et al., 2020). HPP is particularly useful in beverages that require heat sensitivity because of their possible degradation through heat. One of them is the fortified or vitamin and antioxidant compounds beverages.

Cold plasma technology is a new nonthermal technology, which involves the use of ionized gas to inactivate microorganisms on the surfaces of beverages and packaging materials. This technique acts on atmospheric pressure and can reduce the number of microbes by a long margin without affecting the chemical quality of the product (Charoux et al., 2021). Reactive species formed during the cold plasma process have the potential to cause damage to microbial cell membranes and inactivate pathogens, which places it as an option to enhance food safety (Munekata, Dominguez, Budaraj, et al., 2020). Cold plasma use in the beverage industry is gaining more and more popularity because of the effectiveness of the method to combat surface contamination. Moreover, studies have revealed that cold plasma treatment does not modify sensory characteristics of drinks and thus a good option among the beverage manufacturers who would not like to compromise quality and safety simultaneously.

The PEF technology entails the effective application of high-voltage electric field on the liquid to permeabilize the cell wall of the microbes, and inactivate the pathogens without destroying the food. It performs at ambient temperatures and is a safe nonthermal alternative, which does not lead to the degradation of nutritional and sensory properties of beverages (Ganessingh et al., 2018; Sehrawat et al., 2021). The safety attribute of PEF is quite significant in the sense that it can be used in inactivating a wide range of microorganisms, in no fewer than, molds, yeasts, or bacteria, without the harmful consequences that come with thermal treatment. Studies have established that PEF can help in maintaining the quality of heat-sensitive substances, including vitamins and antioxidants, which are critical in drinks whose primary characteristic is health.

Besides this, PEF has been associated with increased recovery of bioactive compounds from vegetables and fruits and higher nutritional attributes of beverages. Application of the technology of PEF has been accomplished in the juice processing of fruit and smoothies and dairy beverages where it has been able to prolong shelf life while ensuring quality of the end-product (Ganessingh et al., 2018; Munekata, Domínguez, Pateiro, *et al.*, 2020). The efficiency of the process in microbial inactivation and retention of nutrients renders it a strong candidate for future applications in beverages processing.

The differences between nonthermal processing technologies, such as high-pressure processing (HPP), cold plasma, and pulsed electric fields (PEF), and thermal processes, strong and similar, are compared. Thermal processing can destroy microorganisms, but at a high temperature, there is high loss of constituent nutrients and sensory properties (Eunice & Chidinma Ezinne, 2020; Mieszczakowska-Frąc et al., 2021). On the contrary, nonthermal technologies can help retain the nutritional quality of beverages by allowing us to preserve vitamins, some antioxidants, and other bioactive compounds that benefit health (López-Gámez et al., 2021). Nonthermal technologies are also frequently mandated for shorter processing time and lower intensity requirements than thermal technologies and therefore become preferred environmentally friendly alternatives for the manufacturing of beverages (Ganessingh et al., 2018). Nonthermal technologies' retention of the quality of a component while facilitating the assurance of its safety makes them popular choices for the progressive age of food processing. All in all, it can be concluded that the nonthermal processing technologies used in the beverage industry enhance product safety and quality. HPP, cold plasma, and PEF provide unique benefits which enhance the safety and nutritional quality of beverages and oppose the adverse effect of traditional thermal processes (Table 8.1). As consumers increasingly chose for healthier and safer beverages, beverage processors will need to introduce these new technologies to stay ahead of the curve.

8.4 Filtration and separation technologies

The beverage sector employs various filtration and separation technologies to guarantee product safety. Juices and soft drinks are produced using microfiltration and ultrafiltration membrane separation principles. Microfiltration usually works through pores sized between 0.1 and 10 μm. As a result, it removes larger particles such as yeast, bacteria, and suspended solids but preserves the remaining ingredients' nutrients and flavors (Castro-Muñoz, 2019). UF has a smaller size range of the pores, which can range from 010 to 0.1 μm to separate smaller lighter molecules like protein and some dissolved solids making the final product clearer and more stable. It has been found that the use of these technologies in juice production enhances the quality of the product by lowering the microbial load and more shelf-life without using any chemical preservatives. In one study, juice can be concentrated using UF such that undesired components will be removed. For instance, the turbidity component and all the flavor compounds that can impact off-flavors (Podolak et al., 2020). MF and UF processes can be used for products that need clarity and stability like clear juices and soft drinks in the beverages industry.

And the other important beverage technology in the industry is activated carbon filtration that is used to purify and remove impurities. This is done at the expense of the porous characteristics of activated carbon to trap myriad organic compounds like chlorine, volatile organic compounds (VOCs), and other unwanted taste and safety risks to beverages (Pepin et al., 2019). Its adsorption capacity is extremely high, and it has been determined that not only organic contaminants can be adsorbed by use of activated carbon, but also some metal ions can be adsorbed by up to 90% or more when using activated carbon. Activated carbon filtration is commonly used in producing juice to eliminate off-flavors and odors that way, the end product will be expected to be tasting and quality-wise satisfactory to the consumer. Also, it is possible to use this technology to decolourize the juices, which will improve the appearance of the final product. Activated carbon filtration depends on the following parameters including contact time, temperature, and the character of contaminants and therefore there are conditions that the soft drinks manufacturers must correct to attain a better performance (Pepin et al., 2019).

Reverse osmosis (RO) and nanofiltration (NF) are membrane filtering technologies that are important in beer clarification and purification of drinks. These procedures employ the semipermeable membranes to segregate components on the basis of size and charges, so that unwanted products can be selectively eliminated while desirable flavors and nutrients are being retained (Castro-Muñoz et al., 2019). For example, RO is common in the concentration of fruit juices (i.e., removing water and concentrating), which intensifies flavor and reduces shipping costs. Membrane filtration in another important use in the processing of beverage has contributed to improving product consistency and quality.

Membrane technology is viewed as a very effective method for the removal of pathogens and spoilage microorganisms thus it is, by all means, a major contributor to the overall beverages' safety. Plus, maintenance of the vitamins and bioactive compounds, which are considered important for the health of the consumers, is done through the operation of the process under lower temperatures than those of the standard thermal (Podolak et al., 2020).

The method of centrifugation separates the particles based on their density by applying centrifugal force. This method is noted for the juice extraction where pulp and sediment are separated from the liquids leading to a beverage that is much clearer (Castro-Muñoz, 2019). Moreover, centrifugation can eliminate the need to filter repeatedly thus making the production quicker and less expensive (Podolak et al., 2020). A comprehensive comparison of different filtration and separation methods is presented in Table 8.2. The major features, together with the pros and cons of each method, are clearly stated. The recent research proves that the usage of filtration and separation methods is essential to prevent the beverage industry to maintain the safety and quality of products and the qualities they want. Microfiltration and ultrafiltration absorb the good and reject the bad; activated carbon filters provide taste and safety; membrane filtration helps in product uniformity; centrifugation provides clarity of the liquid. Therefore, the importance of such technologies in the manufacturing of beverages will be greater as the demand toward the high-quality products is ever-growing.

8.5 Fermentation and biotechnology in beverage production

When sugars are made into acids, gases, and/or drinks, when no air is present, this can be done through fermentation which is using small life forms such as yeasts and/or bacteria. Key to its making is a lot of drinks like beer, wine, cider, and other more traditional drinks such as kefir or kombucha. The varying fermentation options may alter the typical taste, smell, and sensory of beverages that cause consumers to like and purchase them (Cuvas-Limon et al., 2020; Liszkowska & Berlowska, 2021). The primary form of the yeast that is utilized in producing a beverage containing alcohol is Saccharomyces

Table 8.2 Comparison of filtration and separation technologies.

Technology	Description	Pros	Cons	References
Mechanical filtration	Uses physical barriers (e.g., screens and membranes) to separate particles from fluids.	- High efficiency for large particles. - Low operational cost. - Simple to operate.	- Clogging can occur - Limited effectiveness for fine particles or dissolved substances	Cosio et al. (2023); Jihill et al. (2025)
Centrifugation	Utilizes centrifugal force to separate components based on density differences.	- Effective for separating liquids and solids. - Fast processing time. - Scalable.	- High energy consumption - Expensive equipment - Not suitable for all mixtures	Chiozzi et al. (2022); Huang et al. (2022); Vasquez-Rojas et al. (2023)
Ultrafiltration	Membrane-based process to separate macromolecules and suspended solids.	- Removes bacteria and viruses. - Operates at low pressure. - Environmentally friendly.	- Membrane fouling - High initial cost - Limited to specific particle sizes	Haghighi Enayat et al. (2024); Schulze et al. (2022); Zachariah et al. (2024)
Adsorption	Uses adsorbent materials (e.g., activated carbon) to capture contaminants.	- Effective for removing dissolved impurities. - Versatile applications. - Regenerable.	- Adsorbent saturation requires replacement - Can be expensive - Slow process	Baig et al. (2023); Cheng et al. (2022); Haghighi Enayat et al. (2024)

cerevisiae that assists in transforming sugars into carbon dioxide and ethanol. It is a favorite yeast as it is effective and produces alcohol in great quantities. The process of fermentation is conditional on temperature and pH level and other microbial content that lead to the variation of flavor and quality of the product (Walker et al., 2019, pp. 477–512). Nonalcoholic beverages fermentation process needs to be modified to limit alcohol formation but allow it to produce desirable taste and smell compounds. The immobilization of yeasts and controlled parameters of fermentation make the creation of desired results in fermentation processes possible (Ignat et al., 2020). The manipulation of the fermentation conditions is crucial toward the safety of the products, as well as the consistency of production in beverage production. This is because the nutrient availability, oxygen level, and temperature are strictly monitored to prevent the spoilage organisms and pathogens. There is a need to ensure anaerobic conditions to prevent the unwanted microbial contamination in the alcoholic fermentation. The process of fermentation allows the use of certain yeast and bacterial strains that contribute to the creation of safer and higher-quality end-products since the microorganisms compete with harmful pathogens (Behera et al., 2018). In combination with hazard analysis critical control points (HACCP) systems, proper management tools that regulate fermentation processes are the implementation of good manufacturing practices (GMP) to ensure the safety of products (Valero-Cases et al., 2020). Consumption of probiotics has been embraced in the beverage industry through the manufacture of kefir and kombucha products as the microorganism's present health benefits to consumers. Probiotics are living mini organisms which present health benefits to individuals when consumed in large quantities. They maintain gut health, enhance the body immunity to illness, and can even improve mood through the connection of the gut to the brain (Maciel & Souza, 2020). The proper handling of these small life forms in probiotic drinks is important since otherwise, it can have health risks because of unmitigated proliferation of microorganisms. The effectiveness of probiotics depends on the survival of probiotics during the storage period and their capacity to achieve adequate gut levels (Molero & Briñez, 2018). Probiotic products have to be carefully produced under quality control measures to cleanse the product of pathogenic strains (Cottet et al., 2020). Newer biotechnology has come up with new approaches to fermentation operations that are safe and more productive. To come up with improved fermentation processes that generate improved products, scientists research on genetically modified microorganisms (GMMs) and microbial consortia. Genetic modification is employed by scientists to produce GMMs that are capable of performing diverse functions, such as increasing the yield of alcohol and producing flavors. Microbial consortia are complex collections of microorganisms that fill complex taste and scent profiles due to the synergistic interactions of different microorganisms (Aldrete-Tapia et al., 2019; Moreno-García et al., 2018). Studies have shown that microorganisms listed in GRAS form useful compounds by the production of siderophores and its ability to increase iron intake and bacterial growth during processing of the beverages (Makris et al., 2022). Bioreactors that have controlled fermentation systems allow the precise control of fermentation parameters that lead to better consistency of the product and safety (Castro-Muñoz, 2019). The fermentation process affects the formation of flavor and, therefore, the quality and safety of alcoholic and nonalcoholic drinks. Besides probiotics providing health benefits to the consumers, it is necessary to regulate the fermentation conditions to ensure the product safety and quality. Advances in biotechnology continue to perfect the process of fermentation, creating innovative and safe ways of making drinks. With the increasing demand of the functional drinks by the customers, the beverage industry has to meet their demands without compromising the quality and safety of the products available.

8.6 Chemical additives and preservatives in beverage production

The use of preservatives is crucial in food and beverage industry. They inhibit the growth of microbes and inhibit various forms of spoilage. Knowing the different preservatives and their purposes, manufacturers could make superior decisions (Fig. 8.1).

According to Fig. 8.1, the principal categories of additives used in nonalcoholic beverages to preserve and maintain sensory properties are shown (Silva et al., 2019). In addition, the quality and safety are ensured by the adherence to beverage legislation. Lastly, the new consumer trends influence the trend toward natural additives. With the industry evolving on a continuous basis, exploring new solutions will increase products. Therefore, ensuring safety and customer satisfaction is one of the priorities of the beverage industry (Silva et al., 2019). Preservatives in beverage processing are used as a critical component in the shelf life and after-growth of microorganisms. Both natural and synthetic preservatives are used to inhibit the growth of microorganisms and pathogens that cause spoilage of beverages, and in the process, they increase the quality and safety of beverages. The use of the synthetic preservatives such as sodium benzoate and potassium sorbate also plays a key role in the food preservation by reducing microbial growth and extending shelf life. Their use has created agendas, however. Likewise, the consumer awareness has led to increased dystopia about synthetic food

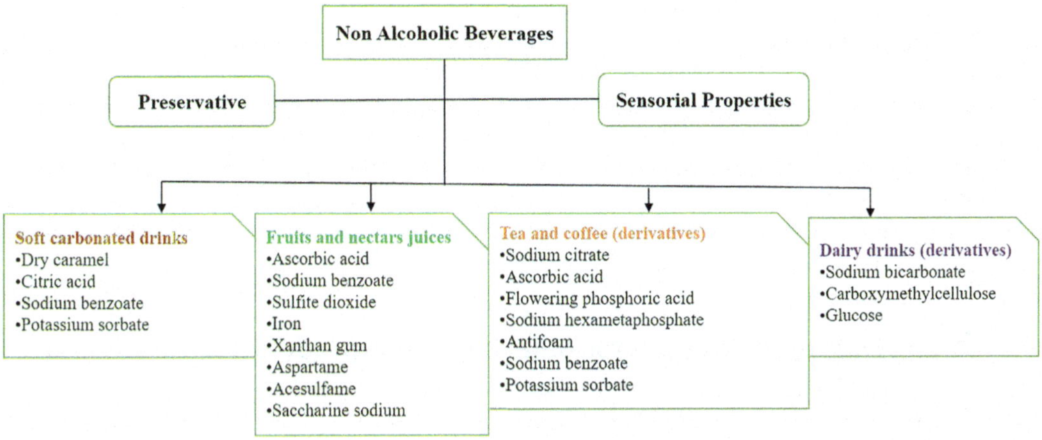

FIGURE 8.1

Main types of additives used in non-alcoholic beverages for the preservation and/maintenance of sensory characteristics.

Silva, Marselle MN, K. S. Pereira, and M. A. Z. C. (2019). Food additives used in non-alcoholic water-based beverages – a review. Journal of Nutritional Health & Food Engineering, 9(3), 109–121. https://doi.org/10.15406/jnhfe.2019.09.00335 no date, permission link: http://lattes.cnpq.br/3348345023065192.

additives (Hassoun et al., 2020; Quinto et al., 2019). Natural antimicrobials found in plants, animals, microbes, algae, and fungi provide an alternative multifaceted way of preserving food (Khunsee et al., 2024). Their bactericidal effect together with the proven antioxidant effect presents a massive potential in improving food safety and quality management. The unique characteristics of herbs and spices are the focus of this discipline. With suitable extraction methods and increased knowledge about the mechanisms of fermentation, we shall be able to realize their potentials. A merge of these aspects might create healthier and more nutritious food and beverages. The change to natural preservation processes not only guarantees health, but also guarantees environmentally friendly practices. The process of antioxidants is involved when the beverages are processed. They have high inhibition of oxidative degradation, which is an aspect that preserves flavor, aroma, and nutritive value of food. Consumer satisfaction is ensured by food safety and quality control. Therefore, there is a need to embrace antioxidants in the new future of the industry. Fruits and vegetables are also natural antioxidants that are getting more and more popular in the preparation of beverages to add to stability and flavor without the adverse effects of the synthetic ones (Lourenço et al., 2019). In addition, other acids like citric and ascorbic acid are mostly used not only due to their preservative properties but also a result of their ability to modify flavors (Pérez-Lamela et al., 2021). Additive safety codes and regulatory mechanisms are required to ensure consumer protection and maintenance of the health of citizens. Various departments, including the Food and Drug Administration (FDA) and the European Food Safety Authority (EFSA) provide the guidelines to be followed in the use of food additives, including preservatives. Such rules provide the allowed levels of some additives to make it possible to use them safely in food and beverage products (D'Amore et al., 2020). New additives can be approved only after a severe safety assessment, including toxicological tests, and evaluation of health hazard risks. As the consumer demands are shifting toward natural products, the guideline of the regulating agencies is also changing to suit the increasing demand for natural preservatives and additives (Luzardo-Ocampo et al., 2021; Wang et al., 2019). There is also an impressive change in the preferences of the beverage market in terms of preservatives usage, which is propagated by the necessity of people to use natural products and their increasing knowledge about food safety.

The producers are faced with a complex task of satisfying the demand for longer shelf life and safety without compromising on the flavor. As the regulatory environment evolves, the industry will move toward more natural preservatives, reduce the use of synthetic additives, and respond to the needs of consumers to have safer and healthier beverages.

8.7 Packaging technologies for safe beverage production

The choice of packaging material is very important in beverage processing. Different materials presented create various safety concerns. Therefore, it is also important to learn all the types of packaging. The advantages of using aseptic package are many; it helps in preservation of the beverages and blocking their contamination during their shelf life. The vacuum sealing of foods eliminates air in the package and in the case, it preserves the spoilage of food stuffs in foods and prolongs the shelf life of food products. One of the factors that has a significant impact on food safety is modified atmosphere packaging (MAP), which alters the environment in which a product is kept to preserve it. And the tamper-proof packaging will also ensure that the consumer is assured that the product will be safe to use. These packages deter tampering through the application of visual cues. The kind of beverage packaging is also extremely valuable since each of them represents a dissimilar safety concern. Plastic packaging more so Polyethylene terephthalate (PET) is commonly used because it is light and inexpensive. However, there are some concerns about the toxicity of certain plastics since some of them cause a leaching of toxic substances such as bisphenol A (BPA) and phthalates into beverages, which are potentially dangerous to health (Sarioglu et al., 2018). Glass packaging is not very dangerous, but in an inattentive manner, it can be both dangerous and contaminated because of its breakage and contamination. Moreover, a large amount of glass may increase transportation costs and carbon emissions (Guillard et al., 2018). Metal cans (including aluminum) are preferred as well, as they are recyclable and solid (Guillard et al., 2018). However, there have been reports on the problem of the potential leaching of metal, particularly aluminum, into beverages, which casts a shadow of doubt on long-term health effects (Guillard et al., 2018). Durability of beverage packaging has become a matter of serious concern due to the massive environmental effect created by plastic waste.

These are different studies, which present alarming statistics. As an example, a recent report has reported that only 44.11% of beverage companies have established measurable targets of reducing, reusing, and recycling packaging containers (özenir et al., 2023). The resultant effect is that the societies are confronted with strict environmental problems. The global shift to sustainable packaging options is compulsory. This change affects different industries, primarily, beverage processing. Eco-packaging is not only the expression of environmental consciousness but also needs of consumers. In this way, a market needs to transform its packaging habits (Esturo et al., 2023). Moreover, composite packaging (BPCP) is also difficult to recycle and reuse due to the multiplicity of the product since it consists of many layers that complicate the recovery process (Chen et al., 2023). The beverage industry is changing due to the innovations in the packaging technology. Such innovations as smart packaging systems are putting safety and quality control in the front seat. Consumers are getting safer and better quality of beverages with the manufacturers adopting such technologies. Also, smart solutions are very critical in the current innovation of the beverage processing. The future of enhancing the quality of food safety and beverages, therefore, is a very promising matter. In addition, nanotechnology has emerged as an innovative technology in packaging food. As shown in Fig. 8.2, the food packaging technologies of manufacturing safe beverages incorporate imagining the most critical ingredients and operations required to make beverages safe and of high quality using high-tech packaging. Its ability to enhance resistance to rancidity as well as shelf life is invaluable. However, this innovation has serious problems associated with food safety. The risks of engineered nanomaterials in foodstuffs are questionable (Yang et al., 2021). The beverage packages life cycle assessment (LCA) of package material is significant because it demonstrates the environmental effects of various packaging. Based on the influence of each type of packaging on the environment, manufacturers will be able to make right decisions.

This paper presents types of beverage packaging, as well as explores their effects on the environment (Brock & Williams, 2020). LCA studies are focused on the complexity of the interactions of different packaging materials within the beverage industry. Despite the fact that both glass and aluminum are the best in recycling, the light nature of PET reduces the impact of transportation emissions. These complexities require that beverage processors address them, and their focus should be on food safety and quality control during the manufacturing process (Schneider et al., 2025). The contact between the design of packaging and consumer preferences is the most important. Sustainability, health claims, and quality control determine how decisions are made when buying. These trends require companies to be aware of them to remain in line with the competition. Finally, a good packaging might enhance brand loyalty and sales (Shibata et al., 2022). The functional and esthetic value of the packaging are essential qualities that can impact purchasing, and there should be a balance between the functional necessity and the marketing necessity (Pratiwi et al., 2023). Deposit Return System (DRS) is an economic policy that has been incorporated in the context of a circular economy to encourage the reuse or recycling of used beverage containers (bottles and cans) by levying a small amount of money as a refund to consumers at the point of purchase. This deposit is refunded upon returning the container to a point of returning. The current level of success in reducing waste, maximizing recycling rates, and promoting environmentally friendly consumption makes DRS a generally accepted best practice. It has been demonstrated that the creation of DRS is best practice. Such systems make recycling a paid exercise thus maximizing consumer engagement. The positive

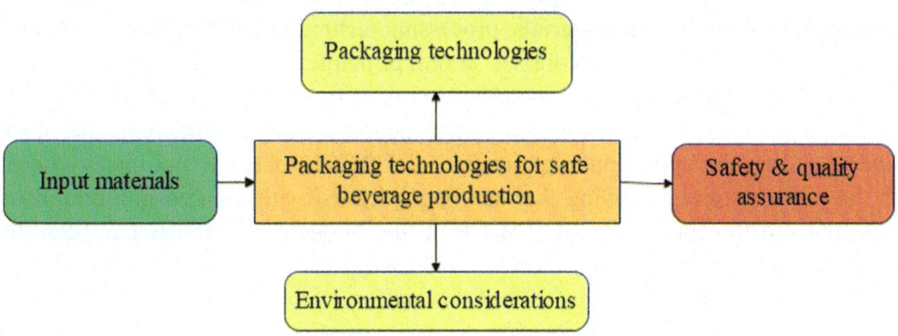

FIGURE 8.2

F packaging technologies for safe beverage production.

impact on the environment cannot be disputed either. Lastly, programs like DRS are relied upon to transition to a circular economy. We can have a brighter future that is more sustainable with a mass implementation. It is not just necessary but our duty to switch to better recycling and waste management (Görgün et al., 2021). Regulatory compliance is the key to quality management in the complex world of the beverage industry with safety as the first and foremost consideration. On top of that, the beverage producers must put a complete consideration on food safety and packaging. Experience of the effect of fermentation and extraction method will improve the quality of the product. Lastly, the significance of these matters ensures consumer safety (Schmid & Welle, 2020). The regulatory bodies usually request a lot of testing of the packaging to determine their safety and ability to meet the required standards. The last couple of years have seen the use of biodegradable and compostable packaging gaining momentum at an impressive pace. The increasing interest of consumers and their inclination toward eco-friendly packaging alternatives have resulted in the rise of this trend. The transformation is primarily with the use of polylactic acid (PLA) blends, as the suppliers are making the transition to environmentally friendly substitutes for plastics packaging. It is a considerable trend in various industries (Han, 2023). In the general sense, the movement of packaging technologies in the direction of ecology is observed. Green alternatives to conventional plastics are within reach. Moreover, material science and environmental sustainability are attaining a breakthrough in the industry. Eventually, packaging technology, which is always being invented is, the heart of the future beverage industry. The new technologies imply the things to be safe, the things to be higher quality, and the things to be green in production. By placing food safety, quality control, fermentation, and extraction process on top priority, the industry can truly welcome a sustainable future.

8.8 Quality control and assurance in beverage processing

Quality control refers to a practice used in the food and beverages sector to maintain the quality of the products to meet the expected quality and regulatory standards as quality assurance incorporates all the code of conduct, standards, and requirement to enable the stake holders in the food supply chain to ensure compliance standard to make them safe to be consumed (Okpala & Korzeniowska, 2023). HACCP is abbreviated as Hazard Analysis Critical Control Point, which is an approach of scientific prevention that identifies, evaluates, and controls the risks that are very important in food safety. In the processing of drinks, this approach is important because it gives a platform where numerous contaminants may be brought about by raw materials, processing techniques, and storing (Dlamini & Adetunji, 2023, pp. 243–262). The HACCP comprises seven principles of implementation that include the following: Conducting a hazard analysis, identification of critical control points (CCPs), setting critical limits, monitoring critical control points, corrective actions, system validation, and documentation. Research indicates that the appropriate application of HACCP makes a significant contribution to a decrease in the cases of food poisoning that can be associated with the consumption of drinks (Levy et al., 2022). Indicatively, application of HACCP in the production of juices has been discovered to minimize microbial contamination and therefore enhancing safety of products. Good Manufacturing Practice (GMP) are good principles that ensure that uniform production of safe and quality drinks is done. The concept of GMP covers all the raw materials used in the manufacturing environment and equipment. To prevent contamination and make certain that the drinks are in a safe range, there should be compliance with GMP (Owusu-Apenten & Vieira, 2022). The microbiological analysis process is an inseparable component of quality control in beverage processing to determine the presence of pathogens and microorganisms responsible for food spoilage, which can make it unsafe (Kyaw et al., 2024).

Some of the methods that are employed in microbiological analysis include culture, polymerase chain reaction (PCR), and quick test kits. As an example, the use of Petrifilm plates has been reported as an efficient and convenient method to analyze the beverages microbiologically to be able to quickly detect the microbial contamination (Papkovsky & Kerry, 2023). The regular microbiological testing not only gives an assurance of safety standards but also helps in detecting potential sources of contamination, therefore, enabling corrective action to be taken. Testing Shelf-life testing is essential to determining beverages safety and quality during storage.

Such testing involves determining the effect of such factors as temperature, light, and packaging on the stability of drinks in the long-term (Ghosh et al., 2022). Shelf-life testing is usually a combination of sensory testing, chemical testing, and microbiological testing to establish viability of the product in regard to its shelf life. As an example, beverages that have been subjected to high temperatures are subjected to a special shelf-life test to determine the results of their stability in standard conditions of storage over time. Quality shelf-life testing may lead to superior product formulations, therefore, customer satisfaction, which is caused by superior flavor and freshness (Lohita & Srijaya, 2024). The awareness of the shelf life of soft drinks is also vital in inventory management and minimization of food waste, which is a major problem in the soft drink industry. Overall, quality assurance and control in the soft drink processing are complicated and involve the integration of a variety of methodologies and practices. The use of HACCP and GMP and rigorous microbiological and shelf-life analysis is essential in ensuring the safety, quality, and uniformity of beverage products. As the beverage industry changes in the dynamics, the necessity of such quality control measures will increase as well, and the research and development of food safety controls and consumer confidence must be enhanced continuously (Owusu-Apenten & Vieira, 2022).

8.9 Sanitation and hygiene in beverage production

Sanitary and hygiene in the food beverage production industry is paramount in ensuring quality and safety of the products. Avoiding contamination during the processing requires proper cleaning and sanitation plans, but more than ever, the food and drink industries require hygiene routines due to the outbreak of the COVID-19 pandemic (Telukdarie et al., 2020). There should be good cleaning practices, including Clean-in-Place (CIP) systems, that are significant in the beverages production process. Such measures allow cleaning equipment without it being disinfected, therefore, reducing the chances of contamination (Karuppuchamy et al., 2024; Pant et al., 2023). The performance of any type of sanitizer in the prevention of microbes depends on various factors such as the type of sanitizer, concentration, contact time, and the organism (Silva et al., 2019). For example, the fact that the effectiveness of sanitizers is species-dependent is the reason for the need for improvement in the sanitation efforts (Alonso et al., 2023). Also, biofilms are communities of microorganisms sticking to surfaces, and these are the biggest issues in the food processing sector since they are not easily removed by disinfectants. Thus, there should be a better understanding of biofilm dynamics and the use of disassembling methods to achieve better sanitation. HACCP is a systematized methodology for detecting and minimizing possible risks in the beverage manufacturing process.

Beverage corporations can measure and control sources that may result in contamination; therefore, they can certify safety in products through the designated critical control points (Dubey et al., 2022; Magdovitz et al., 2020).

HACCP adopted together with new technology such as computational fluid dynamics (CFD) can contribute more to maximizing cleaning processes as they would model fluid interactions as well as the effectiveness of cleaning agents. Moreover, introduction of novel sanitization technologies such as ozonation has demonstrated tremendous potential in improving food safety through the reduction in microbial loads in a drink by a significant margin. To conclude, the problems of sanitation and hygiene connected with beverage manufacturing industry mainly should be addressed with the implementation of the overall cleaning processes, the successful use of sanitizers, and the observance of the principles of HACCP. New technologies and their introduction, with continued research and implementation, are a critical factor that would be utilized in the quest to deal with the dynamics of contamination and safety of beverage products.

8.10 Advances in beverage processing technologies

Automation, digitalization, and the Internet of Things (IoT) have been major contributors to innovation in the technologies of beverage processing. These technologies are essential in enhancing efficiency in its operations, safety of its products and remain abreast with evolving consumer needs (see Table 8.3). The drink industry has been progressively automating and going digital in an attempt to streamline production.

The manufacturing processes can be real-time monitored and controlled by automation technologies such as Industrial Internet of Things, which reduces the impact of human error and improves the productivity of the operations. As an example, one of the studies mentions that an Industrial Internet of Things-based production monitoring system can optimize industrial operations by enabling the automated collection of data and analytics as well as improve the overall quality and efficiency of production (Maulana et al., 2023). Moreover, the digital supply chain has significantly enhanced the performance of the food and beverage industry, particularly the reduction in the cost and quality (Saryatmo & Sukhotu, 2021). The shift to digital platforms not only improves operational actions but also helps the industry to be sustainable and resilient during the times of setbacks such as the COVID-19 pandemic (Memon et al., 2021). The IoT technologies allow installing the sensors that continuously observe various parameters, such as temperature, humidity, and water quality, which are the primary concerns of the product quality and safety. Indicatively, a smart water quality monitoring system based on IoT can provide real-time data on the use and quality of water, which is crucial in the production of beverages that rely on water (Jan et al., 2021). Moreover, predictive maintenance due to the integration of IoT into monitoring systems helps to avoid equipment failures as well as minimize downtime, therefore, leading to the further increase in the production efficiency. This is because the possibility of monitoring processes remotely and in real-time not only improves the operations management but also contributes to the achievement of safety regulations to facilitate safe production of beverages.

8.11 Emerging trends and future of beverage processing

The beverage processing industry is undergoing radical transformation whose pace is being fed by the forthcoming trends that focus on quality management, sustainability, consumer preferences, and emerging processing technologies (Awuchi, 2023). These trends are changing the manner in which beverages are produced, marketed, and consumed, embodiment of the current health, safety, and

Table 8.3 Advances in beverage processing technologies.

Technology	Description	Benefits	Applications	References
High-pressure processing	Uses high pressure to inactivate pathogens and spoilage microorganisms.	Extends shelf life, preserves nutrients, and maintains fresh taste.	Juices, smoothies, cold-pressed beverages.	Donda Zbinden et al. (2024); Yusuf et al. (2023)
Pulsed electric field	Applies short electric pulses to disrupt microbial cell membranes.	Retains flavor, color, and nutrients; energy-efficient.	Fruit juices, milk, and plant-based beverages.	Prakasha et al. (2024); Trzyniec et al. (2022)
Ultraviolet (UV) treatment	Uses UV light to disinfect beverages by damaging microbial DNA.	Chemical-free, effective against bacteria and viruses.	Water, juices, and dairy beverages	Lanrewaju et al. (2022); Pravallika et al. (2024)
Membrane filtration	Separates particles based on size using semipermeable membranes.	Improves clarity, removes microorganisms, and concentrates flavors.	Beer, wine, dairy, and plant-based beverages.	Genova et al. (2025); Krstanović et al. (2024); Seidel et al. (2024)
Ohmic heating	Heats beverages by passing electric current through them.	Uniform heating, preserves sensory and nutritional quality.	Juices, soups, and liquid dairy products	Murakami et al. (2023); Tavares-Filho et al. (2024)
Ultrasound technology	Uses high-frequency sound waves to disrupt microbial cells and enhance extraction.	Improves extraction efficiency, reduces processing time.	Fruit juices, tea, and functional beverages.	Baiano et al. (2024)
Cold plasma technology	Uses ionized gas to inactivate pathogens and enzymes.	Nonthermal, preserves sensory properties, and extends shelf life.	Juices, dairy, and alcoholic beverages	Li et al. (2024); Sruthi et al. (2022)
Nanotechnology	Incorporates nanoparticles for improved filtration, packaging, and nutrient delivery.	Enhances nutrient bioavailability and improves packaging efficiency.	Functional and fortified beverages	Prakash et al. (2024); Yadav et al. (2024)
Fermentation technology	Uses microbial cultures to produce bioactive compounds and enhance flavors.	Improves gut health, enhances flavor, and increases shelf life.	Probiotic drinks, kombucha, and alcoholic beverages	Facchin et al. (2024)
Advanced packaging solutions	Utilizes smart and active packaging to monitor and extend beverage quality.	Reduces spoilage, enhances safety, and provides real-time quality monitoring.	All beverage types, especially perishable and functional beverages	Guo et al. (2024); Kadirvel et al. (2025)

environmental responsibilities expectations. Fig. 8.3 represents the core of the structure, and the stemming branches lead to the future trends and the tendencies of the future.

Quality monitoring and safety in beverage processing is being transformed by integrating smart technologies and especially sensors and artificial intelligence (AI). Real-time monitoring systems will allow watching vital parameters such as temperature, pH, and levels of microbes throughout the production process (da Costa et al., 2023). Regulatory compliance is also ensured by this technology. Indicatively, AI algorithms have the ability to predict possible quality issues in advance, which makes it possible to implement preemptive countermeasures and reduce waste and inefficiency (Onyijen et al., 2024, pp. 183–200). Also, the intelligent systems are capable of providing batch traceability in the supply chain, a feature that supports manufacturers in the process of detecting and amending the safety issues associated with certain product batches easily.

Sustainability has emerged as a primary concern of the beverage processing sector, and the environmental impact of production processes has been assigned a high priority. The beverage processing industry is gradually introducing energy-efficient and waste-reduction technologies. As an example, the new technologies like HPP and PEF, which are proving to be more effective than traditional methods in energy savings are also preserving the nutritional quality of beverages better (Sharma et al., 2024). On top of that, the embodiment of the principles of the circular economy like recycling, and reuse of manufacturing by-products of beverages, is being of great importance which is indeed the case. This approach that creates and opens up the business opportunities for the producers also allows them to have a new business opportunity (Lemaire, 2020).

The processing technology advance which is very important is the increase in the food safety and the lessening of energy consumption in the beverage production (Lisboa et al., 2024). The stability and shelf life of beverages are boosted using techniques such as high-pressure homogenization and nonthermal processing technologies without impairing the sensory properties. These methods are particularly useful in the case of plant-based beverages, which are prone to emulsification and other stability-related problems (Rani et al., 2024, pp. 169–185). The use of microbial enzymes in beverages

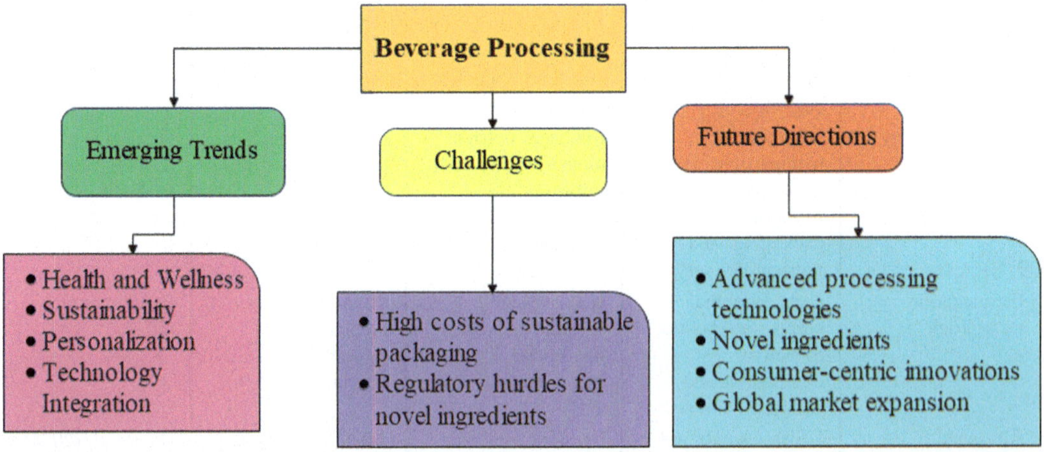

FIGURE 8.3

Emerging trends and future of beverage processing.

production to speed up the fermentation process, introduce new flavors, and overall product quality improvement has been really impressive. While the operation continues, the main subject about integrating those newest systems will be a determinant issue in the process of realization of customer needs and compliance with the laws.

The prospects of the drinks processing are promising to make great breakthroughs with the momentum of smart technologies, sustainability initiatives, changed consumer behavior, and new processing methods (Farmer, 2013, pp. 1–21). As the industry moves toward these emerging trends, quality, security, and environmental sustainability will play a critical role in shaping the face of the drink-making industry. The manufacturers welcoming change will probably gain a competitive edge in the dynamically evolving market, which will eventually result in a healthier world and the cleaner planet.

8.12 Conclusion

The processing technologies applied in the beverage industry are the most significant in ensuring safety and quality of end products. The elimination of pathogens, preservation of nutritional value, and shelf life of the beverages are due to the most important technologies such as pasteurization, filtration, and fermentation as well as state-of-the-art packaging methods. Such processes enhance safety of drinks in addition to enhancing sensory characteristics of the drinks, which are the determinant of consumer acceptance.

Some of the challenges that face the drinks industry in the future entail adapting to the changing consumer demands toward healthier drinks, increased demands on transparency in the origin of the ingredients and environmental footprint. There are opportunities, such as using the recent technologies such as smart packaging that can monitor the quality of products in real-time and natural preservatives, which are in line with the changes in the consumer toward clean label products. Furthermore, the development of fermentation and biotechnology can give possibilities to develop functional beverages with a health-promoting effect that is not limited to nutrition. Safety and consumer protection are dependent on the dynamic role of technology in the beverages industry. With the stricter nature of the regulatory requirements, it will be essential to deploy the more advanced technologies to create the compliance and to develop the consumer confidence. Continuing research and development in processing technology will not only be a reaction to the current safety concerns but will also preempt future demands thereby making the sector of beverages more robust and sustainable.

References

Aldrete-Tapia, J. A., Miranda-Castilleja, D. E., Arvizu-Medrano, S. M., Martínez-Peniche, R.Á., Soto-Muñoz, L., & Hernández-Iturriaga, M. (2019). Pursuing the perfect performer of fermented beverages. *GMMs vs. Microbial Consortium*. https://doi.org/10.5772/intechopen.81616

Alonso, V. P. P., Gonçalves, M. P. M. B. B., de Brito, F. A. E., Barboza, G. R., Rocha, L.d. O., & Silva, N. C. C. (2023). Dry surface biofilms in the food processing industry: An overview on surface characteristics, adhesion and biofilm formation, detection of biofilms, and dry sanitization methods. *Comprehensive Reviews in Food Science and Food Safety, 22*(1), 688–713. https://doi.org/10.1111/1541-4337.13089. Available from: http://onlinelibrary.wiley.com/journal/10.1111/(ISSN)1541-4337.

Amini, R., Palupi, E., & Ekayanti, I. (2024). Physical and chemical properties of boba beverages as a source of fiber made from red seaweed (Eucheuma cottonii). *IOP Conference Series: Earth and Environmental Science, 1359*(1), Article 012025. https://doi.org/10.1088/1755-1315/1359/1/012025

Aqib, A., Ijaz, M., Anjum, A., Kulyar, M., Shoaib, M., & Farooqi, S. (2019). *Reconnoitering milk constituents of different species, probing and soliciting factors to its soundness*. IntechOpen. https://doi.org/10.5772/intechopen.82852

Areti, H. A., Muleta, M. D., Abo, L. D., Hamda, A. S., Adugna, A. A., Edae, I. T., Daba, B. J., & Gudeta, R. L. (2024). Innovative uses of agricultural by-products in the food and beverage sector: A review. *Food Chemistry Advances, 5*. https://doi.org/10.1016/j.focha.2024.100838. Available from: https://www.sciencedirect.com/science/journal/2772753X.

Arruda, H. S., Silva, E. K., Pastore, G. M., & Marostica Junior, M. R. (2023). Non-Thermal supercritical carbon dioxide processing retains the quality parameters and improves the kinetic stability of an araticum beverage enriched with inulin-type dietary fibers. *Foods, 12*(13). https://doi.org/10.3390/foods12132595. Available from: www.mdpi.com/journal/foods.

Avîrvarei, A. C., Salanță, L. C., Pop, C. R., Mudura, E., Pasqualone, A., Anjos, O., Barboza, N., Usaga, J., Dărab, C. P., Burja-Udrea, C., Zhao, H., Fărcas, A. C., & Coldea, T. E. (2023). Fruit-based fermented beverages: Contamination sources and emerging technologies applied to assure their safety. *Foods, 12*(4). https://doi.org/10.3390/foods12040838. Available from: www.mdpi.com/journal/foods.

Awuchi, C. G. (2023). HACCP, quality, and food safety management in food and agricultural systems. *Cogent Food & Agriculture, 9*(1). https://doi.org/10.1080/23311932.2023.2176280. Available from: www.tandfonline.com/action/journalInformation?journalCode=oafa20.

Bahmani, M., O'Lone, C. E., Juhász, A., Nye-Wood, M., Dunn, H., Edwards, I. B., & Colgrave, M. L. (2021). Application of mass spectrometry-based proteomics to barley research. *Journal of Agricultural and Food Chemistry, 69*(31), 8591–8609. Available from: http://pubs.acs.org/journal/jafcau. doi: 10.1021/acs.jafc.1c01871.

Baiano, A., De Pilli, T., & Fiore, A. (2024). Green and sustainable techniques to increase the extraction of phenolic compounds from turnip greens by-products. *Journal of Food Process Engineering, 47*(5). https://doi.org/10.1111/jfpe.14617. Available from: http://onlinelibrary.wiley.com/journal/10.1111/(ISSN)1745-4530.

Baig, N., Khan, N. A., Salhi, B., Abdulazeez, I., Abu-Zahra, N., Abdelazem, S., & Aljundi, I. H. (2023). Highly permeable sulfonated polydopamine integrated MXene membranes for efficient surfactant-stabilized oil-in-water separation. *Langmuir, 39*(39), 13953–13967. Available from: http://pubs.acs.org/journal/langd5. doi: 10.1021/acs.langmuir.3c01651.

Balakrishna, A. K., Abdul Wazed, Md, & Farid, M. (2020). A review on the effect of high pressure processing (HPP) on gelatinization and infusion of nutrients. *Molecules, 25*(10), 2369. https://doi.org/10.3390/molecules25102369

Behera, S. S., Ray, R. C., & Zdolec, N. (2018). Lactobacillus plantarum with functional properties: An approach to increase safety and shelf-life of fermented foods. *BioMed Research International, 2018*, 1–18. https://doi.org/10.1155/2018/9361614

Brock, A., & Williams, I. (2020). Life cycle assessment of beverage packaging. *Detritus, 13*, 47–61. https://doi.org/10.31025/2611-4135/2020.14025

Castro-Muñoz, R. (2019). Pervaporation-based membrane processes for the production of non-alcoholic beverages. *Journal of Food Science and Technology, 56*(5), 2333–2344. https://doi.org/10.1007/s13197-019-03751-4

Charoux, C. M. G., Patange, A., Lamba, S., O'Donnell, C. P., Tiwari, B. K., & Scannell, A. G. M. (2021). Applications of nonthermal plasma technology on safety and quality of dried food ingredients. *Journal of Applied Microbiology, 130*(2), 325–340. https://doi.org/10.1111/jam.14823

Chen, J., Mu, X., Tu, C., & Hu, G. (2023). Evaluation index system for the implementation of extended producer responsibility system: Chinese beverage paper-based composite packaging manufacturers. *Packaging Technology and Science, 36*(3), 195–210. https://doi.org/10.1002/pts.2704

Cheng, Y., Datta, S. J., Zhou, S., Jia, J., Shekhah, O., & Eddaoudi, M. (2022). Advances in metal-organic framework-based membranes. *Chemical Society Reviews, 51*(19), 8300–8350. https://doi.org/10.1039/d2cs00031h

Chiozzi, V., Agriopoulou, S., & Varzakas, T. (2022). Advances, applications, and comparison of thermal (pasteurization, sterilization, and aseptic packaging) against non-thermal (ultrasounds, UV radiation, ozonation, high hydrostatic pressure) technologies in food processing. *Applied Sciences, 12*(4), 2202. https://doi.org/10.3390/app12042202

Codina-Torrella, I., Gallardo-Chacón, J. J., Juan, B., Guamis, B., & Trujillo, A. J. (2023). Effect of ultra-high pressure homogenization (UHPH) and conventional thermal pasteurization on the volatile composition of tiger nut beverage. *Foods, 12*(4). https://doi.org/10.3390/foods12040683. Available from: www.mdpi.com/journal/foods.

Cosio, M. S., Pellicanò, A., Gardana, C., & Fuenmayor, C. A. (2023). Debittering of grape juice by electrospun nylon nanofibrous membranes: Impact of filtration on physicochemical, functional, and sensory properties. *Polymers, 15*(1). https://doi.org/10.3390/polym15010192. Available from: http://www.mdpi.com/journal/polymers.

Cosme, F., Ines, A., & Vilela, A. (2022). *Incorporating microbial and commercial enzymes into beverage manufacturing procedures*. Vide Leaf. https://doi.org/10.37247/afs.1.23.35

Cottet, C., Ramirez-Tapias, Y. A., Delgado, J. F., la Osa, O. D., Salvay, A. G., & Peltzer, M. A. (2020). Biobased materials from microbial biomass and its derivatives. *Materials, 13*(6). https://doi.org/10.3390/ma13061263. Available from: https://res.mdpi.com/d_attachment/materials/materials-13-01263/article_deploy/materials-13-01263.pdf.

Cuvas-Limon, R. B., Nobre, C., Cruz, M., Rodriguez-Jasso, R. M., Ruíz, H. A., Loredo-Treviño, A., Texeira, J. A., & Belmares, R. (2020). Spontaneously fermented traditional beverages as a source of bioactive compounds: An overview. *Critical Reviews in Food Science and Nutrition*, 1–23. https://doi.org/10.1080/10408398.2020.1791050. Available from: https://www.tandfonline.com/loi/bfsn20.

D'Amore, T., Di Taranto, A., Berardi, G., Vita, V., Marchesani, G., Chiaravalle, A. E., & Iammarino, M. (2020). Sulfites in meat: Occurrence, activity, toxicity, regulation, and detection. A comprehensive review. *Comprehensive Reviews in Food Science and Food Safety, 19*(5), 2701–2720. https://doi.org/10.1111/1541-4337.12607. Available from: http://onlinelibrary.wiley.com/journal/10.1111/(ISSN)1541-4337.

da Costa, T. P., Gillespie, J., Cama-Moncunill, X., Ward, S., Condell, J., Ramanathan, R., & Murphy, F. (2023). A systematic review of real-time monitoring technologies and its potential application to reduce food loss and waste: Key elements of food supply chains and IoT technologies. *Sustainability, 15*(1), 614. https://doi.org/10.3390/su15010614

Darwish, A., Ricci, M., Tobon Vasquez, J. A., Migliaccio, C., & Vipiana, F. (2024). Near-field microwave sensing technology enhanced with machine learning for the non-destructive evaluation of packaged food and beverage products. *Scientific Reports, 14*(1). https://doi.org/10.1038/s41598-024-62287-6. Available from: https://www.nature.com/srep/.

Dhar, R., & Chakraborty, S. (2024). Enhancing shelf-life of Bael beverage through various pasteurization techniques: A comparative study at 25°C and 4°C with thermal, pulsed light, and microwave treatments. *Journal of Food Process Engineering, 47*(11). https://doi.org/10.1111/jfpe.14776

Dlamini, B. C., & Adetunji, A. I. (2023). *Hazard analysis and critical control point (HACCP) and food safety management systems food safety and toxicology: Present and future perspectives*. South Africa: De Gruyter. https://doi.org/10.1515/9783110748345-011

Donda Zbinden, M., Schmidt, M., Vignatti, C. I., Pirovani, M.É., & Böhm, V. (2024). High-pressure processing of fruit smoothies enriched with dietary fiber from carrot discards: Effects on the contents and bioaccessibilities of carotenoids and vitamin E. *Molecules, 29*(6). https://doi.org/10.3390/molecules29061259. Available from: http://www.mdpi.com/journal/molecules.

Dosoky, N. S., & Setzer, W. N. (2018). Biological activities and safety of citrus spp. essential oils. *International Journal of Molecular Sciences, 19*(7). https://doi.org/10.3390/ijms19071966. Available from: http://www.mdpi.com/1422-0067/19/7/1966/pdf.

Dubey, P., Singh, A., & Yousuf, O. (2022). Ozonation: An evolving disinfectant technology for the food industry. *Food and Bioprocess Technology, 15*(9), 2102–2113. https://doi.org/10.1007/s11947-022-02876-3

Ehtesham, A. M., Filipello, V., Fernandèz Escàmez, P. S., & Perez, A. G. (2024). Training in modern statistical methodologies and software tools for the definition and analysis of (stochastic) quantitative microbial risk assessment models with relevant food products for the Italian and Spanish food supply chains. *EFSA Journal, 22*(1). https://doi.org/10.2903/j.efsa.2024.e221103. Available from: efsa.onlinelibrary.wiley.com/journal/18314732/.

Eunice, U., & Chidinma Ezinne, O. (2020). *Effect of pasteurization on chemical and sensory properties of fruit pulps-based smoothie with added coconut milk.* Vide Leaf. https://doi.org/10.37247/afs.1.2020.10

Esturo, A., Lizundia, E., & Sáez de Cámara, E. (2023). Fruit juice industry's transition towards sustainability from the viewpoint of the producers. *Sustainability, 15*(4), 3066. https://doi.org/10.3390/su15043066

Facchin, S., Bertin, L., Bonazzi, E., Lorenzon, G., De Barba, C., Barberio, B., Zingone, F., Maniero, D., Scarpa, M., Ruffolo, C., Angriman, I., & Savarino, E. V. (2024). Short-chain fatty acids and human health: From metabolic pathways to current therapeutic implications. *Life, 14*(5). https://doi.org/10.3390/life14050559. Available from: www.mdpi.com/journal/life/.

Farmer, N. (2013). *Present status and trends in innovations in packaging for food, beverages and other fast-moving consumer goods trends in packaging of food, beverages and other fast-moving consumer goods (FMCG).* United Kingdom: Elsevier Inc.. https://doi.org/10.1533/9780857098979.1. Available from: http://www.sciencedirect.com/science/book/9780857095039.

Fentie, E. G., Emire, S. A., Demsash, H. D., Dadi, D. W., & Shin, J. H. (2020). Cereal-and fruit-based ethiopian traditional fermented alcoholic beverages. *Foods, 9*(12). https://doi.org/10.3390/foods9121781. Available from: https://www.mdpi.com/2304-8158/9/12/1781/pdf.

Görgün, E., Adsal, K., Mısır, A., Aydin, E., Ergün, Ç., Keskin, N., Acar, A., & Ergenekon, S. (2021). Deposit refund system for beverage containers as a best practice example for recycling maximization. *Environmental Research and Technology, 4*(3), 199–205. https://doi.org/10.35208/ert.862611

Ganessingh, V., Sahibdeen, R., & Maharaj, R. (2018). *An evaluation of the impact of novel processing technologies on the phytochemical composition of fruits and vegetables.* IntechOpen. https://doi.org/10.5772/intechopen.77730

Genova, J., Dencheva-Zarkova, M., Yankov, D., & Tsibranska, I. (2025). Influence of transmembrane pressure on the retention of bioactive compounds and alcohol content in red wine nanofiltration. *WSEAS Transactions on Biology and Biomedicine, 22*, 67–71. https://doi.org/10.37394/23208.2025.22.7

Ghosh, T., Raj, G. V. S. B., & Dash, K. K. (2022). A comprehensive review on nanotechnology based sensors for monitoring quality and shelf life of food products. *Measurement: Food, 7*. https://doi.org/10.1016/j.meafoo.2022.100049. Available from: https://www.journals.elsevier.com/measurement-food.

Govaris, A., & Pexara, A. (2021). Inactivation of foodborne viruses by high-pressure processing (HPP). *Foods, 10*(2), 215. https://doi.org/10.3390/foods10020215

Guillard, V., Gaucel, S., Fornaciari, C., Angellier-Coussy, H., Buche, P., & Gontard, N. (2018). The next generation of sustainable food packaging to preserve our environment in a circular economy context. *Frontiers in Nutrition, 5*. https://doi.org/10.3389/fnut.2018.00121

Guo, S., Hu, Y., Zhao, C., Li, Y., Zhang, Z., Wang, W., Bai, Y., Zhou, J., Xue, Y., Zou, L., & Ren, G. (2024). Effects of enzymatic hydrolysis technology on the physicochemical properties and biological activities of American ginseng beverages. *Food Science and Nutrition, 12*(5), 3674–3687. https://doi.org/10.1002/fsn3.4038

Haghighi Enayat, M., Azami, H., Tapak, L., Reza Borzou, S., & Gholyaf, M. (2024). Impact of ultrafiltration profiling compared to conventional methods on blood pressure regulation among hemodialysis patients. *Nephro-Urology Monthly, 16*(1). https://doi.org/10.5812/numonthly-138699

Han, G. (2023). An aging study of PLA-PBAT blends in commercial beverages. *Journal of Physics: Conference Series, 2539*(1), Article 012012. https://doi.org/10.1088/1742-6596/2539/1/012012

Hassoun, A., Carpena, M., Prieto, M. A., Simal-Gandara, J., Özogul, F., Özogul, Y., Çoban, Ö. E., Guðjónsdóttir, M., Barba, F. J., Marti-Quijal, F. J., Jambrak, A. R., Maltar-Strmečki, N., Kljusurić, J. G., & Regenstein, J. M. (2020). Use of spectroscopic techniques to monitor changes in food quality during application of natural preservatives: A review. *Antioxidants, 9*(9), 1–30. https://doi.org/10.3390/antiox9090882

Hetika, H., Ayu Khasanah, R., & Yasmin, A. (2022). *The analysis of survival strategies for micro small and medium enterprises (MSMEs) food and beverages in the time of the Covid-19 pandemic*. Atlantis Press SARL. https://doi.org/10.2991/978-2-494069-09-1_44

Huang, H., Song, Y., Zhang, Y., Li, Y., Li, J., Lu, X., & Wang, C. (2022). Electrospun nanofibers: Current progress and applications in food systems. *Journal of Agricultural and Food Chemistry, 70*(5), 1391–1409. https://doi.org/10.1021/acs.jafc.1c05352

Ignat, M. V., Salanță, L. C., Pop, O. L., Rodica Pop, C., Tofană, M., Mudura, E., Coldea, T. E., Borsa, A., & Pasqualone, A. (2020). Current functionality and potential improvements of non-alcoholic fermented cereal beverages. *Foods, 9*(8), 1031. https://doi.org/10.3390/foods9081031

Jan, F.nullah, Min-Allah, N., & Düstegör, D. (2021). IoT based smart water quality monitoring: Recent techniques, trends and challenges for domestic applications. *Water, 13*(13), 1729. https://doi.org/10.3390/w13131729

Jihill, A. A. A., Hushim, M. F., Madon, R. H., Kosnin, H., & Mohamed Nazar, M. I. S. (2025). Selection of filtration systems to improve the quality of beverage and paste production. *Journal of Engineering Research and Education (JERE), 16*, 1–8. https://doi.org/10.58915/jere.v16.2024.1654

Kadirvel, V., Palanisamy, Y., & Ganesan, N. (2025). Active packaging System—An overview of recent advances for enhanced food quality and safety. *Packaging Technology and Science, 38*(2), 145–162. https://doi.org/10.1002/pts.2863. Available from: http://onlinelibrary.wiley.com/journal/10.1002/(ISSN)1099-1522.

Karuppuchamy, V., Heldman, D. R., & Snyder, A. B. (2024). A review of food safety in low-moisture foods with current and potential dry-cleaning methods. *Journal of Food Science, 89*(2), 793–810. https://doi.org/10.1111/1750-3841.16920. Available from: http://onlinelibrary.wiley.com/journal/10.1111/(ISSN)1750-3841.

Khunsee, A., Kaewsritong, J., & Srikaeo, K. (2024). Clean label approach for condiment sauces: A case in Thai style sauces. *Multidisciplinary Science Journal, 6*(12), Article 2024255. https://doi.org/10.31893/multiscience.2024255

Kraak, V. I., Patiño, S. R.-G., & Sacks, G. (2019). An accountability evaluation for the international food & beverage alliance's global policy on marketing communications to children to reduce obesity: A narrative review to inform policy. *Obesity Reviews, 20*(S2), 90–106. https://doi.org/10.1111/obr.12859

Krstanović, V., Mastanjević, K., Košir, I. J., Jurić, M., & Habschied, K. (2024). The influence of milling granulation on the proportion of fermentable and non-fermentable ingredients in mash obtained from mixed endosperm wheat. *Applied Sciences, 14*(14), 5985. https://doi.org/10.3390/app14145985

Kyaw, K. S., Adegoke, S. C., Ajani, C. K., Nwabor, O. F., & Onyeaka, H. (2024). Toward in-process technology-aided automation for enhanced microbial food safety and quality assurance in milk and beverages processing. *Critical Reviews in Food Science and Nutrition, 64*(6), 1715–1735. https://doi.org/10.1080/10408398.2022.2118660

López-Gámez, G., Elez-Martínez, P., Martín-Belloso, O., & Soliva-Fortuny, R. (2021). Recent advances toward the application of non-thermal technologies in food processing: An insight on the bioaccessibility of health-related constituents in plant-based products. *Foods, 10*(7), 1538. https://doi.org/10.3390/foods10071538

Lafarga, T., Bobo, G., Viñas, I., Collazo, C., & Aguiló-Aguayo, I. (2018). Effects of thermal and non-thermal processing of cruciferous vegetables on glucosinolates and its derived forms. *Journal of Food Science and Technology, 55*(6), 1973–1981. https://doi.org/10.1007/s13197-018-3153-7

Lanrewaju, A. A., Enitan-Folami, A. M., Sabiu, S., & Swalaha, F. M. (2022). A review on disinfection methods for inactivation of waterborne viruses. *Frontiers in Microbiology, 13*. https://doi.org/10.3389/fmicb.2022.991856. Available from: https://www.frontiersin.org/journals/microbiology#.

Lemaire, A. (2020). *Circular economy: Best practices and future perspectives for the beer brewing industry.* Prom.: Truyens, Vincent: Louvain School of Management, Université Catholique de Louvain, Article 24674. Available in: Http://Hdl. Handle. Net/2078.1/Th e Sis.

Levy, N., Hashiguchi, T. C. O., & Cecchini, M. (2022). Food safety policies and their effectiveness to prevent foodborne diseases in catering establishments: A systematic review and meta-analysis. *Food Research International, 156*, Article 111076. https://doi.org/10.1016/j.foodres.2022.111076

Li, B., Peng, L., Cao, Y., Liu, S., Zhu, Y., Dou, J., Yang, Z., & Zhou, C. (2024). Insights into cold plasma treatment on the cereal and legume proteins modification: Principle, mechanism, and application. *Foods, 13*(10), 1522. https://doi.org/10.3390/foods13101522

Liao, H., Asif, H., Huang, X., Luo, Y., & Xia, X. (2023). Mitigation of microbial nitrogen-derived metabolic hazards as a driver for safer alcoholic beverage choices: An evidence-based review and future perspectives. *Comprehensive Reviews in Food Science and Food Safety, 22*(6), 5020–5062. https://doi.org/10.1111/1541-4337.13253

Lisboa, H. M., Pasquali, M. B., dos Anjos, A. I., Sarinho, A. M., de Melo, E. D., Andrade, R., Batista, L., Lima, J., Diniz, Y., & Barros, A. (2024). Innovative and sustainable food preservation techniques: Enhancing food quality, safety, and environmental sustainability. *Sustainability, 16*(18). https://doi.org/10.3390/su16188223. Available from: http://www.mdpi.com/journal/sustainability/.

Liszkowska, W., & Berlowska, J. (2021). Yeast fermentation at low temperatures: Adaptation to changing environmental conditions and formation of volatile compounds. *Molecules, 26*(4), 1035. https://doi.org/10.3390/molecules26041035

Lohita, B., & Srijaya, M. (2024). Novel technologies for shelf-life extension of food products as a competitive advantage: A review. *Food Production, Diversity, and Safety Under Climate Change*, 285–306.

Lourenço, S. C., Moldão-Martins, M., & Alves, V. D. (2019). Antioxidants of natural plant origins: From sources to food industry applications. *Molecules, 24*(22). https://doi.org/10.3390/molecules24224132. Available from: https://www.mdpi.com/1420-3049/24/22/4132/pdf.

Luzardo-Ocampo, I., Ramírez-Jiménez, A. K., Yañez, J., Mojica, L., & Luna-Vital, D. A. (2021). Technological applications of natural colorants in food systems: A review. *Foods, 10*(3). https://doi.org/10.3390/foods10030634. Available from: https://www.mdpi.com/2304-8158/10/3/634/pdf.

Maciel, M. I. S., & Souza, M. M. B. D. (2020). *Prebiotics and probiotics - Potential benefits in human nutrition and health* https://doi.org/10.5772/intechopen.89155

Madilo, F. K., Parry-Hanson Kunadu, A., Tano-Debrah, K., Saalia, F. K., & Kolanisi, U. (2024). Diversity of production techniques and microbiology of African cereal-based traditional fermented beverages. *Journal of Food Quality, 2024.* https://doi.org/10.1155/2024/1241614. Available from: https://www.hindawi.com/journals/jfq/.

Magdovitz, B. F., Gummalla, S., Thippareddi, H., & Harrison, M. A. (2020). Evaluating environmental monitoring protocols for Listeria spp. and Listeria monocytogenes in frozen food manufacturing facilities. *Journal of Food Protection, 83*(1), 172–187. https://doi.org/10.4315/0362-028X.JFP-19-190. Available from: https://jfoodprotection.org/doi/pdf/10.4315/0362-028X.JFP-19-190.

Makris, C., Carmichael, J. R., Zhou, H., & Butler, A. (2022). C-Diazeniumdiolate graminine in the Siderophore Gramibactin is photoreactive and originates from arginine. *ACS Chemical Biology, 17*(11), 3140–3147. https://doi.org/10.1021/acschembio.2c00593

Maulana, G. G., Aminah, S., & Aji Nugraha, B. (2023). Implementation of a production monitoring system using IIoT based on Mobile application. *Jurnal RESTI (Rekayasa Sistem dan Teknologi Informasi), 7*(5), 1077–1087. https://doi.org/10.29207/resti.v7i5.5221

Memon, S. U. R., Pawase, V. R., Soomro, M. A., & Pavase, T. R. (2021). Investigation of covid-19 impact on the food and beverages industry: China and India perspective. *Foods, 10*(5). https://doi.org/10.3390/foods10051069. Available from: https://www.mdpi.com/2304-8158/10/5/1069/pdf.

Mieszczakowska-Frąc, M., Celejewska, K., & Płocharski, W. (2021). Impact of innovative technologies on the content of vitamin C and its bioavailability from processed fruit and vegetable products. *Antioxidants, 10*(1), 54. https://doi.org/10.3390/antiox10010054

Molero, M. S., & Briñez, W. J. (2018). *Probiotics consumption increment through the use of Whey- based fermented beverages*. IntechOpen. https://doi.org/10.5772/intechopen.72362

Morata, A., & Guamis, B. (2020). Use of UHPH to obtain juices with better nutritional quality and healthier wines with low levels of SO2. *Frontiers in Nutrition, 7*. https://doi.org/10.3389/fnut.2020.598286. Available from: journal.frontiersin.org/journal/nutrition.

Moreno-García, J., García-Martínez, T., Mauricio, J. C., & Moreno, J. (2018). Yeast immobilization systems for alcoholic wine fermentations: Actual trends and future perspectives. *Frontiers in Microbiology, 9*. https://doi.org/10.3389/fmicb.2018.00241. Available from: https://www.frontiersin.org/articles/10.3389/fmicb.2018.00241/full.

Munekata, P. E. S., Domínguez, R., Budaraju, S., Roselló-Soto, E., Barba, F. J., Mallikarjunan, K., Roohinejad, S., & Lorenzo, J. M. (2020). Effect of innovative food processing technologies on the physicochemical and nutritional properties and quality of non-dairy plant-based beverages. *Foods, 9*(3). https://doi.org/10.3390/foods9030288. Available from: https://www.mdpi.com/2304-8158/9/3/288.

Munekata, P. E. S., Domínguez, R., Pateiro, M., & Lorenzo, J. M. (2020). Influence of plasma treatment on the polyphenols of food products-A review. *Foods, 9*(7). https://doi.org/10.3390/foods9070929. Available from: https://www.mdpi.com/2304-8158/9/7/929.

Murakami, K., Matsuno, M., & Shimoyamada, M. (2023). Investigating thermal denaturation kinetics of 7S and 11S proteins and lipoxygenase in soymilk through ohmic heating. *Journal of Food Process Engineering, 46*(12). https://doi.org/10.1111/jfpe.14493

Nesterova, E., Morozova, P., Gladkikh, M., Kazemzadeh, S., & Syromyatnikov, M. (2024). Molecular methods for detecting microorganisms in beverages. *Federation Beverages, 10*(2). https://doi.org/10.3390/beverages10020046. Available from: www.mdpi.com/journal/beverages.

Özenïr, Ç., Kaçar, M., Berk, G., & Kayhan, B. (2023). Evaluation of energy and nutrient content of fruit juices and similar beverages in Türkiye and their investigation in terms of sustainability. *International Journal of Agriculture Environment and Food Sciences, 7*(4), 818–827. https://doi.org/10.31015/jaefs.2023.4.12

Okpala, C. O. R., & Korzeniowska, M. (2023). Understanding the relevance of quality management in agro-food product industry: From ethical considerations to assuring food hygiene quality safety standards and its associated processes. *Food Reviews International, 39*(4), 1879–1952. https://doi.org/10.1080/87559129.2021.1938600

Onyijen, O. H., Oyelola, S., & Ogieriakhi, O. J. (2024). *Food manufacturing, processing, storage, and marketing using artificial intelligence A Biologist's guide to artificial intelligence: Building the foundations of artificial intelligence and machine learning for achieving advancements in life sciences*. Nigeria: Elsevier. https://doi.org/10.1016/B978-0-443-24001-0.00012-9. Available from: https://www.sciencedirect.com/book/9780443240010.

Owusu-Apenten, R., & Vieira, E. (2022). Food safety management, GMP & HACCP. In *Elementary food science* (pp. 217–236). Springer.

Pérez, P., Hashemi, S., Cano-Lamadrid, M., Martínez-Zamora, L., Gómez, P. A., & Artés-Hernández, F. (2023). Effect of ultrasound and high hydrostatic pressure processing on quality and bioactive compounds during the shelf life of a broccoli and carrot By-Products beverage. *Foods, 12*(20), 3808. https://doi.org/10.3390/foods12203808

Pérez-Lamela, C., Franco, I., & Falqué, E. (2021). Impact of high-pressure processing on antioxidant activity during storage of fruits and fruit products: A review. *Molecules, 26*(17), 5265. https://doi.org/10.3390/molecules26175265

Pant, K. J., Cotter, P. D., Wilkinson, M. G., & Sheehan, J. J. (2023). Towards sustainable cleaning-in-place (CIP) in dairy processing: Exploring enzyme-based approaches to cleaning in the cheese industry. *Comprehensive*

Reviews in Food Science and Food Safety, 22(5), 3602–3619. https://doi.org/10.1111/1541-4337.13206. Available from: http://onlinelibrary.wiley.com/journal/10.1111/(ISSN)1541-4337.

Papkovsky, D. B., & Kerry, J. P. (2023). Oxygen sensor-based respirometry and the landscape of microbial testing methods as applicable to food and beverage matrices. *Sensors, 23*(9). https://doi.org/10.3390/s23094519. Available from: http://www.mdpi.com/journal/sensors.

Pepin, A., Stanhope, K. L., & Imbeault, P. (2019). Are fruit juices healthier than sugar-sweetened beverages? A review. *Nutrients, 11*(5), 1006. https://doi.org/10.3390/nu11051006

Pinto, C. A., Moreira, S. A., Fidalgo, L. G., Inácio, R. S., Barba, F. J., & Saraiva, J. A. (2020). Effects of high-pressure processing on fungi spores: Factors affecting spore germination and inactivation and impact on ultrastructure. *Comprehensive Reviews in Food Science and Food Safety, 19*(2), 553–573. https://doi.org/10.1111/1541-4337.12534. Available from: http://onlinelibrary.wiley.com/journal/10.1111/(ISSN)1541-4337.

Podolak, R., Whitman, D., & Black, D. G. (2020). Factors affecting microbial inactivation during high pressure processing in juices and beverages: A review. *Journal of Food Protection, 83*(9), 1561–1575. https://doi.org/10.4315/JFP-20-096

Prakash, S. P., Yoha, K. S., Leena Michael, M., Moses, J. A., & Anandharamakrishnan, C. (2024). Emerging applications of electrospun nanofiber membranes for liquid foods. *ACS Food Science & Technology, 4*(8), 1805–1816. https://doi.org/10.1021/acsfoodscitech.4c00226

Prakasha, R., Pandey, H., & Vinay, G. M. (2024). Enhancing nutritional quality and color stability of tomato juice through low-intensity pulsed electric field treatment. *European Journal of Nutrition & Food Safety, 16*(4), 123–131. https://doi.org/10.9734/ejnfs/2024/v16i41414

Pratiwi, K., Taufan Andreyanto, M., & Asrol, M. (2023). Taufik, herbal beverage packaging product design using kansei engineering. *JENIUS: Jurnal Terapan Teknik Industri, 4*(1), 12–21. https://doi.org/10.37373/jenius.v4i1.365

Pravallika, K., Shaik, L., Alzahrani, K. J., Misra, N. N., & Chakraborty, S. (2024). Pulsed light processing of low sugar, added fiber RTD mango beverage. *Journal of Food Process Engineering, 47*(3). https://doi.org/10.1111/jfpe.14539. Available from: http://onlinelibrary.wiley.com/journal/10.1111/(ISSN)1745-4530.

Quinto, E. J., Caro, I., Villalobos-Delgado, L. H., Mateo, J., De-Mateo-silleras, B., & Redondo-Del-río, M. P. (2019). Food safety through natural antimicrobials. *Antibiotics, 8*(4). https://doi.org/10.3390/antibiotics8040208. Available from: https://www.mdpi.com/2079-6382/8/4/208/pdf.

Rani, R., Solanki, K., Kulshrestha, R., & Rehal, J. (2024). *Non-thermal processing techniques for enhancing quality and stability of functional beverages non-thermal processing of functional foods*. India: CRC Press. https://doi.org/10.1201/9781003436560-9. Available from: https://www.routledge.com/Non-Thermal-Processing-of-Functional-Foods/Pattanayek-Dutta-Singh/p/book/9781032557588.

Sarioglu, E., Kaynak, H. K., Çelik, H., & Vuruskan, D. (2018). The tensile and bursting strength evaluation of linear low density polyethylene (LLDPE) spunbond fabrics. In *Conference: ICETI 2018, July.*

Saryatmo, M. A., & Sukhotu, V. (2021). The influence of the digital supply chain on operational performance: A study of the food and beverage industry in Indonesia. *Sustainability, 13*(9), 5109. https://doi.org/10.3390/su13095109

Schmid, P., & Welle, F. (2020). Chemical migration from beverage packaging materials—A review. *Beverages, 6*(2), 37. https://doi.org/10.3390/beverages6020037

Schneider, J. M., Ghannadzadeh, A., & van der Meer, Y. (2025). Material flow analysis of a post-consumer plastic packaging recycling system in the Netherlands: A focus on beverage carton. *Clean Technologies and Environmental Policy, 27*(11), 6099–6110. https://doi.org/10.1007/s10098-022-02342-w

Schulze, P. C., Bogoviku, J., Westphal, J., Aftanski, P., Haertel, F., Grund, S., Von Haehling, S., Schumacher, U., Möbius-Winkler, S., & Busch, M. (2022). Effects of early empagliflozin initiation on diuresis and kidney function in patients with acute decompensated heart failure (EMPAG-HF). *Circulation, 146*(4), 289–298. https://doi.org/10.1161/CIRCULATIONAHA.122.059038

Sehrawat, R., Kaur, B. P., Nema, P. K., Tewari, S., & Kumar, L. (2021). Microbial inactivation by high pressure processing: Principle, mechanism and factors responsible. *Food Science and Biotechnology, 30*(1), 19–35. https://doi.org/10.1007/s10068-020-00831-6

Seidel, L., Runkel, K., Albuquerque, W., Happel, K., Ghezellou, P., Spengler, B., Zorn, H., Gand, M., Freund, M., Will, F., & Schweiggert, R. (2024). Investigations into the protein stabilization of musts and wines by Aspergillopepsin under different enzymatic and thermal treatments. *ACS Food Science & Technology, 4*(9), 2124–2133. https://doi.org/10.1021/acsfoodscitech.4c00308

Serna-Hernandez, S. O., Escobedo-Avellaneda, Z., García-García, R., Rostro-Alanis, M.d. J., & Welti-Chanes, J. (2021). High hydrostatic pressure induced changes in the physicochemical and functional properties of milk and dairy products: A review. *Foods, 10*(8). https://doi.org/10.3390/foods10081867. Available from: https://www.mdpi.com/2304-8158/10/8/1867/pdf.

Sharma, M., Vidhya, C. S., Sunitha, N. H., Sachan, P., Singh, B., Santhosh, K., & Shameena, S. (2024). Emerging food processing and preservation approaches for nutrition and health. *European Journal of Nutrition & Food Safety, 16*(1), 112–127. https://doi.org/10.9734/ejnfs/2024/v16i11382

Shibata, N., Sihong, C., Nagamatsu, A., & Sakurai, S. (2022). An analysis of the effects of package design alterations for tea-based beverages. *International Journal of Japan Association for Management Systems, 14*(1), 13–17. https://doi.org/10.14790/ijams.14.13

Silva, Marselle, M. N., Pereira, K. S., & Marie, A. Z. C. (2019). Food additives used in non-alcoholic water-based beverages – A review. *Journal of Nutritional Health & Food Engineering, 9*(3), 109–121. https://doi.org/10.15406/jnhfe.2019.09.00335

Sivamaruthi, B. S., Kesika, P., & Chaiyasut, C. (2018). Impact of fermented foods on human cognitive function—A review of outcome of clinical trials. *Scientia Pharmaceutica, 86*(2), 22. https://doi.org/10.3390/scipharm86020022

Sruthi, N. U., Josna, K., Pandiselvam, R., Kothakota, A., Gavahian, M., & Khaneghah, A. M. (2022). Impacts of cold plasma treatment on physicochemical, functional, bioactive, textural, and sensory attributes of food: A comprehensive review. *Food Chemistry, 368*, Article 130809. https://doi.org/10.1016/j.foodchem.2021.130809

Tavares-Filho, E. R., Hidalgo, L. G. S., Lima, L. M., Spers, E. E., Pimentel, T. C., Esmerino, E. A., & Cruz, A. G. (2024). Impact of animal origin of milk, processing technology, type of product, and price on the Boursin cheese choice process: Insights of a discrete choice experiment and eye tracking. *Journal of Food Science, 89*(1), 640–655. https://doi.org/10.1111/1750-3841.16859. Available from: http://onlinelibrary.wiley.com/journal/10.1111/(ISSN)1750-3841.

Telukdarie, A., Munsamy, M., & Mohlala, P. (2020). Analysis of the impact of COVID-19 on the food and beverages manufacturing sector. *Sustainability, 12*(22), 9331. https://doi.org/10.3390/su12229331

Trzyniec, K., Skorupa, K., & Stachurska, M. (2022). Impact of pulse electric field on the level of photon emission in selected soft fruits. *Journal of Physics: Conference Series, 2408*(1), Article 012014. https://doi.org/10.1088/1742-6596/2408/1/012014

Udayakumar, S., Rasika, D. M. D., Priyashantha, H., & Vidanarachchi, J. K. (2022). Chaminda senaka ranadheera, probiotics and beneficial microorganisms in biopreservation of plant-based foods and beverages. *Applied Sciences, 12*(22), Article 11737. https://doi.org/10.3390/app122211737

Valero-Cases, E., Cerdá-Bernad, D., Pastor, J. J., & Frutos, M. J. (2020). Non-dairy fermented beverages as potential carriers to ensure probiotics, prebiotics, and bioactive compounds arrival to the gut and their health benefits. *Nutrients, 12*(6). https://doi.org/10.3390/nu12061666. Available from: https://www.mdpi.com/2072-6643/12/6/1666/pdf.

Vasquez-Rojas, W. V., Martín, D., Fornari, T., & Cano, M. P. (2023). Brazil nut (Bertholletia excelsa) beverage processed by high-pressure homogenization: Changes in main components and antioxidant capacity during cold storage. *Molecules, 28*(12). https://doi.org/10.3390/molecules28124675. Available from http://www.mdpi.com/journal/molecules.

Vilas-Boas, A. A., Magalhães, D., Campos, D. A., Porretta, S., Dellapina, G., Poli, G., Istanbullu, Y., Demir, S., San Martín, Á. M., García-Gómez, P., Mohammed, R. S., Ibrahim, F. M., El Habbasha, E. S., & Pintado, M. (2022). Innovative processing technologies to develop a new segment of functional citrus-based beverages: Current and future trends. *Foods, 11*(23). https://doi.org/10.3390/foods11233859. Available from: www.mdpi.com/journal/foods.

Vilela, A., Bacelar, E., Pinto, T., Anjos, R., Correia, E., Gonçalves, B., & Cosme, F. (2019). Beverage and food fragrance biotechnology, novel applications, sensory and sensor techniques: An overview. *Foods, 8*(12), 643. https://doi.org/10.3390/foods8120643

Walker, G. M., Lappe-Oliveras, P., Moreno-Terrazas, R. C., Kirchmayr, M., Arellano-Plaza, M., & Gschaedler-Mathis, A. C. (2019). *Yeasts associated with the production of distilled alcoholic beverages yeasts in the production of wine*. New York, United Kingdom: Springer. https://doi.org/10.1007/978-1-4939-9782-4_16

Wang, P. L., Xie, L. H., Joseph, E. A., Li, J. R., Su, X. O., & Zhou, H. C. (2019). Metal-organic frameworks for food safety. *Chemical Reviews, 119*(18), 10638–10690. Available from: http://pubs.acs.org/journal/chreay. doi: 10.1021/acs.chemrev.9b00257.

Wiesner, A., Gajewska, D., & Paśko, P. (2021). Levothyroxine interactions with food and dietary Supplements–A systematic review. *Pharmaceuticals, 14*(3), 206. https://doi.org/10.3390/ph14030206

Yadav, N., Nath, A., Singh, P. P., Bohidar, H. B., Callahan, D. L., Dujon, A. M., Afonso, L. O. B., & Schultz, A. G. (2024). Influence of humic acid and UV-irradiation on iron-based nanoparticle toxicity in Girardia tigrina. *Environmental Science: Nano, 12*(1), 325–339. https://doi.org/10.1039/d4en00449c

Yang, T., Paulose, T., Redan, B. W., Mabon, J. C., & Duncan, T. V. (2021). Food and beverage ingredients induce the formation of silver nanoparticles in products stored within nanotechnology-enabled packaging. *ACS Applied Materials and Interfaces, 13*(1), 1398–1412.

Yusuf, E. H., Wojdyło, A., & Nowicka, P. (2023). Possibility to use the different sizes and colors of carrots for the production of juices – Comparison of bioactive compounds, nutritional quality, pro-health properties, and sensory evaluation. *Journal of the Science of Food and Agriculture, 103*(2), 933–943. https://doi.org/10.1002/jsfa.12206. Available from: http://onlinelibrary.wiley.com/journal/10.1002/(ISSN)1097-0010.

Zachariah, V. K., Sunitha, V. C., Ramachandran, N., Vairappan, B., Parameswaran, S., & Priyamvada, P. S. (2024). Does lung ultrasound-guided ultrafiltration lead to better outcomes in acute kidney injury requiring intermittent hemodialysis: A randomized control trial. *Hemodialysis International, 28*(4), 435–443. https://doi.org/10.1111/hdi.13170. Available from: http://onlinelibrary.wiley.com/journal/10.1111/(ISSN)1542-4758.

Zhou, M., Rincón-Gallardo Patiño, S., Hedrick, V. E., & Kraak, V. I. (2020). An accountability evaluation for the responsible use of celebrity endorsement by the food and beverage industry to promote healthy food environments for young Americans: A narrative review to inform obesity prevention policy. *Obesity Reviews, 21*(12). https://doi.org/10.1111/obr.13094. Available from: http://onlinelibrary.wiley.com/journal/10.1111/(ISSN)1467-789X.

CHAPTER

Role of packaging in contaminant migration in beverages

9

Crisiana de Andrade Nobre[1, 2], Felipe Sousa da Silva[1], Tiago Rocha Nogueira[1], Fuad Pereira Nogueira Filho[1, 3], Luana Guabiraba Mendes[1, 4], Kelvi Wilson Evaristo Miranda[5], Andrêssa Maria Medeiros Theóphilo Galvão[6], Andréa Cardoso de Aquino[2], Gleyde Anny Cruz Barros[2], Maria Aparecida Liberato Milhome[4], Jesus Fernando Ayala-Zavala[7] and Luciana de Siqueira Oliveira[2]

[1]*Nucleus of Technology and Industrial Quality of Ceará (NUTEC), Fortaleza, Ceará, Brazil;* [2]*Postgraduate Program in Food Science and Technology (PPGCTA), Federal University of Ceará (UFC), Fortaleza, Ceará, Brazil;* [3]*Graduate Program in Development and Environment, Federal University of Ceará, Fortaleza, Ceará, Brazil;* [4]*Postgraduate Program in Food Technology (PPGTA), Federal Institute of Education, Science and Technology of Ceará (IFCE), Limoeiro do Norte, Ceará, Brazil;* [5]*Laboratory of Research and Innovation in Plant Products and Packaging, Federal University of Ceará (UFC), Fortaleza, Ceará, Brazil;* [6]*University of International Integration of Afro-Brazilian Lusophony (UNILAB), Institute of Rural Development (IDR), Food Engineering Course, Redenção, Ceará, Brazil;* [7]*Secretariat of Science, Humanities, Technology and Innovation, Center for Research in Food and Development (CIAD), Sonora, Mexico*

9.1 Introduction

Packaging plays a pivotal role in maintaining the safety, quality, and stability of beverages, functioning not only as a protective physical barrier but also as a crucial component in the preservation of chemical and sensory properties throughout the product's life cycle. Beyond its practical and esthetic attributes, packaging directly influences food safety by modulating the interaction between the beverage and external environmental factors, such as oxygen, moisture, and light, as well as by limiting the migration of potentially harmful substances from the packaging into the product (Ramos et al., 2016).

With growing scientific and regulatory concerns regarding the transfer of chemical compounds from packaging materials to beverages, the food industry has increasingly embraced the development of active, smart, and sustainable packaging technologies. These systems—such as oxygen scavengers, antimicrobial layers, and sensor-integrated packages—are designed not only to preserve product integrity but also to enhance consumer safety by actively interacting with the internal and external conditions of the product (Bledsoe & Rasco, 2018; Petrović, 2024).

Chemical migration from packaging remains one of the most critical safety challenges in beverage production. Compounds such as plasticizers (e.g., phthalates), antioxidants, and bisphenol A (BPA) are known to leach from certain materials, particularly plastics, and have been associated with adverse health effects, including endocrine disruption, chronic diseases, and reproductive toxicity

The Science and Safety of Beverages. https://doi.org/10.1016/B978-0-443-36536-2.00007-7

(Agarwal et al., 2025; Muncke, 2021). These risks are exacerbated in packaging derived from recycled materials, where chemical residues may accumulate or become more bioavailable, demanding stringent control and assessment measures (Geueke et al., 2018).

More recently, microplastics have emerged as a new class of contaminants in the food chain, including beverages. These particles, often originating from packaging degradation or wear, are not only capable of migrating into the product but can also act as vectors for other environmental contaminants, such as heavy metals and pesticides. Their presence in beverages–particularly in high-fat or acidic matrices-raises concerns about their bioavailability and potential impact on human health, including intestinal inflammation and oxidative stress (Miao et al., 2024).

To address these challenges, packaging innovation must be guided by integrated approaches that combine toxicological risk assessment, materials science, and compliance with evolving regulatory frameworks. Furthermore, life cycle assessments (LCAs) are essential to ensure that the transition to biodegradable, compostable, or reusable packaging alternatives does not compromise food safety in the pursuit of sustainability (Coles & Kirwan, 2011; Sazdovski et al., 2021).

This chapter explores the mechanisms by which contaminants migrate from packaging into beverages and the implications for food safety and public health. The discussion encompasses fundamental processes such as diffusion, permeation, sorption, desorption, and leaching of additives and byproducts. It also addresses the various types of contaminants, including chemical substances like bisphenol A (BPA), phthalates, heavy metals, PFAS, residual monomers, and antioxidants, as well as microbial agents, and examines how beverage composition, storage conditions, and the use of recycled or bio-based packaging materials influence migration dynamics. Analytical techniques used to detect and quantify contaminant migration will be reviewed alongside current toxicological assessments and international regulatory frameworks. Finally, the chapter highlights emerging trends and innovations in packaging technologies aimed at minimizing contaminant transfer and promoting safety and sustainability in the beverage industry.

9.2 Microplastics and nanoplastics in beverages

Plastic particles with diameters between 5 mm and 1 μm represent a fraction known as microplastics (MPs). Accordingly, several procedures are employed to select the particle size for analysis, as well as methodologies to reduce or eliminate matrices that may interfere with analytical results. However, the diversity of beverages and the complexity of their compounds pose significant challenges to both the development of analytical methods and the standardization of these procedures.

Beverages can be classified as alcoholic (fermented and distilled) or nonalcoholic (refreshing, stimulating, and nutritious) and are subjected to various processing and packaging technologies. These processes often involve the use of plastic materials, which can serve as a potential source of plastic particles. Several beverage types have already been studied with the aim of quantifying microplastics (Table 9.1), using digestion processes with hydrogen peroxide to oxidize organic matter. Heating may be applied to accelerate the decomposition of carbohydrates, proteins, lipids, fibers, and pigments, or to facilitate the removal of carbon dioxide. Finally, membrane filtration is performed. However, some beverages may not require the digestion step due to the low concentration of suspended solids.

Imaging-based analytical methods may require the removal of the matrix to facilitate the visualization of MP particles. In quantification studies conducted by Ramaremisa et al. (2025) on alcoholic

Table 9.1 Analytical methods for the quantification of microplastics.

Study	Beverage	MPs value (Particles per L)	MPs type	Flask type	Analysis: Sample Treatment	Analysis: Instrument
Hassan et al. (2025)	Carbonated drink	63–216	PET, PP, and HDPE	Plastic, glass, and aluminum bottles	1000 mL + H_2O_2 30% 3 days of digestion Filtration w/0.45 μm glass fiber	Estereomicroscope, FTIR, and SEM
Ramaremisa et al. (2025)	Nonalcoholic drinks	2.0–38	PP, PE, PU, PA, PET, and PBT	Plastic, glass, and aluminum bottles	Sample + $FeSO_4/H_2O_2$ add Rose Bengal (corant) Filtration w/0.7 μm glass fiber	Estereomicroscope and Micro-Raman
	Alcoholic drinks	4.0–29				
Ahmad et al. (2025)	Bottled water	4.36–77.55	PP, PE, PET, PVC, and PC	Plastic bottle	1000 mL of sample Filtration w/0.45 μm glass fiber	SEM and FTIR
	Carbonated soft drinks	2.63–56.25				
	Juice	3.6–76.6			1000 mL + H2O2 33% 3 days of digestion Filtration w/0.45 μm glass fiber	
Soca-Hernánd (2024)	Water	42.4	PET, PE, PES, PP, and PA	Plastic and glass bottles	Filtration w/0.45 μm stainless-steel mesh filter	Estereomicroscope and Micro-FTIR
	Beer	22.0–281.8				
	Wine	4.0–283.3				
	Soft drinks	1.0–57.6				
Prata et al. (2020)	Wine	2563–5857	–	Glass bottle	350–750 mL of sample, add Nile Red (corant) Filtration 0.7 μm glass fiber	Fluorescence microscopy and Micro-Raman
Wang and Wang (2024)	Soda	51–371	PVC	Plastic bottle	Filtration w/0.45 μm PTFE membrane	LDIR and FTIR
Chakraborty et al. (2024)	Milk	95–250	PA, PET, PS, PP, PE, and Nylon-6	Plastic bottle	200 mL heated at 60°C Filtration w/glass fiber	Microscope and FTIR
Shruti et al. (2020)	Soft drinks	ND-7	PA, PEA, and PET	Plastic and glass bottles	Filtration w/11 μm glass fiber	SEM, EDX, and Micro-Raman
	Cold tea	1–6				
	Energy drinks	ND-6				
	Beer	ND-28				

Particles—fiber, films, tangled messes and foams; ND—Not detected.
Source: Author (2025).

and nonalcoholic beverages packaged in aluminum, glass, or plastic bottles, Fenton's reagent ($FeSO_4$/H_2O_2) was used during the digestion stage to break down beverage constituents while preserving the microplastics. The samples were then filtered using glass fiber membranes and subsequently analyzed by stereomicroscopy and micro-Raman spectroscopy, identifying particles of PP, PE, PU, PA, PET, and PBT.

In fermented alcoholic beverages such as wine and beer, the determination of MPs may not require a digestion step. In such cases, filtration is performed using stainless steel sieves or glass fiber membranes. Microplastics can then be identified through micro-FTIR and micro-Raman spectroscopy, and their structures can be analyzed using stereomicroscopy, SEM-EDX, and fluorescence microscopy with Nile Red staining (GVR, 2024; Prata et al., 2020; Shruti et al., 2020; Socas-Hernández et al., 2024). For nonalcoholic beverages, although some studies apply digestion—even for similar sample types such as soft drinks—membrane filtration remains the predominant sample preparation method. This approach enables further analysis using FTIR, Raman, optical microscopy, SEM, and EDX techniques (Ahmad et al., 2025; Chakraborty et al., 2024; Hassan et al., 2025; Shruti et al., 2020).

While micro-FTIR and micro-Raman systems are most commonly used for the analysis of microplastics—due to their ability to process small samples and capture sequential images—the LDIR system has emerged as a promising alternative. Its application in the detection of MPs in soft drinks and mineral water has made it possible to identify up to 30 different types of plastics (Nizamali et al., 2023; Wang & Wang, 2024). In summary, current evidence confirms that micro- and nanoplastics are already present across a wide spectrum of beverages and that reliable quantification hinges on meticulous sample preparation and high-resolution analytical platforms. Yet, identifying these particles is only the first step toward safeguarding consumer health. To predict and ultimately mitigate their entry into the drink itself, we must understand the complex physicochemical forces that drive migration from packaging materials.

9.3 Factors influencing contaminant migration

Packaging materials (PMs) can interact with food, altering its quality and allowing the migration of harmful chemical compounds, which poses a risk to consumers' health (Wani et al., 2024). During production, food may contain micronutrients, flavorings, antimicrobials, pesticides, and mycotoxins. Materials such as plastic, paper, metal, and Styrofoam use compounds such as plasticizers, monomers, and oligomers, which can be transferred to food through the migration process (Alamri et al., 2021; Wani et al., 2024).

The factors that influence migration are temperature, storage time, contact surface/food volume ratio, type of material used, nature of the food, and chemical and physical properties of the FCMs. The total or global migration test analyzes the total mass transfer of an FCM to food, providing a qualitative assessment of the inertness of a packaging material. Migration analysis is performed to identify the risk to human health of a chemical compound ingested with food (Gupta et al., 2024; Geuekeet al., 2018).

The total migration test is a relevant analytical tool for assessing the safety of food contact materials (FCMs). The test determines the total transfer of substances (expressed as total mass) that migrate from the material to the food simulant under controlled conditions, which represent the actual use of the food/beverage. This total migration reflects the inertness of the material, that is, its ability not to release compounds at levels that could compromise food safety (Beneventi et al., 2020). The assessment of total migration does not identify specific compounds but provides a quantitative measure of the sum of all substances that can migrate, including both intentional additives and unintentionally added compounds (NIAs). The latter may include impurities, reaction byproducts, or contaminants formed during manufacturing, and their presence is especially concerning because they are often not properly characterized toxicologically (Geueke and Muncke, 2018).

The analysis of the total mass of chemical components faces methodological challenges due to the complexity of food matrices and the actual conditions of use of the materials. Foods present a wide variety of physical and chemical compositions—such as variations in pH, fat content, alcohol content, and the presence of water—that directly influence the rate and type of migration that may occur. According to Mercea et al. (2020), this variability makes it difficult to perform accurate and reproducible laboratory tests that faithfully simulate all possible situations of contact between food and packaging. To overcome these limitations, European and Brazilian health legislation establishes the use of standardized food simulants, which represent groups of foods with similar characteristics.

Another factor that contributes to migration is the size of the contact surface between the packaging and the food, which is an important factor since the larger this area, the higher the rate of migration of the components. In addition, the size of the packaging and the migratory movement within the material also play a role in the amount of migration that occurs, thus influencing the safety and quality of the packaged food (Gupta et al., 2024).

9.3.1 Beverage composition and its interaction with packaging

One of the factors that influence the migration of compounds is the characteristics of the food itself, such as lipid content, alcohol content, moisture level, and pH, which can have a significant impact on permeation, migration, and sorption (Fig. 9.1). Beverages with low pH, such as soft drinks and citrus

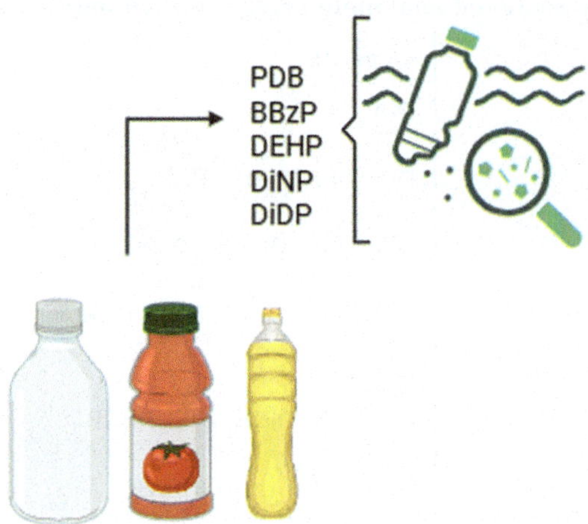

FIGURE 9.1

Illustrative image of phthalate migration in food, PDB (dibutyl phthalate), BBzP (butyl benzyl phthalate), DEHP (diethylhexyl phthalate), DiNP (di-isononyl phthalate) e DiDP (di-iso-decyl phthalate).

juices, are highly corrosive and can damage the internal coating of packaging and solubilize plastic components.

According to Calcaterra et al. (2024), foods with high fat or acidity content can promote the release of certain compounds, such as bisphenol A (BPA) and phthalates, substances associated with potential adverse health effects. In addition, the permeation of gases, moisture, and volatile compounds from the packaging can intensify oxidative reactions, in addition to causing loss of flavor and nutritional value, further compromising the quality of the food (Table 9.2) (Gupta et al., 2024).

Foods with high-fat content are more susceptible to the migration of lipophilic compounds present in packaging materials, such as plasticizers (e.g., phthalates) and stabilizers. This occurs due to the high chemical affinity between the lipid matrix of the food and hydrophobic substances present in the polymers used in plastic packaging, which favors their solubilization and diffusion (Fankhauser-Noti & Grob, 2006). Studies show that the migration of phthalates, such as di(2-ethylhexyl) phthalate (DEHP), is significantly higher in fatty foods, such as cheeses, processed meats, and vegetable oils, especially when stored for long periods or at high temperatures (Fierens et al., 2013).

The acidity of beverages is one of the main factors that influence packaging stability and contaminant migration. Beverages with low pH, such as soft drinks and citrus juices, have corrosive potential, especially when packaged in metal packaging with coating defects. This can lead to the release of metals such as aluminum and tin into the product, posing a toxicological risk to the consumer (Veríssimo & Gomes, 2008). In addition, high acidity can accelerate the degradation of polymers in plastic packaging, promoting the migration of additives such as phthalates and bisphenol A (BPA). Studies also indicate that migration is intensified in beverages with high bottling and storage temperatures, which increases the diffusion of compounds through the polymer matrix (Geueke et al., 2018; Santillana et al., 2011).

Table 9.2 Data from international food monitoring research indicate plasticizing compounds.

Sample	Phthalate	Study
Beverage	DBP	Kato et al. (2002) Yano et al. (2002)
Bottled water	DEP, DBP, DiBP, DEHP	Cao (2008) Montuori et al. (2008)
Human Milk	DEP, DBP, BBzp, DOP, DEHP	Högberg et al. (2008) Zhu et al. (2006)
Milk, raw Yogurt with fruit	DBP, BBzP, DEHP, DiNP, DiDP	Sørensen (2006)
Vegetable oils	DEHP	Fierens et al. (2013)
Wine	DEP, DBP, DEHP, DBP, DEHP	Carrillo et al. (2007) Yano et al. (2002)
Vodka, run, whiskey, gin, and brandy	DEHP, DEHA, DOP, BBzP	He et al. (2024)

BBzP, *Butyl benzyl phthalate;* DBP, *di-n-butyl phthalate;* DEP, *diethyl phthalate;* DiBP, *Di-iso-butyl phthalate;* DEHP, *Di-2-ethylhexyl phthalate;* DOP, *Di-n-octyl phthalate;* DiNP, *Di-iso-nonyl phthalate;* DiDP, *Di-iso-decyl phthalate;* DEHA, *bis(2-etilhexil)adipate.*

The alcohol content of beverages is a critical factor in the interaction with packaging materials, especially plastics. Ethanol acts as an organic solvent, promoting the extraction of additives present in the polymer matrix, such as phthalates, antioxidants, and thermal stabilizers (Cao, 2010).

Research shows that alcoholic beverages, such as wine, cachaça and liquors, can induce the migration of plasticizers and polyethylene terephthalate (PET) oligomers when stored for prolonged periods, especially under high-temperature conditions (Konieczna et al., 2015). Glass packaging continues to be the best option from a toxicological and chemical point of view, due to its high inertia and resistance to interaction with the content. However, accessories such as polyethylene stoppers or metal lids with internal coatings can represent secondary sources of contaminant migration, especially when there is prolonged contact with the alcoholic beverage (Bach et al., 2013).

The studies by He et al. (2024) investigated the presence of bisphenols, phthalates, and other plastic-derived compounds in several distilled products sold in Canada. The targeted analysis did not detect bisphenols in any of the samples evaluated ($n = 37$); however, the plasticizers DEHP and DEHA were detected. For the first time, the compound DPP was identified in vodka samples, while BBzP was detected in brandy, and DEHA was identified in several beverages, including vodka, rum, whiskey, whisky, gin, and cognac. Therefore, the type of packaging did not significantly influence the profile of chemical contaminants present in alcoholic beverages; however, the type of product and the particularities of the production process were shown to play a relevant role in the composition and variation of these contaminants.

Basaran et al., (2024) conducted a study evaluating microplastic contamination in water, natural mineral water, and spring water, carbonated soft drinks, iced tea, and some traditional beverages sold in Turkey. The research findings indicate that most of the beverages evaluated contained microplastics. The estimated daily and annual exposure to microplastics from beverage consumption for the general population over 15 years of age was 5.22 particles/mL/day and 1907 particles/mL/year. The physical and chemical characteristics of the microplastics present in the beverages examined indicate that the packaging material may be a significant source of microplastics.

9.3.2 Effect of storage conditions on contaminant migration

Storage conditions play a fundamental role in the rate at which contaminants migrate from packaging to food. Factors such as temperature, storage time, type of food, and exposure to light are determining factors in this process (Fig. 9.2). Studies show that increased temperature accelerates the molecular mobility of additives present in polymers, favoring the diffusion of compounds such as phthalates, bisphenol A (BPA), and aromatic amines (Muncke et al., 2020).

Storing food at temperatures above 30°C, a common situation during inadequate transportation, storage in places without adequate refrigeration, or direct exposure to solar radiation, represents a critical factor in intensifying the migration of contaminants from packaging to food. Increased temperature promotes greater molecular mobility of polymers, accelerating the diffusion and solubilization processes of chemical compounds present in packaging materials, such as plasticizers (phthalates), antioxidants, residual monomers, and other additives (Bach et al., 2013; Khokhar & Pawar, 2025).

In addition to temperature, prolonged contact time intensifies migration, since diffusion is a cumulative process. Another relevant factor is exposure to ultraviolet light, which can degrade the polymer structure, releasing degradation products that were not initially present in the material

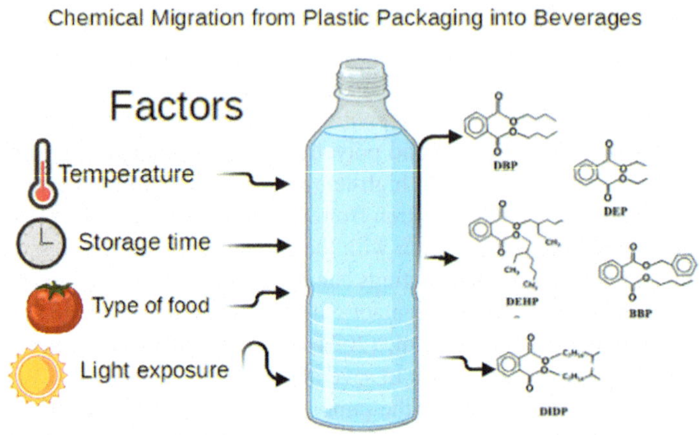

FIGURE 9.2

Chemical migration from plastic packaging into beverages.

(Pivnenko et al., 2016). Therefore, strict control of storage conditions—maintaining adequate temperature, avoiding exposure to light, and reducing storage time—is essential to minimize risks to public health resulting from contaminant migration.

During heating processes, the temperature to which plastic packaging is exposed can accelerate material degradation, leading to an increase in the release of nanoplastics into food (Hussain et al., 2023). Understanding these temperature limits is essential to assess potential risks and establish effective control measures during food storage and processing (Table 9.3).

For example, in the study conducted by Kida and Koszelnik (2021), it was observed that the chemical leaching of Polycyclic Aromatic Hydrocarbons (PAH) and Phthalic Acid Esters (PAE)

Table 9.3 Research on storage conditions in the migration of microplastics into beverages.

Study	Technique	Packaging material	Temperature (°C)	Exposure time	Microplastics
Kida and Koszelnik (2021)	GC–MS	PVC; PS; PP	20°C, 40°C, and 60	24 h	DMP; DEP; DBP; DEHP; PHE; FLU; PYE
Isci and Dagdemir (2024)	LC-MS/MS	PET	4°C, 25°C, and 40	90, 180, and 365 days	DEP; DEHP; DIDP; DNOP; DBP; DINP
Duric et al., (2024)	GC-MS		−18	3 and 6 months	DMP; DEP; DiBP; DBP; DEHP.
Allafi (2020)	ICP-MS	PET	−5°C, 25°C e 50°C	24 h	DEHP

BBP, *Benzyl butyl phthalate;* BB, *Benzyl Benzoate;* DMP, *Dimetil phthalate;* DEP, *Dietil phthalate;* DBP, *di-n-butyl phthalate;* DEHP, *Di-2-ethylhexyl phthalate;* DiDP, *Di-iso-decyl phthalate;* DNOP, *di-n-octyl phthalate;* DiNP, *Di-iso-nonyl phthalate;* DiBP, *diisobutyl phthalate;* HDPE, *high-density polyethylene;* LDPE, *low-density polyethylene;* PP, *polypropylene (PP);* PAPE, *polyamide polyethylene;* PET, *polyethylene terephthalate;* PVC, *polyvinyl chloride;* PS, *polystyrene;* PHE, *phenanthrene;* FLU, *fluoranthene;* PYE, *Pyrene.*

groups occurs more efficiently at higher temperatures, with this influence being more pronounced for the PAE group. For PAHs, increasing the temperature to 60°C did not bring about a significant difference in leaching. Furthermore, leaching of DEPs from PVC and PP at lower temperatures, such as 60°C, was not even detected.

The research analyzed the storage conditions that affect the migration of phthalate esters (PAEs) from polyethylene terephthalate (PET) bottles into various beverages sold in Turkey, including drinking water, mineral water, cola, carbonated drinks, and lemonade. A deterministic model was used to assess the health risks associated with this migration, with analyses performed by LC-MS/MS instruments. The analysis identified the presence of PAEs in various concentrations, with emphasis on diisodecyl phthalate (DIDP) and diisononyl phthalate (DINP), especially in mineral waters, which presented the highest levels of migration. In addition, temperature (4°C, 25°C, and 40°C) and storage time (365 days) influenced the release of substances (Isci & Dagdemir, 2024).

Studies by Duric (2024) show that the migration of phthalates from plastic packaging, storage time, and composition, especially their fat content, evaluated the influence of six different types of plastic packaging on the migration of phthalate residues in food stored at −18°C for three and 6 months. The results demonstrated that phthalates, such as diisobutyl phthalate (DIBP) and dibutyl phthalate (DBP), migrated in greater quantities to food packaged in polyamide polyethylene after 6 months. The highest concentrations of bis(2-ethylhexyl) phthalate (DEHP) were detected in polyamide polyethylene packaging (253.56 μg/kg), while the lowest was observed in polypropylene (157.72 μg/kg). In general, phthalate levels were significantly higher after three and 6 months of storage compared with control samples.

Allafi (2020) evaluated the effect of storage and temperature on the release of antimony in bottled water. Storage at 25°C showed no significant increase, but at 50°C, the levels rose to 16.8 ppb in 24 h. Although the levels are below the WHO limit (6 ppb) at 25°C, inadequate storage at high temperatures can exceed this limit. The study suggests the need to define safe temperatures for the storage of PET bottles. This scenario highlights the importance of continuous monitoring of phthalate levels in food, especially given the absence of specific regulations regarding maximum permitted limits (Coltro et al., 2021).

Taken together, the evidence reviewed in Sections 9.3, 9.3.1 and 9.3.2 demonstrates that contaminant migration is not an isolated packaging flaw but the result of a dynamic triad: (i) the intrinsic chemistry of the beverage (pH, ethanol, lipid fraction), (ii) the polymer architecture and additive load of the packaging, and (iii) the external storage environment, where time–temperature histories and light exposure amplify diffusion pathways. These variables act synergistically—acidic or alcoholic drinks accelerate polymer swelling, high-fat matrices solubilize lipophilic additives, and transient thermal spikes multiply diffusion coefficients—so that even low-level migrants such as phthalates, bisphenols, heavy metals, or micro/nanoplastics can surpass toxicological thresholds over shelf life. Quantifying that risk now hinges on analytical tools capable of capturing trace concentrations amid complex liquid matrices.

9.4 Analytical techniques for detecting contaminant migration

Monitoring the migration of contaminants from packaging into food and beverages has become an increasingly important requirement in the context of food safety, demanding the use of highly sensitive and selective analytical techniques. In this regard, it is essential to develop methods capable of identifying a wide range of chemical substances, even at low concentrations.

Over the past decades, there has been a significant shift from conventional methods—such as visual inspections and simple chemical reactions—to high-precision instrumental approaches, including gas and liquid chromatography, mass spectrometry, Raman spectroscopy, and coupled techniques (such as HPLC-MS/MS and UHPLC-MS/MS). These tools represent a substantial advancement in the detection and monitoring of migratory contaminants, playing a critical role in ensuring quality control throughout the food supply chain.

9.4.1 Chromatographic and spectroscopic methods

With the aim of enhancing food safety and complying with regulatory requirements, professionals in the field have increasingly adopted sophisticated methods for contaminant detection. Over the past decades, a significant shift has occurred from classical techniques—such as visual inspections and low-sensitivity chemical reactions—to more precise instrumental approaches, including spectrophotometry and chromatography (Ziani et al., 2025).

Within this context, traditional thin-layer chromatography has been progressively replaced by faster and more sensitive techniques such as gas chromatography (GC) and high-performance liquid chromatography (HPLC), which have become essential tools in the analysis of food contaminants. Technological advancements have further enabled the development of refined methods, including wide-line surface-enhanced Raman spectroscopy (WL-SERS), nuclear magnetic resonance (NMR) spectroscopy, inductively coupled plasma mass spectrometry (ICP-MS), and conventional mass spectrometry, all capable of detecting compounds at extremely low concentrations (Beecher, 2024).

More recently, the integration of liquid chromatography with mass spectrometry has evolved into high-performance configurations such as HPLC-MS/MS and UHPLC-MS/MS, which are distinguished by their ability to analyze complex molecular structures and detect contaminants at levels as low as nanograms per milliliter (ng/mL) (Pandey et al., 2023). In parallel, high-resolution chromatographic techniques, such as two-dimensional liquid chromatography (2D-LC) and multidimensional gas chromatography (MDGC), have expanded the depth of both qualitative and quantitative analyses, allowing for the discrimination of structurally similar compounds (Ziani et al., 2025).

Furthermore, Kokesch-Himmelreich et al. (2022) demonstrated the use of mass spectrometry imaging (MSI) to spatially map ion distribution in food matrices, achieving quantification at parts per million (ppm) levels and providing crucial metabolic information for assessing food safety.

9.4.2 Mass spectrometry and emerging analytical technologies

In recent years, numerous studies have highlighted the effectiveness of mass spectrometry as a key analytical tool for detecting contaminants associated with food and beverage packaging. This technique has been widely employed to identify compounds that migrate from packaging materials, such as bisphenol A (BPA), heavy metals, phthalates, plasticizers, perfluoroalkyl, and poly-fluoroalkyl substances, as well as residual compounds from the manufacturing process itself. It has also proven effective in identifying external contaminants that penetrate packaging barriers, including pesticides, microorganisms, and toxins.

Pereira et al. (2023) applied gas chromatography coupled with tandem mass spectrometry (GC-MS/MS) to quantify phthalates and di(2-ethylhexyl) adipate (DEHA) in beer samples. Six out of seven target compounds were detected, with concentrations ranging from 1.77 to 205.40 μg/L, and DEHA being the most prevalent. Conversely, Lestido Cardama et al. (2017) employed high-performance liquid chromatography with fluorescence detection (HPLC-FLD), confirmed by LC-MS/MS, and found no evidence of BPA migration in canned beverages such as beers and energy drinks.

Schaider et al. (2017) investigated beverages from fast-food restaurants in the United States using high-resolution liquid chromatography-mass spectrometry (LC-HRMS). They detected perfluoro-carboxylates, perfluoro-sulfonates, and polyfluorinated compounds in 5% of the samples, with total fluorine levels exceeding 200 nmol/cm^2. Sujana et al. (2024) assessed the migration of heavy metals from plastic bottles using inductively coupled plasma mass spectrometry (ICP-MS), identifying 28 ng/L of cadmium (Cd) and 636 ng/L of lead (Pb) in virgin PET, along with 469 ng/L of mercury (Hg) and 5042 ng/L of antimony (Sb) in recycled PET (R-PET).

Using the same technique, Shen et al. (2025) reported elevated levels of benzene and acetaldehyde in plastic beverage packaging during storage. Meanwhile, Arigò et al. (2021) applied HPLC-MS/MS to detect bioactive compounds such as furocoumarins, coumarins, and poly-methoxyflavones in citrus-based drinks, successfully quantifying 35 of the targeted analytes.

In addition to mass spectrometry, biosensors, and nanosensors have emerged as promising tools for the sensitive and selective detection of food and beverage contaminants. Ouyang et al. (2023) developed a cobalt-porphyrin-based fluorescence nanosensor for the detection of N-nitrosodimethylamine (NDMA), achieving recovery rates between 84.0% and 101.4%. Similarly, Verma et al. (2021) utilized green-synthesized silver nanoparticles (AgNPs) anchored to a reduced graphene oxide (RGO) composite to detect BPA in milk and water, reporting concentrations ranging from 1.9×10^{-10} to 0.820 μM.

Recent advances have integrated these analytical approaches with intelligent detection systems, incorporating machine learning algorithms. Tools such as convolutional neural networks (CNNs), support vector machines (SVMs), radial basis function neural networks (RBFNNs), and other ML models have been applied for ultrasensitive tracking, predictive modeling, and real-time contaminant detection at concentrations as low as parts per billion (ppb), as demonstrated by Liu et al. (2025) and Ziani et al. (2025) combined Raman spectroscopy with CNNs to analyze contaminants in PET and PE bottles, achieving 100% accuracy. Wang et al. (2022) further enhanced the analytical framework by integrating sensors with multiple ML algorithms to evaluate alcoholic beverages, resulting in notable improvements in detection accuracy and efficiency—facilitating informed decisions regarding packaging, transportation, and shelf life.

9.4.3 Methods for microplastic and nanoplastic detection

Beverage consumption has increased across various population groups worldwide (Hu et al., 2023). Consequently, plastic bottles and packaging—primarily composed of polyethylene terephthalate (PET) have become widely used due to their lightweight, durability, and cost-effectiveness (Wagner & Oehlmann, 2009). However, this widespread usage has raised growing concerns regarding the contamination of beverages with plastic microparticles (GVR, 2024; Lam et al., 2024; Zaki & Shoeib, 2018).

In view of this problem, it is important to investigate and detect the presence of plastic particles in packaged beverages. Nevertheless, the identification and quantification of micro- and nanoplastics (MNPs) represent significant analytical challenges due to their minute size, the broad range of plastic chemical compositions, and their potential interactions with components of the food matrix. To address these limitations, a variety of detection techniques are employed, which differ depending on particle size and sample complexity.

A fundamental step in understanding this issue is differentiating between microplastics (MPs) and nanoplastics (NPs). MPs are defined as plastic particles smaller than 5 mm, whereas NPs measure less than 1 μm. Both types of particles may result from environmental degradation processes—such as UV radiation, microbial activity, and mechanical fragmentation—as well as anthropogenic activities (Liu et al., 2020; Song et al., 2017; Utetiwabo et al., 2020).

To detect these contaminants, several analytical methods are commonly employed, including Raman spectroscopy, optical and scanning electron microscopy, Fourier-transform infrared spectroscopy (FTIR), and pyrolysis coupled with gas chromatography-mass spectrometry (Py-GC-MS). Each technique offers distinct advantages and limitations in terms of sensitivity, specificity, and suitability for various types of matrices (Table 9.4).

As revised, the analytical toolkit has evolved from classical chromatography to high-resolution, multihyphenated platforms, fluorescence nanosensors, and AI-assisted spectroscopy—each pushing detection limits from the ppm down to the sub-ppb and even single-particle scale. This technological leap converts what were once "background-level" migrants into quantifiable, regulatory-relevant targets, enabling real-time surveillance of everything from phthalate traces to nanoplastics. Yet generating ever finer data is only half the equation; translating those insights into preventive action at the design stage of beverage packaging is the next imperative.

9.5 Emerging trends and innovations in safe beverage packaging

The accelerated modernization of society is one of the main contemporary social phenomena that, linked to economic development, allows the emergence of environmental changes in the food sectors (production, storage, and distribution) (Buss & Henkes, 2014). Such changes aim to meet this new society's demands for safe and quality food (Nicoletti & Serrone, 2017). According to a report presented by "Grand View Research," the size of the global food and beverage market is estimated at approximately 564.0 billion dollars by 2030, with an annual growth rate of almost 14.0% between (GVR, 2024).

According to data from FAO—Food and Agriculture Organization of the United Nations—the amount of food lost and wasted could provide relief to one-eighth of the world's population in a state of nutritional vulnerability and achieve one of the global objectives of promoting increased demand and accessibility for healthy food (FAO, 2014; Ishangulyyev et al., 2019). Between 2000 and 2015, the eight Millennium Development Goals (MDGs) were created during the Sustainable Development Summit by the United Nations (UN), which are part of the so-called 2030 Agenda, which has as its central axis the so-called Sustainable Development Goals (SDGs) that seek to create a global model to, for example, end hunger—SDG-2—with a total of 17 SDGs and 169 targets stimulating feasible actions by 2030 in crucial areas of importance and impact to humanity and the planet (FAO-WFP, 2022) (Fig. 9.3).

Table 9.4 Characteristics of methods for detection of microplastics and nanoplastics.

Technique definition	Main application	Advantages	Limitations	Analysis method	References
Method:	**Fourier transform infrared spectroscopy (FTIR)**				
Nondestructive analytical technique that detects the absorption of mid-infrared radiation (2.5–25 μm) by polymers, allowing their chemical characterization with high specificity.	Identification and characterization of microplastics (MPs) in food matrices.	- High chemical specificity. - Nondestructive method. - Minimal sample preparation. - Absence of chemical reagents (environmentally friendly). - Ability to analyze a wide range of MP sizes.	- Interference of water molecules in spectral readings. - Limited resolution due to diffraction, making it difficult to detect very small particles. - Challenge in differentiating between synthetic and natural plastics.	- Transmission: Uses transparent filters (aluminum oxide or silicon oxide). - Reflection: Faster analysis, but sensitive to particle morphology. - Attenuated Total Reflection (ATR): Direct analysis of the sample with minimal contact.	Cunsolo et al. (2021) Xu et al. (2019) Ivleva et al. (2017) Sridhar et al. (2022) Lee and Chae (2021)
Method:	**Benchtop Raman spectrometers**				
Highly sophisticated instruments, designed exclusively for laboratory use, used Raman scattering for chemical characterization of micro and nanoplastics (MNPs).	Accurate identification of microplastics and nanoplastics (MNPs) at low concentrations in diverse matrices.	- High sensitivity and accuracy. - Capable of detecting MNPs at low concentrations. - Flexibility in the choice of analytical parameters (laser, power, integration time).	- Large size and complex operation (restricted to the laboratory environment). - High acquisition and maintenance costs. - Need for elaborate sample preparation.	- Raman spectroscopy based on light scattering, with the ability to adjust: - Laser wavelength. - Laser power. - Integration time, allowing optimization for different types and sizes of particles.	Pilot (2018) Liu, Ahmed, et al. (2021) Caldwell et al. (2022) Schmitt and Popp (2006) Jarvis and Goodacre (2004)
Method:	**Raman Spectroscopy**				
Technique based on inelastic light scattering (Raman Scattering), which generates characteristic spectra of polymeric materials, allowing their	Identification of micro and nanoplastics (MNPs) in food and environmental matrices, with high precision and resolution.	- Detection of particles up to 1 μm. - Less water interference compared with FTIR. - Nondestructive method.	- May require specific sample preparation protocols. - Spectral interference in complex matrices (e.g., food). - Problems with	- Based on inelastic light scattering. - Generation of unique spectral fingerprints for each polymer. - It is possible to optimize parameters	Chakraborty et al. (2023)

Continued

Table 9.4 Characteristics of methods for detection of microplastics and nanoplastics.—cont'd

Technique definition	Main application	Advantages	Limitations	Analysis method	References
identification with high specificity.		- Minimal sample preparation. - Sustainable and efficient techniques for analysis of MPs and NPs.	fluorescence generated by organic residues or microorganisms present in the particles.	(such as laser and integration time) to improve resolution and reduce interference.	
Method:	**Portable Raman Spectrometers**				
Compact and lightweight devices that use Raman spectroscopy for field analysis, allowing real-time detection of micro and nanoplastics (MNPs) without the need to transport samples to the laboratory.	Rapid and real-time monitoring of MNPs in diverse environments, including food matrices, water, and soil.	- Direct analysis in the field, without transporting samples. - Fast analytical response. - Operation possible by nonspecialists. - Relatively lower cost than benchtop models.	- Lower sensitivity and spectral resolution compared with benchtop models. - Difficulty in detecting low concentrations of MNPs. - Susceptible to environmental interference (light, temperature).	Raman spectroscopy is applied directly on site. - Fast detection with fewer parameter customization options. - Prioritizing portability and speed over analytical resolution.	Guo et al. (2021) Liu, Ahmed, et al. (2021), (2022) Pilot (2018)
Method:	**Fluorescence Spectroscopy**				
Method based on fluorescent staining of microplastics (MPs) using specific dyes that bind to the surfaces of the polymers, allowing their visualization and identification by fluorescence emission under appropriate light.	Rapid and economical detection of microplastics, mainly in preliminary analyses of environmental and food matrices.	- Fast and low-cost method. - Strong fluorescence emission. - Possibility of rapid visual analysis. - Nile Red allows a broad classification of polymers due to its solvate-chromic properties.	- Dyes are physically adsorbed to the surface of plastics and can easily desorb. - Ineffective for polymers with low hydrophobicity, such as PVC, polycarbonate, and PET. - Does not provide detailed chemical characterization.	- Staining of MPs with fluorescent dyes. - Visualization under UV or blue light. - Manual analysis or image processing software for quantification.	Maes et al. (2017) Lv et al. (2019) Karakolis et al. (2019) Prata et al. (2020) Shim et al. (2016) Gagné et al. (2019) Erni-Cassola et al. (2017)

Method:	**Laser-Induced Fluorescence (LIF) Spectroscopy**				
Technique that uses the intrinsic fluorescence of polymers, induced by laser excitation, for the detection and analysis of microplastics (MPs).	In situ and real-time detection of microplastics without the need for extensive sample preparation or external dyes.	- Less dependence on expensive spectrometers. - Potential for field and real-time monitoring. - Fast and low-cost method. - The operation is more straightforward compared with other spectroscopic techniques.	- There is a spectrum overlap between different polymers, making accurate identification difficult. - Lower capacity for detailed chemical differentiation between types of plastics.	- Excitation of MPs by laser, generating intrinsic fluorescence. - Detection and analysis of emitted spectra. - Rapid assessment of the presence of MPs, with limitations in the exact identification of polymer types due to spectral overlap.	Asamoah et al. (2021)
Method:	**Matrix-assisted laser desorption ionization time-of-flight mass spectroscopy (MALDI-TOF-MS)**				
Mass spectrometry technique that uses a laser to ionize and desorb analytes, generating ions that are separated based on the mass/charge (m/z) ratio by time of flight. Adapted for microplastic analysis due to its high sensitivity and speed.	Identification and chemical characterization of microplastics, including composition analysis through oligomers generated from polymer fragmentation.	- Fast and relatively low-cost technique. - Capable of generating mass spectra with periodic patterns ("barcodes") that facilitate the identification of polymers. - Operational simplicity without the need for chromatographic separation in most cases.	- Matrix interferences may compromise the analysis. - Limitations for in situ application due to the need for matrix preparation and possible interferences. - Lower efficacy in the absence of preconcentration or separation of components.	- Matrix-assisted laser ionization. - Time-of-flight (TOF) analysis of ions generated based on mass-to-charge ratio. - Interpretation of spectral patterns for identification of polymers and their oligomers. - Suitable for detailed structural characterization.	Wu et al. (2020) Luo et al. (2020) Zhang et al. (2024)
Method:	**Microscopic Methods**				
Set of methods based on microscopy techniques for visualization, morphological characterization, and, in some cases, compositional analysis of microplastics. Includes optical microscopy, scanning electron microscopy	- Optical microscopy: Initial screening and morphological analysis of particles. - SEM: Analysis of morphology, surface texture, and elemental composition (coupled with EDS). - AFM: Analysis of	- Optical microscopy: Simple, accessible, and fast. - SEM: High resolution, three-dimensional analysis of morphology and texture; EDS allows elemental analysis. - AFM: Very high	- Optical: Risk of false identification due to visual similarity with other materials (organic/inorganic); low resolution for microscopic particles. - SEM: Need for coating with conductive material (e.g., gold),	- Direct observation of morphology and size. - SEM-EDS allows evaluation of elemental composition. - AFM allows evaluation of properties such as roughness, hydrophobicity, rigidity, and	Gniadek and Dąbrowska (2019) Enyoh et al. (2019) Nolasco Banegas et al. (2023) Huang et al. (2023) Chen et al., (2020)

Continued

Table 9.4 Characteristics of methods for detection of microplastics and nanoplastics.—cont'd

Technique definition	Main application	Advantages	Limitations	Analysis method	References
(SEM), transmission electron microscopy (TEM), and atomic force microscopy (AFM).	physicochemical properties of surfaces (hydrophobicity, rigidity, conductivity, etc.) and high-resolution 3D images, especially useful for nonconductive materials.	resolution, 3D images, no need for metalization, detailed analysis of physical-chemical properties of surfaces.	increasing preparation time. - AFM: Possibility of contamination, generation of artifacts, detachment of fragments during analysis.	conductivity, in addition to three-dimensional topographic images. - Integration with spectroscopy (Raman, FTIR) increases identification reliability.	
Method:	**Chromatographic Method**				
A technique that combines pyrolysis (Py) — controlled thermal decomposition — with gas chromatography (GC) and mass spectrometry (MS). It allows the separation and identification of compounds resulting from the thermal degradation of polymers, offering a detailed analysis of the chemical composition of microplastics.	- Accurate quantification of the chemical composition of microplastics, especially in low-fat food matrices ($<3\%$). - Identification of different types of polymers present in the samples. - Robust technique for quantitative assessment of MPs.	- High chemical sensitivity and specificity. - Provides detailed quantitative analysis of polymers. - The robust technique is considered the gold standard for chemical characterization of MPs. - Effective for complex matrices, such as food.	- Destructive method, with no possibility of recovering the particles. - It does not provide physical information (color, shape, size) on the MPs. - Lower sensitivity for polar polymers. - Time-consuming analysis. - Small sample quantities and manual transfer of the particles to the pyrolysis crucible are needed. - High-cost equipment and specialized operation.	- Pyrolysis: Thermal decomposition of MPs. - GC: Separation of the volatile compounds formed. - MS: Identification based on the mass/charge ratio (m/z) of the fragments. - Analysis of chromatographic peaks and mass spectra to identify the polymers present.	Tian et al. (2023) Rauert et al. (2022) Ribeiro et al. (2020) Vitali et al. (2022)

Source: Author (2025).

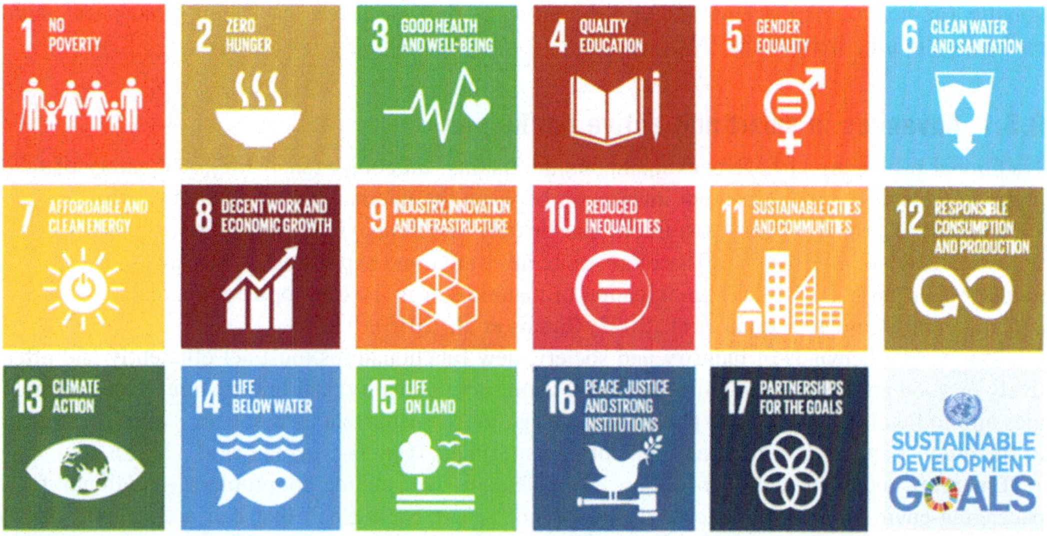
1 NO POVERTY
2 ZERO HUNGER
3 GOOD HEALTH AND WELL-BEING
4 QUALITY EDUCATION
5 GENDER EQUALITY
6 CLEAN WATER AND SANITATION
7 AFFORDABLE AND CLEAN ENERGY
8 DECENT WORK AND ECONOMIC GROWTH
9 INDUSTRY, INNOVATION AND INFRASTRUCTURE
10 REDUCED INEQUALITIES
11 SUSTAINABLE CITIES AND COMMUNITIES
12 RESPONSIBLE CONSUMPTION AND PRODUCTION
13 CLIMATE ACTION
14 LIFE BELOW WATER
15 LIFE ON LAND
16 PEACE, JUSTICE AND STRONG INSTITUTIONS
17 PARTNERSHIPS FOR THE GOALS
SUSTAINABLE DEVELOPMENT GOALS

FIGURE 9.3

Outline of the SDGs—sustainable development goals—by the united Nations.

Source: U. N. Transforming our world: The 2030 agenda for sustainable development department of economic and social affairs. Available at: https://sdgs.un.org/2030agenda. Accessed at 29 april, 2025

Packaging plays an intrinsic role in the safety, shelf life, and maintenance of the sensory quality of food and beverages (fresh, refrigerated, and/or frozen). They act as barrier agents and are considered excellent alternatives to prevent or reduce the susceptibility of food to different degradation reactions. In addition, they can promote a high barrier to interaction between the internal environment (food) and the external environment (environment) (KuswandI, 2020), ensuring a longer shelf life and maintaining the product's natural characteristics (Wikström et al., 2019).

The search for emerging technological innovations for packaging is studied to promote intentional food-packaging-environment interactions. The industrial sector has been presenting itself as a great ally and motivator for strengthening these actions, using arguments from the so-called "sustainable industrial ecology" (Haghighi et al., 2019; Zore et al., 2018). Thus, through new eco-friendly materials, emerging technologies called smart packaging emerge, which can present direct action (active packaging) and indirect action (smart and interactive packaging), demonstrating a promising future in the industrial sector.

Packaging involves fundamental steps to ensure the preservation of beverages throughout the postproduction chain process, involving storage, transportation, distribution, sale, and consumption (García-Guzmán et al., 2022). In 2020, the juice industry recorded a significant reduction of 23.0% in global sales (Neves et al., 2020). This may be related to the relevance of the data on the packaging and affect consumers' sensory expectations and acceptance of the new product. In addition, the relationship between scientific research and practical application of beverage packaging has sought new technologies to meet different forms of interaction between packaging and beverage, that is, by diffusion of volatile (or nonvolatile) agents and/or desorption at the interfaces: packaging-headspace and/or packaging-liquid (Arabi et al., 2012).

9.5.1 Advances in smart and active packaging

Traditional packaging of beverages maintains the quality, durability (shelf-life), and safety of food, promoting barrier action to prevent interaction between the internal and external environment (Kuswandi et al., 2020). However, most traditional flexible and nonflexible packaging is limited to functionalities and barrier properties. Therefore, more innovative and expanding studies are needed for new trends, either through structural modification of materials or in the development of emerging systems and strategies (García-Guzmán et al., 2022; Ramos et al., 2015).

To meet the demands of industry and society, new functionalities must act efficiently and effectively on food and beverages, promoting protection, safety, quality, and information. Such technologies aim to functionally improve packaging through mechanisms that enhance the sensory properties of the product and/or provide health benefits to consumers (García-Guzmán et al., 2022).

Emerging technological innovations for packaging are studied to promote intentional food-packaging-environment interactions, the so-called "smart packaging" that can act directly (active packaging) or indirectly (smart and interactive packaging) (Fig. 9.4).

Fig. 9.4 illustrates the action of emerging packaging. Active packaging releases or absorbs substances to extend shelf life through antioxidant, antimicrobial, ethylene, or moisture absorption actions. Smart and interactive packaging has sensors or indicators that change color in response to changes in pH, temperature, humidity, gases, or contamination, in addition to providing information on the origin, traceability, and condition of the product. These technologies are trends that add value, safety, and reliability (Martins et al. 2022; Boonsiriwit et al., 2021; Veeraiyan et al., 2022). These packages emerge as promising trends, whose technologies can add value, reliability, and safety, and can be used with different technologies, as shown in Table 9.5.

Table 9.5 shows different types of indicators, sensors, and biosensors that provide qualitative or semiqualitative information through visual changes, such as color variation or some type of detectable change in the packaging. Smart packaging aims to act as a surveillance element over the packaged or bottled product. It also monitors the external factors surrounding the product, such as storage and transportation within the supply chain. Therefore, ensuring traceability, automation, and protection against counterfeiting, storing and transmitting essential information (Abekoon et al., 2024).

Veeraiyan et al. (2022) observed the growing existence of smart devices that are integrated into food packaging to promote direct communication with the consumer and act synchronously with the indicators and materials used in the packaging. In addition, the authors corroborate the importance of packaging as one of the determining agents of the quality and freshness of finished food products.

Yekta et al. (2023) highlight that dynamic systems drive both research and the creation of smart packaging for the market, although there are still few products commercialized or with production ended. To be effective, these systems must avoid false negatives, have few false positives, and be tested under different conditions. Thus, they allow the consumer to know whether the food is suitable for consumption without opening the packaging. In addition, there is a growing search for natural raw materials from agro-industrial waste, reinforcing the sustainable appeal.

Among the bioactives used in packaging, anthocyanin stands out, known for its ability to change color depending on pH. In an acidic medium ($pH < 3$), it presents red, purple, or orange hues due to

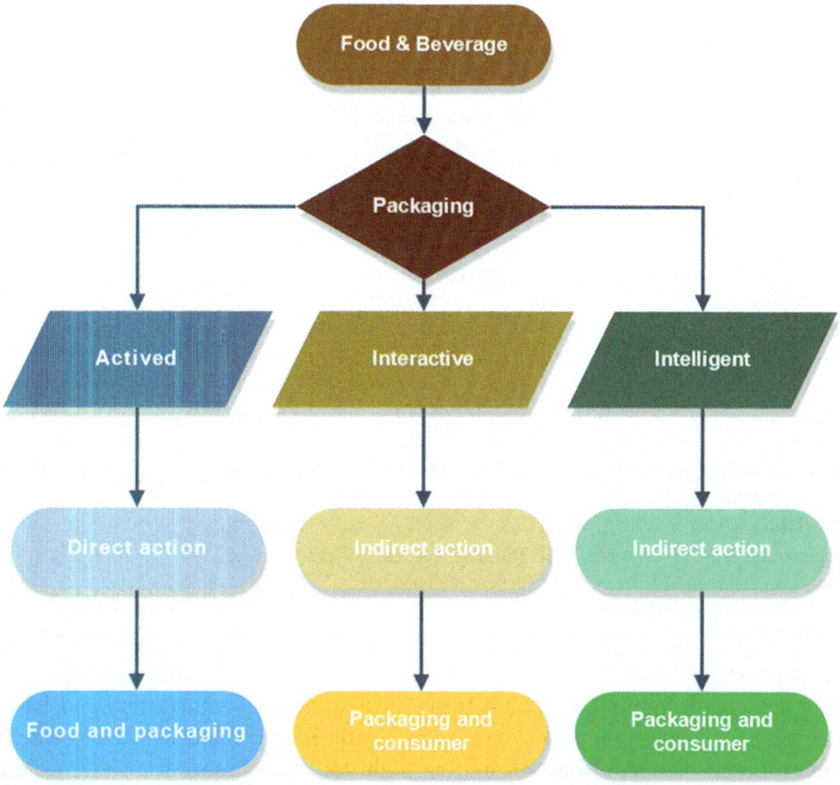

FIGURE 9.4

Types of packaging and their interactions, whether with food and/or consumer.

the formation of flavylium cations. As the pH increases (7–9), the color changes to green, and at pH 11, to yellow, because of the deprotonation of molecules and oxidation of polyphenols (Table 9.6) (Li et al., 2024; Liu et al., 2020; Roy & Rhim, 2021).

Interactive packaging is considered an extremely new and versatile technology (Khair et al., 2022; Li et al., 2024; Rotsios et al., 2022; Zuo et al., 2022). Furthermore, it is considered an inevitable trend in the food technology innovation sector when associated with coding technology (Yang et al., 2021). However, many challenges hinder the potential use of this packaging: consumer engagement, high technical cost, high marginal cost, information overload, and technical barriers (Li et al., 2024).

Packaging can influence consumer perception of food, especially in the purchasing decision, and is considered an industrial business with global demand (Ahmed et al., 2022). Table 9.7 presents studies on active packaging in different polymeric and biopolymeric matrices with bioactive compounds.

Table 9.7 presents different active packaging systems, which have a wide range of applications and innovations, due to the use of bioactive compounds extracted from alternative sources, the so-called agro-industrial waste. The use of this waste minimizes environmental problems, adding value to compounds that would otherwise be discarded, producing a sustainable product.

Table 9.5 Intelligent packaging examples.

Technology/Active	Action	References
Polymeric nanofibers	Time-temperature indicator	Forghani et al. (2021)
Anthocyanins	Freshness indicator	Becerril et al. (2021)
Calcium hydroxide/bromothymol blue	Ripeness indicator	Lee et al. (2023)
Methylcellulose/polyethylene glycol-400/bromothymol blue	Integrity gas indicator (CO_2)	Noiwan et al. (2022)
Cellulose/glycerol/polyethylene glycol nanocrystals-10kDa	Moisture indicator	Babaei-Ghazvini and Acharya (2021)
Poly(ε-caprolactone)/bromothymol blue nanofibers	Halochromic sensor—volatile acidity	Miranda et al. (2020)
Hydroxypropyl methyl cellulose/ microcrystalline cellulose/anthocyanin	Halochromic sensor—Selective colorimetric detection of hydrogen sulfate (HSO_{4-})	Boonsiriwit et al. (2021)
Chitosan hydrogel (80% deacetylated)/ acetic acid/hexamethylene 1,6-diisocyanate (HMDI)	Sensor—biosensor for pH variation (meat and chicken)	El-Mekawy et al. (2021)
Thin and nanostructured film of noble metals (gold—Au, silver—Ag, platinum—Pt, or palladium—Pd)	Biogenic biosensor—detection of genes, bacteria, etc.	Balbinot et al. (2021)

Packaging made with biopolymers tends to be biodegradable. Sethulakshmi and Saravanakumar (2024) formulated films based on potato starch and gelatin incorporated with green tea. The authors demonstrated, through biodegradability tests, the high decomposition rate of the packaging in the period of 5–20 days. In addition to this ability to be biodegradable, biopolymer-based packaging, to be compatible with commercial polymer packaging, must present tear and tensile strength, lower water vapor permeability, low solubility, control over quality and safety during storage and transportation of products, and increased shelf life of food (Abedi-Firoozjah et al., 2023).

Table 9.6 Interactive packaging examples.

Technology/Active	Action	References
RFID—Radio-Frequency Identification	Active and passive tags	Khair et al. (2022) Zuo et al. (2022)
Thermoresponsive hydrogel of poly (N-isopropyl acrylamide) (PNIPAM)	Printing (gravure and screen printing)	Choe et al. (2018) Hu et al. (2019)
QR code—traceability	QR code—product and producer information	Li et al. (2024) Rotsios et al. (2022)
PEGS—electrical gas sensors (paper)/ 90% conductive carbon/10% diluent	Wireless gas sensor—NFC—Near Field Communication	Naik et al. (2024)

Table 9.7 Active packaging studies in polymeric matrix difference.

(Bio)Polymer	Active	Properties	References
ε-Polylysine	–	Antimicrobials	Yang et al. (2024)
Polyvinyl alcohol	Carbon and clay	Antioxidants and antibacterials	Mao et al. (2025)
Polyvinyl alcohol	Itaconic acid and chitosan	Antimicrobials	Szabo et al. (2020)
Polyvinyl alcohol	Graphene quantum	Antimicrobials	Sun et al. (2024)
Polylactic acid and polycaprolactone	Oregano essential oil and β-cyclodextrin	Antibacterial and antifungal	Shi et al. (2022)
Polylactic acid	Graphene oxide and zinc oxide nanocomposites	Antimicrobials	Liew et al. (2023)
Polylactic acid	Clove essential oil and cochineal	Antimicrobials	Mohammadi, Fasihi, 2025
Plasticized polylactic acid	Tea polyphenols	Antioxidants and antibacterials	Ren et al. (2021)
Banana starch	Orange oil and curcumin	Antioxidants and antimicrobials	Sanchez et al. (2022)
Carboxymethylcellulose	Lavender-cotton, mastic and eucalyptus-globe essential oils	Antimicrobials	Simsek et al. (2020)
Chitosan	Pomegranate peel extract	Antioxidants and antimicrobials	Kumar et al. (2021)
Gelatine	Bioactive casein phosphopeptides	Antioxidants and antimicrobials	Khedri et al. (2021)
Corn starch and chitosan	Turmeric	Antimicrobials	Schaefer et al. (2020)
Potato starch and gelatine	Green tea	Antioxidants	Sethulakshmi and Saravanakum (2024)
Chitosan	Orange peel extract	Antioxidants and antimicrobials	Merino et al. (2023)
Methylcellulose	Jambolão skins extract	Antioxidants	da Silva Filipini, Romani and Guimarães Martins (2020)
Chitosan and gelatin	Butterfly pea flower anthocyanin extract	Antioxidants	Li et al. (2024)

The polymers listed in Table 9.7 as poly(vinyl alcohol) (PVOH), poly(lactide) (PLA), and poly (ε-caprolactone) (PCL) are commercially used in food packaging because they have good oxygen barrier, water solubility, mechanical strength, chemical stability, and transparency. However, packaging made only with these polymers is not considered active because it does not have active functional properties, such as antioxidants and/or antimicrobials. Therefore, for these packages to be considered active, they must incorporate compounds that present antimicrobial properties, such as carbon (Mao et al., 2025), chitosan (Szabo et al., 2020), graphene (Sun et al., 2024), zinc oxide (Liew et al., 2023), oregano essential oil (Shi et al., 2022), clove essential oil (Mihammadi et al., 2025), and tea polyphenols (Ren et al., 2022). In these studies, the antimicrobial property was confirmed by the inhibition of *Escherichia coli, Staphylococcus aureus, Pseudomonas aeruginosa, Bacillus cereus, Saccharomyces cerevisiae, Listeria monocytogenes.*

Biopolymer-based packaging mentioned in Table 9.6 may have antioxidant and antimicrobial properties because it contains bioactives in its composition, such as chitosan. In addition, it is possible to add bioactivity to biopolymer matrices by incorporating essential oils (Sanchez et al., 2022; Simsek et al., 2020) and plant extracts (Kumar et al., 2021; Merino et al., 2023; Filipini et al., 2020).

Studies in the food area seek to develop active packaging for beverages. In the studies by Naderi Bab Anari et al. (2022), active packaging for yogurt was developed based on UV-modified low-density polyethylene (LDPE) incorporated with natamycin. In the results, the authors observed that yogurts with this packaging presented antimicrobial properties capable of controlling the growth of *Rhodotorula mucilaginosa* and *Candida parapsilosis*. In addition, they extended their shelf life by up to 23 days.

Polylactic acid (PLA) packaging with nitrilotriacetic acid (NTA) has the potential to package dairy, protein, sports drinks, juices, coconut water, and smoothies, which are sensitive to oxidative degradation due to the presence of vitamins and natural colors. NTA acts as an antioxidant, scavenging free radicals through electron transfer, which improves product stability (Kay et al., 2022). Beverages such as juices can change flavor and aroma during storage due to exposure to oxygen, light, and heat, and the use of inert atmospheres (N_2 or CO_2) helps to preserve their nutritional and sensory characteristics (Kopuncová et al., 2018, 2022); Tobolová et al. (GVR, 2024). These changes may be related to packaging that allows exposure to oxygen, light, and high temperatures. One alternative to minimize these changes is the use of an atmosphere with inert gas (N_2 or CO_2), which can improve the nutritional and aromatic quality of juices (Kopuncová et al., 2018, 2022; Tobolová et al. (GVR, 2024).

The use of inert gases can increase product costs and not contribute to sustainability and the circular economy. In view of this, new packaging options for beverages are being explored. Chakraborty et al. (2023) and Shaik & Chakraborty (2023) studied the use of packaging produced with coextruded ethylene vinyl alcohol copolymer (EVOH) and multilayer polyethylene terephthalate (ML-PET) films for lemon juice. The authors observed that the juices stored in ML-PET packaging showed better nutrient retention, maintaining the sensory and vitamin C profile after 37 days of storage, and, consequently, a longer shelf life than in the EVOH bag.

9.5.2 Development of sustainable and biodegradable packaging solutions

Urbanization associated with the accelerated modernization of society is one of the main contemporary social phenomena that, linked to economic development, has allowed the emergence of environmental changes with the modernization of the food industry (Spadotto & Ribeiro, 2006; Buss & Henkes, 2014). Such changes aim to meet the needs of the new society that is consumerist, mainly regarding fast food, safe food, and excellent quality. In addition, the market's exposure to globalized competitiveness has motivated the food industry to develop efficient and effective actions, becoming synonymous with survival or permanence in business, relating exclusively to the production system of safe food, for example, the food packaging sector (Wissmann et al., 2013).

In many situations, packaging goes unnoticed by consumers during the process of society's evolution, given that the main objective in the act of "purchasing" is directed at the internal content and not the wrapping (Mourad & Tavares, 2020). However, such wrapping plays an intrinsically important role in food safety, shelf life, maintenance of sensory qualities, and in natura characteristics when related to fresh, refrigerated, and/or frozen food. However, postconsumer packaging management is deficient and insufficient, requiring actions that aim to balance production and reuse (Mourad & Tavares, 2020).

Packaging must feature materials that guarantee food quality and safety without generating an impact on the environment (Yin et al., 2023). This concern for the environment boosts research on the development of packaging, such as biodegradable films, based on alternative materials of renewable origin (proteins, polysaccharides, and lipids) (Bhatia et al., 2022; García-Guzmán et al., 2022; Kasaai, 2022; Xiaojia Liu, Guo, et al., 2021). For packaging materials, in addition to the vision related to sustainable development and sustainability, a term that has been presented to society is the so-called "circular economy" (cradle-to-cradle), relating to "zero" waste, transforming waste into valuable resources (Zore et al., 2018). However, applying and evaluating the performance of this circularity has shown great economic, political, and social difficulties, generating complex and decentralized actions regarding the use of indicators to monitor products throughout their life cycle and the value chain (Geissdoerfer et al., 2017).

Over the years, nonbiodegradable polymers have been the greatest precursors of environmental impact due to the high amount of solid waste accumulated in landfills and dumps. This level of impact promotes the generation of crises not only in the environment but also in the economic and social spheres (Landim et al., 2016). Packaging made of plastic for beverages can produce a large volume of plastic waste annually (Ye et al., 2022); according to Kwon et al. (2023), it increased the plastic market share by approximately 4.7% compared to 2019. If the current trend of plastic waste production continues without changes in its management, it is estimated that by 2050, global plastic production should reach between 902 million metric tons (Mt) and 1124 Mt, which could become plastic waste and be introduced into global aquatic ecosystems (Dokl et al., 2024). Analyzing this global issue, one solution that can reduce this waste production is the development of biodegradable plastics produced from renewable biomass waste (Shen et al., 2020).

The trend toward sustainability has generated a focus on beverage packaging produced with postconsumer recycled polyethylene terephthalate (PET-PCR) (Bharadwaj et al., 2024; Marcelino et al., 2025). Legislation is applied to minimize the accumulation of waste and make the packaging production flow more sustainable.

In Brazil, these packages must follow Collegiate Board Resolution (RDC) No. 20, which determines the Technical Regulation on food-grade postconsumer recycled polyethylene terephthalate (PET) packaging (food-grade PET-PCR) intended to come into contact with food (Brasil, 2008). In Europe, by 2030, Pepsico has assured that it will use 50.0% recycled plastic in its bottles. By 2025, the Coca-Cola company has committed to collecting packaging and using 50.0% recycled plastic in PET bottles sold in Western Europe (Mordor, 2025b).

The United Kingdom applies a plastic tax as an alternative to achieving the goal of net zero plastic waste emissions into the environment by 2050 (Walker et al., 2020). Other countries, such as China, Morocco, India, and Kenya, have banned the use of single-use plastic and thin plastic bags (Knoblauch & Mederake, 2021). These government laws are challenges for the packaging industries; other adversities faced by these industries are the shortage of raw materials and the increase in the costs of these raw materials (Esaki et al., 2024). This increase in the cost of packaging raw materials may be related to the war in Ukraine, which generated instability in energy markets and increased the prices of petroleum-based products (Dure, 2022). An example of a shortage in the market is low-carbon aluminum packaging for beverages, as the demand for this raw material has increased to comply with sustainability legislation (Moreira et al., 2023). However, the search for environmentally friendly materials requires practical changes, assessment of quality, material cost, and the impact of this material's waste on the environment (Mudgal et al., 2024).

The search for new environmentally friendly materials has shown a promising future in the industrial sector, which has been presenting itself as a great ally and motivator for the strengthening of these actions, using arguments from the so-called "sustainable industrial ecology" (Haghighi et al., 2019; Zore et al., 2018). Given the major environmental impacts of nonbiodegradable materials from destructive extractive processes, through petrochemical sources and the imminent shortage of oil and the high price (in relation to the process and product), research centers have been motivated to search for alternative materials (Table 9.8).

According to the World Economic Forum (WEF), in 2019, environmental impacts were classified as "investment risks" for companies, which must include so-called "environmental sustainability" in their business plans and not just profit maximization (stalkehouder capitalism) (ABIPLAST (2019)). Estimates point to a possible doubling in the production of plastic packaging by 2040, highlighting the urgent need to seek sustainable options (Sabet, 2025). Biopolymers and biodegradable polymers may be this alternative due to their ability to degrade, that is, short life cycle, through biological processes and/or decomposition into sustainable co-products, such as water, biomass, and carbon dioxide (Ghosh et al., 2021). The main sources for obtaining these biopolymers are shown in Fig. 9.5.

The search for packaging with sustainable characteristics for beverages has aroused interest in studies such as the replacement of polyethylene terephthalate-based packaging with bio-polyethylene terephthalate (Nath et al., 2023). Polyethylene terephthalate (PET) is widely used as packaging for beverages and is produced through the polymerization of ethylene glycol and terephthalic acid.

Table 9.8 Research seeking alternative materials for beverage packaging.

Study	Study description	Potential advantages
ABIPLAST (2019)	Discussion on the environmental impact of the improper disposal of plastic packaging derived from petroleum.	Reduction of environmental impacts and encouragement of the circular economy.
Brito et al. (2011)	Approach to the need for sustainable alternatives in the packaging industry, highlighting the challenges of replacing synthetic polymers.	Develop sustainable packaging that performs similarly to conventional packaging.
Landim et al. (2016)	Study on the expansion of biopolymers and bioplastics in industry, highlighting the advantages of renewable sources, clean technologies, and economic viability.	High industrial viability, reduced environmental impact, use of clean technologies, and better acceptance in the sustainable market.

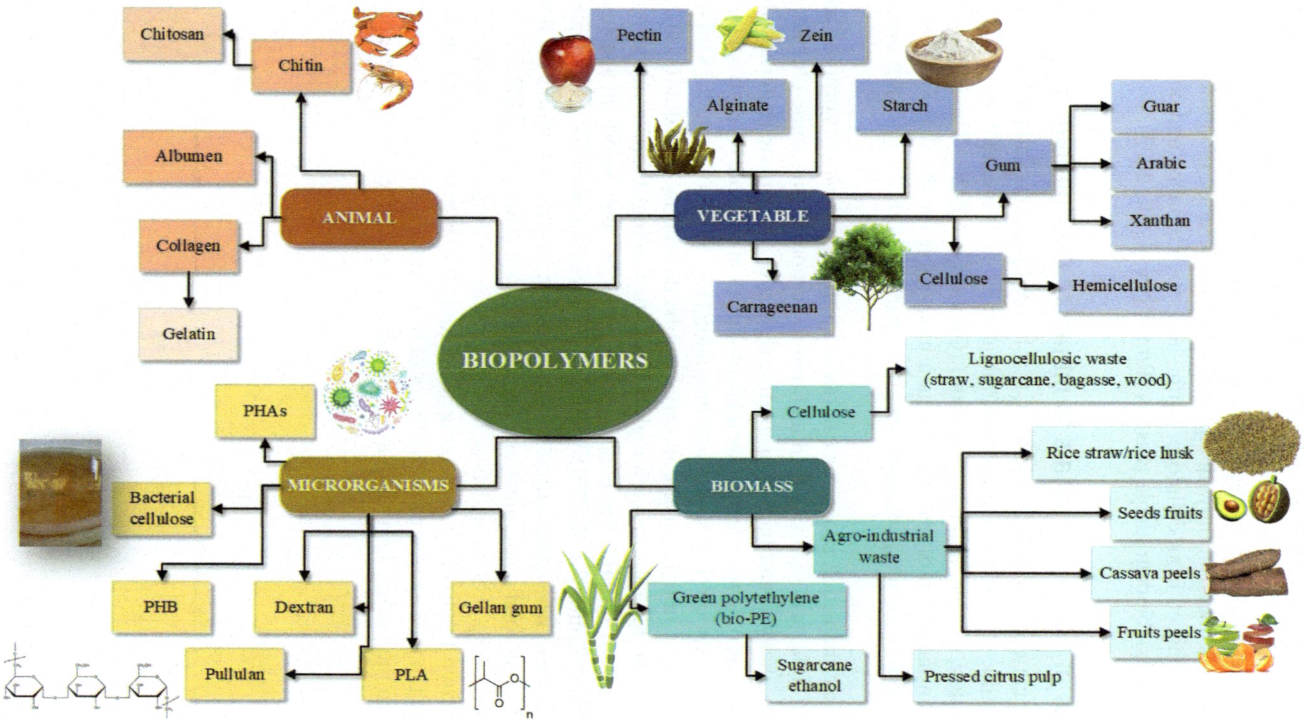

FIGURE 9.5

Sources of biopolymers. PHA: poly(hydroxyalkanoates); PHB: poly(hydroxybutyrate); PLA: poly(lactic acid).

However, its main disadvantage is that it takes many years for its complete degradation by nature (Rossa et al., 2022). However, bio-polyethylene terephthalate (bio-PET) can be produced partially or totally from renewable sources, which makes it a sustainable option (Rossa et al., 2022). Bio-PET can be produced from the fermentation of lignocellulosic materials, which involves the processes of oxidation of p-xylene and condensation with ethylene glycol-generating monomers (Sharif & Hoque, 2019). Bioplastics are produced from cellulose, lignin, and starch biomass and become alternatives to replace fossil-based and nonbiodegradable plastics (Rahardiyan et al., 2023).

9.5.3 Innovations in barrier materials to minimize contaminant migration

The direct interaction between food and packaging, that is, food products and packaging materials, has proven to be complex due to the potential for contamination by additives that may migrate during the supply chain (production, storage, and transportation) (Gupta et al., 2024). The increased demand for healthy foods with "in natura" profiles emerges as a motivation for the development of new technologies and new materials for the packaging sector, in parallel with the growing evolution of food systems.

The packaging-food interaction processes can occur through permeation, sorption, and migration. Such interactions can influence each other, in addition to compromising some characteristics of the packaging, such as mechanical and barrier properties (Fig. 9.6). Polymeric materials allow the phenomenon of mass transport of low molecular weight substances at variable levels from the processes of permeation (Fig. 9.6A), sorption (Fig. 9.6B), and migration (Fig. 9.6C) (Caner, 2018). The permeation process (Fig. 9.6A) of a gas in a polymeric material can be defined by the solution diffusion model, where molecules from the highest-pressure region of the packaging dissolve in the polymer of the packaging material, diffuse through the concentration gradient, and desorb in the lowest-pressure region of the packaging (Santoro et al., 2016). Thus, the packaging must have adequate water vapor permeability to prevent internal condensation in the packaging, which can inhibit the development of microorganisms and delay food contamination and deterioration (Hu et al., 2024).

The sorption process (Fig. 9.6B) consists of the absorption of components such as aromas, flavors, moisture, and lipids from the food by packaging. Consequently, diffusion occurs through this packaging, which can result in the loss of aroma and flavor of this food (Caner, 2018). Therefore, the choice of material to produce the packaging is important because it can influence the sorption process and,

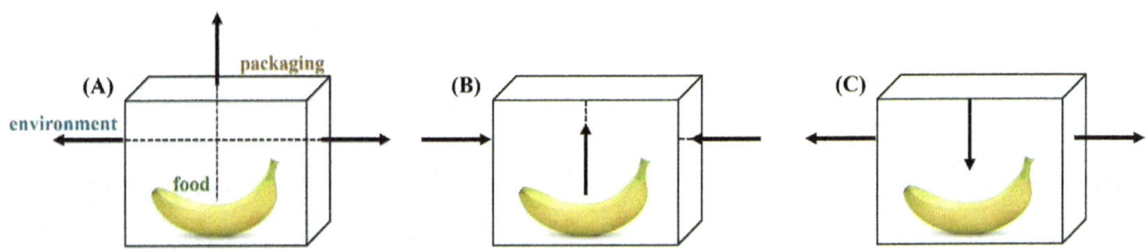

FIGURE 9.6

Illustration of the different types of interaction between food-packaging-environment, being (A) permeation, (B) sorption, and (C) migration.

Source: modified from Azevedo, H. M. C. (2012). Fundamentos de estabilidade de alimentos. Vol 2. ed. Brasília, DF: (Técnica)

consequently, the behavior of the packaging-food interaction and affect the long-term stability of this food (Akbar et al., 2025). Evaluating the processes of permeation and sorption of water in the materials to produce packaging is important to define the best application and to understand the behavior of this packaging under different humidity conditions inside and/or outside the food-packaging relationship (Table 9.9) (Lara et al., 2020).

To ensure food safety, human health, and reduce environmental impacts without compromising the advancement of research into new materials and technologies, regulatory bodies such as the FDA—Food and Drug Administration (USA) and EFSA—European Food Safety Authority—implement regulations that allow or restrict the use of certain polymeric materials for packaging composition and chemical agents/components that come into direct contact with food. In addition, they establish migration limits for components, whether specific (SML) or global (SML) (Gupta et al.,

Table 9.9 Studies of different types of packaging and their functional properties.

Study	Packaging material	Main results
Akbar et al. (2025)	- Polietileno de baixa densidade (PEBD)	- LDPE: Increased moisture content during storage. - Suitable for food and environments with water activity (Aw) < 0.75.
Lara et al. (2020)	- Film based on whey protein isolate and polyvinyl alcohol (PVA)	- The thermodynamic study of water sorption showed limitations in environments with high humidity.
Geng et al. (2024)	- Films with nanoscale metal-organic frameworks (MOFs) added for sleeves	- Obtained antibacterial activity. - Presented selective permeation of CO_2 and O_2. - The mangoes maintained good appearance and freshness for up to 7 days. - Gas selectivity contributed to preserving the quality of the fruits.
Wang et al. (2025)	- Carboxymethyl cellulose (CMC) and gelatin film with resveratrol and candelilla wax	- Candelilla wax: Reduced water vapor permeability due to its high hydrophobicity. - Gelatin: Contributed to the moisture barrier. - Resveratrol: Provided a barrier to visible and UV light, in addition to possible antioxidant properties. - The vapor transport mechanism occurs through sorption, diffusion, and desorption of the material.

2024). Other countries implement national regulations if they are available, as is the case in Brazil, through ANVISA—National Health Surveillance Agency (Fig. 9.7).

Fig. 9.7 illustrates the numerous laws, regulations, and guidelines in effect worldwide. These regulations present a long list of compounds that may come into contact with food. However, there is a lack of information regarding the migratory power of the components and a lack of standardization of analytical quantification methods. In addition, there are problems with equipment limitations and practical implementation issues (Gupta et al., 2024; Ilyas et al., 2021). According to Regulation (EC) No. 1935/2004 of the European Parliament and of the Council, materials and objects intended to come into contact with food must be inert to prevent the transfer of large quantities of substances to food that could endanger consumer health or cause unacceptable changes to food. European Commission. Directive (EU) (no date). The European Parliament and the Council establish the fundamental principles and rules of food law, create the European Food Safety Authority, and define procedures related to food safety. The Food Contact Materials and Articles Regulations 2012 (England) state that consumer health must be protected against the consumption of foods that contain harmful levels of chemicals that may migrate from materials that are in contact with these foods (European Commission, 2012).

In Brazil, the Board of Directors Resolution (RDC) No. 51 of November 26, 2010, sets out the regulations on the migration of components present in plastic materials, packaging, and equipment that are in contact with food (Ministério da Saúde, 2010). RDC No. 56, issued on November 16, 2012, establishes the monomers, substances, and polymers permitted for use in the production of plastic packaging and equipment intended for use with food (Minsitério da Saúde, 2012). Another resolution that regulates the migration of compounds into food is RDC No. 88, approved on June 29, 2016. It establishes a technical regulation for cellulosic materials, as well as for packaging and equipment coated or treated with waxes, paraffins, mineral oils, and mineral pigments that come into contact with food or food-related materials (Ministério da Saúde, 2016).

These global regulations and the high volume of food waste drive the demand for more sustainable and safe food packaging systems. Therefore, the food industry is looking for technological and material innovations whose solutions are sustainable, combined with simpler and less complex processes (Ahari et al., 2025). Materials based on biopolymers, polysaccharides, and proteins have an effective barrier action against gases (CO_2 and O_2) (Azeredo, 2012; Rocha et al., 2014). However, they have high permeability to water vapor due to their hydrophilic nature, which may limit their application as packaging (Azeredo, 2012; Brito et al. 2011). Such limitations have motivated numerous research into the modification of biopolymers, to enable processing, usability, and applicability, such as blends (Giteru et al., 2019; Miranda et al., 2025), composite films (Barbato et al., 2023), multilayer films (Haghighi et al., 2019), composites (Maalige, et al., 2021). In addition to the use of nanotechnology: nanocomposites (Jamróz et al., 2020), bio-nanocomposites (Alizadeh-Sani et al., 2018), and nanobiocomposites (Diañez et al., 2020).

Nanotechnology has been standing out within science and technology as a multifaceted emerging technological innovation, given the ramifications of application in various areas of research, mainly to obtain new materials for biomedicine (Haque et al., 2018), civil construction (Azevedo & Gleize, 2018), agribusiness (Prasad et al., 2017), cosmetics (Gupta et al., 2022), pharmacology (Zhang et al., 2018), functional materials for food (Durán & Marcato, 2013; Miranda et al., 2019). To be considered a nanomaterial, one or more dimensions of the material must be on a nanometric scale; that is, one or more external dimensions must be between 1 and 100 nm (Thakur & Thakur, 2024). However, this

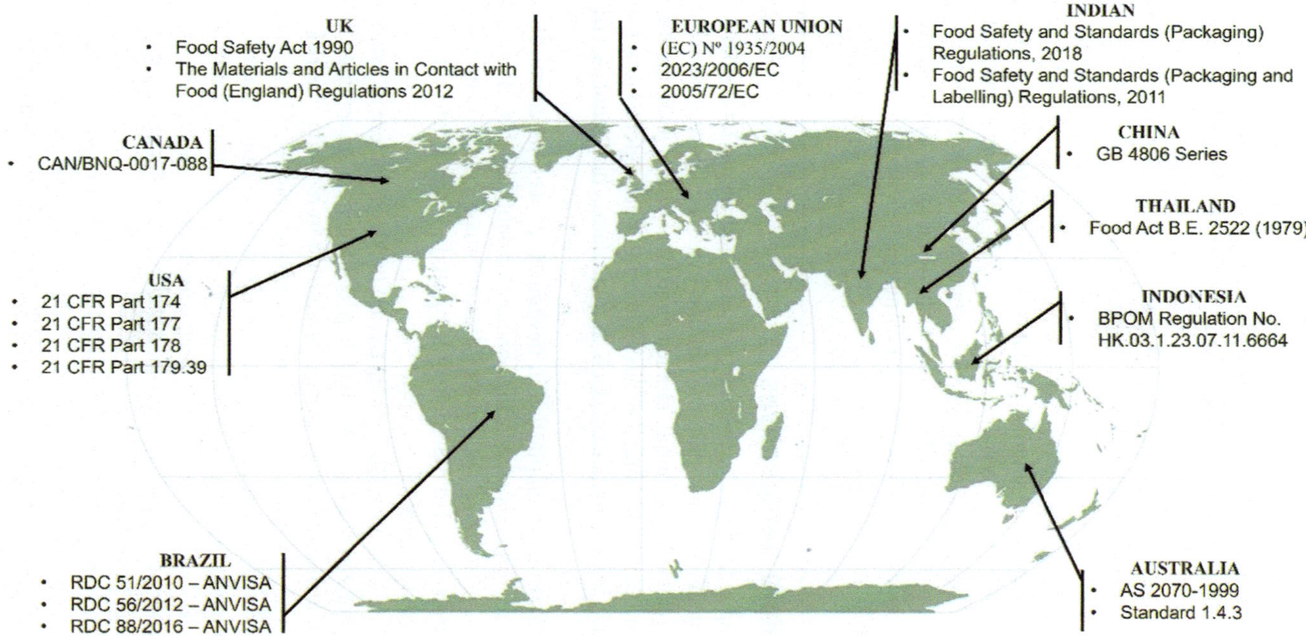

FIGURE 9.7

Major global regulations, guidelines, and legislation for food contact packaging materials.

Source: modified from Gupta, D., Lall, A., Kumar, S., Patil, T.D., Gaikwad, K.K. (2024). Plant-based edible films and coatings for food-packaging applications: Recent advances, applications, and trends. Sustainable Food Technology, *2(5), 1428–1455. https://doi.org/10.1039/d4fb00110a; Gupta, R.K., Pipliya, S., Karunanithi, S., Eswaran G.M., Kumar, U, S., Mandliya, S., Srivastav, P.P., Suthar, T., Shaikh, A.M., Harsányi, E., Kovács, B. (2024). Migration of chemical compounds from packaging materials into packaged foods: Interaction, mechanism, assessment, and regulations.* Foods *13 (19). Available from: http://www.mdpi.com/journal/foods. https://doi.org/10.3390/foods13193125.*

definition can be adapted according to the organization, agency, and committees to which the product is intended (Rasmussen et al. 2014).

According to researchers, nanomaterials can be classified according to the variation in the nanoscale and/or in the number of dimensions related to the structural elements of the nanomaterial: (i) "zero-dimensional" (0D): nanoparticles and nanodispersions; one-dimensional (1D): nanofibers and nanotubes; two-dimensional (2D): films and coatings with nanometric thickness; and three-dimensional (3D): formation of interfaces between the other dimensions (Cerqueira, 2018).

For the food sector, nanostructures can be applied as stabilizing material, improving hydrophobic or hydrophilic characteristics, promoting an increase in the bioavailability of compounds that may improve the sensory characteristics of the food or promoting the controlled release of certain substances that may promote the safety of the internal product (Alizadeh-Sani et al., 2018; Cerqueira, 2018; Cui et al., 2020). Studies with nanomaterials applied to packaging have gained prominence in recent years to increase shelf life and improve barrier properties (Hasaannezhad et al., 2025). Nanotechnology in the packaging area can contribute to protection and improvements in the flavor and texture of food, the controlled release of bioactives such as nutrients, vitamins, minerals, and food safety (Hasaannezhad et al., 2025).

9.6 Conclusion and future perspectives

Advances in beverage packaging technology have been crucial in addressing food safety challenges, particularly those related to contaminant migration. Scientific evidence shows that factors such as beverage composition, type of packaging material, storage conditions (time, temperature, and exposure to light), and physical and chemical characteristics of the food are determining factors in the migration process of potentially toxic substances, such as phthalates, bisphenol A (BPA), heavy metals, and microplastics.

The growing presence of micro and nanoplastics in beverages, as well as chemical compounds derived from plastic packaging, represents an emerging concern for public health, given their capacity for bioaccumulation and the risks associated with endocrine, inflammatory, and toxic effects. Studies indicate that packaging made from recycled materials or subjected to inadequate storage conditions intensifies the release of these contaminants.

Considering this scenario, there is a strong movement toward the development of smart, active, and sustainable packaging. These not only act as physical barriers but also incorporate features that monitor, preserve, and extend the shelf life of products, in addition to reducing the risk of contamination. Technologies such as gas detection sensors, freshness indicators, biodegradable packaging, and materials with antimicrobial and antioxidant properties stand out as promising solutions.

Despite the advances, significant challenges remain, including the standardization of analytical methods for detecting micro and nano contaminants, the definition of safe limits for compound migration, and the need for stricter public policies that encourage the circular economy and the use of materials with low environmental impact.

Therefore, the future of safety in beverage packaging lies in the integration of technological innovation, sustainability, regulatory rigor, and consumer education. Only through this multidisciplinary approach will it be possible to ensure that the search for more sustainable packaging does not compromise the quality, safety, and health of consumers.

9.7 Future directions for safer beverage packaging

In view of the challenges raised, several research fronts need to be explored in greater depth in the coming years:

- Development of more sensitive and standardized analytical methods for detecting microplastics, nanoplastics, and chemical contaminants in complex liquid matrices, such as alcoholic, dairy, and soft drinks;
- In-depth studies on the behavior of biodegradable and recycled materials, evaluating their chemical and microbiological safety throughout the product life cycle, considering different storage conditions;
- Investigation of the effects of exposure to extreme conditions, such as high temperatures, UV radiation, and long storage periods, on the degradation of packaging and the formation of toxic by-products;
- Development and validation of smart packaging with sensors coupled to remote monitoring systems (IoT), allowing real-time monitoring of storage conditions and beverage quality;
- Progress in the harmonization of international legislation and regulations, considering both food safety and environmental sustainability criteria.

AI disclosure

During the preparation of this work, the author(s) used ChatGPT and Napkin to Language review: improving grammar, spelling, clarity, and text style. Translation: converting the manuscript or parts of it into another language. Text generation: creating drafts, suggestions, or specific parts of the content, duly reviewed by the authors. Data or image visualization: assisting in the generation or refinement of figures, graphs, or illustrations. After using this tool/service, the author(s) reviewed and edited the content as needed and take(s) full responsibility for the content of the publication.

References

Abedi-Firoozjah, R., Parandi, E., Heydari, M., Kolahdouz-Nasiri, A., Bahraminejad, M., Mohammadi, R., Rouhi, M., & Garavand, F. (2023). Betalains as promising natural colorants in smart/active food packaging. *Food Chemistry, 424*, Article 136408. https://doi.org/10.1016/j.foodchem.2023.136408

Abekoon, T., Buthpitiya, B. L. S. K., Sajindra, H., Samarakoon, E. R. J., Jayakody, J. A. D. C. A., Kantamaneni, K., & Rathnayake, U. (2024). A comprehensive review to evaluate the synergy of intelligent food packaging with modern food technology and artificial intelligence field. *Discover Sustainability, 5*(1). https://doi.org/10.1007/s43621-024-00371-7

ABIPLAST. (2019). Abiplast: Perfil 2019. http://www.abiplast.org.br/publicacoes/perfil2019. (Accessed 6 November 2020).

Agarwal, A., Gandhi, S., Tripathi, A. D., Gupta, A., Iammarino, M., & Sidhu, J. K. (2025). Food contamination from packaging material with special focus on the Bisphenol-A. *Critical Reviews in Biotechnology, 45*(1), 69–79. https://doi.org/10.1080/07388551.2024.2344571

Ahari, H., Jafari, A., Ozdal, T., Moradi, S., Bahari, H.-R., Wu, Q., & Khaneghah, A. M. (2025). Recent innovations in metal-based nanoparticles for food packaging: A focus on safety and environmental impact. *Applied Food Research, 5*(1), Article 100860. https://doi.org/10.1016/j.afres.2025.100860

Ahmad, M., Ahmad, J., Usama, M., Al-Swadi, H. A., Mousa, M. A., Rafique, M. I., Al-Wabel, M. I., & Al-Farraj, A. S. F. (2025). Microplastic contamination in commercial food and drink products and associated risk of potential human intake in Riyadh, Saudi Arabia. *Environmental Monitoring and Assessment, 197*(3). https://doi.org/10.1007/s10661-025-13680-9

Ahmed, MdW., Azizul Haque, Md, Mohibbullah, M., Sirajul Islam Khan, Md, Islam, M. A., Tarek Mondal, MdH., & Ahmmed, R. (2022). A review on active packaging for quality and safety of foods: Current trends, applications, prospects and challenges. *Food Packaging and Shelf Life, 33*, Article 100913. https://doi.org/10.1016/j.fpsl.2022.100913

Akbar, U., Mondol, Singh, J., Rasane, P., Nanda, V., Abdi, G., & Kaur, S. (2025). Effects of various packaging materials and temperature conditions on the storage stability of Zea mays L. (baby corn) powder. *Applied Food Research, 5*(1), 100913. https://doi.org/10.1016/j.afres.2025.100913

Alamri, M. S., Qasem, A. A. A., Mohamed, A. A., Hussain, S., Ibraheem, M. A., Shamlan, G., Alqah, H. A., & Qasha, A. S. (2021). Food packaging's materials: A food safety perspective. *Journal of Biological Sciences, 28* (8), 4490–4499. https://doi.org/10.1016/j.sjbs.2021.04.047

Alizadeh-Sani, M., Khezerlou, A., & Ehsani, A. (2018). Fabrication and characterization of the bionanocomposite film based on whey protein biopolymer loaded with TiO2 nanoparticles, cellulose nanofibers and rosemary essential oil. *Industrial Crops and Products, 124*, 300–315. https://doi.org/10.1016/j.indcrop.2018.08.001

Allafi, A. R. (2020). The effect of temperature and storage time on the migration of antimony from polyethylene terephthalate (pet) into commercial bottled water in Kuwait. *Acta BioMedica, 91*(4), 1–5. https://doi.org/10.23750/abm.v91i4.8463

Arabi, S., Chen, X., Shen, L., & Lee, D. S. (2012). Flavor-release food and beverage packaging. In K. L. Yam, & D. S. Lee (Eds.), *Book: Emerging food packaging technologies* (pp. 96–108). Woodhead Publishing. https://doi.org/10.1016/B978-1-84569-809-6.50006-3.

Arigò, A., Rigano, F., Russo, M., Trovato, E., Dugo, P., & Mondello, L. (2021). Dietary intake of coumarins and furocoumarins through citrus beverages: A detailed estimation by a HPLC-MS/MS method combined with the linear retention index system. *Foods, 10*(7), 1533. https://doi.org/10.3390/foods10071533

Asamoah, B. O., Uurasjärvi, E., Räty, J., Koistinen, A., Roussey, M., & Peiponen, K. E. (2021). Towards the development of portable and in situ optical devices for detection of micro and nanoplastics in water: A review on the current status. *Polymers, 13*(5), 1–30. https://doi.org/10.3390/polym13050730

Azevedo, N. H.d., & Gleize, P. J. P. (2018). Effect of silicon carbide nanowhiskers on hydration and mechanical properties of a Portland cement paste. *Construction and Building Materials, 169*, 388–395. https://doi.org/10.1016/j.conbuildmat.2018.02.185

Azevedo, H. M. C. (2012). In D. F. Brasília (Ed.), *Fundamentos de estabilidade de alimentos* (Vol 2) (Técnica).

Babaei-Ghazvini, A., & Acharya, B. (2021). Humidity-responsive photonic films and coatings based on tuned cellulose nanocrystals/glycerol/polyethylene glycol. *Polymers, 13*(21), 3695. https://doi.org/10.3390/polym13213695

Bach, C., Dauchy, X., Severin, I., Munoz, J. F., Etienne, S., & Chagnon, M. C. (2013). Effect of temperature on the release of intentionally and non-intentionally added substances from polyethylene terephthalate (PET) bottles into water: Chemical analysis and potential toxicity. *Food Chemistry, 139*(1–4), 672–680. https://doi.org/10.1016/j.foodchem.2013.01.046

Balbinot, S., Srivastav, A. M., Vidic, J., Abdulhalim, I., & Manzano, M. (2021). Plasmonic biosensors for food control. *Trends in Food Science and Technology, 111*, 128–140. https://doi.org/10.1016/j.tifs.2021.02.057

Banegas, M. E. N., Saboia, L., Barros, Y., Lemos, V. A.da S., Henrrique Barbosa de Oliveira, A., Vidal, C. B., & Martins Cavalcante, R. (2023). Microplastics and nanoplastics in the aquatic environment: Contamination, determination and interaction with other contaminants. *PERIÓDICO TCHÊ QUÍMICA, 20*(43), 58–92. https://doi.org/10.52571/ptq.v20.n43.2023_05_cavalcante_pgs_58_92.pdf

Barbato, A., Apicella, A., Malvano, F., Scarfato, P., & Incarnato, L. (2023). High-barrier, biodegradable films with polyvinyl alcohol/polylactic acid + wax double coatings: Influence of relative humidity on transport properties and suitability for modified atmosphere packaging applications. *Polymers, 15*(19), 4002. https://doi.org/10.3390/polym15194002

Basaran, B., Aytan, U., Senturk, Y., Ozicici, Z., & Akçay, H. T. (2024). Microplastic contamination in turkiyl: Characterístics dietary exposure and risk assessment. *Food and Chemical Toxicology, 189*, Article 114730. https://doi.org/10.1016/j.fct.2024.114730

Becerril, R., Nerín, C., & Silva, F. (2021). Bring some colour to your package: Freshness indicators based on anthocyanin extracts. *Trends in Food Science & Technology, 111*, 495–505. https://doi.org/10.1016/j.tifs.2021.02.042

Beecher, G. R. (2024). Evolution of food composition knowledge in the United States from its beginning. *Journal of Food Composition and Analysis, 126*, Article 105802. https://doi.org/10.1016/j.jfca.2023.105802

Beneventi, E., Tietz, T., & Merkel, S. (2020). Risk assessment of food contact materials. *EFSA Journal, 18*(Suppl. 1). https://doi.org/10.2903/j.efsa.2020.e181109

Bharadwaj, C., Purbey, R., Bora, D., Chetia, P., Maheswari R, U., Duarah, R., Dutta, K., Sadiku, E. R., Varaprasad, K., & Jayaramudu, J. (2024). A review on sustainable PET recycling: Strategies and trends. *Materials Today Sustainability, 27*, Article 100936. https://doi.org/10.1016/j.mtsust.2024.100936

Bhatia, S., Al-Harrasi, A., Al-Azri, M. S., Ullah, S., Makeen, H. A., Meraya, A. M., Albratty, M., Najmi, A., & Anwer, M. K. (2022). Gallic acid crosslinked gelatin and casein based composite films for food packaging applications. *Polymers, 14*(19). https://doi.org/10.3390/polym14194065

Bledsoe, G., & Rasco, B. (2018). Recent advances on intelligent and active packaging in food and beverage technology. *Foods, 1*(2). Available at: http://www.dscc.dla.mil/downloads/packaging/pkghistory.pdf.

Boonsiriwit, A., Lee, M., Kim, M., Inthamat, P., Siripatrawan, U., & Lee, Y. S. (2021). Hydroxypropyl methylcellulose/microcrystalline cellulose biocomposite film incorporated with butterfly pea anthocyanin as a sustainable pH-responsive indicator for intelligent food-packaging applications. *Food Bioscience, 44*, Article 101392. https://doi.org/10.1016/j.fbio.2021.101392

Brasil. (2008). *Ministério da Saúde Agência Nacional de Vigilância Sanitária. Resolução - RDC N° 20, de 26 de março de 2008. Dispõe sobre o Regulamento Técnico sobre embalagens de polietilenotereftalato (PET) pós-consumo reciclado grau alimentício (PET-PCR grau alimentício) destinados a entrar em contato com alimentos. Diário Oficial da União, Poder Executivo, de 18 de março de 2008.* Available at: https://bvsms.saude.gov.br/bvs/saudelegis/anvisa/2008/rdc0020_26_03_2008.html.

Brito, G. F., Araújo, E. M., Jeferson, I., & Agrawal, P. (2011). Biopolímeros, Polímeros Biodegradáveis e Polímeros Verdes. *Revista Eletrônica de Materiais e Processos, 6*(2), 127–139.

Buss, D. A., & Henkes, J. A. (2014). Estudo dos impactos ambientais causados por laticínios com foco no reaproveitamento dos resíduos gerados. *Revista Gestão & Sustentabilidade Ambiental, 3*(2), 384. https://doi.org/10.19177/rgsa.v3e22014384-395

Calcaterra, V., Cena, H., Loperfido, F., Rossi, V., Grazi, R., Quatrale, A., De Giuseppe, R., Manuelli, M., & Zuccotti, G. (2024). Evaluating phthalates and bisphenol in foods: Risks for precocious puberty and early-onset obesity. *Nutrients, 16*(16), 2732. https://doi.org/10.3390/nu16162732

Caldwell, J., Taladriz-Blanco, P., Lehner, R., Lubskyy, A., Diego Ortuso, R., Rothen-Rutishauser, B., & Petri-Fink, A. (2022). The micro-, submicron-, and nanoplastic hunt: A review of detection methods for plastic particles. *Chemosphere, 293*, Article 133514. https://doi.org/10.1016/j.chemosphere.2022.133514

Caner, C. (2018). Fundamentals of the sorption (scalping) phenomena in packaged foods. In *Reference module in food science* (p. 12). Elsevier. https://doi.org/10.1016/B978-0-08-100596-5.22346-9

Cao, X. L. (2008). Determination of phthalates and adipate in bottled water by headspace solid-phase microextraction and gas chromatography/mass spectrometry. *Journal of Chromatography A, 1178*(1–2), 231–238. https://doi.org/10.1016/j.chroma.2007.11.095

Cao, X. L. (2010). Phthalate esters in foods: Sources, occurrence, and analytical methods. *Comprehensive Reviews in Food Science and Food Safety, 9*(1), 21–43. https://doi.org/10.1111/j.1541-4337.2009.00093.x

Cardama, A. L., Rodríguez-Bernaldo de Quirós, A., & Sendón, R. (2017). Analysis of bisphenol A in beverages and food packaging by High- performance liquid chromatography. *Food & Nutrition Journal, 5*(5). https://doi.org/10.29011/2575-7091.100043

Carrillo, J. D., Salazar, C., Moreta, C., & Tena, M. T. (2007). Determination of phthalates in wine by headspace solid-phase microextraction followed by gas chromatography–mass spectrometry: Fibre comparison and selection. *Journal of Chromatography A, 1164*(1–2), 248–261. https://doi.org/10.1016/j.chroma.2007.06.059

Cerqueira, M. A., Vicente, A. A., & Pastrana, L. M. (2018). Chapter 1 - Nanotechnology in food packaging: Opportunities and challenges. In *Micro and nano technologies, cerqueira.*

Chakraborty, I., Banik, S., Biswas, R., Yamamoto, T., Noothalapati, H., & Mazumder, N. (2023). Raman spectroscopy for microplastic detection in water sources: A systematic review. *International Journal of Environmental Science and Technology, 20*(9), 10435–10448. https://doi.org/10.1007/s13762-022-04505-0

Chakraborty, T. K., Hasan, M. J., Netema, B. N., Rayhan, M. A., Asif, S. M. H., Biswas, A., Sarker, S., Ahmmed, M., Nice, M. S., Islam, K. R., Debnath, P. C., Chowdhury, P., Rahman, M. S., Zaman, S., Ghosh, G. C., & Hasibuzzaman, M. (2024). Microplastics in the commercially available branded milk in Bangladesh: An emerging threat for human health. *Journal of Hazardous Materials, 477.* https://doi.org/10.1016/j.jhazmat.2024.135374

Chen, Y., Wen, D., Pei, J., Fei, Y., Ouyang, D., Zhang, H., & Luo, Y. (2020). Identification and quantification of microplastics using Fourier-transform infrared spectroscopy: Current status and future prospects. *Current Opinion in Environmental Science & Health, 18*, 14–19. https://doi.org/10.1016/j.coesh.2020.05.004

Choe, A., Yeom, J., Shanker, R., Kim, M. P., Kang, S., & Ko, H. (2018). Stretchable and wearable colorimetric patches based on thermoresponsive plasmonic microgels embedded in a hydrogel film. *NPG Asia Materials, 10*(9), 912–922. https://doi.org/10.1038/s41427-018-0086-6

Coles, R., & Kirwan, M. (2011). *Food and beverage packaging technology.* Wiley. https://doi.org/10.1002/9781444392180

Coltro, L., Saron, E. S., Pessoa, T. I., Morandi, J., & Silva, B. S. (2021). Migration of phthalates and 2,6-diisopropylnaphthalene from cellulose food packaging. *Polimeros, 31*(2). https://doi.org/10.1590/0104-1428.02321

Cui, H., Surendhiran, D., Li, C., & Lin, L. (2020). Biodegradable zein active film containing chitosan nanoparticle encapsulated with pomegranate peel extract for food packaging. *Food Packaging and Shelf Life, 24.* https://doi.org/10.1016/j.fpsl.2020.100511

Cunsolo, S., Williams, J., Hale, M., Read, D. S., & Couceiro, F. (2021). Optimising sample preparation for FTIR-Based microplastic analysis in wastewater and sludge samples: Multiple digestions. *Analytical and Bioanalytical Chemistry, 413*(14), 3789–3799. https://doi.org/10.1007/s00216-021-03331-6

da Silva Filipini, G., Patrícia Romani, V., & Martins, V. G. (2020). Biodegradable and active-intelligent films based on methylcellulose and jambolão (Syzygium cumini) skins extract for food packaging. *Food Hydrocolloids, 109*, Article 106139. https://doi.org/10.1016/j.foodhyd.2020.106139

Diañez, I., Martínez, I., & Gómez, P. A. (2020). Effect of plasticiser on the morphology, mechanical properties and permeability of albumen-based nanobiocomposites. *Food Packaging and Shelf Life, 24*, Article 100499. https://doi.org/10.1016/j.fpsl.2020.100499

Dokl, M., Copot, A., Krajnc, D., Fan, Y. V., Vujanović, A., Aviso, K. B., Tan, R. R., Kravanja, Z., & Čuček, L. (2024). Global projections of plastic use, end-of-life fate and potential changes in consumption, reduction, recycling and replacement with bioplastics to 2050. *Sustainable Production and Consumption, 51*, 498–518. https://doi.org/10.1016/j.spc.2024.09.025

Dube, N. (2022). *Potential packaging costs increase in wake of war.* Available at: https://www.industrialpackaging.com/blog/war-increases-packaging-cost.

Durán, N., & Marcato, P. D. (2013). Nanobiotechnology perspectives. Role of nanotechnology in the food industry: A review. *International Journal of Food Science and Technology, 48*(6), 1127–1134. https://doi.org/10.1111/ijfs.12027

Duric, B., Kartalovic, B., Habschied, K., Novakov, N., Vranesevic, J., Brkic, B., & Mastanjevic, K. (2024). Effects of packaging material type, storage time and lipid content on phthalate migration in smoked fish meat. *Applied Sciences, 14*(4), 1660. https://doi.org/10.3390/app14041660

El-Mekawy, R. E., Elhady, H. A., & Al-Shareef, H. F. (2021). Highly stretchable, smooth, and biodegradable hydrogel films based on chitosan as safety food packaging. *Polymers and Polymer Composites, 29*(6), 563–573. https://doi.org/10.1177/0967391120926892

Enyoh, C. E., Verla, A. W., Verla, E. N., Ibe, F. C., & Amaobi, C. E. (2019). Airborne microplastics: A review study on method for analysis, occurrence, movement and risks. *Environmental Monitoring and Assessment, 191*(11). https://doi.org/10.1007/s10661-019-7842-0

Erni-Cassola, G., Gibson, M. I., Thompson, R. C., & Christie-Oleza, J. A. (2017). Lost, but found with nile red: A novel method for detecting and quantifying small microplastics (1 mm to 20 μm) in environmental samples. *Environmental Science and Technology, 51*(23), 13641–13648. https://doi.org/10.1021/acs.est.7b04512

Esaki, Y., Fukuda, O., Yeoh, W. L., Okumura, H., & Yamaguchi, N. (2024). Strawberry packaging support system based on image recognition. In *2024 IEEE/SICE International Symposium on System Integration, SII 2024* (pp. 496–501). https://doi.org/10.1109/SII58957.2024.10417558. http://ieeexplore.ieee.org/xpl/mostRecentIssue.jsp?punumber=10417130

2619 European Commission. (2012). *The materials and articles in contact with food (England) regulations.*

European Commission. Directive (EU) 2019/904. Directive (EU) 2019/of the European Parliament and of the Council of 5 June 2019 on the reduction of the impact of certain plastic products on the environment. .

Fankhauser-Noti, A., & Grob, K. (2006). Migration of plasticizers from PVC gaskets into oily foods: Amount of gasket material and diffusion constants. *Trends in Food Science & Technology, 17*(3), 105–112. https://doi.org/10.1016/j.tifs.2005.10.013

FAO. (2014). In *Food wastage foodprint: Full-cost accounting ; final report*. Rome: FAO.

FAO-WFP. (2022). *Hunger hotspots: FAO-WFP early warnings on acute food insecurity: October 2022 to January 2023 outlook*. União Européia: Global Network Against Food Crises. Available at: https://www.fao.org/3/cc2134en/cc2134en.pdf.

Fierens, T., Van Holderbeke, M., Willems, H., De Henauw, S., & Sioen, I. (2013). Transfer of eight phthalates through the milk chain — A case study. *Environment International, 51*, 1–7. https://doi.org/10.1016/j.envint.2012.10.002

Forghani, S., Alamasi, H., & Moradi, M. (2021). Electrospun nanofibers as food freshness and time-temperature indicators: A new approach in food intelligent packaging. *Innovative Food Science & Emerging Technologies, 73*, Article 102804. https://doi.org/10.1016/j.foodhyd.2020.106139

Gagné, F., Auclair, J., & Quinn, B. (2019). Detection of polystyrene nanoplastics in biological samples based on the solvatochromic properties of Nile red: Application in *Hydra attenuata* exposed to nanoplastics. *Environmental Science and Pollution Research, 26*(32), 33524–33531. https://doi.org/10.1007/s11356-019-06501-3

García-Guzmán, L., Cabrera-Barjas, G., Soria-Hernández, C. G., Castaño, J., Guadarrama-Lezama, A. Y., & Rodríguez Llamazares, S. (2022). Progress in starch-based materials for food packaging applications. *Polysaccharides, 3*(1), 136–177. https://doi.org/10.3390/polysaccharides3010007

Geissdoerfer, M., Savaget, P., Bocken, N. M. P., & Hultink, E. J. (2017). The circular economy – A new sustainability paradigm? *Journal of Cleaner Production, 143*, 757–768. https://doi.org/10.1016/j.jclepro.2016.12.048

Geng, C., Jiang, Y., Bian, H., & Huang, G. (2024). Selective gas-permeation films with nanoMOFs as gas “switches” for mango preservation. *Chemical Engineering Journal, 481*, Article 148757. https://doi.org/10.1016/j.cej.2024.148757

Geueke, B., Groh, K., & Muncke, J. (2018). Food packaging in the circular economy: Overview of chemical safety aspects for commonly used materials. *Journal of Cleaner Production, 193*, 491–505. https://doi.org/10.1016/j.jclepro.2018.05.005

Ghosh, T., Das, M., Katiyar, Y., & Aji, M. M. (2021). Biopolymer nanocomposites in edible food packaging: Opportunity and applications. In V. Katiyar, & T. Ghosh (Eds.), *Nanotechnology in edible food packaging: Food preservation practices for a sustainable future* (pp. 233–257). Singapore: Springer. https://doi.org/10.1007/978-981-33-6169-0_9

Giteru, S. G., Ali, M. A., & Oey, I. (2019). Solvent strength and biopolymer blending effects on physicochemical properties of zein-chitosan-polyvinyl alcohol composite films. *Food Hydrocolloids, 87*, 270–286. https://doi.org/10.1016/j.foodhyd.2018.08.006

Gniadek, M., & Dąbrowska, A. (2019). The marine nano- and microplastics characterisation by SEM-EDX: The potential of the method in comparison with various physical and chemical approaches. *Marine Pollution Bulletin, 148*, 210–216. https://doi.org/10.1016/j.marpolbul.2019.07.067

Guo, Y., O'Brien, A. M., Lins, T. F., Shahmohamadloo, R. S., Almirall, X. O., Rochman, C. M., & Sinton, D. (2021). Effects of hydrogen peroxide on Cyanobacterium microcystis aeruginosa in the presence of nanoplastics. *ACS ES&T Water, 1*(7), 1596–1607. https://doi.org/10.1021/acsestwater.1c00090

Gupta, V., Mohapatra, S., Mishra, H., Farooq, U., Kumar, K., Ansari, M. J., Aldawsari, M. F., Alalaiwe, A. S., Mirza, M. A., & Iqbal, Z. (2022). Nanotechnology in cosmetics and cosmeceuticals—A review of latest advancements. *Gels, 8*(3). https://doi.org/10.3390/gels8030173

Gupta, D., Lall, A., Kumar, S., Patil, T. D., & Gaikwad, K. K. (2024). Plant-based edible films and coatings for food-packaging applications: Recent advances, applications, and trends. *Sustainable Food Technology, 2*(5), 1428–1455. https://doi.org/10.1039/d4fb00110a

Gupta, R. K., Pipliya, S., Karunanithi, S., Eswaran U, G. M., Kumar, S., Mandliya, S., Srivastav, P. P., Suthar, T., Shaikh, A. M., Harsányi, E., & Kovács, B. (2024). Migration of chemical compounds from packaging materials into packaged foods: Interaction, mechanism, assessment, and regulations. *Foods, 13*(19). https://doi.org/10.3390/foods13193125

GVR. (2024). Organic food and beverages market size, share & trends analysis report by product (organic food, organic beverages), by distribution channel (convenience stores, specialty stores), by region, and segment forecasts, 2024–2030. Available at: https://www.grandviewresearch.com/industry-analysis/organic-foods-beverages-market.

Haghighi, H., De Leo, R., Bedin, E., Pfeifer, F., Siesler, H. W., & Pulvirenti, A. (2019). Comparative analysis of blend and bilayer films based on chitosan and gelatin enriched with LAE (Lauroyl arginate ethyl) with antimicrobial activity for food packaging applications. *Food Packaging and Shelf Life, 19*, 31–39. https://doi.org/10.1016/j.fpsl.2018.11.015

Haque, F., Pi, F., Zhao, Z., Gu, S., Hu, H., Yu, H., & Guo, P. (2018). RNA versatility, flexibility, and thermostability for practice in RNA nanotechnology and biomedical applications. *Wiley Interdisciplinary Reviews: RNA, 9*(1). https://doi.org/10.1002/wrna.1452

Hasannezhad, H., Bakshi, A., Mozafari, M. R., & Naghib, S. M. (2025). A review of chitosan role in milk bioactive-based drug delivery, smart packaging and biosensors: Recent advances and developments. *International Journal of Biological Macromolecules, 294*, Article 139248. https://doi.org/10.1016/j.ijbioma

Hassan, MdA., Islam, R., Shammi, M., & Tareq, S. M. (2025). Microplastics contamination in carbonated beverage: An emerging threat to human health in Bangladesh. *Journal of Food Composition and Analysis, 141*, Article 107312. https://doi.org/10.1016/j.jfca.2025.107312

He, N., Yargeau, V., Liu, L., & Bayen, S. (2024). Development of a targeted and non-targeted direct-injection analysis of plastic-related contaminants in liquor products. *Food Control, 162*, Article 110424. https://doi.org/10.1016/j.foodcont.2024.110424

Högberg, J., Hanberg, A., Berglund, M., Skerfving, S., Remberger, M., Calafat, A. M., Filipsson, A. F., Jansson, B., Johansson, N., Appelgren, M., & Håkansson, H. (2008). Phthalate diesters and their metabolites in human breast milk, blood or serum, and urine as biomarkers of exposure in vulnerable populations. *Environmental Health Perspectives, 116*(3), 334–339. https://doi.org/10.1289/ehp.10788Sweden

Hu, L., Zhang, Q., Li, X., & Serpe, M. J. (2019). Stimuli-responsive polymers for sensing and actuation. *Materials Horizons, 6*(9), 1774–1793. https://doi.org/10.1039/c9mh00490d

Hu, H., Song, J., MacGregor, G. A., & He, F. J. (2023). Consumption of soft drinks and overweight and obesity among adolescents in 107 countries and regions. *JAMA Network Open, 6*(7). https://doi.org/10.1001/jamanetworkopen.2023.25158

Hu, J., Yun, X., Zheng, Y., Sun, T., Song, L., Pan, P., & Dong, T. (2024). Development of ultra-thin poly(L-lactic acid)-based films integrating toughness, barrier properties, and gas selectivity: Towards gas-permeation controllable green food packaging. *Food Chemistry, 449*, Article 139218. https://doi.org/10.1016/j.foodchem.2024.139218

Huang, Z., Hu, B., & Wang, H. (2023). Analytical methods for microplastics in the environment: A review. *Environmental Chemistry Letters, 21*(1), 383–401. https://doi.org/10.1007/s10311-022-01525-7

Hussain, K. A., Romanova, S., Okur, I., Zhang, D., Kuebler, J., Huang, X., Wang, B., Fernandez-Ballester, L., Lu, Y., Schubert, M., & Li, Y. (2023). Assessing the release of microplastics and nanoplastics from plastic containers and reusable food pouches: Implications for human health. *Environmental Science & Technology, 57*(26), 9782–9792. https://doi.org/10.1021/acs.est.3c01942

Ilyas, R. A., Sapuan, S. M., Megashah, L. N., Ibrahim, R., Atikah, M. S. N., Ainun, Z. M. A., Aung, M. M., Saifulazry, S. O. A., & Lee, C. H. (2021). Regulations for food packaging materials. In *Bio-based packaging: Material, environmental and economic aspects* (pp. 467–494). Malaysia: wiley. https://doi.org/10.1002/9781119381228.ch27

Isci, G., & Dagdemir, E. (2024). Human health risk assessment of phthalate esters and antimony levels in beverages packaged in polyethylene terephthalate under different storage conditions. *Journal of Food Composition and Analysis, 126*, Article 105922. https://doi.org/10.1016/j.jfca.2023.105922

Ishangulyyev, R., Kim, S., & Lee, S. (2019). Understanding food loss and waste—why are we losing and wasting food? *Foods, 8*(8), 297. https://doi.org/10.3390/foods8080297

Ivleva, N. P., Wiesheu, A. C., & Niessner, R. (2017). Microplastic in aquatic ecosystems. *Angewandte Chemie, International Edition, 56*(7), 1720–1739. https://doi.org/10.1002/anie.201606957

Jamróz, E., Khachatryan, G., Kopel, P., Juszczak, L., Kawecka, A., Krzyściak, P., Kucharek, M., Bębenek, Z., Zimowska, M., & nanocomposite films, F. (2020). The effect of nanofillers on the structural, thermal, mechanical and antimicrobial properties of biopolymer films. *Carbohydrate Polymers, 240*, Article 116244. https://doi.org/10.1016/j.carbpol.2020.116244

Jarvis, R. M., & Goodacre, R. (2004). Discrimination of bacteria using surface-enhanced Raman spectroscopy. *Analytical Chemistry, 76*(1), 40–47. https://doi.org/10.1021/ac034689c

Karakolis, E. G., Nguyen, B., You, J. B., Rochman, C. M., & Sinton, D. (2019). Fluorescent dyes for visualizing microplastic particles and fibers in laboratory-based studies. *Environmental Science and Technology Letters, 6* (6), 334–340. https://doi.org/10.1021/acs.estlett.9b00241

Kasaai, M. R. (2022). Bio-nano-composites containing at least two components, chitosan and zein, for food packaging applications: A review of the nano-composites in comparison with the conventional counterparts. *Carbohydrate Polymers, 280*, Article 119027. https://doi.org/10.1016/j.carbpol.2021.119027

Kato, K., Yoshimura, Y., Nakazawa, H., Ito, Y., & Oka, H. (2002). Preparation of samples for gas chromatography/mass spectrometry analysis of phthalate and adipate esters in plasma and beverages by steam distillation and extraction. *Journal of AOAC International, 85*(3), 719–723. https://doi.org/10.1093/jaoac/85.3.719

Kay, I. P., Herskovitz, J. E., & Goddard, J. M. (2022). Interfacial behavior of a polylactic acid active packaging film dictates its performance in complex food matrices. *Food Packaging and Shelf Life, 32*. https://doi.org/10.1016/j.fpsl.2022.100832

Khair, N. S., Yusof, N. B. A. T., Ariff, M. H. M., & Wahab, Y. A. (2022). Recent advances and open challenges in RFID antenna applications. In: Enabling industry 4.0 through advances in mechatronics. In I. M. Khairuddin, et al. (Eds.), *Lecture notes in electrical engineering* (pp. 507–517). Singapore: Springer Nature. https://doi.org/10.1007/978-981-19-2095-0_43

Khedri, S., Sadeghi, E., Rouhi, M., Delshadian, Z., Mortazavian, A. M., de Toledo Guimarães, J., fallah, M., & Mohammadi, R. (2021). Bioactive edible films: Development and characterization of gelatin edible films incorporated with casein phosphopeptides. *LWT, 138*, Article 110649. https://doi.org/10.1016/j.lwt.2020.110649

Khokhar, P., & Pawar, K. (2025). Chemical migration from packaging materials into consumable food matrices: A mini review. *Journal of Agriculture and Food Science, 7*(1), 21–25. https://doi.org/10.33545/2664844X.2025.v7.i1a.233

Kida, M., & Koszelnik, P. (2021). Investigation of the presence and possible migration from microplastics of phthalic acid esters and polycyclic aromatic hydrocarbons. *Journal of Polymers and the Environment, 29*(2), 599–611. https://doi.org/10.1007/s10924-020-01899-1

Knoblauch, D., & Mederake, L. (2021). Government policies combatting plastic pollution. *Current Opinion in Toxicology, 28*, 87–96. https://doi.org/10.1016/j.cotox.2021.10.003

Kokesch-Himmelreich, J., Wittek, O., Race, A. M., Rakete, S., Schlicht, C., Busch, U., & Römpp, A. (2022). MALDI mass spectrometry imaging: From constituents in fresh food to ingredients, contaminants and additives in processed food. *Food Chemistry, 385*, Article 132529. https://doi.org/10.1016/j.foodchem.2022.132529

Konieczna, A., Ruthowska, A., & Rachón, D. (2015). Health risk of exposure to Bisphenol A (BPA). *Roczniki Panstwowego Zakladu Higieny, 66*(1), 5–11.

Kopuncová, M., Sádecká, J., Kolek, E., Polovka, M., Durec, J., & Blaško, J. (2018). Impact of inert gas atmosphere application on the complex profile of commercial Orange juice volatiles during four-month storage. *Journal of Food and Nutrition Research, 57*(4), 373–383.

Kopuncová, M., Sádecká, J., Kolek, E., Dimitrov, F., Tobolková, B., Durec, J., & Blaško, J. (2022). Aroma stability and sensory aspects of commercially produced Orange juice: Gas chromatography–olfactometry study. *Chemical Papers, 76*(8), 4941–4953. https://doi.org/10.1007/s11696-022-02198-w

Kumar, A., Gupta, V., Singh, S., Saini, S., & Gaikwad, K. K. (2021). Pine needles lignocellulosic ethylene scavenging paper impregnated with nanozeolite for active packaging applications. *Industrial Crops and Products, 170*, Article 113752. https://doi.org/10.1016/j.indcrop.2021.113752

KuswandI, B.,J. (2020). 12 - Active and intelligent packaging, safety, and quality controls. In M. W. Siddiqui (Ed.), *Fresh-cut fruits and vegetables* (pp. 243–294). Academic Press.

Kwon, G., Cho, D. W., Park, J., Bhatnagar, A., & Song, H. (2023). A review of plastic pollution and their treatment technology: A circular economy platform by thermochemical pathway. *Chemical Engineering Journal, 464*. https://doi.org/10.1016/j.cej.2023.142771

Lam, T. W. L., Chow, A. S. Y., & Fok, L. (2024). Human exposure to microplastics via the consumption of nonalcoholic beverages in various packaging materials: The case of Hong Kong. *Journal of Hazardous Materials, 472*, Article 134575. https://doi.org/10.1016/j.jhazma

Landim, A. P. M., Bernardo, C. O., Martins, I. B. A., Francisco, M. R., Santos, M. B., & melo, N. R. (2016). Sustainability concerning food packaging in Brazil. *Polímeros, 26*, 82–92. https://doi.org/10.1590/0104-1428.1897

Lara, B. R. B., Dias, M. V., Guimarães Junior, M., de Andrade, P. S., de Souza Nascimento, B., Ferreira, L. F., & Yoshida, M. I. (2020). Water sorption thermodynamic behavior of whey protein isolate/polyvinyl alcohol blends for food packaging. *Food Hydrocolloids, 103*. https://doi.org/10.1016/j.foodhyd.2020.105710

Lee, J., & Chae, K.-J. (2021). A systematic protocol of microplastics analysis from their identification to quantification in water environment: A comprehensive review. *Journal of Hazardous Materials, 403*, Article 124049. https://doi.org/10.1016/j.jhazmat.2020.124049

Lee, H.-G., Jeong, S., & Yoo, S. R. (2023). Development of a calcium hydroxide–dye kimchi ripening indicator and its application in kimchi packaging. *Food Chemistry, 400*, Article 134039. https://doi.org/10.1016/j.foodchem.2022.134039

Li, P., Yang, J., Jiménez-Carvelo, A. M., & Erasmus, S. W. (2024). Applications of food packaging quick response codes in information transmission toward food supply chain integrity. *Trends in Food Science and Technology, 146*. https://doi.org/10.1016/j.tifs.2024.104384

Liew, W. C., Muhamad, I. I., Chew, J. W., & Karim, K. J. A. (2023). Synergistic effect of graphene oxide/zinc oxide nanocomposites on polylactic acid-based active packaging film: Properties, release kinetics and antimicrobial efficiency. *International Journal of Biological Macromolecules, 253*. https://doi.org/10.1016/j.ijbiomac.2023.127288

Liu, Y., Zhang, X., Li, C., Qin, Y., Xiao, L., & Liu, J. (2020). Comparison of the structural, physical and functional properties of κ-carrageenan films incorporated with pomegranate flesh and peel extracts. *International Journal of Biological Macromolecules, 147*, 1076–1088. https://doi.org/10.1016/j.ijbiomac.2019.10.075

Liu, X., Guo, J., Li, Y., Wang, B., Yang, S., Chen, W., Wu, X., Guo, J., & Xing, M. (2021). SERS substrate fabrication for biochemical sensing: Towards point-of-care diagnostics. *Journal of Materials Chemistry B, 9* (40), 8378–8388. https://doi.org/10.1039/d1tb01299a

Liu, Y., Ahmed, S., Sameen, D. E., Wang, Y., Lu, R., Dai, J., Li, S., & Qin, W. (2021). A review of cellulose and its derivatives in biopolymer-based for food packaging application. *Trends in Food Science and Technology, 112*, 532–546. https://doi.org/10.1016/j.tifs.2021.04.016

Liu, C., Xu, Di, Dong, X., & Huang, Q. (2022). A review: Research progress of SERS-Based sensors for agricultural applications. *Trends in Food Science & Technology, 128*, 90–101. https://doi.org/10.1016/j.tifs.2022.07.012

Liu, X., Wang, L., Li, W., & Wan, J. (2025). Rapid identification of plastic beverage bottles by using raman spectroscopy combined with machine learning algorithm. *Journal of Raman Spectroscopy, 56*(5), 381–388. https://doi.org/10.1002/jrs.6778

Luo, H., Xiang, Y., Zhao, Y., Li, Y., & Pan, X. (2020). Nanoscale infrared, thermal and mechanical properties of aged microplastics revealed by an atomic force microscopy coupled with infrared spectroscopy (AFM-IR) technique. *Science of the Total Environment, 744*, Article 140944. https://doi.org/10.1016/j.scitotenv.2020.140944

Lv, L., Qu, J., Yu, Z., Chen, D., Zhou, C., Hong, P., Sun, S., & Li, C. (2019). A simple method for detecting and quantifying microplastics utilizing fluorescent dyes - Safranine T, fluorescein isophosphate, Nile red based on thermal expansion and contraction property. *Environmental Pollution, 255*(Pt 2), Article 113283. https://doi.org/10.1016/j.envpol.2019.113283

Maalige R, N., Aruchamy, K., Polishetti, V., Halakarni, M., Mahto, A., Mondal, D., & Sanna Kotrappanavar, N. (2021). Restructuring thin film composite membrane interfaces using biopolymer as a sustainable alternative to prevent organic fouling. *Carbohydrate Polymers, 254*. https://doi.org/10.1016/j.carbpol.2020.117297

Maes, T., Jessop, R., Wellner, N., Haupt, K., & Mayes, A. G. (2017). A rapid-screening approach to detect and quantify microplastics based on fluorescent tagging with Nile Red. *Scientific Reports, 7*. https://doi.org/10.1038/srep44501

Mao, L., Wang, C., Dong, Z. Y., Jin, Y., Fang, D., & Dai, X. (2025). Fabrication of polylactic acid bilayer composite films using polyvinyl alcohol based coatings containing functionalized carbon dots and layered clay for active food packaging. *Industrial Crops and Products, 225*, Article 120460. https://doi.org/10.1016/j.indcrop.2025.120460

Marcelino, C. S., Souza Gomes, V. E.de, & Marangoni Júnior, L. (2025). Post-consumer recycled PET: A comprehensive review of food and beverage packaging safety in Brazil. *Polymers, 17*(5), 594. https://doi.org/10.3390/polym17050594

Martins, D., Migliorini, F. L., Teodoro, K. B. R., Facure, M. H. M., & Correa, D. S. (2022). Capítulo 4 - Nanocompósitos poliméricos. In *Nanocompósitos poliméricos. 1. 1* (Vol 1, pp. 133–168). São Paulo, Brasil: Edgard Blücher.

Mercea, P. V., Losher, C., Herburger, M., Piringer, O. G., Tosa, V., Cassart, M., Dawkins, G., & Faust, B. (2020). Repeated migration of additives from a polymeric article in food simulants. *Polymer Testing, 85*, Article 106436. https://doi.org/10.1016/j.polymertesting.2020.106436

Merino, D., Bellassi, P., Paul, U. C., Morelli, L., & Athanassiou, A. (2023). Assessment of chitosan/pectin-rich vegetable waste composites for the active packaging of dry foods. *Food Hydrocolloids, 139*, Article 108580. https://doi.org/10.1016/j.foodhyd.2023.108580

Miao, S., Wang, X., Zhu, Q., Liao, C., & Jiang, G. (2024). Migration patterns of organophosphate esters from plastic food packaging simulants to foods: Donors, behaviours, and influencing factors. *Science of the Total Environment, 954*, Article 176272. https://doi.org/10.1016/j.scitotenv.2024.176272

Mihammadi, M., & Fasihi, M. (2025). Eco-friendly polylactic acid/modified thermoplastic starch films enhanced with clove essential oil and cochineal for dual-functional active and intelligent food packaging. *Carbohydrate Polymers, 354*, Article 123320. https://doi.org/10.1016/j.carbpol.2025.123320

Ministério da Saúde, A. (2010). *Resolução - RDC No 51, de 26 de novembro de 2010. Dispõe sobre os requisitos mínimos para a análise, avaliação e aprovação dos projetos físicos de estabelecimentos de saúde no Sistema Nacional de Vigilância Sanitária (SNVS) e dá outras providências*. Available at: https://bvsms.saude.gov.br/bvs/saudelegis/anvisa/2011/res0051_06_10_2011.html.

Ministério da Saúde, A. (2016). Resolução da Diretoria Colegiada – RDC No° 88, de 29 de junho de 2016. In *Aprova o regulamento técnico sobre materiais, embalagens e equipamentos celulósicos destinados a entrar em contato com alimentos e dá outras providências*. . (Accessed 6 May 2025).

Minsitério da Saúde, A. (2012). *Resolução - RDC No 56, de 16 de novembro de 2012. Dispõe sobre a lista positiva de monômeros, outras substâncias iniciadoras e polímeros autorizados para a elaboração de embalagens e equipamentos plásticos em contato com alimentos*. Available at: https://bvsms.saude.gov.br/bvs/saudelegis/anvisa/2012/rdc0056_16_11_2012.html.

Miranda, K. W. E., Mattoso, L. H. C., Bresolin, J. D., Hubinger, S. Z., Medeiros, E. S., & de Oliveira, J. E. (2019). Polystyrene bioactive nanofibers using orange oil as an ecofriendly solvent. *Journal of Applied Polymer Science, 136*(15). https://doi.org/10.1002/app.47337

Miranda, K. W. E., Natarelli, C. V. L., Thomazi, A. C., Ferreira, G. M. D., Frota, M. M., Bastos, M.d. S. R., Mattoso, L. H. C., & Oliveira, J. E. (2020). Halochromic polystyrene nanofibers obtained by solution blow spinning for wine pH sensing. *Sensors, 20*(2). https://doi.org/10.3390/s20020417

Miranda, K. W. E., Frota, M. M., Mattos, A. L. A., Araújo, A. W. O., Alves Júnior, F. T., Vasconcelos, L. B., Bastos, M.d. S. R., & Souza, T. M. (2025). Eco-friendly bionanocomposite based on a ternary blend reinforced with bacterial cellulose for application in packaging materials. *Food Packaging and Shelf Life, 48*. https://doi.org/10.1016/j.fpsl.2025.101442

Montuori, P., Jover, E., Morgantini, M., Bayona, J. M., & Triassi, M. (2008). Assessing human exposure to phthalic acid and phthalate esters from mineral water stored in polyethylene terephthalate and glass bottles. *Food Additives & Contaminants: Part A, 25*(4), 511–518. https://doi.org/10.1080/02652030701551800

Mordor. (2025b). *Packaging market size & share analysis - Growth trends & forecasts (2025–2030)*. Available at: https://www.mordorintelligence.com/industry-reports/global-packaging-market.

Moreira, S., Laing, T., & Saavedra, A. U. (2023). *Cost-competitive, low-carbon aluminum is key to the energy transition*. Available at: https://blogs.worldbank.org/en/energy/cost-competitive-low-carbon-aluminum-key-energy-transition.

Mourad, A. L., & Tavares, M. P. F. (2020). A responsabilidade compartilhada das embalagens pós-consumo. *Boletim de Tecnologia e Desenvolvimento de Embalagens, 32*(1), 1–4.

Mudgal, D., Pagone, E., & Salonitis, K. (2024). Selecting sustainable packaging materials and strategies: A holistic approach considering whole life cycle and customer preferences. *Journal of Cleaner Production, 481*, Article 144133. https://doi.org/10.1016/j.jclepro.2024.144133

Muncke, J., Andersson, A. M., Backhaus, T., Boucher, J. M., Carney Almroth, B., Castillo Castillo, A., Chevrier, J., Demeneix, B. A., Emmanuel, J. A., Fini, J. B., Gee, D., Geueke, B., Groh, K., Heindel, J. J.,

Houlihan, J., Kassotis, C. D., Kwiatkowski, C. F., Lefferts, L. Y., Maffini, M. V., … Scheringer, M. (2020). Impacts of food contact chemicals on human health: A consensus statement. *Environmental Health: A Global Access Science Source, 19*(1). https://doi.org/10.1186/s12940-020-0572-5

Muncke, J. (2021). Tackling the toxics in plastics packaging. *PLoS Biology, 19*(3). https://doi.org/10.1371/JOURNAL.PBIO.3000961

Naderi Bab Anari, H., Majdinasab, M., Shaghaghian, S., & Khalesi, M. (2022). Development of a natamycin-based non-migratory antimicrobial active packaging for extending shelf-life of yogurt drink (Doogh). *Food Chemistry, 366*, Article 130606. https://doi.org/10.1016/j.foodchem.2021.130606

Naik, A., Lee, H. S., Herrington, J., Barandun, G., Flock, G., Güder, F., & Gonzalez-Macia, L. (2024). Smart packaging with disposable NFC-Enabled wireless gas sensors for monitoring food spoilage. *ACS Sensors, 9* (12), 6789–6799. https://doi.org/10.1021/acssensors.4c02510

Nath, P. C., Sharma, R., Debnath, S., Sharma, M., Inbaraj, B. S., Dikkala, P. K., Nayak, P. K., & Sridhar, K. (2023). Recent trends in polysaccharide-based biodegradable polymers for smart food packaging industry. *International Journal of Biological Macromolecules, 253*. https://doi.org/10.1016/j.ijbiomac.2023.127524

Neves, M. F., Trombin, V. G., Marques, V. N., & Martinez, L. F. (2020). Global Orange juice market: A 16-year summary and opportunities for creating value. *Tropical Plant Pathology, 45*(3), 166–174. https://doi.org/10.1007/s40858-020-00378-1

Nicoletti, M., & Serrone, P. Del (2017). *Intelligent and smart packaging*. IntechOpen. https://doi.org/10.5772/intechopen.68773

Nizamali, J., Mintenig, S. M., & Koelmans, A. A. (2023). Assessing microplastic characteristics in bottled drinking water and air deposition samples using laser direct infrared imaging. *Journal of Hazardous Materials, 441*, Article 129942. https://doi.org/10.1016/j.jhazmat.2022.129942

Noiwan, D., Suppakul, P., & Rachtanapun, P. (2022). Preparation of methylcellulose film-based CO2 indicator for monitoring the ripeness quality of mango fruit cv. Nam Dok Mai Si Thong. *Polymers, 14*(17), 3616. https://doi.org/10.3390/polym14173616

Ouyang, Q., Zhang, M., Wang, B., Ahmad, W., & Chen, Q. (2023). Development of a novel upconversion fluorescence nanosensor based on metalloporphyrin element for sensitive detection of N-nitrosodimethylamine. *Sensors and Actuators B: Chemical, 393*, Article 134260. https://doi.org/10.1016/j.snb.2023.134260

Pandey, A. K., Samota, M. K., & Sanches Silva, A. (2023). Mycotoxins along the tea supply chain: A dark side of an ancient and high valued aromatic beverage. *Critical Reviews in Food Science and Nutrition, 63*(27), 8672–8697. https://doi.org/10.1080/10408398.2022.2061908

Pereira, C., Cunha, S. C., & Fernandes, J. O. (2023). Commercial beers: A source of phthalates and di-ethylhexyl adipate. *Journal of the Science of Food and Agriculture, 19*, Article 100768. https://doi.org/10.1016/j.fochx.2023.100768

Petrović, T. (2024). Beer packaging: Trends for the future. *VII Naučno-Stručni Simpozijum Sa Međunarodnim Učešćem "Pivo, Pivarske Sirovine i Tržište" - Zbornik Radova, 7–8*. https://doi.org/10.5937/PIVOS24003P

Pilot, R. (2018). SERS detection of food contaminants by means of portable Raman instruments. *Journal of Raman Spectroscopy, 49*(6), 954–981. https://doi.org/10.1002/jrs.5400

Pivnenko, K., Eriksen, M. K., Martín-Fernández, J. A., Eriksson, E., & Astrup, T. F. (2016). Recycling of plastic waste: Presence of phthalates in plastics from households and industry. *Waste Management, 54*, 44–52. https://doi.org/10.1016/j.wasman.2016.05.014

Prasad, R., Bhattacharyya, A., & Nguyen, Q. D. (2017). Nanotechnology in sustainable agriculture: Recent developments, challenges, and perspectives. *Frontiers in Microbiology, 8*. https://doi.org/10.3389/fmicb.2017.01014

Prata, J. C., Alves, J. R., da Costa, J. P., Duarte, A. C., & Rocha-Santos, T. (2020). Major factors influencing the quantification of Nile Red stained microplastics and improved automatic quantification (MP-VAT 2.0). *Science of the Total Environment, 719*. https://doi.org/10.1016/j.scitotenv.2020.137498

Rahardiyan, D., Moko, E. M., Tan, J. S., & Lee, C. K. (2023). Thermoplastic starch (TPS) bioplastic, the green solution for single-use petroleum plastic food packaging – A review. *Enzyme and Microbial Technology, 168*. https://doi.org/10.1016/j.enzmictec.2023.110260

Ramaremisa, G., Erasmus, R. M., Tutu, H., & Saad, D. (2025). Occurrence and characteristics of microplastics in South African beverages. *Environmental Pollution, 365*, Article 125388. https://doi.org/10.1016/j.envpol.2024.125388

Ramos, M., Valdés, A., Mellinas, A. C., & Garrigós, M. C. (2015). New trends in beverage packaging systems: A review. *Beverages, 1*(4), 248–272. https://doi.org/10.3390/beverages1040248

Ramos, M., Valdés, A., & Garrigós, M. C. (2016). Packaging for drinks. In *Reference module in food science*. Elsevier. https://doi.org/10.1016/B978-0-08-100596-5.03224-8

Rasmussen, K., et al. (2014). *Towards a review of the EC recommendation for a definition of the term "Nanomaterial".Part 1, compilation of information concerning the experience with the definition. LU*. Publications Office of the European Union.

Rauert, C., Pan, Y., Okoffo, E. D., O'brien, J. W., & Thomas, K. V. (2022). Extraction and Pyrolysis-GC-MS analysis of polyethylene in samples with medium to high lipid content. *Journal of Environmental Exposure Assessment, 1*(2). https://doi.org/10.20517/jeea.2022.04

Ren, Y., Yuan, T. Z., Chigwedere, C. M., & Ai, Y. (2021). A current review of structure, functional properties, and industrial applications of pulse starches for value-added utilization. *Comprehensive Reviews in Food Science and Food Safety, 20*(3), 3061–3092. https://doi.org/10.1111/1541-4337.12735

Ren, J., Li, Y., Lin, Q., Li, Z., & Zhang, G. (2022). Development of biomaterials based on plasticized polylactic acid and tea polyphenols for active-packaging application. *International Journal of Biological Macromolecules, 217*, 814–823. https://doi.org/10.1016/j.ijbiomac.2022.07.154

Ribeiro, F., Okoffo, E. D., O'Brien, J. W., Fraissinet-Tachet, S., O'Brien, S., Gallen, M., Samanipour, S., Kaserzon, S., Mueller, J. F., Galloway, T., & Thomas, K. V. (2020). Quantitative analysis of selected plastics in high-commercial-value Australian seafood by pyrolysis gas chromatography mass spectrometry. *Environmental Science & Technology, 54*(15), 9408–9417. https://doi.org/10.1021/acs.est.0c02337

Rocha, G. O., Farias, M. G., De Carvalho, C. W. P., Ascheri, J. L. R., & Galdeano, M. C. (2014). Biodegradable composite films based on cassava starch and soy protein. *Polimeros, 24*(5), 587–595. https://doi.org/10.1590/0104-1428.1355

Rossa, V., Ferreira, L. E. M., Vasconcelos, S. C., Shimabukuro, E. T., Madriaga, V. G. C., Carvalho, A. P., Pergher, S. B. C., Silva, F. C., Ferreira, V. F., Júnior, C. A. C., & Lima, T. M. (2022). Nanocomposites based on the graphene family for food packaging: Historical perspective, preparation methods, and properties. *RSC Advances, 12*(22), 14084–14111. https://doi.org/10.1039/D2RA00912A

Rotsios, K., Konstantoglou, A., Folinas, D., Fotiadis, T., Hatzithomas, L., & Boutsouki, C. (2022). Evaluating the use of QR codes on food products. *Sustainability, 14*(8), 4437. https://doi.org/10.3390/su14084437

Roy, S., & Rhim, J. W. (2021). Anthocyanin food colorant and its application in pH-responsive color change indicator films. *Critical Reviews in Food Science and Nutrition, 61*(14), 2297–2325. https://doi.org/10.1080/10408398.2020.1776211

Sabet, M. (2025). Exploring biodegradable polymer composites for sustainable packaging: A review on properties, manufacturing techniques, and environmental impacts. *Iranian Polymer Journal, 34*(1), 123–142. https://doi.org/10.1007/s13726-024-01365-y

Sanchez, L. T., Pinzon, M. I., & Villa, C. C. (2022). Development of active edible films made from banana starch and curcumin-loaded nanoemulsions. *Food Chemistry, 371*. https://doi.org/10.1016/j.foodchem.2021.131121

Santillana, M. I., Ruiz, E., Nieto, M. T., Bustos, J., Maia, J., Sendón, R., & Sánchez, J. J. (2011). Migration of bisphenol A from polycarbonate baby bottles purchased in the Spanish market by liquid chromatography and fluorescence detection. *Food Additives & Contaminants: Part A, 28*(11), 1610–1618. https://doi.org/10.1080/19440049.2011.589036

Santoro, S., Moro, A. J., Portugal, C., Crespo, J. G., Lima, J. C., & Coelhoso, I. M. (2016). Monitoring oxygen permeation through polymeric packaging films using a ratiometric luminescent sensor. *Journal of Food Engineering, 189*, 37–44. https://doi.org/10.1016/j.jfoodeng.2016.05.020

Sazdovski, I., Bala, A., & Fullana-i-Palmer, P. (2021). Linking LCA literature with circular economy value creation: A review on beverage packaging. *Science of the Total Environment, 771*, Article 145322. https://doi.org/10.1016/j.scitotenv.2021.145322

Schaefer, E. W., Pavoni, J. M. F., Luchese, C. L., Faccin, D. J. L., & Tessaro, I. C. (2020). Influence of turmeric incorporation on physicochemical, antimicrobial and mechanical properties of the cornstarch and chitosan films. *International Journal of Biological Macromolecules, 148*, 342–350. https://doi.org/10.1016/j.ijbiomac.2020.01.148

Schaider, L. A., Balan, S. A., Blum, A., Andrews, D. Q., Strynar, M. J., Dickinson, M. E., Lunderberg, D. M., Lang, J. R., & Peaslee, G. F. (2017). Fluorinated compounds in U.S. fast food packaging. *Environmental Science and Technology Letters, 4*(3), 105–111. https://doi.org/10.1021/acs.estlett.6b00435

Schmitt, M., & Popp, J. (2006). Raman spectroscopy at the beginning of the twenty-first century. *Journal of Raman Spectroscopy, 37*(1–3), 20–28. https://doi.org/10.1002/jrs.1486

Sethulakshmi, A. G., & Saravanakumar, M. P. (2024). Sustainable papaya plant waste and green tea residue composite films integrated with starch and gelatin for active food packaging applications. *International Journal of Biological Macromolecules, 260*(Pt 1), Article 129153. https://doi.org/10.1016/j.ijbiomac.2023.129153

Shaik, L., & Chakraborty, S. (2023). The impact of storage temperature and packaging material on the quality of ultrasound treated sweet lime juice. *Food and Humanity, 1*, 445–458. https://doi.org/10.1016/j.foohum.2023.06.016

Sharif, A., & Hoque, M. E. (2019). Renewable resource-based polymers Bio-based polymers and nanocomposites. In *Preparation, Processing, Properties & Performance* (pp. 1–28). Bangladesh: Springer International Publishing. https://doi.org/10.1007/978-3-030-05825-8_1

Shen, M., Song, B., Zeng, G., Zhang, Y., Huang, W., Wen, X., & Tang, W. (2020). Are biodegradable plastics a promising solution to solve the global plastic pollution? *Environmental Pollution, 263*(Pt A), Article 114469. https://doi.org/10.1016/j.envpol.2020.114469

Shen, X., Hed, Y., Annfinsen, S., Singh, N., Anwar, H., Mylvaganam, B., Kamfjord, T., & Emmer, Å. (2025). Investigating polyethylene terephthalate beverage packaging: Impact of recycled content on acetaldehyde, benzene, and other contaminants. *Journal of Polymers and the Environment, 33*(5), 2362–2370. https://doi.org/10.1007/s10924-025-03544-1

Shi, C., Zhou, A., Fang, D., Lu, T., Wang, J., Song, Y., Lyu, L., Wu, W., Huang, C., & Li, W. (2022). Oregano essential oil/β-cyclodextrin inclusion compound polylactic acid/polycaprolactone electrospun nanofibers for active food packaging. *Chemical Engineering Journal, 445*, Article 136746. https://doi.org/10.1016/j.cej.2022.136746

Shim, W. J., Song, Y. K., Hong, S. H., & Jang, M. (2016). Identification and quantification of microplastics using Nile Red staining. *Marine Pollution Bulletin, 113*(1–2), 469–476. https://doi.org/10.1016/j.marpolbul.2016.10.049

Shruti, V. C., Pérez-Guevara, F., Elizalde-Martínez, I., & Kutralam-Muniasamy, G. (2020). First study of its kind on the microplastic contamination of soft drinks, cold tea and energy drinks - Future research and environmental considerations. *Science of the Total Environment, 726*, Article 138580. https://doi.org/10.1016/j.scitotenv.2020.138580

Simsek, M., Eke, B., & Demir, H. (2020). Characterization of carboxymethyl cellulose-based antimicrobial films incorporated with plant essential oils. *International Journal of Biological Macromolecules, 163*, 2172–2179. https://doi.org/10.1016/j.ijbiomac.2020.09.075

Socas-Hernández, C., Miralles, P., González-Sálamo, J., Hernández-Borges, J., & Coscollà, C. (2024). Assessment of anthropogenic particles content in commercial beverages. *Food Chemistry, 447.* https://doi.org/10.1016/j.foodchem.2024.139002

Song, Y. K., Sang, H. H., Jang, M., Han, G. M., Jung, S. W., & Shim, W. J. (2017). Combined effects of UV exposure duration and mechanical abrasion on microplastic fragmentation by polymer type. *Environmental Science & Technology, 51*(8), 4368–4376. https://doi.org/10.1021/acs.est.6b06155

Sørensen, L. K. (2006). Determination of phthalates in milk and milk products by liquid chromatography/tandem mass spectrometry. *Rapid Communications in Mass Spectrometry, 20*(7), 1135–1143. https://doi.org/10.1002/rcm.2425

Spadotto, C. A., & Ribeiro, W. C. (2006). In S. P. Botucatu, & v.Ú. FEPAF (Eds.), *Gestão de resíduos na agricultura e agroindústria* (Vol. 1).

Sridhar, A., Kannan, D., Kapoor, A., & Prabhakar, S. (2022). Extraction and detection methods of microplastics in food and marine systems: A critical review. *Chemosphere, 286*(Pt 1), Article 131653. https://doi.org/10.1016/j.chemosphere.2021.131653

Sujana, R. D., Lioe, H. N., & Suyatma, N. E. (2024). Characteristics of heavy metal migration from virgin PET and recycled PET plastic bottles in beverage products. *Food Additives & Contaminants: Part A, 42*(2), 273–280. https://doi.org/10.1080/1944004

Sun, Q., Zhang, L., Huang, M., Ma, M., Zeng, J., & Le, T. (2024). Modification of starch-derived graphene quantum dots as multifunctional nanofillers to produce polymer starch/polyvinyl alcohol composite films for active packaging. *LWT, 198*, Article 115953. https://doi.org/10.1016/j.lwt.2024.115953

Szabo, K., Teleky, B. E., Mitrea, L., Călinoiu, L. F., Martău, G. A., Simon, E., Varvara, R. A., & Vodnar, D. C. (2020). Active packaging-poly (vinyl alcohol) films enriched with tomato by-products extract. *Coatings, 10*(2). https://doi.org/10.3390/coatings10020141

Thakur, P., & Thakur, A. (2024). Introduction to nanotechnology. In A. Thakur, P. Thakur, & S. M. P. Khurana (Eds.), *Synthesis and applications of nanoparticles* (pp. 1–17). Singapore: Springer Nature. https://doi.org/10.1007/978-981-99-6105-4_1

Tian, Z. Y., Mbayachi, V. B., Dai, W. K., Khalil, M., & Ayejoto, D. A. (2023). Gas chromatography/mass spectrometry. In *Advanced diagnostics in combustion science* (pp. 33–69). China: Springer Singapore. https://doi.org/10.1007/9789819905461_2

UN. Transforming our world: The 2030 agenda for sustainable development department of economic and social affairs. Available at: https://sdgs.un.org/2030agenda Accessed at 29 April, 2025.

Utetiwabo, W., Yang, L., Tufail, M. K., Zhou, L., Chen, R., Lian, Y., & Yang, W. (2020). Electrode materials derived from plastic wastes and other industrial wastes for supercapacitors. *Chinese Chemical Letters, 31*(6), 1474–1489. https://doi.org/10.1016/j.cclet.2020.01.003

Veeraiyan, S., et al. (2022). Surface chemistry for intelligent food packaging. In *Biomateriais em Embalagens de Alimentos. 1* (s.l., p. 22). Jenny Stanford Publishing.

Veríssimo, M. I. S., & Gomes, M. T. S. R. (2008). Aluminium migration into beverages: Are dented cans safe? *Science of the Total Environment, 405*(1–3), 385–388. https://doi.org/10.1016/j.scitotenv.2008.05.045

Verma, D., Dhiman, T. K., Das Mukherjee, M., & Solanki, P. R. (2021). Electrophoretically deposited green synthesized silver nanoparticles anchored in reduced graphene oxide composite based electrochemical sensor for detection of bisphenol A. *Journal of the Electrochemical Society, 168*(9). https://doi.org/10.1149/1945-7111/ac218a

Vitali, C., Peters, R. J. B., Janssen, H.-G., Nielen, M. W. F., & Ruggeri, F. S. (2022). Microplastics and nanoplastics in food, water, and beverages, part II. *Methods . TrAC Trends in Analytical Chemistry, 157*, Article 116819. https://doi.org/10.1016/j.trac.2022.116819

Wagner, M., & Oehlmann, J. (2009). Endocrine disruptors in bottled mineral water: Total estrogenic burden and migration from plastic bottles. *Environmental Science and Pollution Research, 16*(3), 278–286. https://doi.org/10.1007/s11356-009-0107-7

Walker, T., Gramlich, D., & Dumont-Bergeron, A. (2020). The case for a plastic tax: A review of its benefits and disadvantages within a circular economy. *Sustainability, 4*, 185–211. https://doi.org/10.1108/S2514-175920200000004010

Wang, Y., & Wang, Y. (2024). Assessing microplastic contamination in soda beverages: A multi-city, multi-container laser direct infrared spectroscopy study. *Heliyon, 10*(12), Article e32805. https://doi.org/10.1016/j.heliyon.2024.e32805

Wang, A., Zhu, Y., Zou, L., Zhu, H., Cao, R., & Zhao, G. (2022). Combination of machine learning and intelligent sensors in real-time quality control of alcoholic beverages. *Food Science and Technology*, 42. https://doi.org/10.1590/fst.54622

Wang, Y., Jiang, L., Liu, T., Qin, R., Xue, J., Wang, L., & Ren, L. (2025). Duck feather inspired hydrophobic carboxymethyl cellulose/gelatin film for intelligent and active food packaging. *International Journal of Biological Macromolecules, 301*, Article 140424. https://doi.org/10.1016/j.ijbiomac.2025.140424

Wani, A. K., Anjli, A., Tripathi, I., & Mir, T. G. (2024). *Carpter 10 - Interaction of food and packaging* (pp. 289–318). Intelligent Packaging. https://doi.org/10.1016/B978-0-443-15388-4.00011-0

Wikström, F., Williams, H., Trischler, J., & Rowe, Z. (2019). The importance of packaging functions for food waste of different products in households. *Sustainability, 11*(9), 2641. https://doi.org/10.3390/su11092641

Wissmann, M. A., Hein, A. F., & Neuls, H. N. H. (2013). Geração de resíduos: uma análise da ecoeficiência nas linhas de produção em uma indústria de laticínios e a influência sobre os custos ambientais. *Custos e agronegócio online, 9*(4), 83–103.

Wu, P., Tang, Y., Cao, G., Li, J., Wang, S., Chang, X., Miao, D., Jin, H., Zheng, C., & Cai, Z. (2020). Determination of environmental Micro(Nano)Plastics by matrix-assisted laser desorption/ionization–time-Of-flight mass spectrometry. *Analytical Chemistry, 92*(21), 14346–14356. https://doi.org/10.1021/acs.analchem.0c01928

Xu, J. L., Thomas, K. V., Luo, Z., & Gowen, A. A. (2019). FTIR and Raman imaging for microplastics analysis: State of the art, challenges and prospects. *TrAC, Trends in Analytical Chemistry, 119*. https://doi.org/10.1016/j.trac.2019.115629

Yang, J., Shen, M., Luo, Y., Wu, T., Chen, X., Wang, Y., & Xie, J. (2021). Advanced applications of chitosan-based hydrogels: From biosensors to intelligent food packaging system. *Trends in Food Science & Technology, 110*, 822–832. https://doi.org/10.1016/j.tifs.2021.02.032

Yang, J., Punia Bangar, S., Khan, M. R., Hammouda, G. A., Alam, P., & Zhang, W. (2024). Biopolymer-based packaging films/edible coatings functionalized with ε-polylysine: New options for food preservation. *Food Research International, 187*, Article 114390. https://doi.org/10.1016/j.foodres.2024.114390

Yano, K., Hirosawa, N., Sakamoto, Y., Katayama, H., Moriguchi, T., Joung, K. E., Sheen, Y. Y., & Asaoka, K. (2002). Phthalate levels in beverages in Japan and Korea. *Bulletin of Environmental Contamination and Toxicology, 68*(4), 463–469. https://doi.org/10.1007/s001280277

Ye, X., Liu, R., Qi, X., Wang, X., Wang, Y., Qi, C., & Gao, X. (2022). Preparation of bioactive gelatin film using semi-refined pectin reclaimed from blueberry juice pomace: Creating an oxidation and light barrier for food packaging. *Food Hydrocolloids, 129*, Article 107673. https://doi.org/10.1016/j.foodhyd.2022.107673

Yekta, R., Abedi-Firoozjah, R., Azimi Salim, S., Khezerlou, A., & Abdolmaleki, K. (2023). Application of cellulose and cellulose derivatives in smart/intelligent bio-based food packaging. *Cellulose, 30*(16), 9925–9953. https://doi.org/10.1007/s10570-023-05520-1

Yin, W., Qiu, C., Ji, H., Li, X., Sang, S., McClements, D. J., Jiao, A., Wang, J., & Jin, Z. (2023). Recent advances in biomolecule-based films and coatings for active and smart food packaging applications. *Food Bioscience, 52*, Article 102378. https://doi.org/10.1016/j.fbio.2023.102378

Zaki, G., & Shoeib, T. (2018). Concentrations of several phthalates contaminants in Egyptian bottled water: Effects of storage conditions and estimate of human exposure. *Science of the Total Environment, 618*, 142–150. https://doi.org/10.1016/j.scitotenv.2017.10.337

Zhang, R. X., Li, J., Zhang, T., Amini, M. A., He, C., Lu, B., Ahmed, T., Lip, H., Rauth, A. M., & Wu, X. Y. (2018). Importance of integrating nanotechnology with pharmacology and physiology for innovative drug delivery and therapy - An illustration with firsthand examples. *Acta Pharmacologica Sinica, 39*(5), 825–844. https://doi.org/10.1038/aps.2018.33

Zhang, J., Fu, D., Feng, H., Li, Y., Zhang, S., Peng, C., Wang, Y., Sun, H., & Wang, L. (2024). Mass spectrometry detection of environmental microplastics: Advances and challenges. *TrAC, Trends in Analytical Chemistry, 170*, Article 117472. https://doi.org/10.1016/j.trac.2023.117472

Zhu, J., Phillips, S. P., Feng, Y. L., & Yang, X. (2006). Phthalate esters in human milk: Concentration variations over a 6-month postpartum time. *Environmental Science and Technology, 40*(17), 5276–5281. https://doi.org/10.1021/es060356w

Ziani, I., Bouakline, H., El Guerraf, A., El Bachiri, A., Fauconnier, M.-L., & Sher, F. (2025). Integrating AI and advanced spectroscopic techniques for precision food safety and quality control. *Trends in Food Science & Technology, 156*, Article 104850. https://doi.org/10.1016/j.tifs.2024.104850

Zore, Ž., Čuček, L., & Kravanja, Z. (2018). Synthesis of sustainable production systems using an upgraded concept of sustainability profit and circularity. *Journal of Cleaner Production, 201*, 1138–1154. https://doi.org/10.1016/j.jclepro.2018.07.150

Zuo, J., Feng, J., Gameiro, M. G., Tian, Y., Liang, J., Wang, Y., Ding, J., & He, Q. (2022). RFID-Based sensing in smart packaging for food applications: A review. *Future Foods, 6*. https://doi.org/10.1016/j.fufo.2022.100198

CHAPTER

Analytical techniques for beverage analysis 10

Luana Guabiraba Mendes[1,2], Jéssica Roberta Pereira Martins[1], Magnólia Carneiro de Oliveira[1], José Leitão Sena Lima Filho[1], Felipe Sousa da Silva[2], Crisiana de Andrade Nobre[2,3], Tiago Rocha Nogueira[2], Tatiana Sainara Maia Fernandes[4], Mayara Salgado Silva[1], Luciana de Siqueira Oliveira[3], Ronaldo Ferreira do Nascimento[4] and Maria Aparecida Liberato Milhome[1]

[1]Postgraduate Program in Food Technology (PPGTA), Federal Institute of Education, Science and Technology of Ceará (IFCE), Limoeiro do Norte, Ceará, Brazil; [2]Nucleus of Technology and Industrial Quality of Ceará (NUTEC), Fortaleza, Ceará, Brazil; [3]Universidade Federal do Ceará, Departamento de Engenharia de Alimentos, Campus do Pici, Fortaleza, Ceará, Brazil; [4]Universidade Federal do Ceará, Departamento de Química Analítica e Físico-Química, Campus do Pici, Fortaleza, Ceará, Brazil

10.1 Introduction

Quality control of beverages has been increasingly required by current legislation. As a result, concerns regarding the compliance of the components used in beverages, the production processes and packaging of the items, have been growing. The industry has sought to identify and mitigate the risks associated with contamination, generally caused by deterioration, fermentation or even the use of prohibited chemicals in the formulations.

Alcoholic and non-alcoholic beverages have diverse compositions, involving complex matrices, requiring modern techniques of high sensitivity and selectivity. This has resulted in the advancement of analytical methodologies that can enable the monitoring of different chemical substances in foods (Nascimento et al., 2018).

Choosing the analytical methodology for controlling contaminants in beverages is a crucial step in ensuring the quality of the final product. The technique must be capable of analyzing different classes of chemical substances at different concentration levels, in addition to being efficient, fast, low-cost, reliable and environmentally friendly.

New analytical methods have been developed with the aim of promoting the qualitative and quantitative determination of toxic residues, nutrients and aditives in food, replacing traditional methods with eco-friendly/green methods. Spectrophotometric and chromatographic methods, such as gas chromatography (GC) and high performance liquid chromatography (HPLC) associated with different detectors are capable of analyzing a wide variety of compounds in beverages, such as volatile compounds, higher alcohols, fatty acids, bioactives and contaminants.

The Science and Safety of Beverages. https://doi.org/10.1016/B978-0-443-36536-2.00013-2

In this context, the chapter presents an approach to the main instrumental techniques for the analysis of: Volatile compounds (VCs) in functional beverages (juices and mixed drinks); Aldehydes, ketones and higher alcohols in distilled alcoholic beverages (spirits); additives (in juices, soft drinks, mixed drinks, teas, alcoholic beverages); fatty acids in fermented beverages (dairy, kefir); bioactives in fruit juices; pesticides in beverages and processed fruit and vegetable products. The text describes the main sample preparation methods and detection systems used in research over the last decade for the analysis of constituents and contaminants in beverages.

10.2 Trends in methods for analyzing beverage composition

10.2.1 VCs in functional beverages

VCs are substances that have the ability to evaporate easily at room temperature and are widely used in the food and beverage industry to impart flavor, aroma and fragrance. These compounds are often found in essential oils, extracts and other natural or synthetic substances that characterize a food or beverage, playing a major role in the quality, not only of the sensory aspect of the product, but also in ensuring that the food is safe (Fretwell, 2020; Ramos et al., 2021).

In view of the growing demand for food, VCs have gained prominence for providing sensory pleasure and health benefits. These compounds encompass a wide variety of chemical substances responsible for essential sensory characteristics, such as the aroma and flavor of foods. The sensory quality of food products is directly related to the presence, concentration and interaction of these compounds, which influence the perception of flavor and intensity, playing a crucial role in consumer acceptance (Ramos et al., 2021).

Although fruits and vegetables can synthesize hundreds of VCs, only a small fraction of these substances play an essential role in consumer preference for functional beverages. For a volatile compound to effectively contribute to sensory perception, it must have a high vapor pressure, allowing its release and olfactory recognition. In addition, its solubility in water and adequate concentration are determining factors for interacting effectively with olfactory receptors. The concentration of these VCs is generally low and can be influenced by several factors. Agronomic aspects, such as plant variety, climatic conditions and ripening stage, directly impact the volatile composition. Technological factors, such as harvesting methods, post-harvest treatment, storage and processing conditions, also play a crucial role in preserving or modifying the aromatic profile of foods (Table 10.1) (Beltrame et al., 2021; Dudareva et al., 2004).

Each fruit and vegetable (other vegetables) has a unique profile of VCs, which directly influences the sensory characteristics (flavor) (Fig. 10.1). The composition and concentration vary according to genetic, environmental and technological factors. The qualitative and quantitative analysis of these compounds is essential for quality control, allowing the detection of changes during storage, processing and marketing. In addition, the identification of these compounds enables the development of new applications, such as in the formulation, improvement and innovation of functional beverages (Felipe & Bicas, 2017).

The chemical class of terpenes stands out due to its diverse structural and functional characteristics. These substances are made up of isoprene units, organized in polymer chains that can be linear or cyclic. In addition, they can present different oxygenated functional groups, such as alcohols, ethers, aldehydes, ketones and lactones. After their formation, terpenes can undergo condensation processes,

Table 10.1 Main VCs in the food industry.

Compounds	Description
Terpenes	Citrus fruits, herbs and spices
Esters	Fruity and sweet flavors
Alcohols	Herbaceous and floral flavors
Aldehydes	Fresh and green flavors
Ketones	Buttery and caramel notes
Carboxylic acids	Sour and rancid flavors
Sulfurated	Pungent and characteristic flavors
Phenolics	Smoky and woody notes

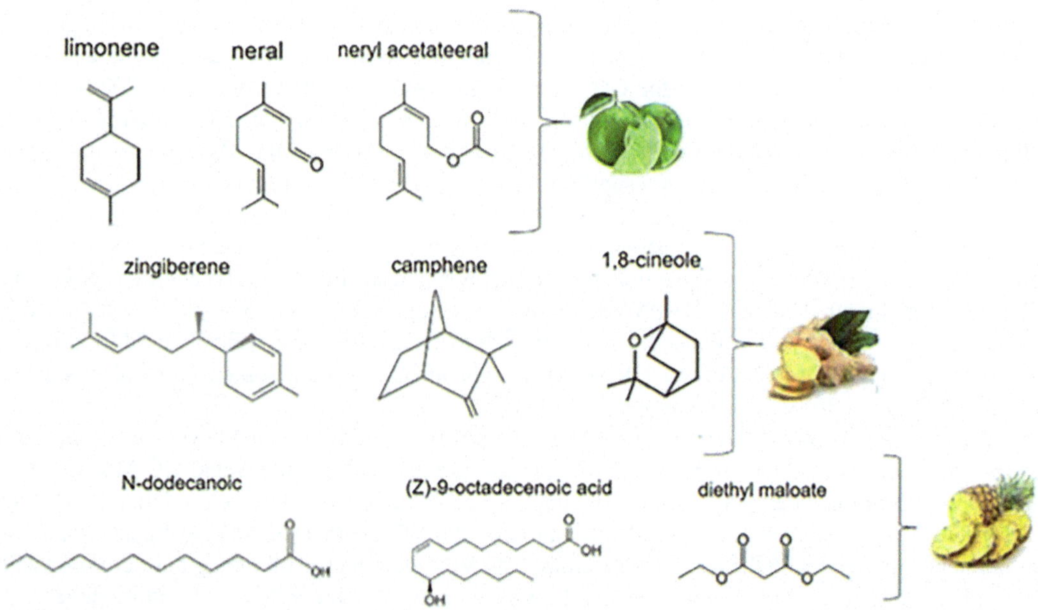

FIGURE 10.1

Structure of some chemical compounds, attributed to the flavor of fruits and roots.

reacting with other chemical groups and producing compounds with more complex structures, such as carbonates, thus expanding their diversity and applications in different areas of food (Fig. 10.1) (Rodrigues et al., 2021; Santos et al., 2020).

Currently, several sample preparation methods are used to extract VCs from food matrices. In addition, several efficient techniques are available for detecting and identifying these compounds. Among the most commonly used procedures in the food industry are *headspace*-solid phase microextraction (*HS*-SPME) and GC-MS (Nascimento et al., 2018). These methodologies have been applied in research focused on different products, such as mixed fruit and vegetable soft drinks (Da Silva et al., 2023), beers (Pina et al., 2022), dairy drinks (da Silva Rocha et al., 2023), black teas (Aminianfar et al., 2024; Liao et al., 2024) and probiotic fruit drinks (Marnpae et al., 2022). Its use is essential for monitoring food quality and safety, ensuring the maintenance of sensory characteristics and meeting market demands.

SPME is a technique that allows the rapid extraction and concentration of volatile and semi-volatile compounds without the need for organic solvents. The process involves the adsorption or absorption of analytes present in solid or liquid matrices onto a fused silica fiber or a fiber coated with a non-volatile polymer. This fiber is coated with a polymeric layer (stationary phase), where the compounds are retained and subsequently desorbed in the chromatographic system (Mariano et al., 2022; Nascimento et al., 2018).

The *HS* technique is widely used in the evaluation of VCs in foods, especially in simple, mixed, and functional beverages. There are two common types of extraction treatment: Static Headspace (SHS) and Dynamic Headspace (DHS). In SHS, it occurs directly in a vial containing the sample equilibrated under static conditions (agitation, time, and temperature). In contrast, DHS consists of purging the vial with a continuous flow of inert gas, removing the analytes, which are then adsorbed by a fiber for subsequent (thermal) desorption in the GC system (Chapko & Seo, 2019; Pua et al., 2022). SHS is widely used for the analysis of volatile and semi-VCs in food samples (Fig. 10.2), mainly due to its ability to capture low molecular weight or highly VCs (Abdelwareth et al., 2021; Pua et al., 2022).

The silica fiber SPME consists of a capillary filament protected by a retractable hypodermic tube, which connects to a device known as a holder, similar to a syringe and widely used in various analyses. Regarding the extraction of VCs, fibers with different types of coating stand out, such as polydimethylsiloxane (PDMS), polydimethylsiloxane/divinylbenzene (PDMS/DVB) and divinylbenzene/carboxen/polydimethylsiloxane (DVB/CAR/PDMS). The selection of the fiber type is determined by the properties of the desired analytes; for example, PDMS-coated fibers are typically used for nonpolar compounds, while PDMS/DVB and DVB/CAR/PDMS fibers are more suitable for polar and VCs (Toffoli & Lanças, 2015; Nascimento et al., 2018).

The study by Da Silva et al. (2023) analyzed the flavor profile of a mixed beverage composed of fruits, roots, and vegetables, using HS-SPME (85 μm polyacrylate-PA fiber) and GC-MS detection. The Kovats retention index (RI_{Kovats}) was obtained for each VC identified in the food matrix. The HS-SPME/GC-MS technique was able to identify a total of 90 VCs, with 15 main constituents, including D-limonene and citral with the largest peak areas. The VCs identified in this study have commercially recognized aftertaste, with functional and biological activities (caprylic acid, D-limonene, etc.) (Fig. 10.3).

VCs can be separated on a chromatographic column and detected by GC with different detectors, with mass spectrometry (MS) being the most widely used. MS fragments the analyte molecules eluted on the column, allowing identification of the components based on their mass-to-charge (m/z) ratios and comparison with reference mass spectral libraries. GC-MS consists of a technique in which a chemically inert gas flow (mobile phase) is used to transport the components of the mixture to be analyzed in the form of gas or vapor, after interacting with a stationary phase conditioned internally in the column. The separation of analytes in mixed beverages should result from the physical and chemical properties of the components and their interaction with the stationary phase inside the column. Coupling allows the separation and elucidation of the most diverse types of mixtures, without the need for analyte standards for identification, which are only necessary for quantification. In

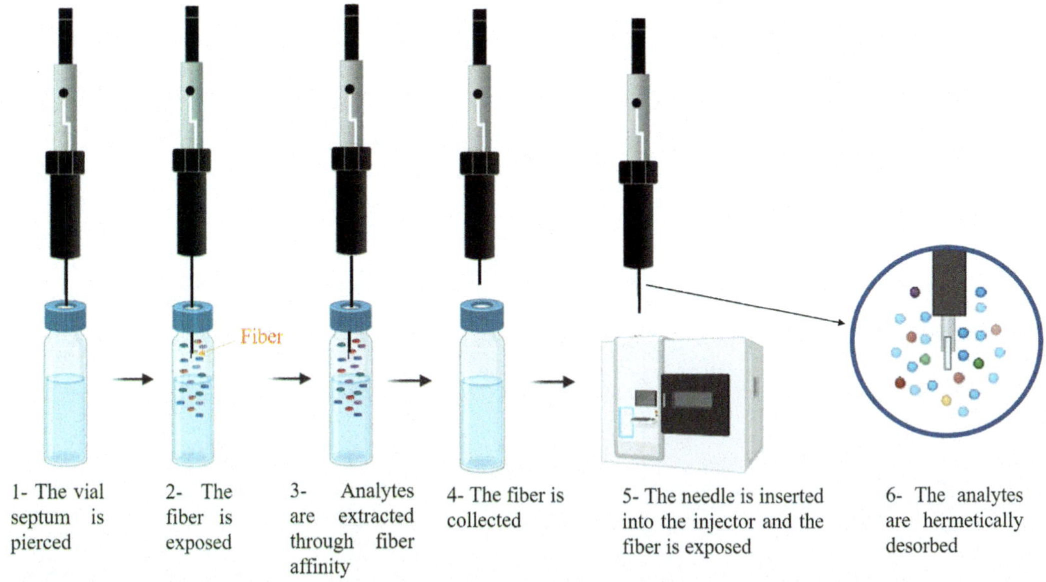

FIGURE 10.2

Representation of the solid or liquid phase microextraction procedure in static headspace mode. (1) Selection of the silica fiber; (2) Insertion of the needle into the vial; (3) Exposure of the silica fiber; (4) Adsorption of analytes (volatile and semivolatile); (5) Reclusion of the fiber in the needle and (6) Desorption of analytes in the gas chromatograph.

addition, coupling the techniques offers easy operation, higher sensitivity, faster analysis and excellent results with high precision and accuracy, as well as moderate cost (Ali et al., 2023; Nascimento et al., 2018), contributing significantly to the quality control and authentication of food products.

The identification of VCs was performed by Da Silva et al. (2023) by GC-MS, in *full scan* acquisition mode (35–400 m/z), allowing a comprehensive analysis of the components presente mixed beverages. National Institute of Standards and Technology Mass Spectral Library -NIST version 2.0 was used for identification of compounds, based on the evaluation of the area percentage and the similarity percentage of the mass spectra obtained, ensuring greater precision in the characterization of the volatiles present in the beverage (Table 10.2).

Some of the VCs identified have great commercial relevance for the food industry and other industrial sectors. According to the Food and Agriculture Organization (FAO), the Food and Drug Administration (FDA) and the Flavor and Extract Manufacturers Association (FEMA), these compounds are recognized as flavorings and/or aroma fixatives, playing an essential role in the formulation of sensory products.

Among these compounds, (Z)-hex-3-enal and (Z)-hex-3-en-1-ol stand out for providing herbaceous, fruity and green leafy notes, and are widely used in the food industry to create natural aromatic profiles in beverages, juices and fresh products. Esters, such as methyl hexanoate and neryl acetate, provide fresh, fruity, citrus and sweet sensations, desirable characteristics in products such as soft drinks, sweets, ice cream and artificial flavors (TGSC, 2021).

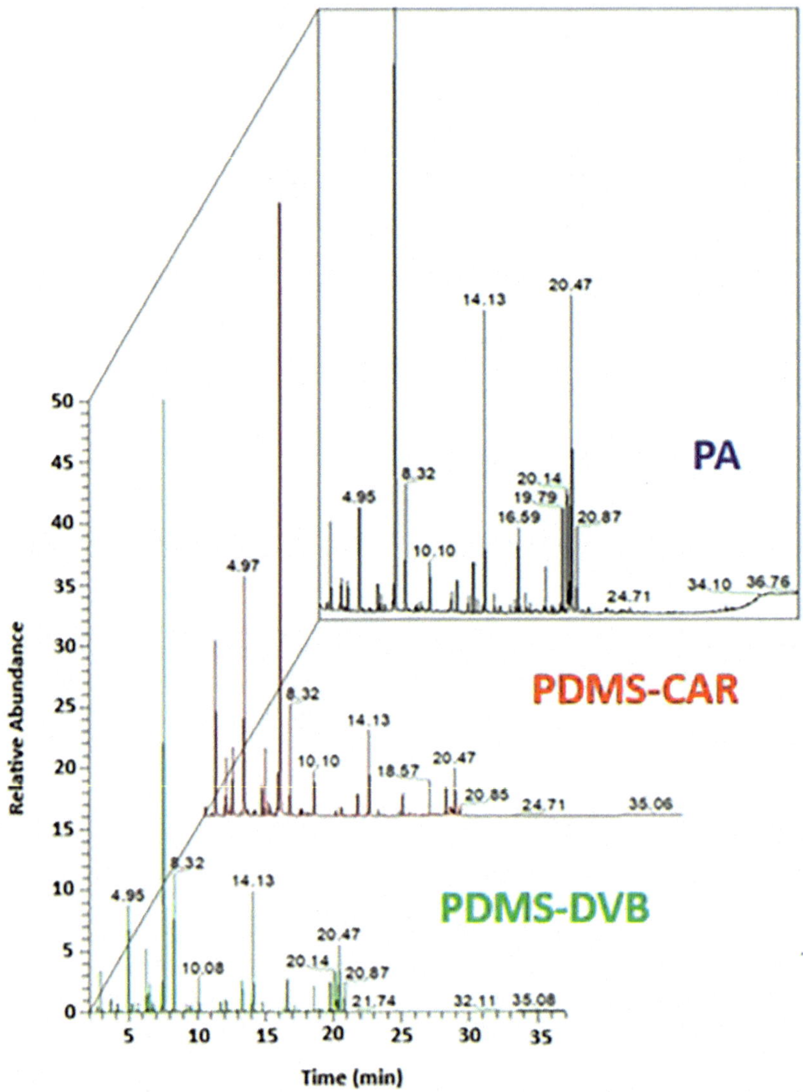

FIGURE 10.3

Comparative overlay of chromatograms of VCs of mixed fruit and vegetable soft drink, using three fibers polyacrylate (PA), polydimethylsiloxane-carboxen (PDMS-CAR) and polydimethylsiloxane-divinylbenzene (PDMS-DVB).

The compound 3-isothiocyanatoprop-1-ene is responsible for the characteristic spicy flavor of mustard, horseradish and wasabi. Isothiocyanates are natural metabolites found in several plants and are widely recognized for their antimicrobial properties. Several studies have confirmed their potent antimicrobial properties. Scientific evidence indicates that these compounds reduce oxygen

Table 10.2 Main, VCs present in mixed fruit and vegetable drinks.

RT (min)	RI $_{Kovats}$	VCs Iupac nomenclature	Ions (m/z)	Flavor characteristics
2.84	801	*cis*-3-Hexenal/(Z)-hex-3-enal	41(100), 39(49), 42(46), 27(44), 55(43), 69(40), 29(26)	Green fatty grassy weedy Fruity apple
3.65	857	*cis*-3-Hexen-1-ol/(Z)-hex-3-en-1-ol	67(100), 41(77), 39(42), 55(41), 82(35)	Green grassy, melon rind Pungent
4.10	887	Allyl isothiocyanate/3-isothiocyanatoprop-1-ene	99(100), 41(63), 39(63), 72(41)	Pungent mustard
4.95	916	Methyl hexanoate/methyl hexanoate	74(100), 87(34), 43(32), 99(20), 41(18)	Fruity pineapple, apricot, fruit Tropical, banana
6.28	934	α-pinene/2,6,6-trimethylbicyclo[3.1.1] hept-2-ene	93(100), 92(37), 91(35), 77(30), 79(25)	Fresh camphor, sweet, pine, earthy, woody
7.56	1036	D-limonene/(4R)-1-methyl-4-prop-1-en-2-Ylcyclohexene	68(100), 93(41), 39(34), 67(33), 41(28)	Citrus, orange, fresh, sweet
8.32	1195	α-terpineol/2-[(1R)-4-methylcyclohex-3-en–yl]propan-2-ol	59(100), 93(69), 121(60), 136(50), 81(39)	Pine, woody, lilac, citrus, floral
10.10	1249	Caprylic acid/octanoic acid	60(100), 73(67), 43(42), 41(27), 55(25)	Fatty, rancid oily vegetable, cheesy
14.13	1254	Citral/(2E)-3,7-dimethylocta-2,6-dienal	69(100), 41(75), 84(28), 39(26), 94(16)	Lemon, sweet
16.59	1365	Neryl acetate/[(2Z)-3,7-dimethylocta-2,6-dienyl] acetate	69(100), 41(62), 43(44), 68(40), 93(40)	Floral, rose, lavender, green waxy
18.57	1435	(E)-α-bergamotene/2,6-dimethyl-6-(4-Methylpent-3-enyl)bicyclo[3.1.1]hept-2-ene	93(100), 41(91), 119(87), 91(48), 69(46)	Woody, warm tea
19.79	-	(E)-Nuciferol/(E)-2-methyl-7-(4-methylphenyl)hept-2-en-1-o	119(100), 132 (63), 105(39), 91(38), 43(30)	Sandalwood oil
20.14	1495	(−)-Zingiberene/2-methyl-5-(6-methylhept-5-en-2-yl)cyclohexa-1,3-diene	93(100), 119(80), 41(45), 69(43), 77(28)	Spice, fresh, ginger
20.36	-	-(Z,E)-α-farnesene/(3Z,6E)-3,7,11-Trimethyldodeca-1,3,6,10-tetraene	41(100), 93(85), 119(64), 69(45), 55(44)	Spice, fresh, ginger
20.47	1604	β-atlantol/6-methyl-2-[(1R)-4-methylcyclohex-3-en-1-yl]hepta-1,5-dien-4-one	119(100), 91(92), 41(86), 105(82), 131(66)	Spice, fresh, ginger

From the study by Da Silva et al. (2023).

consumption by microorganisms, directly interfering in their metabolic processes, inducing oxidative stress. In addition to the food sector, isothiocyanates have potential application in agriculture, being researched a natural alternative for the control of phytopathogenic fungi and agricultural pests, including insects (Vilela et al., 2021; Yadav et al., 2022). Caprylic acid, also known as octanoic acid, is a medium-chain fatty acid characterized by its unpleasant and rancid taste (TGSC, 2021).

Despite this, it has wide industrial and commercial applications, being used in perfumery and in the manufacture of dyes for various sectors. In addition to industrial use, lipid compounds have been studied as more effective applications of medicines, contributing to innovative advances in pharmaceutical science, such as strategic approaches to formulations using lipids as carriers to improve the solubility and bioavailability of medications (Kaiser et al., 2017; Preeti et al., 2023). And studies such as that of Vandenberghe et al. (2017) highlighted its role in clinical nutrition, being an efficient source of energy for malnourished people, premature children and individuals with specific metabolic conditions. D-Limonene[(4R)-1-methyl-4-prop-1-en-2-ylcyclohexene] is a monoterpene widely found in citrus fruits and has several industrial applications and bioactive properties. *D*-Limonene is used as a precursor in the synthesis of compounds such as α-terpineol and perillyl alcohol. Studies demonstrate that the acidic hydration of D-limonene, catalyzed by beta zeolites, results in the formation of α-terpineol, a compound valued in the fragrance and food industries due to its sensory properties and antimicrobial, insecticidal, and antifungal activities (Lin et al., 2013; Zítová et al., 2021). The compound has been investigated as a natural alternative to synthetic pesticides due to its strong insecticidal potential. Research indicates that it is active against several pests, including the German cockroach (*Blattella germanica*), the housefly (*Musca domestica*), the rice weevil (*Sitophilus oryzae*) and the western corn root beetle (*Diabrotica virgifera virgifera*), showing moderate topical toxicity and being (Da Silva et al., 2023) potentiated by the use of piperonyl butoxide (de Brito et al., 2021; Viegas Júnior, 2003).

Some terpenes and terpenoids present in fruits, roots and vegetables have great biological relevance, being related to several therapeutic and pharmacological activities. (E)-nuciferol, for example, acts directly on the central nervous system, being indicated for elevating mood, relieving anxiety, reducing agitation and relaxing the mind, in addition to being widely used in cases of depression (Wu et al., 2021). (E)-α-bergamotene stands out as an important intermediate in the biosynthesis of natural antibiotics and in the formulation of pharmaceutical products due to its antimicrobial potential (Da Silva et al., 2023; Van, 2021; Zhou et al., 2017).

Another terpene with broad biological activity is α-pinene, found in several plant species, and recognized for its anti-inflammatory, antitumor, antimicrobial, bronchodilator, and antioxidant actions (Da Silva et al., 2023; Tolentino et al., 2024). Citral, a compound formed by a mixture of geranial and neral isomers, has calming, hypotensive, and diuretic effects, in addition to enhancing the efficacy of antibiotics against multidrug-resistant bacteria (Gutiérrez-Pacheco et al., 2023).

Other VCs, such as (−)-zingiberene, α-farnesene, and β-atlantol, are mainly responsible for the characteristic flavor of ginger (*Zingiber officinale*). In addition to their sensory importance, several studies highlight the biological properties of these compounds, with anti-inflammatory actions, promoting relief of symptoms associated with inflammatory diseases, such as ulcerative colitis and rheumatoid arthritis. Antioxidant, bactericidal, and antiviral activities are also reported, in addition to the potential effect on controlling blood glucose and cholesterol levels. These volatiles can also act in the treatment of muscle pain, sore throat, cramps, constipation, indigestion, vomiting, fever and infectious diseases (Rufino et al., 2023; Da Silva et al., 2023).

10.2.2 Aldehydes, ketones and higher alcohols in distilled alcoholic beverages

In Brazil, Decree No. 12,709, of October 31, 2025, defines distilled alcoholic beverages as alcoholic beverages obtained by a fermentation process followed by distillation or by lowering the alcoholic content of alcoholic distillate (Brazil, 2025). Distilled alcoholic beverages are food products that represent an important point of sale for the agricultural industry worldwide. This is mainly due to the quality of flavor and the reputation that these products have acquired in the world market over hundreds of years (Christoph & Bauer-Christoph, 2007). Distilled alcoholic beverages represent the largest segment of the market, approximately 36.5% of the global alcoholic beverage market, with a value of US$408.8 billion in 2023. Distilled alcoholic beverages can be marketed with or without aging (Oliveira-Alves et al., 2024).

In the production of distilled alcoholic beverages, the raw material is fermented in a liquid or solid state and then distilled at a high temperature, resulting in a high content of alcohol and other compounds (Oliveira do Nascimento et al., 2022). The minor compounds responsible for the beverage's bouquet are produced in small quantities. These compounds (volatile, semi-volatile or non-volatile) are present in low concentrations and are formed mainly during alcoholic fermentation and selected by the distillation process. Some VCs are already formed even before the fermentation process (Reis & Dos Santos, 2022). For a pleasant and harmonious impression of the beverages (sensory acceptance), all the compounds present need to be in balance with each other. Therefore, all stages of the production process must be carried out carefully, from the selection of the raw material, through crushing and introduction into fermentation, fermentation conditions, distillation and, finally, aging and storage (Stanzer et al., 2023).

More than 500 individual chemical compounds can be present in a distilled alcoholic beverage matrix. This complex mixture contains very different chemical classes, such as alcohols, esters, acids, volatile phenols, sulfur compounds, terpenes, aldehydes, and ketones (Stanzer et al., 2023). The chemical and sensory qualities of distilled alcoholic beverages depend on the presence of secondary compounds, also defined as congeners. Sensory perception depends mainly on the abundance and activity of the odor, thus it is worth noting that some congeners even at trace levels can have a much greater impact on sensory perception than much more abundant congeners. The congener profile of a distilled beverage will depend on the type of raw material used in its preparation and each stage of the process, such as malting, mashing, fermentation, distillation and barrel maturation (Kelly et al., 2023). The presence of volatile congeners formed during the fermentation process depends on the distillation method used (Alcarde et al., 2014). In the production of a purified distillate, to achieve the desired alcohol concentration and congener level, a multiple distillation process using a continuous multi-column system is typically employed (Balcerek et al., 2024). Examples of congeners include aldehydes and ketones (Kelly et al., 2023).

Since the generation of unique aromas in distilled beverages depends on the aging time, the increase or decrease in the concentration of chemical components due to aging directly influences the undesirable characteristics often present in fresh distillates, such as green, spicy and raw. A well-balanced and harmonious flavor is created during long-term storage, where several physical and chemical reactions alter the concentration of compounds in the distilled beverage (Wang et al., 2023). Wood is a rich source of phenolic aldehydes and phenolic ketones, and their concentration depends on the botanical origin, the part of the tree from which it comes and the degree of toasting (burning). In oak and chestnut wood, phenolic aldehydes and phenolic ketones are some of the predominant compounds. Generally, the presence of phenolic compounds confers smoky, woody and vanilla flavors to beverages (Tarko et al., 2023). The highest concentrations of important volatiles such as phenylketones and aldehydes (syringaldehyde, coniferaldehyde, and vanillin) are created by the initiation of lignin degradation through stronger and longer toasting (Kelly et al., 2023). In several distilled beverages, aldehyde concentrations increase significantly during the aging process. Most aldehydes are characterized by fruity, sweet, and fresh odors. During the aging process of distilled beverages, ketones slowly increase due to decarboxylation and β-oxidation of long-chain fatty acids. Several methyl ketones have been used as inherent aging markers of cognacs (Wang et al., 2023).

Aldehydes represent one of the categories of CVs with boiling points up to 260°C (Catalano et al., 2024). Aldehydes are chemically categorized into different groups, including aromatic aldehydes (e.g., benzaldehyde, furfural, and vanillin), highly reactive aldehydes (e.g., alkenals, hydroxyalkenals, and dialdehydes), and saturated aldehydes (e.g., alkanals). Furthermore, there is a subclassification of aldehydes based on the nature of their side chains (El-Maghrabey et al., 2024). The presence of the polarized carbon-oxygen double bond in the structure of aldehydes makes them a particular group of potentially reactive organic compounds. Examples of fatty aldehydes include hexanal, decanal, and octanal, whose odors are, respectively, of fresh apple, orange peel, and citrus, while aromatic aldehydes include benzaldehyde, whose odor is of cinnamon and almond, and terpenoid aldehydes, which include safranal and citral, have aromas of saffron and lemon, respectively (Catalano et al., 2024). Among the aldehydes, acetaldehyde, formaldehyde, furfural, and 5-hydroxymethylfurfural stand out (Oliveira do Nascimento et al., 2023).

A low aldehyde content in beverages is often associated with improved quality (Nascimento et al., 1997). Generally, aldehydes such as acetaldehyde, formaldehyde, acrolein, benzaldehyde and furfural have penetrating and nauseating aromas, being considered undesirable in distilled beverages, and therefore constitute negative notes for aroma and flavor (Alcarde et al., 2014). In the case of distilled alcoholic beverages, acetaldehyde is the major compound that gives the beverage spicy characteristics (Oliveira do Nascimento et al., 2023).

Higher alcohols present in distilled beverages can be partially oxidized to aldehydes and subsequently to short-chain carboxylic acids because yeast requires oxygen for growth at the beginning of fermentation. Aldehydes can also be produced by fatty acids and amino acids from barley malt (Kelly et al., 2023). Aldehydes formed in alcoholic fermentation during the production of distilled beverages are mostly undesirable due to their toxicity, high volatility, and intense odor that impairs the aroma of the beverages. Aldehyde concentrations in distilled beverages should be monitored, since ingestion of high concentrations can cause malaise the next day, headaches, nasal discomfort, malaise, and watery eyes. Aldehyde poisoning can also cause changes in the central nervous system (Reis & Dos Santos, 2022). Numerous critical health problems related to aldehydes have led to the emergence of several methods for their detection, especially for highly volatile aliphatic aldehydes such as formaldehyde, acetaldehyde and furfural (Catalano et al., 2024).

Ketone formation occurs in secondary fermentation or by contamination during the production process (Reis & Dos Santos, 2022). Although methyl ketones such as 2-heptanone, 2-nonanone, 2-undecanone, and 2-tridecanone are probably not the exclusive contributors, they are the main compounds responsible for the rancid character in the beverage (Wang et al., 2023). Some ketones in distilled spirits are classified as vicinal diketones (VDKs) and are key flavor congeners (Kelly et al., 2023). VDKs strongly affect beverage quality, as they are responsible for off-flavors and spoilage markers. Therefore, their determination is necessary both in the production process and in the final beverage (Gomes et al., 2024). VDKs can be produced during amino acid metabolism, with key examples of VDKs that can be produced at this stage being diacetyl (2,3-butanedione) and acetylpropionyl (2,3-pentanedione), which are associated with a pleasant and strong caramel aroma (Kelly et al., 2023). However, when in excess, these compounds can cause an unpleasant taste. During the fermentation process, monitoring diacetyl and acetylpropionyl is crucial. Diacetyl (sweet, buttery) modifies the perception of trigeminal and textural sensations in foods, causes nasal pungency and can be an irritant in high concentrations (Lester et al., 2021).

The main ketone found in alcoholic beverages is acetoin (3-hydroxybutan-2-one). Acetoin is present in almost all alcoholic beverages and is essential for contributing to their flavors. Acetoin is a desirable compound in cachaça and is often found in wines. In low concentrations, it does not affect the sensory quality of the alcoholic beverage; however, in high concentrations, it can modify the bouquet and body of the beverage due to its slightly bitter taste and viscosity (Reis & Dos Santos, 2022).

Insight into the age-related effects of odorant compounds in different types of distilled beverages can be provided by understanding the changes in ketone levels during the aging process, as well as analyzing their aroma characteristics (Wang et al., 2023). Even though they are present in small concentrations in distilled alcoholic beverages, ketones are known to be important in determining the aroma and flavor of the beverage. However, prolonged inhalation of ketones can cause confusion, narcotic effects, irritation of mucous membranes, headaches, and can also lead to coma (Cardoso et al., 2003).

The authenticity of distilled beverages is of utmost importance to consumers, producers, the agri-food sector and government authorities (Oliveira-Alves et al., 2024). The presence of aldehydes and ketones (low molecular weight carbonyls), normally found in alcoholic beverages, is not desirable because some of them are responsible for unpleasant organoleptic properties (Wardencki et al., 2003). Distilled beverages represent a matrix with a complex composition, considered difficult to analyze, where gas chromatography techniques are usually chosen as the method of analysis (Wiśniewska et al., 2015). Although aldehydes and ketones in different types of distilled beverages can be analyzed by HPLC, a derivatization step is necessary (Oliveira do Nascimento et al., 2023). Among the various types of gas chromatographic analysis used in quality control in the production of distilled beverages, gas chromatography coupled to mass spectrometry (GC/MS) and gas chromatography coupled to flame ionization detector (GC/FID) have been used as traditional analysis techniques for VOCs. However, the analysis of VOCs in distilled beverages in GC-FID generates some problems, since direct injection (simple and easy) is the technique used to analyze the samples (Fig. 10.4). The presence of large amounts of water ends up reducing the useful life of the chromatographic column, resulting in signal disturbances in the FID. In addition, the liner becomes dirty quickly, a fact due to the heating of the organic matter present in the sample (sugar compounds) (Oliveira do Nascimento et al., 2022).

GC/MS has rapidly established itself as an essential analytical technique for detecting VOCs in commercial beverages. In GC, HS analysis is the most effective technique for evaluating VOCs, and can be performed in three ways: static, dynamic, and headspace -SPME. The determination of VOCs using static HS to determine VOCs has several advantages, such as short sample preparation and analysis times, allowing continuous sampling (Petre et al., 2024). The ideal is to protect people and the environment from the potentially harmful consequences that can be caused by activities that occur in analytical chemistry laboratories, such as the use of organic solvents and reagents (El-Maghrabey et al., 2024). Thus, HS-SPME is a solvent-free technique that circumvents many problems and

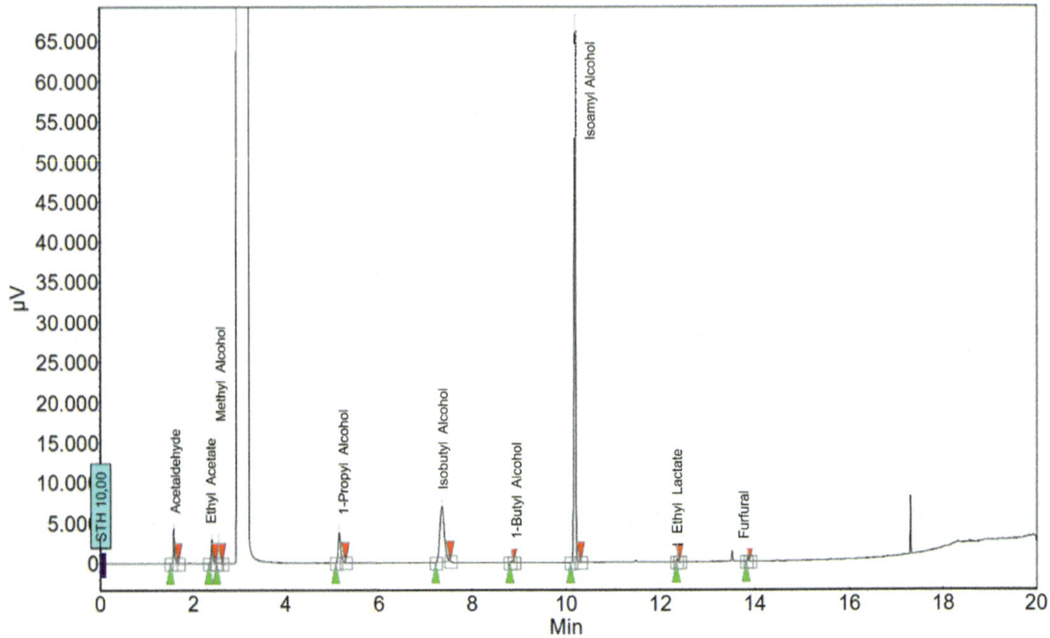

FIGURE 10.4

Qualitative and quantitative chromatogram of honey spirit by gas chromatography-flame ionization detector (GC-FID).

provides better precision, accuracy, and more information on the volatile composition of beverage samples. The DVB/CAR/PDMS (divinylbenzene-carboxene-polydimethylsiloxane) fiber is usually chosen because it combines the characteristics of three different stationary phases, being able to adsorb a wide range of CVs with different polarities, such as alcohols, esters, terpenes, aldehydes and ketones, better than other fibers (Kokoti et al., 2023).

Thus, the identification of VOCs that arise during the fermentation, distillation and storage processes of distilled alcoholic beverages is of great importance, not only to determine the flavor characteristics of the beverage, but also to detect illicit beverages and identify anomalies that are indicative of inconsistent manufacturing practices (Dragone et al., 2009).

Duan et al. (2024) used the HS–SPME–GC–MS analysis method to determine VCs in spine grape brandies aged with wood chips from different species. The research shows that 38 VCs were found, among them, isoamyl alcohol, isobutanol, 1-propanol and ethyl acetate. A study conducted by Xiang et al. (2020) characterized odor-active compounds in samples of the head, heart and tail fractions of fresh distilled grapevine wine (Vitis davidii Foex), through the gas chromatography-olfactometry-mass spectrometry (GC-O-MS) technique associated with Aroma Extract Dilution Analysis (AEDA). These two techniques combined have allowed significant advances in the identification of the main odor-active compounds responsible for the general odor or unpleasant taste in alcoholic beverages. Although there are numerous VCs in beverages, only a small number of odor-active compounds are detected by the human brain. The AEDA results showed the presence of 34, 45 and 37 odor-active compounds in the head, heart and tail fractions, respectively. Furthermore, 20, 22 and 17 quantified compounds, respectively, presented odor activity (OAV) values > 1.

Gas Chromatography using Flame Ionization Detector (GC-FID) has been the most common technique for analyzing higher alcohols in distilled beverages, such as brandy. Fig. 10.4 shows the chromatogram obtained by GC-FID in the analysis of honey brandy. According to the Regulation EU 2019/787 EU Commission (2019), honey brandy can be characterized as a distilled beverage that is produced exclusively by fermentation and distillation of honey mash, whose distillate presents the sensory characteristics of the raw material used. The minimum alcoholic content of honey brandy is 35%, and there may be no addition of alcohol, diluted or pure, and it is free of flavorings, with the exception of caramel coloring. It may be sweetened with honey to improve the final flavor of the product and may not exceed more than 20 g/L of sweeteners expressed as invert sugar. Since European legislation does not provide details on the physical and chemical characteristics of honey brandy, it is necessary to compare them with sugar cane brandy, typically called *Cachaça* in Brazil. Legislation establishes that sugar cane brandy is a beverage with an alcohol content of 38%–54% by volume, at 20°C, obtained by lowering the alcohol content of simple alcoholic distillate or by distilling fermented must, and will be named after the raw material of origin, and sugars may be added (Brazil, 2008, 2011, 2022, 2025). The Standards of Identity and Quality of sugar cane brandy are established in Brazil by MAPA Ordinance N°. 539/2022, as shown in Table 10.3.

10.2.3 Food additives

Food additives are substances incorporated during the preparation or processing of food to modify or preserve sensory characteristics, such as flavor, aroma, texture and appearance. Additives can be classified into categories such as acidity regulators, colorants, preservatives, sweeteners and others (WHO, 2023).

Table 10.3 MAPA Ordinance No. 539/2022– establishes the standards of identity and quality of sugar cane brandy.

Parameter	Min	Max
Alcohol content, expressed in %, in v/v, at 20,0°C	38,0	54,0
Volatile acidity, expressed as acetic acid, in mg/100 mL of anhydrous alcohol	-	150
Total esters, expressed as ethyl acetate, in mg/100 mL of anhydrous alcohol	-	200
Total aldehydes, in acetaldehyde, in mg/100 mL of anhydrous alcohol	-	30
Sum of furfural and hydroxymethylfurfural, in mg/100 mL of anhydrous alcohol	-	5
Sum of isobutyl (2-methyl propanol), isoamyl (2-methyl-1-butanol and 3-methyl-1-butanol) and n-propyl (1-propanol) alcohols, in mg/100 mL of anhydrous alcohol	-	360
Sum of congener coefficient, in mg/100 mL of anhydrous alcohol	200	650
Total sugars (for cachaça), in g/L (expressed as glucose)	-	≤6,0
Copper	-	5,0

Brazil. (2022). MAPA Ordinance N°. 539, of December 26, 2022. Official Gazette of the Union. https://www.gov.br/mdic/pt-br/assuntos/reg/boas-praticas-regulatorias/selo-de-boas-praticas-regulatorias/2022/selo-ouro/mapa-portaria-mapa-ndeg-539-2022, no date.

Sweeteners can be derived from plant biomass (saccharides), and are classified as natural or synthetic. The analysis of saccharides (monosaccharides, disaccharides and polysaccharides) as totais carbohydrates is commonly performed using UV-Vis methods (Sewwandi et al., 2020). However, these methods detect only monosaccharides, requiring sample hydrolysis steps beforehand (Kurzyna-Szklarek et al., 2022).

According to the World Health Organization (WHO), the Recommended Daily Intake (RDI) of sugar is 25 g (WHO, 2015). Therefore, it is important to control the levels of these compounds in foods. Sewwandi et al. (2020) analyzed the total sugar content of fruit nectar samples by comparing titrimetric and UV-visible spectrophotometric methods. According to the authors, there was no significant difference between the results of the two analytical methods studied ($\alpha = 0.05$). The average sugar content in the samples ranged from 18.38 to 9.17 g/100 mL, therefore, the recommended consumption of approximately 100 mL/day of fruit nectar.

The determination of specific saccharide levels in beverages is typically conducted using high-performance liquid chromatography (HPLC), with ion-exchange (IC) or reversed-phase (RP) columns employed for carbohydrate separation. Detectors such as refractive index detection (RID) or evaporative light scattering detector (ELSD) facilitate the identification of saccharides such as sucrose, glucose, fructose, and rafinose (Araujo Filho et al., 2023; Araujo Filho et al., 2023; Li et al., 2007) used HPLC with an infrared refractive index detector (RID-10A) and a Kromasil NH_2 column (4.6×150 mm; 5 μm particle size) to determine the sugar content (sucrose, glucose, fructose, and raffinose) in fermented beverage samples (kombucha and kefir). The method used a mobile phase consisting of 85% acetonitrile and 15% MilliQ water, with a flow rate of 1 mL/min.

Liquid chromatography remains the most widely used approach, with the main distinction being the integration of mass spectrometry (MS) detectors for the identification of synthetic sweeteners such as acesulfame, alitame, aspartame, cyclamate, dulcoside A, neohesperidin DC, neotame, neohesperidin dihydrochalcone (NHDC), rebaudioside A, rebaudioside C, saccharin, steviol, steviolbioside, stevioside, and sucralose (Ferrer & Thurman, 2010; Lorenzo et al., 2015; Ordoñez et al., 2015). When comparing mass spectrometry detectors, triple quadrupole (TSQ) achieves a higher limit of quantification (LOD, 0.05–13.56 μg/L) than time-of-flight (TOF) systems (0.20–5.00 mg/L). Furthermore, other detectors such as charged aerosol detection (CAD) and photodiode array (PDA), as well as alternative analytical systems such as capillary electrophoresis (CE) and direct analysis real-time (DART) QTRAP mass spectrometry, are also reported in the literature (Cheng et al., 2024; Kubica et al., 2016; Le et al., 2017).

Acidity regulators are essential ingredients for maintaining the balance between sweetness and acidity in beverages (Tireki, 2021). They are commonly measured using acid value through titrimetric methods. However, fermentation processes during beverage preparation can produce various acids, and identification and quantification of these compounds are typically performed using liquid chromatography. This method employs ion exchange or reversed-phase columns, along with detectors such as conductivity detectors (CD) or PDA, to measure organic acids such as acetic, citric, formic, fumaric, galacturonic, gluconic, glycolic, isocitric, lactic, malic, propionic, pyruvic, quinic, shikimic, and succinic, as well as anions such as chloride, bromide, bromate, nitrite, nitrate, sulfate, phosphate, and oxalate (Andrés et al., 2015; Uzhel et al., 2021). Furthermore, other analytical systems reported in the literature include capillary zone electrophoresis with indirect UV detection (CZE-UV), desorption electrospray ionization mass spectrometry (DESI-MS), and Fourier transform ion cyclotron resonance (FTICR) tandem mass spectrometry (MS/MS) (Yoshikawa et al., 2011).

Preservatives are substances that help maintain the characteristics of beverages, such as color, aroma, and flavor. Some acids used as acidity regulators also function as preservatives, including acetic, citric, malic, and formic acids. In addition, other additives such as sorbic and benzoic acids can be incorporated. Antioxidant compounds are also used as preservatives to neutralize free radicals, examples being ascorbic acid, butylated hydroxyanisole (BHA), butylated hydroxytoluene (BHT), propyl gallate (PG), gallic acid (GA), caffeic acid (CA), and tertiary butylhydroquinone (TBHQ). Certain beverages rich in phenolic compounds naturally contain phenolic acids, flavonoids, and tannins, which act as naturais antioxidants (de Araújo et al., 2021). Preservative analysis depends on the compound class: organic acids are typically analyzed using IC-HPLC-CD or RP-HPLC-PDA, while preservatives such as ascorbic, sorbic, and benzoic acids are analyzed via RP-HPLC with a UV-Vis (UV) detector (Adam et al., 2012; Das et al., 2024). Synthetic phenolic compounds such as BHA, BHT, and TBHQ have been analyzed using RP-HPLC-UV or gas chromatography coupled with tandem mass spectrometry (GC-MS/MS) (Zhu et al., 2023; Žnideršič et al., 2019). Natural phenolic acids such as GA, CA, and PG are typically analyzed with RP-HPLC-UV, while flavonoids and tannins are analyzed via ultra-high-performance liquid chromatography (UPLC) with MS/MS detection or high-resolution mass spectrometry (HRMS) (Grassino et al., 2024; Huang et al., 2024; Lin et al., 2024; Yu et al., 2022). Alternative analytical methods reported in the literature include capillary zone electrophoresis with UV detection (CZE-UV), paper spray mass spectrometry (PS-MS), and flow injection analysis with UV-VIS photometric detection (FIA-UV) (de Faria et al., 2020; Yu et al., 2018).

Food dyes are substances with chromophore groups that produce color in the ultraviolet and visible region. Whether of natural or synthetic origin, dyes have acceptable daily intake (ADI) values stablished by the Joint FAO/WHO Expert Committee on Food Additives (JECFA) (Pôrto & Arisseto-Bragotto, 2024), and must be monitored to allow safe intake. RP-HPLC-UV or RP-HPLC-PDA systems are the most widely used in the determination of dyes in food, and it is possible to monitor up to 40 dyes at wavelengths of 450, 490, 520 and 620 nm with an analysis time of 20 min (Tamer et al., 2024). However, with the prohibition of some substances, sample preconcentration techniques have shown promise to achieve lower detection limits, such as solid phase extraction (SPE) or the use of high-resolution mass detectors (UPLC-HRMS) (Chen et al., 2022).

Extraction techniques used for additive analysis are crucial to achieving the required quantification limits, with multiple methods employed to access compounds of interest. New techniques have been developed to facilitate analysis using simpler systems; however, limitations persist due to matrix interference in samples and detector sensitivity. Among the available options, MS detectors stand out, as they often eliminate the need for extensive extraction and cleanup steps in sample preparation (Table 10.4).

10.2.4 Fatty acids in fermented beverages

Fatty acids (FAs) can be defined as macromolecules of lipid origin. They are part of a group of important substances in the human diet known as saturated and unsaturated fats. Structurally, they have short or long chains, have single bonds or some double bonds, between some carbon atoms. FAs with no double bonds are referred to as saturated, with one double bond as monounsaturated, and with two or more double bonds as polyunsaturated fatty acids (Young, 1985).

FAs are considered the main components of the biological membrane of animals, plants and microorganisms, in the form of phospholipids and glycolipids. In addition, they circulate in the blood in the form of free FAs such as triacylglycerols. Free FAs can be processed into signaling compounds

Table 10.4 Conventional and unconventional methods of analysis of additives in beverages.

Additive class	Compound	Sample	Sample preparation	System	References
Conventional methods of analysis of food additives					
Sweetness	Total sugar level	Fruit nectar	Samples centrifuged and diluted	UV-visible Spectrophotometer	Sewwandi, et al. (2020)
Sweetness	Aspartame, Saccharin, and Sucralose	Soft drinks and liquid syrups	Diluted by deionized water and filtered through 0.2 μm filters	RP-HPLC-TOF/MS	Ferrer and Thurman (2010)
		Water	Solid-phase Extration Cartridge (SPE)		
Sweetness	Acesulfame, alitame, aspartame, cyclamate, Neohespiridine dihydrochalcone, neotame, saccharin, stevioside and sucralose	Sparkling soft drinks, nectars, and mixed drinks	Ultrasonic bath, diluted by deionized water and filtered	RP-LC-MS/MS	Ordoñez et al. (2015)
Sweetness	Aspartame, Neohesperidine dihydrochalcone, neotame, Potassium acesulfame, saccharin, Sodium cyclamate and sucralose	Soft and powdered drinks, juices, teas, soy beverages, dairy-based drinks, beers, and spirit alcoholic drinks	Ultrasonic bath, diluted by deionized water and filtered	RP-UPLC-DAD RP-LC-MS/MS	Lorenzo et al. (2015)
Sweetness	Alitame, aspartame, cyclamate, dulcoside A, Neohespiridine dihydrochalcone, neotame, Potassium acesulfame, rebaudioside A, rebaudioside C, saccharin, steviol, steviolbioside, stevioside, and sucralose	Alcoholic drinks, non-alcoholic drinks and instant drink powders	Ultrasonic bath, spiked w/IS, diluted by mobile phase and centrifuged at 7000 rpm	RP-LC-MS/MS HILIC-MS/MS	Kubica et al. (2016)
Sweetness	Acesulfame potassium, alitame, aspartame, Erythritol, Mannitol, neotame, saccharin sodium salt, Sodium cyclamate, Sorbitol, stevioside, sucralose and Xylitol	Sugar-free drinks	Ultrasonic bath, diluted by deionized water and filtered through 0.45 μm Nylon filters	RP-UHPLC-CAD	Cheng et al. (2024)
Sweetness and acidulants	Fructose, glucose, raffinose, sucrose, acetic acid, citric acid, D-Glucuronic acid lactic acid	Cashew nut beverage	Filtration in PVDF 0.45 and 0.22 μm filters	HPLC-RID/UV-Vis	Araujo Filho et al. (2023)
Acidulants	Acetic acid, citric acid, formic acid, fumaric acid, galacturonic acid, gluconic acid, glycolic acid, isocitric acid, lactic acid, malic acid, Oxalic acid, propionic acid, pyruvic acid, quinic acid, shikimic acid and succinic acid	Mango, blueberry, grape juices, red wine and light beer	Ultrasonic bath, diluted by deionized water and filtered through 0.45 μm Polyamide filters	IC-LC-CD	Uzhel et al. (2021)

Sweetness and acidulants	Fructose, glucose, Lactose, sucrose, citric acids, L-malic acids and L-Tartaric acids	Milk- and soy-fruit juice beverages	Solid-phase Extration Cartridge (SPE)	RP-HPLC-RID	Andrés et al. (2015)
Preservative	Benzoic acid, sorbic acid, and Methylparaben	Beverage, cake, ketchup and therapeutic products	Ultrasonic bath, diluted by deionized water and filtered through 0.45 μm PTFE filters	RP-HPLC-PDA	Das et al. (2024)
Preservative	L-ascorbic acid	Ice tea, orange, apple and mixed juice	Microextraction by packed sorbent (MEPS)	RP-HPLC-UV	Adam et al. (2012)
Preservative	BHA, BHT and TBHQ	Mineral water, cola, orange juice and rice wine	Ultrasonic bath, diluted by deionized water, centrifuged at 4000 rpm and filtered through 0.45 μm PTFE filters	RP-HPLC-UV	Zhu et al. (2023)
Preservative	Methyl paraben, ethyl paraben, propyl paraben, Butyl paraben, TBHQ, NBBS, TBEP, BHT, BHA and dBHT	Alcoholic beverages and vinegars	SPME	GC-MS/MS	Žnideršič et al. (2019)
Preservative	(−)-catechin gallate, (−)-epicatechin gallate, (−)-epicatechin, (−)-epigallocatechin gallate, (−)-epigallocatechin, (−)-gallocatechin gallate, (−)-gallocatechin, (+)-catechin, caffeine, citric acid, gallic acid, malic acid, quinic acid theogallin	Black tea	Tea infusion (water extraction), lyophilized and extracted w/methanol 70%	RP-UPLC-MRM-MS	Yu et al. (2022)
Preservative	Caffeic acid, caffeine, chlorogenic acid, ferulic acid, gallic acid and p-coumaric acid	Coffee	SPME	GC-MS RP-UPLC-MS/MS	Grassino et al. (2024)
Dyes	Azo Rubine, Ponceau 4R, Quinoline Yellow, Tartrazine and yellow orange S	Soft drinks		RP-HPLC-UV-Vis	García-Falcón and Simal-Gándara (2005)
Dyes	Acid blue 1, acid green 9, acid red 52, acid violet 7, Allura red AC, Amaranth, Amido black 10B, Azorubine, Benzyl violet 4B, Brilliant	Soft drinks	Ultrasonic bath, Ethanol removed in hot plate and pH adjusted to 3	RP-LC-PAD	Yoshioka and Ichihashi (2008)

Continued

Table 10.4 Conventional and unconventional methods of analysis of additives in beverages.—cont'd

Additive class	Compound	Sample	Sample preparation	System	References
	black PN, Brilliant blue FCF, Chrysoine, Eosine, Erythrosine, fast green FCF, fast red E, fast yellow AB, green S, Indigotine, Martius yellow, Naphthol yellow S, orange G, orange I, orange II, orange RN, Patent blue V, Phloxine B, Ponceau 2R, Ponceau 3R, Ponceau 4R, Ponceau 6R, Ponceau SX, Quinoline yellow, Red 10 B, Red 2G, Rose Bengal, Sunset yellow FCF, Tartrazine, Uranine and Yellow 2G				
Dyes	Allura red AC, Brillant blue FCF, Erythrosine B, Patent blue V, Ponceau 4R, Sunset yellow and Tartrazine	Tablets-medicine, syrups-medicine, confectionaries and beverages	Dissolved/diluted by deionized water and filtered through 0.45 μm PTFE filters	RP-HPLC-PAD	Tamer et al. (2024)
Dyes	Allura red AC, Amaranth, Brilliant blue FCF, Erythrosine, Sunset yellow FCF and Tartrazine	Juice drinks, breakfast cereals, frozen desserts, ice cream cones, soft drinks, frostings & icings, fruit snacks/candy, decoration chips, water enhancers, and powder drink mix	Homogenized, sieved and vortexed	RP-HPLC-PAD	Lehmkuhler et al. (2022)
Unconventional methods of analysis of food additives					
Sweetness and acidulants	Acesulfame potassium, aspartame, cyclamate sodium, acetic acid, Butyric acid, citrate sodium, formic acid, Oxalic acid, propionic acid and Tartaric acid	Orange juice, wine, alcohol, beverages, vinegar, coffee sachets, tea bags, black bean sweet soup	Ultrasonic bath, diluted by deionized water and filtered through 0.45 μm PTFE filters	CE-C^4D	Le et al. (2017)
Sweetness	Fructose, glucose and sucrose	Carbonated drink and fruit juice	Ultrasonic bath, diluted by deionized water and filtered through 0.45 μm Nylon filters	IC-HPLC-ELSD	Li et al. (2007)

Acidulants and preservatives	Acetate, Adipate, Ascorbate, citrate, Gluconate, Lactate, Malate, Succinate, Tartrate, Benzoate, Dehydroacetate, Propionate and Sorbate	Red, white wine, health drink, yogurt and pickled ginger	Diluted by deionized water, centrifuged at 1200 g and filtered through 0.45 μm filters	CZE-UV	Yoshikawa et al. (2011)
Preservatives	Ascorbic acid and benzoic acid	Fruit juice	Ultrasonic bath, diluted by deionized water, centrifuged at 3000 rpm and filtered through 0.22 μm filters	PS-MS	Yu et al. (2018)
Preservatives	Ascorbic acid	Multivitamin drink, three milk, fermented milk and chocolate milk	Diluted by supporting electrolyte solution and buffer	Cyclic voltammetry FIA-AMP UFLC-UV-Vis	de Faria et al. (2020)

Column type: RP, *reversed phase;* IC, *ionic-exchange chromatography. Analysis system:* CE, *capillary electrophoresis;* CZE, *capillary zone electrophoresis;* DART, *direct analysis real-time;* DESI, *desorption electrospray ionization;* FIA, *flow injection analysis;* FTICR, *fourier transform ion cyclotron resonance;* GC, *gas chromatography;* HILIC, *hydrophilic interaction chromatography;* HPLC, *high performance liquid chromatography;* LC, *liquid chromatography;* PS, *paper spray;* UFLC, *ultra fast liquid chromatography;* UPLC, *ultra performance liquid chromatography. Detectors:* AMP, *amperometric detector;* C4D, *capacitively coupled contactless conductivity detection;* CAD, *charged aerosol detection;* CD, *conductivity detectors;* ELSD, *evaporative light scattering detector;* HRMS, *high resolution mass spectrometer;* MRM, *multiple reaction monitoring;* MS, *Mass spectrometer detector;* PAD, *pulsed amperometric detection;* PDA, *photodiode array;* RID, *refractive index detection;* TOF/MS, *time of fly mass spectrometer;* UV or UV-VIs, *ultrviolet-visible detector.*

such as eicosanoids, acting as an energy reserve in the form of adipose tissue, and can be considered a good source of nutrients with high caloric value and an essential source of energy (Strzałkowska et al., 2010). In addition, they can influence the structure, stability, flavor, aroma, storage quality, sensory and visual characteristics of foods and beverages, especially fermented beverages. Fermented beverages are beverages that undergo a fermentation process, a traditional method initially used for food preservation and storage (Yuan et al., 2024).

Fermented beverages can be non-dairy, such as those made from fruit, or dairy-based beverages such as kefir and yogurt. They can contain different types of fatty acids, such as saturated, unsaturated, monounsaturated and polyunsaturated. Fermented fruit or vegetable juices have a distinct flavor. In the fruit fermentation process, FAs are produced through the hydrolysis of fats, carbohydrates and other compounds present in the raw material (Al-Madboly et al., 2023).

The FA profile is commonly determined using GC-FID. The technique consists of analyzing VCs, in which the analyte present in the gaseous state is burned in a hydrogen and oxygen flame, producing ions that are collected, forming an electric current that generates the signal. GC-FID is a robust, easy-to-use system with high sensitivity for organic compounds, such as fatty acids.

Kefir is a beverage produced from the fermentation of pasteurized or boiled milk. The raw material used in the production of kefir significantly affects the levels of saturated fatty acids produced in the fermentation process. A study developed by Arda et al. (2025) analyzed fatty acids in kefir samples produced with sheep's milk compared to kefir produced with cow's milk. In the study, the fatty acids of the oil samples converted to methyl esters were analyzed in a GC-FID instrument (Shimadzu GC-2025) and an HP-Innovax capillary column (poly 5% diphenyl/95% dimethyl siloxane phase; 30 m × 0.25 mm × 0.25 μm). The results presented by the authors showed that the omega-6/omega-3 ratios in sheep's milk kefirs ranged from 1.46 to 1.67, while significantly higher values between 5.57 and 7.54 were found in cow's milk kefirs. No significant difference was observed in the omega-6/omega-3 ratio of sheep's milk kefirs produced with grains or starter culture. The results showed that the fatty acid profile and conjugated linoleic acid content found in kefir reduce the synthesis of cholesterol and triglycerides, actinga protector against neurodegenerative diseases.

Another fermented beverage well known for its nutritional value is yogurt. The fatty acid composition of yogurt depends on the type of milk used in its production (Sharma & Ramanathan, 2023). Fruit-based yogurts are widely available and varied dairy products on the market. Yogurt consists of the product obtained by coagulating milk through fermentation by the action of bacteria, which is transformed into lactic acid (Nguyen et al., 2018). The category of concentrated yogurts, which have higher total solids and protein contents, stands out among the yogurts available worldwide, named differently according to their origin (Aryana & Olson, 2017; Uduwerella et al., 2017; Pinto, 2022) identified fatty acids in six fruit pulp yogurt samples. The fatty acid analysis was performed using a gas chromatograph with a flame ionization detector GC-FID (Focus CG-Finnigan model). To separate cis and trans fatty acids, they used a capillary column SP-2560 (poly biscyanopropyl siloxane, 100 m × 0.25 mm × 0.2 μm). The results obtained showed approximately 18 different fatty acids present in the six (6) samples evaluated, ranging from 0.01% to 0.89% (Fig. 10.5).

Sharma and Ramanathan (2023) evaluated the difference in the fatty acid profile present in cow and goat yogurts using GC-FID. The FA profile revealed 38 FA in yogurt produced with goat milk and 31 FA in yogurt produced with cow milk. Goat yogurt had a higher content of myristic acid, in addition to polyunsaturated fatty acids and conjugated linoleic acid, the relative content of capric acid (C10:0) and lauric acid (C12:0) was 75% and 45% higher, respectively. The ratio of n-6/n-3 fatty acids in goat

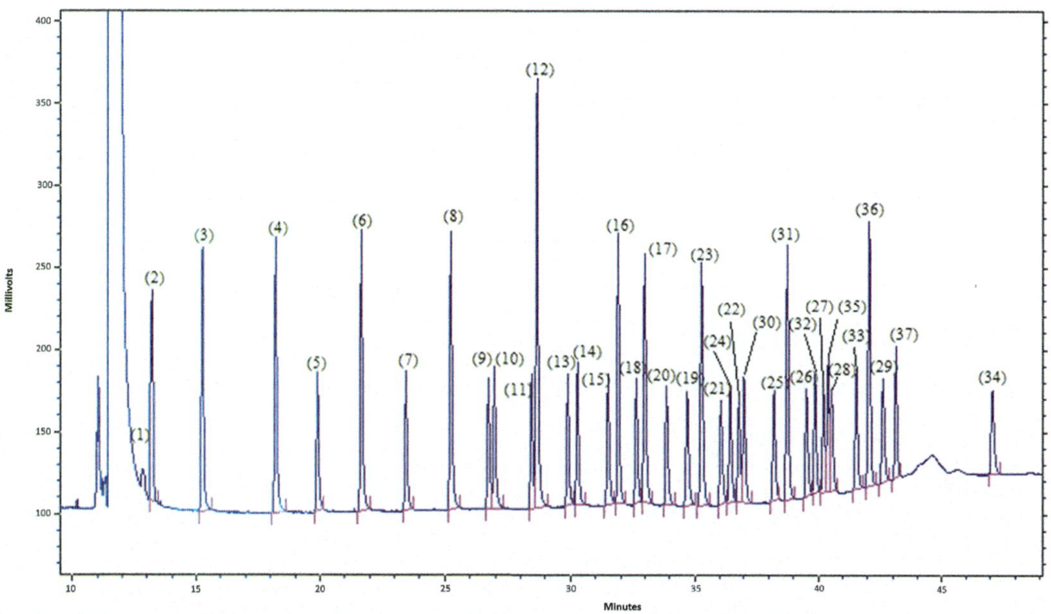

1. Butyric acid methyl ester (C4:0)	**20.** Linolelaidic acid methyl ester (C18:2n6t)
2. Caproic acid methy0)	**21.** y- Linolenic acid methyl ester (C18:3n6)
3. Caprylic acid methyl ester (C8:0)	**22.** α - Linolenic acid methyl ester (C18:3n3)
4. Capric acid methyl ester (C10:0)	**23.** Arachidic acid methyl ester (C20:0)
5. Undecanoic acid methyl ester (11:0)	**24.** *cis*-11- Eicosenoic acid methyl ester (C20:1n9)
6. Lauric acid methyl ester (C12:0)	**25.** *cis*-11,14- Eicosadienoic acid methyl ester (C20:2)
7. Tridecanoic acid methyl ester (C13:0)	**26.** *cis*-8,11,14- Eicosatrienoic acid methyl ester (C20:3n6)
8. Myristic acid methyl ester (C14:0)	**27.** *cis*-11,14,17- Eicosatrienoic acid methyl ester (C20:3n3)
9. Myristoleic acid methyl ester (C14:1)	**28.** Arachidonic acid methyl ester (C20:4n6)
10. Pentadecanol acid methyl ester (C15:0)	**29.** *cis*-5,8,11,14,17- Eicosapentaenoic acid methyl ester (C20:5n3)
11. *cis*-10 Pentadecenoic acid methyl ester (C15:1)	**30.** Heneicosanoic acid methyl ester (C21:0)

FIGURE 10.5

Chromatogram of the standard solution of FAME MIX 37-component fatty acids.

12. Palmitic acid methyl ester (C16:0)	**31.** Behenic acid methyl ester (C22:0)
13. Palmitoleic acid methyl ester (C16:1)	**32.** Erucic acid methyl ester (C22:1n9)
14. Heptadecanoic acid methyl ester (C17:0)	**33.** *cis*-13,16- Docosadienoic acid methyl ester (C22:2)
15. *cis*-10 Heptadecanoic acid methyl ester (C17:1)	**34.** *cis*-4,7,10,13,16,19-Docosahexaenaic acid methyl ester (C22:6n3)
16. Stearic acid methyl ester (C18:0)	**35.** Tricosanoic acid methyl ester (C23:0)
17. Oleic acid methyl ester (C18:1n9c)	**36.** Lignoceric acid methyl ester (C24:0)
18. Elaidic acid methyl ester (C18:1n9t)	**37.** Nervonic acid methyl ester o (C24:1n9)
19. Linoleic acid methyl ester (C18:2n6c)	

FIGURE 10.5

Cont'd

yogurt (4.13) was close to the recommended ratio in the human diet (2:1 to 4:1). Cow yogurt contained erucic acid, nervosoc acid, docosadienoic acid, docosahexaenoic acid, *trans*-10, *cis*-12 conjugated linoleic acid and *cis*-9, *cis*-11 conjugated linoleic acid. Goat yogurt contained higher relative content of medium-chain saturated fatty acids (0.31–8.05 g $100\ g^{-1}$) than cow yogurt (0.207–4.59 g $100\ g^{-1}$), while the relative content of long-chain saturated fatty acids was almost similar in cow yogurt (0.03–28.54 g $100\ g^{-1}$) and goat yogurt (0.04–28.78 g $100\ g^{-1}$) samples. Principal component analysis revealed a clear separation between groups depending on the type of milk used to prepare the yogurt.

10.2.5 Analysis of bioactives

Bioactive compounds have several properties, including antioxidant, antimicrobial, anti-inflammatory, antidiabetic and immunomodulatory action, contributing to the prevention and treatment of several conditions. The importance of quantifying and identifying bioactives is related to their potential health benefits, as well as to assessing the quality and preference of a food by the consumer market.

In vitro methods are widely used for the analysis of bioactive compounds in foods in general, such as beverages, among which include total phenolic content (TPC), total flavonoid content (TFC), total anthocyanins content (TAC) and antioxidant activity assays such as 2,2′-azinobis-(3-ethylbenzothiazoline-6-sulfonate) (ABTS), which evaluates the antioxidant capacity through the reduction of the ABTS + radical, 2, 2-diphenyl-1-picrylhydrazyl (DPPH), which measures the antioxidant activity by scavenging the DPPH radical, ferric reducing antioxidant power (FRAP), which evaluates the antioxidant capacity through the reduction of Fe^{3+} to Fe^{2+}, and oxygen radical absorbance capacity (ORAC), which evaluates the ability to neutralize peroxyl radicals (ROO•).

The use of conventional spectrophotometric methods in the quantification of TPC, TFC and TAC, as well as in the determination of total antioxidant activity, is considered routine analyses, due to their simplicity and reduced cost, with the determination being based on the different structures of each class of the bioactive compound resulting from the separation processes (Ramirez-Sanchez et al., 2010).

In a study carried out by Chomphoosee et al. (2025), the antioxidant potential of the fermented beverage produced from coffee husks was determined by quantifying TPC, verifying an increase to 4214.58 ± 8.51 μg gallic acid equivalents (GAE)/mL with the fermentation process, and the use of DPPH, ABTS and FRAP assays that demonstrated high antioxidant activity of the beverage (2067.28 ± 3.76, 2410.28 ± 5.01, and 3691.09 ± 5.48 μg TE/mL, respectively). These authors also correlated the antimicrobial action of the beverage with its bioactive compounds. Salman et al. (2025) also observed the antioxidant potential of concentrated pomegranate juice by determining the total phenolic content, 3551 mg gallic acid equivalent (GAE)/L, and antioxidant activity by the DPPH (371.0 mM Trolox equivalent (TE)/L) and ABTS (464.0 mM TE/L) methods. Zhou et al. (2025) demonstrated the antioxidant potential of fermented star fruit juice based on the total antioxidant activity of the beverage determined through the ABTS+, DPPH, and CUPRAC methods, measuring the antioxidant capacity through the reduction of cupric ions (Cu^{2+}) to cupric ions (Cu^{+}) and FRAP. These authors associated the antioxidant capacity and potential hypoglycemic activity of the beverage with its antioxidant compounds.

However, these methods have limitations, as they are nonspecific and susceptible to several interferents. Non-phenolic compounds, such as proteins and sugars, can influence the results, leading to the overestimation of the real content of bioactives, such as polyphenols (Ramirez-Sanchez et al., 2010; Silva et al., 2022). In general, conventional methods are destructive to samples, are time-and labor-intensive, require advanced laboratory expertise, and generate potentially harmful chemical residues. Consequently, these limitations compromise their applicability in high-throughput analyses, especially when there is a need to process a large volume of samples in a short time interval (Matos et al., 2024).

In the identification and quantification of bioactive compounds, such as polyphenols, continuous improvement of robust, effective, and cost-effective analytical techniques is required to ensure food safety, quality and traceability, in compliance with consumer-oriented requirements and legislation. Consequently, it is crucial to develop rapid, low-cost, and chemical-free methods for the rapid quantification of bioactive components to meet future demands for nutrition and sustainability.

Specific bioactive compounds such as vitamin C, ferulic acid, gallic acid, caffeine, and catechin can be extracted and quantified by modern methods such as nuclear magnetic resonance spectroscopy, near-infrared spectroscopy, and chromatographic techniques including high- and ultra-HPLC, electrospray ionization, and quadrupole reversed-phase ultra-HPLC (Patra et al., 2022). In addition, chromatographic methods such as high-performance liquid chromatography (HPLC), gas chromatography (GC), countercurrent chromatography (CCC), and capillary electrophoresis (CE) can be applied for both qualitative and quantitative analysis of bioactives. The instruments used to detect signals in chromatography are based on variations in physical and chemical characteristics between the eluents and the analyte, through mass spectrometers (MS), diode arrays (DAD) and fluorescence detectors (FLD) (Ilyas et al., 2024).

The quantification of bioactive compounds in beverages by chromatographic methods allows evaluating the potential of these components during or after processing, in addition to observing the presence of compounds related to the sensory characteristics of the product. In a study carried out by Canedo-Reis et al. (2021), a rapid method was developed and validated for the simultaneous measurement of 16 phenolic compounds present in grape juice by UPLC-MS. The execution took 4.5 min and the method proved to be selective, linear ($r > 0.9961$), precise, accurate, with LOD and LOQ in the range of 0.45–35.34 μg L^{-1} and 1.35–107.08 μg L^{-1}, respectively. The authors reported that anthocyanins were the most abundant compounds in the juices, highlighting the BRS-Violeta cultivar that exhibited the highest concentration of phenolic compounds.

Yıkmıs et al. (2025) used a chromatograph integrated with a DAD detector to optimize the analysis of bioactive compounds in black carrot juice. In the present study, the flow rate was decreased to 0.80 mL.min^{-1}, while maintaining the column temperature at 30°C. In addition, the presence of the following phenolic compounds was identified: chlorogenic acid, caffeic acid, quercetin, p-coumaric acid, vanillin, t-ferulic acid, and resorcinol. This research examined in detail the effects of different processing techniques (C-BCJ, P-BCJ, and TS-BCJ) employed on black carrot juice samples, considering the diversity, preservation, and concentration of phenolic compounds. The findings showed that thermosonication was the most effective technique for maintaining and increasing the concentration of phenolic compounds. The TS-BCJ sample showed a maximum concentration of 149.26 μg mL^{-1} of chlorogenic acid. Statistically, this value exceeded the levels of 89.75 μg mL^{-1} in the C-BCJ sample and 35.39 μg mL^{-1} in the P-BCJ sample ($P < .05$). Although normally low, caffeic acid concentrations were found at the highest level in the thermally pasteurized group (P-BCJ), reaching 1.90 μg mL^{-1}. This value was determined as 0.42 μg mL^{-1} in the TS-BCJ and 0.10 μg mL^{-1} in the C-BCJ. These variations also showed significant statistical significance. The concentration of quercetin was determined at 5.18 μg/mL in TS-BCJ, 1.33 μg/mL in C-BCJ and 0.76 μg mL^{-1} in P-BCJ. A significant increase in the levels of p-coumaric acid and quercetin was identified after ultrasound treatment. The concentration of vanillin was determined at 2.57 μg mL^{-1} in P-BCJ, 2.47 μg mL^{-1} in TS-BCJ and 0.76 μg mL^{-1} in C-BCJ. These variations in vanillin levels indicate that the pasteurization process may intensify some phenolic compounds. The maximum concentration of t-ferulic acid in TS-BCJ was 3.95 μg mL^{-1}, followed by 3.65 μg mL^{-1} in C-BCJ and 2.38 μg mL^{-1} in P-BCJ. Resveratrol was found to be 0.53 μg mL^{-1} in TS-BCJ, 0.08 μg mL^{-1} in P-BCJ and 0.05 μg mL^{-1} in C-BCJ. The compounds showed notable differences in the statistical analyses ($P < .05$).

Sentkowska and Pyrzyńska (2018) used hydrophilic interaction liquid chromatography coupled with mass spectrometry (HILIC–MS) to identify selected bioactive compounds (polyphenols and B vitamins) in beetroot juice. The improvement of the method allowed the selection of separation criteria and increased the sensitivity of the method compared to the RP mode. ZIC HILIC defined detection limits of 0.01 mg/L for flavonoids and phenolic acids, and 0.03 mg/L for B vitamins. Beetroot juices identified as BJ1, BJ2, and BJ3 come from conventional plantations, while BJeco juice comes from agroecological beetroot cultivation. It is observed that traditional juices present a wide variation in the content of catechin, epicatechin, and rhamnetin. The samples presented the following catechin concentrations: BJ1 0.715 mg/L, BJ2 1.75 mg/L, BJ3 below the detection limit, and BJeco 6.73 mg/L. The BJ3 juice presented the lowest concentration of these compounds; however, it had the highest concentration of pHBA in its composition: 6.73 mg/L. No relevant differences were observed in the pantothenic acid content. However, nicotinamide was identified only in the BJ1 juice, with a concentration of 2.85 mg/L compared to conventional juices. The organic BJeco juice was classified as the main source of catechin, with 6.73 mg/L, and pHBA, with 6.83 mg/L, when compared to other juices. It was observed that the BJ1 juice presented a significantly higher concentration of caffeic acid (2.40 mg/L) and procatechuic acid (4.30 mg/L) compared to the other juices analyzed.

Hydrophilic interaction chromatography coupled to a mass spectrometer (HILIC-MS) is a technique that uses a more polar stationary phase than reversed-phase liquid chromatography (RP-HPLC) and a mobile phase with a low concentration of water or buffer, usually above 70% in organic solvent, such as acetonitrile. In HILIC mode, the mobile phase is a mixture of water and an organic solvent, usually acetonitrile, with a high concentration of organic solvent (5%–40% water). This technique uses more polar stationary phases, which retain polar solutes by hydrophilic interactions based on a partition equilibrium. In addition, hydrogen bonding interactions are believed to occur between the polar functional groups of the analytes and the stationary phase, in addition to electrostatic interactions with ionized groups. Van der Waals interactions may also occur between the hydrophobic part of the stationary phase and nonpolar groups of the analytes, as well as the adsorption of the analytes on the surface of the adsorbent. This allows the study of varied selectivity profiles and their use in two-dimensional liquid chromatography (LC × LC), with less incompatibility between the eluents of the two dimensions compared to orthogonal systems such as liquid chromatography in normal phase mode (NP-HPLC) (Silva et al., 2016). The mass spectrometer (MS) consists of five basic components. First, the sample inlet unit, which brings ionizable samples from atmospheric pressure to a lower pressure. Then, the ionization source transforms the sample into ions in the gas phase. The mass analyzer separates the ions based on the mass/charge ratio (m/z), and the ions are counted by the detector, with the signals recorded and processed by the data system (computer) (Calabrese, 2018).

The HPLC system was employed by Karatepe et al. (2025) to identify the polyphenols present in rhubarb juice. For this purpose, 250 μL of the freshly extracted juice was mixed with 10 mL of a methanol-water solution in the ratio of 85:15 and then subjected to ultrasonication for 10 min. The 20 μL sample was injected into the ODS-3 column (C18, 250 × 0.5 mm × 0.5 μm), with the flow rate set to 1 mL/min (Kürsad İncili et al., 2023). Twenty-three phenolic and flavonoid compounds were identified, including vanillic, gallic, protocatechuic and 4-dihydroxybenzoic acids, in addition to flavonoids such as epicatechin, rutin and quercetin-3-glucoside, with rutin being the most predominant compound.

The analysis of bioactive compounds in food can commonly be performed by High Performance Liquid Chromatography-HPLC, with conventional detectors (UV-VIS, Diode Array Detector-DAD). However, new chromatography technologies such as the use of LC-MS/MS improve the detection, identification and quantification of bioactive compounds, allowing a more detailed understanding of the structures and their bioactive properties, crucial for food consumption and health benefits. Studies such as Novaki et al. (2021) can be mentioned, who performed simultaneous analysis of caffeine and other methylxanthines in energy drinks, in which the technique allowed the identification and quantification of these substances, which are known for their stimulant effects. Han et al. (2022), who identified marker compounds in two types of Chinese dark tea after different post-fermentation processes, between teas fermented with Aspergillus niger and those fermented with Eurotium cristatum. Di Matteo et al. (2022), used HPLC-ESI-MS/MS to analyze the phenolic profile of radler beers, which combine beer with citrus fruit juice. Li et al. (2023) who determined nine bioactive phenolic components commonly found in apple juices.

However, both spectrophotometric and chromatographic methods require prior sample treatment, which includes extraction, cleaning, and concentration, before analysis for the determination of bioactive compounds. This is due to the fact that the concentrations of these compounds in complex matrices are generally very low (Silva et al., 2022). In this context, recent studies show the use of analytical methods based on digital images coupled with chemometric tools as promising alternatives for the development of analytical methodologies in the determination of these food quality parameters.

In a study carried out by Beltrán et al. (2021), total phenolics, anthocyanins, and tannins were quantified based on digital images and pseudo-univariate calibration performed using Independent Component Analysis (ICA). In addition, Principal Component Analysis (PCA) and Multivariate Curve Resolution with Alternating Least Squares (MCR-ALS) were used; however, differences were observed between the analyses, with ICA standing out. In all pseudo-univariate calibration curves, correlation coefficients greater than 0.9 were achieved. The results suggest that digital images coupled to ICA can provide pseudo-univariate calibration models for the determination of bioactive compounds. In addition to speed, the device for obtaining an image is cheaper than most analytical instruments.

10.3 Trends in methods for analyzing contaminants in beverages

10.3.1 Contaminant residues

Pesticides are commonly used in agricultural activities due to their effect in controlling pests and diseases, and are a solution for reducing mites, insects, fungi, and caterpillars in crops, among other things. However, the intensive use of these substances can generate chemical residues in food, and given their toxicity, they need to be controlled (Merhi et al., 2022; Milhome et al., 2019).

Beverages such as teas, beers, ciders and others use food from the field as raw materials, which can result in the production of food with pesticide residues. The composition of beverages depends on several factors, including the agricultural soil where the raw materials are planted, the water used in the preparation of the beverage, as well as the varieties of cereals used, the environmental conditions and the pesticides and fertilizers applied to the soil (González et al., 2023).

To control pests and diseases in crops, several chemical substances are used to minimize the devastating effects of these biological organisms. Pesticides such as neocytotinoids, pyrethroids, carbamates, organophosphate compounds, and organochlorine pesticides have been used for this purpose. Most organochlorine pesticides, in turn, are no longer used due to their high toxicity and resistance to degradation, although they were once widely used in agriculture (Wang et al., 2024). In addition to pesticide residues, beverages are also subject to contamination by some trace metals and mycotoxins, natural compounds produced as secondary metabolites of filamentous fungi. Fungal contamination and the consequent production of mycotoxins, such as aflatoxins, ochratoxins, fumonisins and deoxynivalenol, are of great importance to the food industry due to the carcinogenic, teratogenic and mutagenic activities of these compounds. Several metals, such as mercury, lead, cadmium, aluminum and arsenic, pose health risks above certain concentrations (Alonso González et al., 2024; González et al., 2023; Wang et al., 2024).

10.3.2 Multiresidue methods

Chromatographic techniques are currently widely used in the determination of pesticides, given their high degree of precision and the ability to detect pesticide residues at low concentrations (trace levels). In addition, this methodology can also be combined in different detection systems, which facilitates the determination of several chemical analytes in the same sample, with mass spectrometry being the most widely used system for detecting pesticide residues (Martins et al., 2019).

Chromatography coupled with mass spectrometry combines shared advantages of both processes: high selectivity and separation efficiency, from chromatography, as well as structural information, molar mass and additional increase in selectivity, from mass spectrometry. In addition, it has high selectivity power, sensitivity, identification, quantification, and accuracy of results (qualitative and quantitative), being able to detect pesticide residues in low concentrations (Milhome et al., 2017; Nascimento et al., 2018).

In this way, multiresidue methods are capable of detecting different types of pesticides in the same analysis, in addition to simplifying and reducing operational costs, given that it favors rapid and efficient monitoring of the process. However, due to the low concentrations of these residues in food and the complexity of the matrices, these analyses are considered extremely complex (Guedes et al., 2016).

The most widely used multiresidue methods for determining pesticides in food matrices are those based on gas chromatography and liquid chromatography coupled to mass spectrometry, given that these methods cover a vast number of active ingredients, due to the effective separation, identification and quantification of the analytes in the process (Milhome et al., 2019; Pszczolińska et al., 2022) emphasize that the effectiveness of the analysis is strictly related to the choice of the appropriate sample preparation method.

QuEChERS (Quick, Easy, Cheap, Effective, Rugged and Safe) extraction method is the most widely used for determining multi-residue in food, given that it has the best performance due to its ability to perform analyses on samples of different natures (food, pharmaceutical, environmental, forensic), solid and liquid, in addition to the analysis of a wide range of analytes, such as pesticides, mycotoxins, illicit drugs, pharmaceutical residues, etc. (Alcântara et al., 2019, p. 298)

According to Musarurwa et al. (2019), this technique involves only two sample preparation steps: one with liquid-liquid extraction using acetonitrile and a mixture of salts by partition, and the other where cleaning occurs by dispersive solid phase extraction (d-SPE). Furthermore, the method brings a series of advantages, when compared to other methodologies used for the same purpose, such as effective elimination of the effect matrix, obtaining a high recovery of the target analyte and using a smaller amount of solvent.

In addition, choosing the appropriate solvent for food matrices is extremely important, since these products can have several types of constituents that can cause interference during the analysis, ranging from lipids, sugars, sterols, fats or other acids, to chlorophyll and other pigments, that can affect the accuracy and reliability of the analysis (Pszczolińska et al., 2022).

Acetone, ethyl acetate and acetonitrile are the main solvents used in the multi-residue extraction of pesticides, with acetonitrile being the most widely used solvent in the QuEChERS extraction method. The use of acetonitrile, in turn, has numerous advantages, such as the extraction of polar analytes, a high degree of selectivity and detectability, in addition to being compatible with gas and liquid chromatography coupled with mass spectrometry (Musarurwa et al., 2019).

This method, in turn, emerged to generate extracts that could be analyzed by liquid and/or gas chromatography, being best used for matrices with low fat content, although changes in the original methodology may allow analysis in matrices with high fat content, which can be quite reduced by incorporating a liquid-liquid extraction step using hexane (Musarurwa et al., 2019).

One of the crucial steps in developing the method is sample cleaning, in addition to choosing appropriate reagents to minimize interference in the sample. This step promotes the reduction of co-extractants, reducing the matrix effect. In addition, cleaning improves the performance of the equipment used in the reading, improving detection limits (Pszczolińska et al., 2022).

It is worth noting that the matrix effect affects the quantification of the analysis and can generate unreliable data when the pesticide concentration is very low, given the complexity of food samples. The matrix effect can interfere with both gas chromatography analysis (sample injector, analytical column and detector) as well as liquid chromatography analysis (ionization) (Musarurwa et al., 2019).

The *cleanup* step is performed by means of dispersive solid phase extraction (D-SPE) and aims to reduce the presence of compounds that cause interference in the analysis (Fig. 10.6). In this type of

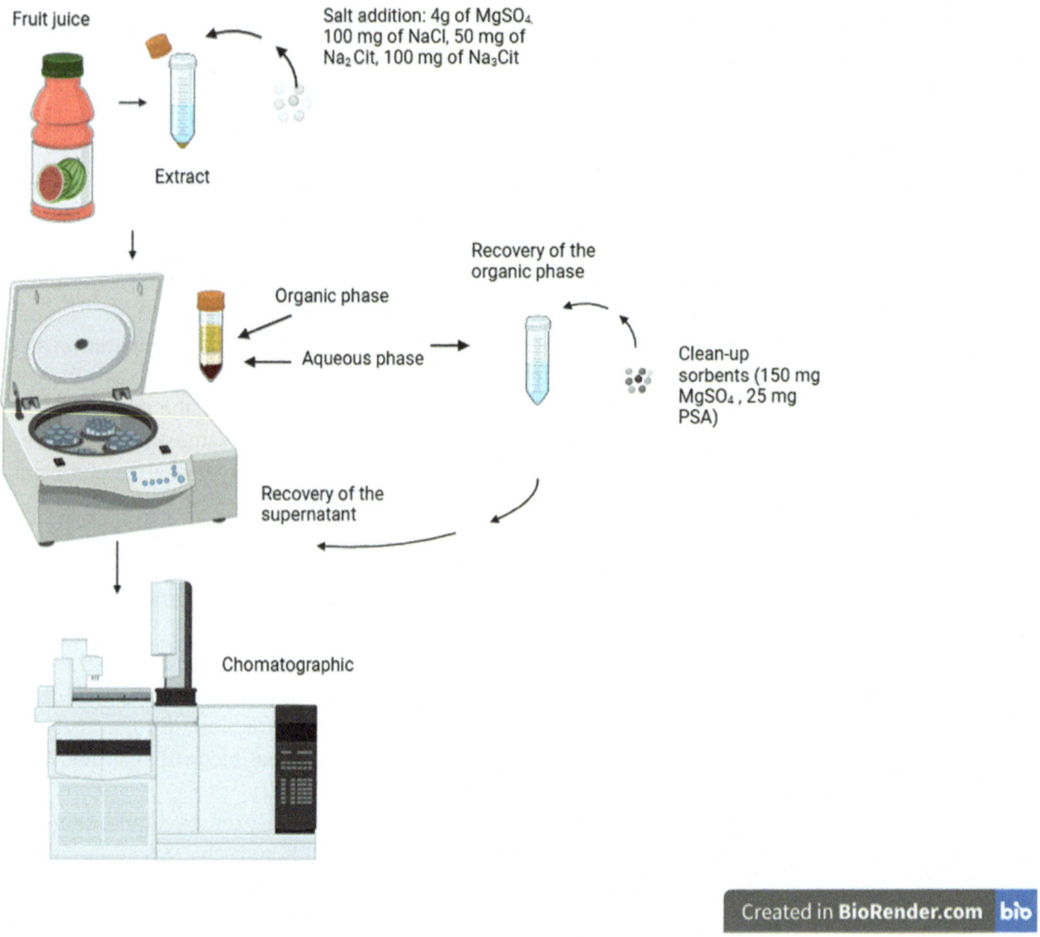

FIGURE 10.6

Steps of the QuEChERS method used for analysis of pesticides in fruit juices.

technique, anhydrous magnesium sulfate is added and mixed with the sample extract, which enhances the salting out effect and has the parallel function of removing water, and the sorbent PSA (primary secondary amine), which promotes a chelating effect. After this step, the extract is subjected to chromatographic analysis (Alcântara et al., 2019, p. 298).

Aiming to overcome the limitations of other multi-residue methods in the detection of pesticide residues, the QuEChERS method has the following advantages: simplicity, low cost, robustness, high precision results, high degree of selectivity and sensitivity, high yield, as well as extraction efficiency.

After the consolidation of the QuEChERS method, other approaches were developed based on the traditional method, with a view to minimizing the influence of sample pH through the addition of other salts to adjust the pH, such as QuEChERS-acetate (developed by Lehotay, Maštovska and Lightfield) and QuEChERS-citrate (developed by Anastassiades and collaborators), as shown in Fig. 10.7. However, the basic steps of the process are the same, that is, a liquid-liquid extraction using a mixture of salts and, subsequently, an aliquot of the organic extract, which was subjected to agitation and centrifugation, is subjected to dispersive solid phase cleaning (d-SPE).

In addition, another difference between the two techniques is related to the *cleanup* step (d-SPE), where in the acetate method 50 mg of PSA is used per milliliter of extract, while in the citrate method 25 mg of PSA is used per milliliter of extract (Musarurwa et al., 2019) Table 10.5.

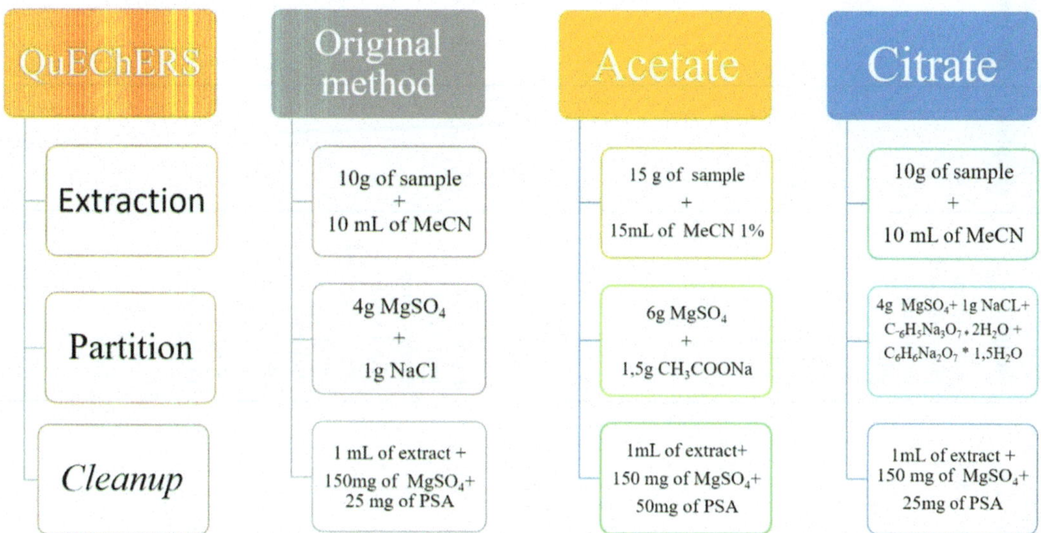

FIGURE 10.7

Steps of the QuEChERS method used for analysis of pesticides in fruit juices: (1) Extraction (2) Partition (3) *Cleanup*.

Table 10.5 Extraction methods and chromatographic systems used for analysis of pesticide residues in beverages.

No.	Sample preparation	Detection system	Sample	No. of real samples	No. of compounds determined	Main compound	References
1	QuEChERS; SPE; SPME	GC–MS	Apple–mango, pineapple and grapefruit juices	4	56	Trifluralin, Atrazine, Hexachlorobenzene, Terbuthylazine, Chlorpyrifos methyl, Alachlor, Chlorpyrifos, Aldrin, Isodrin, Endosulfan I, Endosulfan II, DDE, Dieldrin, Endrin, Bifenthrin	Cherta et al. (2013)
2	Multiplug filtration cleaning	GC–MS	Tomato, tomato juice, ketchup	20	186	Ametryn, Atrazine, Bendiocarb, Bifenthrin, Buprofezin, Carbaryl, Chlorpyrifos, Cyprodinil, Dichlofenthion, Diclobutrazol, Dimethylvinphos, Ethoprophos, Etrimfos, Fenoxycarb, Fluquinconazol, Halfenprox, Isoprothiolane, Kresoxim-methyl, Lactofen, Malathion, Methamidophos, Oxyfluorfen, Parathion, Phosalone, Quinoclamine, Ronnel, Silafluofen, Tebuconazole, Trifluralin, Vinclozolin.	Zhao et al. (2014)
3	MSB-LPME	GC–MS	Lemon, apple, peach and orange juices	4	8	Phorate, Diazinon, Tebupirimfos, Tolclofos-methyl, Pirimiphos-methyl, Fenthion, Fenamiphos, Sulprofos	Wu et al. (2015)
4	Extraction + cleaning (multi-walled carbon nanotubes - MWCNTs/PSA)	GC–MS	Fresh jujube, first and second jujube juice and pomace, jujube wine and jujube vinegar	7	2	Triadimefon, triadimenol.	Zhao et al. (2017)
5	Modified QuEChERS	UHPLC-MS/MS	Orange juice	14	76	Acetamiprid, Azoxystrobin, Bromuconazole, Buprofezin, Carbendazim, Clomazone, Diazinon, Difenoconazole, Epoxiconazole, Etopropho, Fenazaquin, Flusilazole, Imazalil, Linuron, Mecarbam, Mepronil, Omethoate, Penconazole, Propanil, Rotenone, Simazine, Tetraconazole, Thiabendazole, Vamidation.	Rizzetti et al. (2016)
6	Homogeneous liquid-liquid	GC–MS	Grape, sour cherry, mango,	8	10	Bifenthrin, Phenothrin, Tetramethrin, Fenpropathrin, Cyhalothrin,	Torbati et al. (2018)

	microextraction-HLLME		apricot, peach, orange, apple and strawberry juices			Permethrin, Cypermethrin, Cyfluthrin, Flucythrinate, Deltamethrin.	
7	Tissue-phase sorptive extraction-FPSE	GC–MS	Water, apple juice, pomegranate juice and lychee juice	6	19	α-Benzenehexachloride (α-BHC), β-Benzenehexachloride (β-BHC), γ-Benzenehexachloride (γ-BHC), δ-Benzenehexachloride (δ-BHC), Heptachlor, Aldrin, Heptachlorepoxide, *trans* Chlordane, cis Chlordane, p,p Dichlorodiphenyldichloroeth ylene (p, p' DDE), Dieldrin, Endrin, β-Endosulfan, p,p Dichlorodiphenyldichloroeth ane (p,p' DDD), Endrin Aldehyde, Endosulfan sulfate, p,p Dichlorodiphenyltrichloroeth ane (p, p' DDT), Endrin ketone, Methoxychlor.	Kaur et al. (2019)
8	QuEChERS	LC-MS/MS	Canned apricots and peaches and orange juice	3	16	Spinosad, Thiacloprid, Pyridaben, Bupirimate, Flusilazole, Triflumizole, Flonicamid, Imidacloprid, Lambda-cyhalothrin, Cyproconazole, Fludioxinil, Cyprodinil, Abamectin, Chlorpyrifos-methyl, Hexythiazox and Metalaxyl	Cámara et al. (2020)
9	QuEChERS	GC-MS	Potato, apple juice, kale, pear juice, tomato, apricot and peach	7	4	Carbofuron, Mancozeb, Chloropyriphos, Captan.	Naman et al. (2022)
10	TFME coated with HLB/PTFE AF	GC-MS	Apple juice	1	6	Carbaryl, Trifluralin, Chlorpyrifos-methyl, Malathion, methyl-parathion, Diazinon.	Kahremanoğlu et al. (2023)

10.4 Conclusion

Chromatographic methods are a powerful technique for determining different components in beverages. Chromatography coupled with mass spectrometry allows for an increase in the scope of analysis, with greater selectivity and sensitivity. Based on the literature, it was found that several advances have been cited, such as variations in chromatographic columns, in the expansion of detection capacity, as well as in the type of sample preparation. The chapter showed how the techniques have been applied to the analysis of beverages, as well as the main legislation involved.

Acknowledgments

The authors would like to thank Higher Education Personnel Improvement Coordination (CAPES) and National Council for Scientific and Technological Development (CNPQ/INCT-ALIM project) for their financial support for the research.

References

Abdelwareth, A., Ahmed, Z., & Farag, M. A. (2021). Chemometrics-based aroma profiling for revealing origin, roasting indices, and brewing method in coffee seeds and its commercial blends in the Middle East. *Food Chemistry, 349*, Article 129162. https://doi.org/10.1016/j.foodchem.2021.129162

Adam, M., Pavlíková, P., Čížková, A., Bajerová, P., & Ventura, K. (2012). Microextraction by packed sorbent (MEPS) as a suitable selective method for l-ascorbic acid determination in beverages. *Food Chemistry, 135*(3), 1613–1618. https://doi.org/10.1016/j.foodchem.2012.06.039

Al-Madboly, L. A., Yagi, A., Kabbash, A., El-Aasr, M. A., & El-Morsi, R. M. (2023). Microbiota-derived short chain fatty acids in fermented Kidachi aloe promote antimicrobial, anticancer, and immunomodulatory activities. *BMC Microbiology, 23*(1). https://doi.org/10.1186/s12866-023-02981-z. Available from: https://bmcmicrobiol.biomedcentral.com/.

Alcântara, D. B., Fernandes, T. S. M., Nascimento, H. O., Lopes, A. F., Menezes, M. G. G., Lima, A. C. A., Carvalho, T. V., Grinberg, P., Milhome, M. A. L., Oliveira, A. H. B., Becker, H., Zocolo, G. J., & Nascimento, R. F. (2019). *Diagnostic detection systems and QuEChERS methods for multiclass pesticide analyses in different types of fruits: An overview from the last decade*. Elsevier Ltd, Brazil Food Chemistry. Available from: www.elsevier.com/locate/foodchem. doi: 10.1016/j.foodchem.2019.124958.

Alcarde, A. R., Souza, L. M., & Bortoletto, A. M. (2014). Formation of volatile and maturation-related congeners during the aging of sugarcane spirit in oak barrels. *Journal of the Institute of Brewing, 120*, 529–536. https://doi.org/10.1002/jib.165

Ali, S., Rezende, V. T., Ullah, S., de Paiva, E. L., Tonin, F. G., Abdullah, Corassin, C. H., & Oliveira, C. A. F.d. (2023). *Food processing and challenges in the food production and quality: The foodomics approach, 56*. Elsevier Ltd, Brazil Food Bioscience. https://doi.org/10.1016/j.fbio.2023.103217. Available from: http://www.journals.elsevier.com/food-bioscience/.

Alonso González, P., Parga Dans, E., de las Heras Tranche, I., Acosta-Dacal, A. C., Macías Montes, A., Peña, M. Z., Luzardo, O. P., González, P. A., Dans, E. P., de las Heras Tranche, I., Acosta-Dacal, A. C., Montes, A. M., Pena, M. Z., & Luzardo, O. P. (2024). Comparative analyses of pesticide residues, elemental composition and mycotoxin levels in Spanish traditional and novel ciders. *Food Control, 160*(2024), Article 110310. https://doi.org/10.1016/j.foodcont.2024.110310

Aminianfar, A., Fatemi, M. H., & Azimi, F. (2024). Comprehensive characterization of volatile compounds in Iranian black teas using chemometric analysis of GC-MS fingerprints. *Food Chemistry X, 24*, Article 101859. https://doi.org/10.1016/j.fochx.2024.101859

Andrés, V., Tenorio, M. D., & Villanueva, M. J. (2015). *Sensory profile, soluble sugars, organic acids, and mineral content in milk- and soy-juice based beverages, 173* (pp. 1100–1106). Elsevier Ltd, Spain Food Chemistry. https://doi.org/10.1016/j.foodchem.2014.10.136. Available from: www.elsevier.com/locate/foodchem.

Araujo Filho, A. A. L., Sousa, P. H. M.d., Vieira, I. G. P., Fernandes, V. B., Cunha, F. E. T., Magalhaes, F. E. A., & Silva, L. M. R.d. (2023). Kombucha and kefir fermentation dynamics on cashew nut beverage (Anacardium occidentale L.). AZTI-Tecnalia. *Brazil International Journal of Gastronomy and Food Science, 33*. https://doi.org/10.1016/j.ijgfs.2023.100778. Available from: www.journals.elsevier.com/international-journal-of-gastronomy-and-food-science.

Arda, B., Akdeniz, V., Kara, H. H., & Akalın, A. S. (2025). Fatty acid profile, conjugated linoleic acid (CLA) content, microbiological and sensory properties of kefir produced from sheep milk using kefir grains and starter culture in comparison with the respective kefir from cow milk. *International Dairy Journal, 162*. https://doi.org/10.1016/j.idairyj.2024.106157. Available from: https://www.sciencedirect.com/science/journal/09586946.

Aryana, K. J., & Olson, D. W. (2017). A 100-year review: Yogurt and other cultured dairy products. *Journal of Dairy Science, 100*(12), 9987–10013. https://doi.org/10.3168/jds.2017-12981

Balcerek, M., Dziekońska-Kubczak, U., Pielech-Przybylska, K., Oleszczak, A., Koń, M., & Patelski, A. M. (2024). Waste bread as raw material for ethanol production: Effect of mash preparation methods on fermentation efficiency. *Applied Sciences, 14*(20), 9565. https://doi.org/10.3390/app14209565

Beltrán, A. E. E., Salazar, N. A. S., Quezada, R.Á. P., Orozco, G. I. O., Cuéllar, J. L. J., Córdova, M. A. F., Hernández, L. R., Caballero, M. C. S., Moreno, M. N. F., Beltrán, A. E. E., Salazar, N. A. S., Quezada, R.Á. P., Orozco, G. I. O., Cuéllar, J. L. J., Córdova, M. A. F., Hernández, L. R., Caballero, M. C. S., & Moreno, M. N. F. (2021). Perfil de compuestos volátiles y parámetros fisicoquímicos de cuatro variedades de manzana, durante su maduración en árbol. *Interciencia, 46*(4), 140–147.

Beltrame, K. K., Gonçalves, T. R., Gomes, S. T. M., Matsushita, M., Rutledge, D. N., Março, P. H., & Valderrama, P. (2021). Digital images and independent components analysis in the determination of bioactive compounds from grape juice. *LWT*, 152. https://doi.org/10.1016/j.lwt.2021.112308

Brazil. (2008). *Wine and beverage legislation*. Ministry of Agriculture and Livestock (MAPA). https://www.gov.br/agricultura/pt-br/assuntos/inspecao/produtos-vegetal/legislacao-de-produtos-origem-vegetal/bebidas.

Brazil. (2011). *MAPA normative instruction no. 15 of April 01, 2011*. Official Gazette of the Union. https://www.normasbrasil.com.br/norma/instrucao-normativa-15-2011_78327.html.

Brazil. (2022). *MAPA ordinance N°.539, of December 26, 2022*. Official Gazette of the Union. https://www.gov.br/mdic/pt-br/assuntos/reg/boas-praticas-regulatorias/selo-de-boas-praticas-regulatorias/2022/selo-ouro/mapa-portaria-mapa-ndeg-539-2022.

Brazil. (2025). *Decree no. 12,709, of October 31, 2025*. Official Gazette of the Union. https://www.planalto.gov.br/ccivil_03/_Ato2007-2010/2009/Decreto/D6871.htm.

Cámara, M. A., Cermeño, S., Martínez, G., & Oliva, J. (2020). Removal residues of pesticides in apricot, peach and orange processed and dietary exposure assessment. *Food Chemistry, 325*, Article 126936. https://doi.org/10.1016/j.foodchem.2020.126936

Calabrese, B. (2018). Experimental platforms for extracting biological data: Mass spectrometry, microarray, next generation sequencing. *Encyclopedia of Bioinformatics and Computational Biology: ABC of Bioinformatics, 1–3*, 126–129. https://doi.org/10.1016/B978-0-12-809633-8.20412-3

Canedo-Reis, N. A. P., Guerra, C. C., da Silva, L. F., Wetzstein, L. C., Junges, C. H., Ferrão, M. F., & Bergold, A. M. (2021). Fast quantitative determination of phenolic compounds in grape juice by UPLC-MS: Method validation and characterization of juices produced with different grape varieties. *Journal of*

Food Measurement and Characterization, 15(2), 1044–1056. https://doi.org/10.1007/s11694-020-00706-8

Cardoso, D. R., Bettin, S. M., Reche, R. V., Lima-Neto, B. S., & Franco, D. W. (2003). HPLC-DAD analysis of ketones as their 2,4-dinitrophenylhydrazones in Brazilian sugar-cane spirits and rum. *Journal of Food Composition and Analysis, 16*(5), 563–573. https://doi.org/10.1016/S0889-1575(03)00061-9

Catalano, A., Mariconda, A., D'Amato, A., Iacopetta, D., Ceramella, J., Marra, M., Saturnino, C., Sinicropi, M. S., & Longo, P. (2024). Aldehydes: What we should know about them. *Organics, 5*(4), 395–428. https://doi.org/10.3390/org5040021

Chapko, M. J., & Seo, H. S. (2019). Characterizing product temperature-dependent sensory perception of brewed coffee beverages: Descriptive sensory analysis. *Food Research International, 121*, 612–621. https://doi.org/10.1016/j.foodres.2018.12.026. Available from: www.elsevier.com/inca/publications/store/4/2/2/9/7/0.

Chen, S., Li, S., Fang, K., Wang, Y., Yang, Y., Han, C., & Shen, Y. (2022). Rapid determination of 93 banned industrial dyes in beverage, fish, cookie using solid-supported liquid–liquid extraction and ultrahigh-performance liquid chromatography quadrupole orbitrap high-resolution mass spectrometry. *Food Chemistry, 388*, Article 132976. https://doi.org/10.1016/j.foodchem.2022.132976

Cheng, S., Wang, S., Zheng, M., Jin, Y., Li, J., Zhang, M., Li, X.-L., & Min, J. Z. (2024). Simultaneous analysis of natural and artificial sweeteners in sugar-free drinks and urine samples by column-switching UHPLC-charged aerosol detection method. *Journal of Chromatography A, 1713*, Article 464533. https://doi.org/10.1016/j.chroma.2023.464533

Cherta, L., Beltran, J., Pitarch, E., & Hernández, F. (2013). Comparison of simple and rapid extraction procedures for the determination of pesticide residues in fruit juices by fast gas chromatography–mass spectrometry. *Food Analytical Methods, 6*(6), 1671–1684. https://doi.org/10.1007/s12161-013-9578-8

Chomphoosee, T., Seesuriyachan, P., Wattanutchariya, W., Tipbunjong, C., Therdtatha, P., techapun, C., Insomphun, C., Panti, N., & Moukamnerd, C. (2025). A novel beverage of coffee cherry (cascara) water kefir rich in antioxidants, bioactive compounds, and exhibiting promising antibacterial and sensory qualities. *LWT, 219*, Article 117539. https://doi.org/10.1016/j.lwt.2025.117539

Christoph, N., & Bauer-Christoph, C. (2007). *Flavour of spirit drinks: Raw materials, fermentation, distillation, and ageing flavours and fragrances: Chemistry, bioprocessing and sustainability* (pp. 219–239). Berlin Heidelberg: Springer. https://doi.org/10.1007/978-3-540-49339-6_10. Available from: http://www.springerlink.com/openurl.asp?genre=book&isbn=978-3-540-49338-9.

Da Silva, F. S., Maia Pinto, F. V., Amaral, S. M. B., Nobre, C.de A., Silva, V. P.de A., & Milhome, M. A. L. (2023). Extraction of volatile Compounds-VCs from mixed fruit and vegetables refreshment by HS-SPME/GC-MS. *Brazilian Journal of Animal and Environmental Research, 6*(2), 1573–1584. https://doi.org/10.34188/bjaerv6n2-050

da Silva Rocha, R., de Oliveira, L. B., Morais, S. T.d. B., Soutelino, M. E. M., Silva, M. C., de Freitas, M. Q., Junior, S. B., Pimentel, T. C., Esmerino, E. A., & da Cruz, A. G. (2023). Effect of ohmic heating in bioactive peptides, volatile compounds, and fatty acid profile in a high-protein vanilla flavoured milk drink. *International Dairy Journal, 146*. https://doi.org/10.1016/j.idairyj.2023.105733. Available from: www.elsevier.com/inca/publications/store/4/0/5/8/6/0/index.htt.

Das, S., Uddin, M. N., Khaled, A. S. M., Noyon, M. R. O. K., Chakraborty, D., Mostafa, M., Islam, M. S. M. M., Bhattacharjee, S. C., Das, S. K., & Uddin, M. (2024). Health risk assessment of three preservatives in beverage, cake, ketchup, and therapeutic products available in Bangladesh using the new validated HPLC-PDA method. *Journal of Food Composition and Analysis, 126*. https://doi.org/10.1016/j.jfca.2023.105907. Available from: https://www.sciencedirect.com/science/journal/08891575.

de Araújo, F. F., de Paulo Farias, D., Neri-Numa, I. A., & Pastore, G. M. (2021). Underutilized plants of the Cactaceae family: Nutritional aspects and technological applications. *Food Chemistry*, 362. https://doi.org/10.1016/j.foodchem.2021.130196. Available from: www.elsevier.com/locate/foodchem.

de Brito, W. A., Siquieroli, A. C. S., Andaló, V., Duarte, J. G., de Sousa, R. M. F., Felisbino, J. K. R. P., da Silva, G. C., Brito, W. A. D., Siquieroli, A. C. S., Andaló, V., Duarte, J. G., Sousa, R. M. F. D., Felisbino, J. K. R. P., & Silva, G. C. D. (2021). Formulação de inseticida botânico com óleo de nim e D-limoneno para controle da broca-do-café. *Pesquisa Agropecuária Brasileira, 56*, 1–9. https://doi.org/10.1590/S1678-3921.pab2021.v56.02000. Embrapa, Brazil Pesquisa Agropecuaria Brasileira.

de Faria, L. V., Lisboa, T. P., de Farias, D. M., Araujo, F. M., Machado, M. M., de Sousa, R. A., Matos, M. A. C., Muñoz, R. A. A., & Matos, R. C. (2020). Direct analysis of ascorbic acid in food beverage samples by flow injection analysis using reduced graphene oxide sensor. *Food Chemistry*, 319. https://doi.org/10.1016/j.foodchem.2020.126509. Available from: www.elsevier.com/locate/foodchem.

Di Matteo, P., Bortolami, M., Di Virgilio, L., & Petrucci, R. (2022). Targeted phenolic profile of radler beers by HPLC-ESI-MS/MS: The added value of hesperidin to beer antioxidants. *Journal of Food Science and Technology, 59*(11), 4553–4562. https://doi.org/10.1007/s13197-022-05536-8

Dragone, G., Mussatto, S. I., Oliveira, J. M., & Teixeira, J. A. (2009). Characterisation of volatile compounds in an alcoholic beverage produced by whey fermentation. *Food Chemistry, 112*(4), 929–935. https://doi.org/10.1016/j.foodchem.2008.07.005

Duan, B., Chang, W., Zhang, L., Zheng, M., Su-Zhou, C., Merkeryan, H., Xu, M., & Liu, X. (2024). Characterization of volatile compounds and sensory properties of spine grape (Vitis davidii Foex) brandies aged with different toasted wood chips. *Food Chemistry X, 23*, Article 101777. https://doi.org/10.1016/j.fochx.2024.101777

Dudareva, N., Pichersky, E., & Gershenzon, J. (2004). Biochemistry of plant volatiles. *Plant Physiology, 135*(4), 1893–1902. https://doi.org/10.1104/pp.104.049981

El-Maghrabey, M. H., Hashem, H. M., El Hamd, M. A., El-Shaheny, R., Kishikawa, N., Kuroda, N., & Magdy, G. (2024). Comprehensive greenness evaluation of the reported chromatographic methods for aldehydes determination as clinical biomarkers and food quality indicators. *TrAC - Trends in Analytical Chemistry*, 171. https://doi.org/10.1016/j.trac.2024.117548. Available from: https://www.sciencedirect.com/science/journal/01659936.

EU Commission. (2019). Regulation EU 2019/787 (EU) of the European Parliament and of the Council of 17 April 2019 on the definition, description, presentation and labelling of spirit drinks, the use of the names of spirit drinks in the presentation and labelling of other foodstuffs, the protection of geographical indications for spirit drinks, the use of ethyl alcohol and distillates of agricultural origin in alcoholic beverages, and repealing Regulation (EC) no 110/2008008. *Official Journal of the European Union*. https://eur-lex.europa.eu/legal-content/EN/TXT/?uri=CELEX%3A32019R0787&qid=1724175711961.

Felipe, L. O., & Bicas, J. L. (2017). Terpenos, aromas e a química dos compostos naturais. *Química Nova na Escola, 39*(2). https://doi.org/10.21577/0104-8899.20160068

Ferrer, I., & Thurman, E. M. (2010). Analysis of sucralose and other sweeteners in water and beverage samples by liquid chromatography/time-of-flight mass spectrometry. *Journal of Chromatography A, 1217*(25), 4127–4134. https://doi.org/10.1016/j.chroma.2010.02.020

Fretwell, E. (2020). *Sensory experiments: Psychophysics, race, and the aesthetics of feeling*. Duke University Press. https://doi.org/10.2307/j.ctv160btzd

García-Falcón, M. S., & Simal-Gándara, J. (2005). Determination of food dyes in soft drinks containing natural pigments by liquid chromatography with minimal clean-up. *Food Control, 16*(3), 293–297. https://doi.org/10.1016/j.foodcont.2004.03.009

Gomes, W. P. C., Rocha, F. R. P., & Melchert, W. R. (2024). A single-step microdistillation procedure for the determination of total vicinal diketones in beers. *Microchemical Journal, 204*, Article 110969. https://doi.org/10.1016/j.microc.2024.110969

González, P. A., Dans, E. P., Tranche, I.d. L. H., Acosta-Dacal, A. C., Hernández, Á. R., Montes, A. M., Peña, M. Z., & Luzardo, O. P. (2023). Comparative analysis of mycotoxin, pesticide, and elemental content of

Canarian craft and Spanish mainstream beers. *Toxicology Reports, 10*, 389–399. https://doi.org/10.1016/j.toxrep.2023.03.003. Available from: http://www.journals.elsevier.com/toxicology-reports/.

Grassino, A. N., Jerković, I., Pedisić, S., & Dent, M. (2024). Hydrodistillation fractions of coffee (green and roasted) and coffee by-product (silver skin and spent grounds) as a source of bioactive compounds. *Sustainable Chemistry and Pharmacy, 39*, Article 101592. https://doi.org/10.1016/j.scp.2024.101592

Guedes, J. A. C., Silva, R. D. O., Lima, C. G., Milhome, M. A. L., & Do Nascimento, R. F. (2016). Matrix effect in guava multiresidue analysis by QuEChERS method and gas chromatography coupled to quadrupole mass spectrometry. *Brazil Food Chemistry, 199*, 380–386. https://doi.org/10.1016/j.foodchem.2015.12.007. Available from: www.elsevier.com/locate/foodchem.

Gutiérrez-Pacheco, M. M., Torres-Moreno, H., Flores-Lopez, M. L., Velázquez Guadarrama, N., Ayala-Zavala, J. F., Ortega-Ramírez, L. A., & López-Romero, J. C. (2023). Mechanisms and applications of citral's antimicrobial properties in food preservation and pharmaceuticals formulations. *Antibiotics, 12*(11). https://doi.org/10.3390/antibiotics12111608. Available from: http://www.mdpi.com/journal/antibiotics.

Han, Z., Wen, M., Zhang, H., Zhang, L., Wan, X., & Ho, C.-T. (2022). LC-MS based metabolomics and sensory evaluation reveal the critical compounds of different grades of Huangshan Maofeng green tea. *Food Chemistry, 374*, Article 131796. https://doi.org/10.1016/j.foodchem.2021.131796

Huang, Y. B., Zou, C., Gao, Y., Yin, J. F., Contursi, P., Zhang, S., Gong, Y. S., Liu, J. J., & Xu, Y. Q. (2024). Kombucha beverages made from Camellia nitidissima Chi and Camellia sinensis flowers—physicochemical properties, sensory properties and bioactivity. *International Journal of Gastronomy and Food Science, 37*. https://doi.org/10.1016/j.ijgfs.2024.100964. Available from: https://www.sciencedirect.com/science/journal/1878450X.

Ilyas, Z., Nandasiri, R., Redha, A. A., & Aluko, R. E. (2024). High-performance liquid chromatography coupled with associated column and mass spectroscopic methods for honey analysis. In *Advanced techniques of honey analysis* (pp. 259–285). Academic Press. https://doi.org/10.1016/b978-0-443-13175-2.00006-4

Kürsad İncili, G., Akgöl, M., Karatepe, P., Kanmaz, H., Kaya, B., Tekin, A., & Adnan Hayaloğlu, A. (2023). Inhibitory effect of bioactive compounds derived from freeze-dried paraprobiotic of Pediococcus acidilactici against food-borne pathogens: In-vitro and food model studies. *Food Research International*, 170. https://doi.org/10.1016/j.foodres.2023.113045. Available from: www.elsevier.com/inca/publications/store/4/2/2/9/7/0.

Kahremanoğlu, K., Akpınar, Y., & Boyaci, E. (2023). Development of thin film microextraction method for the multi-residue analysis of selected pesticides. *Advances in Sample Preparation, 6*, Article 100061. https://doi.org/10.1016/j.sampre.2023.100061

Kaiser, S. J., Mutters, N. T., Blessing, B., & Günther, F. (2017). Natural isothiocyanates express antimicrobial activity against developing and mature biofilms of Pseudomonas aeruginosa. *Fitoterapia, 119*, 57–63. https://doi.org/10.1016/j.fitote.2017.04.006. Available from: www.elsevier.com/locate/fitote.

Karatepe, P., İncili, G. K., Tekin, A., Çalıcıoğlu, M., Akgöl, M., & Hayaloğlu, A. A. (2025). The impact of rhubarb (*Rheum ribes* L.) juice-based marinade on the quality characteristics and microbial safety of chicken breast fillets during refrigerated storage. *Poultry Science, 104*(2), 104719. https://doi.org/10.1016/j.psj.2024.104719

Kaur, R., Kaur, R., Rani, S., Malik, A. K., Kabir, A., Furton, K. G., & Samanidou, V. F. (2019). Rapid monitoring of organochlorine pesticide residues in various fruit juices and water samples using fabric phase sorptive extraction and gas chromatography-mass spectrometry. *Molecules, 24*(6). https://doi.org/10.3390/molecules24061013. Available from: https://www.mdpi.com/1420-3049/24/6/1013/pdf.

Kelly, T. J., O'Connor, C., & Kilcawley, K. N. (2023). Sources of volatile aromatic congeners in whiskey. *Beverages, 9*(3). https://doi.org/10.3390/beverages9030064. Available from: www.mdpi.com/journal/beverages.

Kokoti, K., Kosma, I. S., Tataridis, P., Badeka, A. V., & Kontominas, M. G. (2023). Volatile aroma compounds of distilled "tsipouro" spirits: Effect of distillation technique. *European Food Research and Technology, 249*(5), 1173–1185. https://doi.org/10.1007/s00217-023-04205-0

Kubica, P., Namieśnik, J., & Wasik, A. (2016). Comparison of hydrophilic interaction and reversed phase liquid chromatography coupled with tandem mass spectrometry for the determination of eight artificial sweeteners and common steviol glycosides in popular beverages. *Journal of Pharmaceutical and Biomedical Analysis, 127*, 184–192. https://doi.org/10.1016/j.jpba.2016.01.006

Kurzyna-Szklarek, M., Cybulska, J., & Zdunek, A. (2022). Analysis of the chemical composition of natural carbohydrates – An overview of methods. *Food Chemistry, 394*, Article 133466. https://doi.org/10.1016/j.foodchem.2022.133466

Le, T. H. H., Nguyen, T. Q. H., Tran, C. S., Vu, T. T., Nguyen, T. L., Cao, V. H., Ta, T. T., Pham, T. N. M., Nguyen, T. A. H., & Mai, T. D. (2017). Screening determination of food additives using capillary electrophoresis coupled with contactless conductivity detection: A case study in Vietnam. *Food Control, 77*, 281–289. https://doi.org/10.1016/j.foodcont.2017.02.020

Lehmkuhler, A., Miller, M. D., Bradman, A., Castorina, R., Chen, M. A., Xie, T., & Mitchell, A. E. (2022). Levels of FD&C certified food dyes in foods commonly consumed by children. *Journal of Food Composition and Analysis, 112*. https://doi.org/10.1016/j.jfca.2022.104649. Available from: http://www.elsevier.com/inca/publications/store/6/2/2/8/7/8/index.htt.

Lester, S., Cornacchia, L., Corbier, C., Taylor, M. A., Ayed, C., Yang, N., Lim, M., Linforth, R., & Fisk, I. (2021). Identification of aroma compounds in a commonly prescribed oral nutritional supplement and associated changes in olfactory abilities with human ageing. *Scientific Reports, 11*(1). https://doi.org/10.1038/s41598-021-95915-6. Available from: www.nature.com/srep/index.html.

Li, Q.-lin, Chen, F.-xin, Luo, Z.-teng, Wang, M.-rang, Han, X., Zhu, J.-feng, Li, J. E., Liu, J., Li, K.-she, & Gong, P. (2023). Determination of nine bioactive phenolic components usually found in apple juice by simultaneous UPLC-MS/MS. *Food Science and Nutrition, 11*(7), 4093–4099. https://doi.org/10.1002/fsn3.3399

Li, J., Chen, M., & Zhu, Y. (2007). Separation and determination of carbohydrates in drinks by ion chromatography with a self-regenerating suppressor and an evaporative light-scattering detector. *Journal of Chromatography A, 1155*(1), 50–56. https://doi.org/10.1016/j.chroma.2007.02.080

Liao, S.y., Yang, S., Li, B.l., Xia, X., Jia, W.b., Zhao, Y.q., Lin, L., Bian, J.l., Bouphun, T., Xu, W., Si-Yu, L., Shu-Ang, Y., Bi-Lin, L., Xue, X., Wen-Bao, J., Yi-Qiao, Z., Ling, L., Jin-Lin, B., Tunyaluk, B., & Wei, X. (2024). Correlation analysis between key volatile compounds and core functional bacterial community during Sichuan black tea processing. *Food Chemistry X, 24*, Article 101969. https://doi.org/10.1016/j.fochx.2024.101969

Lin, C. S. K., Pfaltzgraff, L. A., Herrero-Davila, L., Mubofu, E. B., Abderrahim, S., Clark, J. H., Koutinas, A. A., Kopsahelis, N., Stamatelatou, K., Dickson, F., Thankappan, S., Mohamed, Z., Brocklesby, R., & Luque, R. (2013). Food waste as a valuable resource for the production of chemicals, materials and fuels. Current situation and global perspective. *Energy and Environmental Science, 6*(2), 426–464. https://doi.org/10.1039/c2ee23440h

Lin, Y., Wei, R., Zheng, J. J., Zheng, J., Zhang, W., Yasir, M., Kayama, K., Liu, X., & Su, Z. (2024). Volatile and non-volatile compounds profiling and their role in sensory and antioxidative attributes of two species of "red snow tea" (Lethariella). *Journal of Food Composition and Analysis, 133*. https://doi.org/10.1016/j.jfca.2024.106422. Available from: https://www.sciencedirect.com/science/journal/08891575.

Lorenzo, R. A., Pena, M. T., Fernández, P., González, P., & Carro, A. M. (2015). Artificial sweeteners in beverages by ultra performance liquid chromatography with photodiode array and liquid chromatography tandem mass spectrometry. *Food Control, 47*, 43–52. https://doi.org/10.1016/j.foodcont.2014.06.035

Mariano, A. P. X., Ramos, A. L. C. C., de Oliveira Júnior, A. H., García, Y. M., de Paula, A. C. C. F. F., Silva, M. R., Augusti, R., de Araújo, R. L. B., & Melo, J. O. F. (2022). Optimization of extraction conditions and characterization of volatile organic compounds of Eugenia klotzschiana O. Berg fruit pulp. *Molecules, 27*(3). https://doi.org/10.3390/molecules27030935. Available from https://www.mdpi.com/1420-3049/27/3/935/pdf.

Marnpae, M., Chusak, C., Balmori, V., Kamonsuwan, K., Dahlan, W., Nhujak, T., Hamid, N., & Adisakwattana, S. (2022). Probiotic Gac fruit beverage fermented with Lactobacillus paracasei: Physiochemical properties, phytochemicals, antioxidant activities, functional properties, and volatile flavor compounds. *LWT, 169*, Article 113986. https://doi.org/10.1016/j.lwt.2022.113986

Martins, F. C. O. L., Sentanin, M. A., & De Souza, D. (2019). Analytical methods in food additives determination: Compounds with functional applications. *Food Chemistry, 272*, 732–750. https://doi.org/10.1016/j.foodchem.2018.08.060. Available from: www.elsevier.com/locate/foodchem.

Matos, R. A., Souza, T. L.d., Barreto, L. H. S., Souza e Souza, L. B., Santos, D. C. M. B.d., Brandão, H. N., Santana, D.d. A., & de Freitas Santos Júnior, A. (2024). Sustainable analytical method for determination of bioactive compounds in solid oral formulations (capsules and tablets) containing green tea (Camellia sinensis) marketed in Brazil. *Sustainable Chemistry and Pharmacy, 40*. https://doi.org/10.1016/j.scp.2024.101655. Available from: https://www.sciencedirect.com/science/journal/23525541.

Merhi, A., Taleb, R., Elaridi, J., Hussein, F., & Hassan. (2022). Analytical methods used to determine pesticide residues in tea: A systematic review. *Applied Food Research, 2*(1), Article 100131. https://doi.org/10.1016/j.afres.2022.100131

Milhome, M. A. L., Castro, R. C., Silva, R. O., Nobre, C. A., & Nascimento, R. F. (2017). Advances in liquid chromatography coupled to mass spectrometry for determination of pesticide residues in food. In *Advances in chromatographic analysis* (pp. 2–49). Avid Science.

Milhome, M. A. L., Vieira, S. K. V., Reges, B. M., Fernandes, D. R., Uchoa, M. L. P., Pinheiro, A. I., Castro, R. C., Silva, V. P. A., Nobre, C. A., Menezes, M. G. G., Silva, R. O., & do Nascimento, R. F. (2019). Multiresidue analysis and evaluation of the matrix effect on 20 pesticides in Brazilian maize (Zea mays L.) flour. *Journal of Environmental Science and Health, Part B, 54*(11), 892–897. https://doi.org/10.1080/03601234.2019.1640586

Musarurwa, H., Chimuka, L., Pakade, V. E., & Tavengwa, N. T. (2019). Recent developments and applications of QuEChERS based techniques on food samples during pesticide analysis. *Journal of Food Composition and Analysis, 84*. https://doi.org/10.1016/j.jfca.2019.103314. Available from: http://www.elsevier.com/inca/publications/store/6/2/2/8/7/8/index.htt.

Naman, M., Masoodi, F. A., Wani, S. M., & Ahad, T. (2022). Changes in concentration of pesticide residues in fruits and vegetables during household processing. *Toxicology Reports, 9*, 1419–1425. https://doi.org/10.1016/j.toxrep.2022.06.013. Available from: http://www.journals.elsevier.com/toxicology-reports/.

Nascimento, R. F. D., Lima, A. C. A. D., Barbosa, P. G. A., & Silva, V. P. A. D. (2018). *Cromatografia gasosa: aspectos teóricos e práticos*. Fortaleza: Imprensa universitária.

Nascimento, R. F., Marques, J. C., Lima Neto, B. S., De Keukeleire, D., & Franco, D. W. (1997). Qualitative and quantitative high-performance liquid chromatographic analysis of aldehydes in Brazilian sugar cane spirits and other distilled alcoholic beverages. *Journal of Chromatography A, 782*(1), 13–23. https://doi.org/10.1016/S0021-9673(97)00425-1

Nguyen, H. T. H., Afsar, S., & Day, L. (2018). Differences in the microstructure and rheological properties of low-fat yoghurts from goat, sheep and cow milk. *Food Research International, 108*, 423–429. https://doi.org/10.1016/j.foodres.2018.03.040

Novaki, L. P., Chinelatto, A. M., Silva, V. A. B. B., & El Seoud, O. A. (2021). Analysis of consumer products: Demonstrating the power of LC-MS/MS for the simultaneous analysis of caffeine and other methylxanthines in guaraná fruit powder extract. *Journal of Chemical Education, 98*(6), 2083–2089. Available from: http://pubs.acs.org/loi/jceda8. doi: 10.1021/acs.jchemed.0c01069.

Oliveira do Nascimento, H., Franklin da Silva, M. Z., Alexandre, J. B., Carla, B. V., Vieira Carvalho, T., Ferreira do Nascimento, R., Nascimento, H. O., da Silva, M. Z. F., Alexandre, J. B., Vidal, C. B., Carvalho, T. V., & do Nascimento, R. F. (2022). New HS-SPME-GC-BID method for the determination of volatile constituents in distilled beverages. *Microchemical Journal, 181*. https://doi.org/10.1016/j.microc.2022.107669

Oliveira do Nascimento, H., Franklin da Silva, M. Z., Beserra Alexandre, J., Oliveira, T.Í.da S., de Lima, A. C. A., Ferreira do Nascimento, R., Nascimento, H. O., da Silva, M. Z. F., Alexandre, J. B., da Silva Oliveira, T.Í., de Lima, A. C. A., & Nascimento, R. F. (2023). Chemometric tools associated to chromatographic data to assess the quality and authenticity whiskeys. *Microchemical Journal, 189*. https://doi.org/10.1016/j.microc.2023.108542

Oliveira-Alves, S., Lourenço, S., Fernandes, T. A., & Canas, S. (2024). Coumarins in spirit beverages: Sources, quantification, and their involvement in quality, authenticity and food safety. *Applied Sciences, 14*(3), 1010. https://doi.org/10.3390/app14031010

Ordoñez, E. Y., Rodil, R., Quintana, J. B., & Cela, R. (2015). Determination of artificial sweeteners in beverages with green mobile phases and high temperature liquid chromatography-tandem mass spectrometry. *Food Chemistry, 169*, 162–168. Available from: www.elsevier.com/locate/foodchem. doi: 10.1016/j.foodchem.2014.07.132.

Pôrto, L. B. G., & Arisseto-Bragotto, A. P. (2024). Dietary exposure from food colours by Brazilian adolescents using the ERICA 2013–2014 food consumption database. *Journal of Food Composition and Analysis, 133*. https://doi.org/10.1016/j.jfca.2024.106410. Available from: https://www.sciencedirect.com/science/journal/08891575.

Patra, A., Abdullah, S., & Pradhan, R. C. (2022). Review on the extraction of bioactive compounds and characterization of fruit industry by-products. *Bioresources and Bioprocessing, 9*(1). https://doi.org/10.1186/s40643-022-00498-3

Petre, V. A., Cristea, N. I., Cojocaru, V. C., Pascu, L. F., & Chiriac, F. L. (2024). Analysis of volatile flavor compounds in four commercial beverages using static headspace gas Chromatography/Mass spectrometry: A qualitative approach. *Applied Sciences (Switzerland), 14*(5). https://doi.org/10.3390/app14051910. Available from: www.mdpi.com/journal/applsci/.

Pina, R. L., Cruz, D. C. P., & Cruz Martelli, M. (2022). Avaliação da influência de aromas gerados por leveduras não convencionais utilizadas na produção de cerveja: uma revisão. *Research, Society and Development, 11* (17), Article e43111738868. https://doi.org/10.33448/rsd-v11i17.38868

Pinto, F. V. M. (2022). *Análises cromatográficas do perfil lipídico de polpas de açaí́e produtos lácteos à base de frutas. Trabalho de Conclusão de Curso. (Graduação em Nutrição) - Instituto Federal de Educação Ciência e Tecnologia do Ceará.*

Preeti, S. S., Saharan, R., Narwal, S., Malik, R., Gahlot, V., Khalid, A., Najmi, A., Zoghebi, K., Halawi, M. A., Albratty, M., & Mohan, S. (2023). Exploring LIPIDs for their potential to improves bioavailability of lipophilic drugs candidates: A review. *Saudi Pharmaceutical Journal, 31*(12). https://doi.org/10.1016/j.jsps.2023.101870. Available from: https://www.sciencedirect.com/science/journal/13190164.

Pszczolińska, K., Shakeel, N., & Hanna, B. (2022). A simple approach for pesticide residues determination in green vegetables based on QuEChERS and gas chromatography tandem mass spectrometry. *Journal of Food Composition and Analysis, 114*, Article 104783. https://doi.org/10.1016/j.jfca.2022.104783

Pua, A., Goh, R. M. V., Huang, Y., Tang, V. C. Y., Ee, K. H., Cornuz, M., Liu, S. Q., Lassabliere, B., & Yu, B. (2022). Recent advances in analytical strategies for coffee volatile studies: Opportunities and challenges. *Food Chemistry*, 388. https://doi.org/10.1016/j.foodchem.2022.132971. Available from: www.elsevier.com/locate/foodchem.

Ramirez-Sanchez, I., Maya, L., Ceballos, G., & Villarreal, F. (2010). Fluorescent detection of (−)-epicatechin in microsamples from cacao seeds and cocoa products: Comparison with Folin–Ciocalteu method. *Journal of Food Composition and Analysis, 23*(8), 790–793. https://doi.org/10.1016/j.jfca.2010.03.014

Ramos, S. A., Silva, M. R., Siuves, I. O., Carvalho, M. L. V. G. M., Dias, C. N., Augusti, R., Melo, J. O. F., & Capobiango, M. (2021). Development and characterization of the profile of volatile compounds of ice cream cone produced with Tommy Atkins mango peel and kernel flour. *Research, Society and Development, 10*(3), Article e11310313006. https://doi.org/10.33448/rsd-v10i3.13006

Reis, F. R., & Dos Santos, C. M. E. (2022). *Volatile compounds formation in specialty beverages volatile compounds formation in specialty beverages* (pp. 1–231). Brazil: CRC Press. https://doi.org/10.1201/9781003129462

Rizzetti, T. M., Kemmerich, M., Martins, M. L., Prestes, O. D., Adaime, M. B., & Zanella, R. (2016). Optimization of a QuEChERS based method by means of central composite design for pesticide multiresidue determination in orange juice by UHPLC-MS/MS. *Food Chemistry, 196*, 25–33. https://doi.org/10.1016/j.foodchem.2015.09.010. Available from: www.elsevier.com/locate/foodchem.

Rodrigues, D. B., Mendonça, H. D. O. P., Nogueira, L. A., de Melo, A. C., Reina, L. D. C. B., Silva, M. R., Araujo, R. L. B., Augusti, R., & Melo, J. O. F. (2021). Characterization of volatile compounds and bioactive compounds of pulp and jelly of cagaita by solid phase microextraction in the headspace mode and mass spectrometry by paper spray. *Research, Society and Development, 10*(1), Article e25610111735. https://doi.org/10.33448/rsd-v10i1.11735

Rufino, M. S. M., Nogueira, A. F. A., Silva, A. C., Silva, A. P., Santos, A. C., Costa, C. T. A., Silva, F. M., & Pafo, F. V. V. E. (2023). Estudo dos compostos bioativos do gengibre e suas aplicações na saúde: uma revisão. *International Journal of Development Research, 13*(1), 61101–61105. https://doi.org/10.37118/ijdr.25671.01.2023

Salman, E., Guclu, G., Yaren Pehlivan, Z., Kelebek, H., & Selli, S. (2025). Changes in volatile, key odorants and bioactive properties of pomegranate juice during processing into concentrate. *Food Chemistry, 472*, Article 142856. https://doi.org/10.1016/j.foodchem.2025.142856

Santos, B. O., Augusti, R., Melo, J. O. F., Takahashi, J. A., & de Araújo, R. L. B. (2020). Optimization of extraction conditions of volatile compounds from pequi peel (Caryocar brasiliense Camb.) using HS-SPME. *Research, Society and Development, 9*(7), Article e919974893. https://doi.org/10.33448/rsd-v9i7.4893

Sentkowska, A., & Pyrzyńska, K. (2018). Zwitterionic hydrophilic interaction liquid chromatography coupled to mass spectrometry for analysis of beetroot juice and antioxidant interactions between its bioactive compounds. *LWT, 93*, 641–648. https://doi.org/10.1016/j.lwt.2018.04.023

Sewwandi, S. D. C., Arampath, P. C., Silva, A. B. G., & Jayatissa, R. (2020). Determination and comparative study of sugars and synthetic colorants in commercial branded fruit juice products. *Journal of Food Quality*, 1–11. https://doi.org/10.1155/2020/7406506

Sharma, H., & Ramanathan, R. (2023). Differences and correlation among various fatty acids of cow milk and goat milk probiotic yoghurt: Gas chromatography, PCA and network based analysis. *Food Chemistry Advances, 3*, Article 100430. https://doi.org/10.1016/j.focha.2023.100430

Silva, C. G. A. D., Bottoli, C. B. G., & Collins, C. H. (2016). Cromatografia por interações hidrofilicas (HILIC): Estado da arte e aplicações. *Química Nova, 39*, 210–220. https://doi.org/10.5935/0100-4042.20160003

Silva, A. S. L.da, Silva, A.de J., Latif, A. L. O., Júnior, A.de F. S., & de Jesus Benevides, C. M. (2022). Uso de metodologias analíticas para determinação de compostos fenólicos em alimentos no Brasil: avanços e fragilidades. *Research, Society and Development, 11*(2), Article e1311225193. https://doi.org/10.33448/rsd-v11i2.25193

Stanzer, D., Hanousek Čiča, K., Blesić, M., Murtić, M. S., Mrvčić, J., & Spaho, N. (2023). Alcoholic fermentation as a source of congeners in fruit spirits. *Foods, 12*(10), 1951. https://doi.org/10.3390/foods12101951

Strzałkowska, N., Jóźwik, A., Bagnicka, E., Krzyzewski, J., Horbańczuk, K., Pyzel, B., Słoniewska, D., & Horbańczuk, J. O. (2010). The concentration of free fatty acids in goat milk as related to the stage of lactation, age and somatic cell count. *Animal Science Papers and Reports, 28*(4), 389–395.

Tamer, F. S., Oymak, T., & Dural, E. (2024). Determination of seven synthetic colourants in pharmaceutics, foods, and beverages by a validated HPLC-PDA method: A risk assessment study. *Journal of Food Composition and Analysis, 136*, Article 106797. https://doi.org/10.1016/j.jfca.2024.106797

Tarko, T., Krankowski, F., & Duda-Chodak, A. (2023). The impact of compounds extracted from wood on the quality of alcoholic beverages. *Molecules, 28*(2), 620. https://doi.org/10.3390/molecules28020620

TGSC. (2021). Fragrance and flavor demo formulas. The good scents company information system - Providing information for the flavor, fragrance, food and cosmetic industries. https://www.thegoodscentscompany.com.

Tireki, S. (2021). A review on packed non-alcoholic beverages: Ingredients, production, trends and future opportunities for functional product development. *Trends in Food Science & Technology, 112*, 442–454. https://doi.org/10.1016/j.tifs.2021.03.058

Toffoli, A. L.de, & Lanças, F. M. (2015). Recentes avanços da microextração em fase sólida no tubo (in-tube SPME) e sua aplicação em análises ambientais e alimentícias. *Scientia Chromatographica, 7*(4), 297–315. https://doi.org/10.4322/sc.2016.011

Tolentino Limeira, R. R., De Lima Ramos Júnior, F. J., Limeira, R. R. T., & Júnior, F. J. D. L. R. (2024). Ações FARMACOLÓGICAS DO α-PINENO E β-PINENO. *Revista de Ciências da Saúde Nova Esperança, 22*(3), 373–388.

Torbati, M., Farajzadeh, M. A., Torbati, M., Nabil, A. A. A., Mohebbi, A., & Afshar Mogaddam, M. R. (2018). Development of salt and pH–induced solidified floating organic droplets homogeneous liquid–liquid micro-extraction for extraction of ten pyrethroid insecticides. *Fresh Fruits and Fruit Juices Followed by Gas Chromatography-Mass Spectrometry, 176*, 565–572. https://doi.org/10.1016/j.talanta.2017.08.074

Uduwerella, G., Chandrapala, J., & Vasiljevic, T. (2017). Minimising generation of acid whey during Greek yoghurt manufacturing. *Journal of Dairy Research, 84*(3), 346–354. https://doi.org/10.1017/s0022029917000279

Uzhel, A. S., Borodina, A. N., Gorbovskaya, A. V., Shpigun, O. A., & Zatirakha, A. V. (2021). Determination of full organic acid profiles in fruit juices and alcoholic beverages using novel chemically derivatized hyper-branched anion exchanger. *Journal of Food Composition and Analysis, 95*, Article 103674. https://doi.org/10.1016/j.jfca.2020.103674

Van, H. (2021). Chemical constituents and biological activities of essential oils of amomum genus (Zingiber-aceae). *Asian Pacific Journal of Tropical Biomedicine, 11*(12), 519–526. https://doi.org/10.4103/2221-1691.331267

Vandenberghe, C., St-Pierre, V., Pierotti, T., Fortier, M., Castellano, C. A., & Cunnane, S. C. (2017). Tricaprylin alone increases plasma ketone response more than coconut oil or other medium-chain triglycerides: An acute crossover study in healthy adults. *Canada Current Developments in Nutrition, 1*(4). https://doi.org/10.3945/cdn.116.000257. Available from: https://academic.oup.com/cdn.

Viegas Júnior, C. (2003). Terpenos com atividade inseticida: uma alternativa para o controle químico de insetos. *Química Nova, 26*(3), 390–400. https://doi.org/10.1590/S0100-40422003000300017

Vilela, A.de O., D'Antonino Faroni, L. R., Gomes, J. L., de Sousa, A. H., Paulo, R. C., Vilela, A. D. O., Faroni, L. R. D. A., Gomes, J. L., Sousa, A. H. D., & Cecon, P. R. (2021). Isotiocianato de alilo como fumigante no feijão-caupi e seu efeito nas propriedades físicas dos grãos. *Revista Ciência Agronômica, 52*(2), Article e20207287. https://doi.org/10.5935/1806-6690.20210064

Wang, L., Chen, S., & Xu, Y. (2023). Distilled beverage aging: A review on aroma characteristics, maturation mechanisms, and artificial aging techniques. *Comprehensive Reviews in Food Science and Food Safety, 22*(1), 502–534. https://doi.org/10.1111/1541-4337.13080

Wang, Y., Li, S., Sun, J., Li, Y., Hu, Y., Shen, C., Liu, F., Guo, S., Chen, F., Liu, Q., Ma, J., Ren, F., Yang, F., Zhang, Q., Song, J., Xin, T., & Pu, X. (2024). Comprehensive assessment for species authenticity, pesticide residual, and fungal contamination characteristics of Panax herbal tea. *LWT, 207*, Article 116688. https://doi.org/10.1016/j.lwt.2024.116688

Wardencki, W., Sowiński, P., & Curyło, J. (2003). Evaluation of headspace solid-phase microextraction for the analysis of volatile carbonyl compounds in spirits and alcoholic beverages. *Journal of Chromatography A, 984*(1), 89–96. https://doi.org/10.1016/s0021-9673(02)01741-7

WHO. (2015). *WHO calls on countries to reduce sugars intake among adults and children*. World Health Organization. https://www.who.int/mediacentre/news/releases/2015/sugar-guideline/en/.

WHO. (2023). *Food aditives*. World Health Organization. https://www.who.int/news-room/fact-sheets/detail/food-additives.

Wiśniewska, P., Śliwińska, M., Dymerski, T., Wardencki, W., & Namieśnik, J. (2015). Application of gas chromatography to analysis of spirit-based alcoholic beverages. *Critical Reviews in Analytical Chemistry, 45*(3), 201–225. https://doi.org/10.1080/10408347.2014.904732

Wu, J., Liu, Y., Zhao, H., Huang, M., Sun, Y., Zhang, J., & Sun, B. (2021). Recent advances in the understanding of off-flavors in alcoholic beverages: Generation, regulation, and challenges. *Journal of Food Composition and Analysis, 103*, Article 104117. https://doi.org/10.1016/j.jfca.2021.104117

Wu, L., Song, Y., Hu, M., Zhang, H., Yu, A., Yu, C., Ma, Q., & Wang, Z. (2015). Application of magnetic solvent bar liquid-phase microextraction for determination of organophosphorus pesticides in fruit juice samples by gas chromatography mass spectrometry. *Food Chemistry, 176*, 197–204. https://doi.org/10.1016/j.foodchem.2014.12.055. Available from: www.elsevier.com/locate/foodchem.

Xiang, X. F., Lan, Y. B., Gao, X. T., Xie, H., An, Z. Y., Lv, Z. H., Yin-Shi, Duan, C. Q., & Wu, G. F. (2020). Characterization of odor-active compounds in the head, heart, and tail fractions of freshly distilled spirit from Spine grape (Vitis davidii Foex) wine by gas chromatography-olfactometry and gas chromatography-mass spectrometry. *Food Research International, 137*. https://doi.org/10.1016/j.foodres.2020.109388. Available from: www.elsevier.com/inca/publications/store/4/2/2/9/7/0.

Yıkmıs, S., Türkol, M., Pacal, I., Duman Altan, A., Tokatlı, N., Abdi, G., Tokatlı Demirok, N., & Aadil, R. M. (2025). Optimization of bioactive compounds and sensory quality in thermosonicated black carrot juice: A study using response surface methodology, gradient boosting, and fuzzy logic. *Food Chemistry: X, 25*. https://doi.org/10.1016/j.fochx.2024.102096. Available from: https://www.sciencedirect.com/science/journal/25901575.

Yadav, K., & Dhankhar, J. (2022). Preeti, isothiocyanates – A review of their health benefits anPotential food applications. *Enviro Research Publishers, India Current Research in Nutrition and Food Science, 10*(2), 476–502. https://doi.org/10.12944/CRNFSJ.10.2.6

Yoshikawa, K., Saito, S., & Sakuragawa, A. (2011). Simultaneous analysis of acidulants and preservatives in food samples by using capillary zone electrophoresis with indirect UV detection. *Food Chemistry, 127*(3), 1385–1390. https://doi.org/10.1016/j.foodchem.2011.01.126

Yoshioka, N., & Ichihashi, K. (2008). Determination of 40 synthetic food colors in drinks and candies by high-performance liquid chromatography using a short column with photodiode array detection. *Talanta, 74*(5), 1408–1413. https://doi.org/10.1016/j.talanta.2007.09.015

Young, F. V. K. (1985). Interchangeability of fats and oils. *Journal of the American Oil Chemists' Society, 62*(2), 372–376. https://doi.org/10.1007/bf02541407

Yu, F., Chen, C., Chen, S., Wang, K., Huang, H., Wu, Y., He, P., Tu, Y., & Li, B. (2022). Dynamic changes and mechanisms of organic acids during black tea manufacturing process. *Food Control, 132*, Article 108535. https://doi.org/10.1016/j.foodcont.2021.108535

Yu, M., Wen, R., Jiang, Le, Huang, S., Fang, Z., Chen, B., & Wang, L. (2018). Rapid analysis of benzoic acid and vitamin C in beverages by paper spray mass spectrometry. *Food Chemistry, 268*, 411–415. https://doi.org/10.1016/j.foodchem.2018.06.103

Yuan, Y. H., Mu, D. D., Guo, L., Wu, X. F., Chen, X. S., & Li, X. J. (2024). From flavor to function: A review of fermented fruit drinks, their microbial profiles and health benefits. *Food Research International*, 196. https://doi.org/10.1016/j.foodres.2024.115095. Available from: https://www.sciencedirect.com/science/journal/09639969.

Zítová, K., Vyskočilová, E., & Červený, L. (2021). Preparation of α-terpineol and perillyl alcohol using zeolites beta. *Research on Chemical Intermediates, 47*(10), 4297–4310. https://doi.org/10.1007/s11164-021-04515-6

Žnideršič, L., Mlakar, A., & Prosen, H. (2019). Development of a SPME-GC-MS/MS method for the determination of some contaminants from food contact material in beverages. *Food and Chemical Toxicology, 134*, Article 110829. https://doi.org/10.1016/j.fct.2019.110829

Zhao, P., Huang, B., Li, Y., Han, Y., Zou, N., Gu, K., Li, X., & Pan, C. (2014). Rapid multiplug filtration cleanup with multiple-walled carbon nanotubes and gas Chromatography–triple-quadruple mass spectrometry detection for 186 pesticide residues in tomato and tomato products. *Journal of Agricultural and Food Chemistry, 62*(17), 3710–3725. https://doi.org/10.1021/jf405240j

Zhao, L., Liu, F., Wu, L., Xue, X., & Hou, F. (2017). Fate of triadimefon and its metabolite triadimenol in jujube samples during jujube wine and vinegar processing. *Food Control, 73*, 468–473. https://doi.org/10.1016/j.foodcont.2016.08.039

Zhou, W., Kügler, A., McGale, E., Haverkamp, A., Knaden, M., Guo, H., Beran, F., Yon, F., Li, R., Lackus, N., Köllner, T. G., Bing, J., Schuman, M. C., Hansson, B. S., Kessler, D., Baldwin, I. T., & Xu, S. (2017). Tissue-specific emission of (E)-α-Bergamotene helps resolve the dilemma when pollinators are also herbivores. *Current Biology, 27*(9), 1336–1341. https://doi.org/10.1016/j.cub.2017.03.017

Zhou, X., Zhu, Z., Sun, Z., Xu, J., Meng, X., Wang, H., Wang, R., Chen, F., Hu, X., & Zhang, J. (2025). The fermentation of carambola juice with lactic acid bacteria improves its flavor, bioactive properties, and metabolic composition. *Food Bioscience, 66*, Article 106307. https://doi.org/10.1016/j.fbio.2025.106307

Zhu, W., Jin, P., Yang, H., Li, F., Wang, C., Li, T., & Fan, J. (2023). A green extraction strategy for the detection of antioxidants in food simulants and beverages migrated from plastic packaging materials. *Food Chemistry, 406*, Article 135060. https://doi.org/10.1016/j.foodchem.2022.135060

CHAPTER

Good manufacturing practices and regulation for beverages

11

K.S. Darshan, Rebecca Miranda, Vishal and Roji Waghmare
Department of Food Engineering and Technology, Institute of Chemical Technology, Mumbai, Maharashtra, India

11.1 Introduction

In the highly competitive and scrutinized global beverage market, ensuring product safety and quality is not merely a goal but a foundational, non-negotiable requirement. Good Manufacturing Practices (GMP) present the fundamental system of rules and directions taken throughout the beverage industry in order to ensure this product integrity, uniform quality, and consumer safety. Specifically, international jurisdictions are determined and guided by international regulators, who establish the frameworks necessary to maintain product consistency and reliability in the level of quality control. This comprehensive approach means that GMP attempts to reduce risks by capturing every segment of the production process. This includes the rigorous sourcing, testing, and handling of all raw materials; the appropriate design, installation, calibration, and maintenance of all processing equipment; the thorough and continuous training of all personnel involved in operations; and the final packaging processes that protect the product until it reaches the consumer (Doneski & Dong, 2023). In the beverage industry, a robust GMP system maintains regulatory compliance and enables companies to reinforce their traceability, standardize their operational procedures, and fundamentally reduce the risks of contamination or any lack of quality in production. As a result, organizations that successfully implement GMP increase their credibility with regulators, build sustained interest on the part of consumers who trust the brand, and achieve greater diversification by being loyal in observing the requirements of the GMP standards (Covarrubias et al., 2022).

This is not a static "set it and forget it" system. There is also continuous inspection and audit as a way of strengthening the consistency of compliance and identifying areas that have to be enhanced. These types of checks allow manufacturing firms to maintain high standards of hygiene protocol and quality standards, and, critically, to react to the changing rules and new challenges within the industry. Moreover, the GMP-related tradition of "getting it right the first time" inherently minimizes waste from spoiled batches, decreases the financially devastating recall rates, and streamlines all production processes. These outcomes contribute directly to increased efficiency of operations and significant, measurable cost reduction (Sharma et al., 2023).

The universal implementation of good manufacturing practices did not emerge in a vacuum; it represents a direct reaction to historical public health crises, increased consumer concerns in regards to safety, and the clear necessity to have unifying, enforceable guidelines throughout the food and

The Science and Safety of Beverages. https://doi.org/10.1016/B978-0-443-36536-2.00010-7

beverage sectors (Heir, 1994). This evolution, from early 20th-century food acts to modern, harmonized global standards, is summarized in Table 11.1. This history shows that the constant development of GMP is a dynamic sequence. With manufacturing becoming more and more complex, regulators across the world engage in an endeavor to harmonize GMP guidelines to protect the safety, efficacy, and quality of products patients receive all over the world (Liu, 2014).

At the core of these modern quality-management models, cooperation between preventive and reactive solutions is especially relevant. The fundamental differences between these two quality philosophies are detailed in Table 11.2.

Table 11.1 Key historical milestones in GMP development.

Year	Milestone	Significance and context	References
1906	US Pure Food and Drug Act	This was the pioneering milestone in response to significant regulatory concerns about adulteration and misbranding.	Heir (1994)
1937–1938	Sulfanilamide Tragedy (1937) & US Food, Drug, and Cosmetic Act (1938)	Following the sulphanilamide nightmare which highlighted the dire consequences of poor production, the 1938 Act specified that products had to be proven safe and created systematic factory inspection.	Heir (1994)
1960s	Formalization of GMP in the US	The Food and Drug Administration (FDA) formalized its GMP requirements. These rules contain particular processes, design, structure, and controls to support the identity, strength, quality, and purity of manufactured goods.	Heir (1994)
1968	WHO Publishes First GMP Guidelines	The World Health Organization (WHO) issued its initial guidelines, which allowed for harmonization between countries and provided a standardized approach for nations with less sophisticated regulatory systems.	Patel and Chotai (2011)
1970	Emergence of the PIC/S	The Pharmaceutical Inspection Co-operation Scheme (PIC/S) was founded and has since played a central role in harmonizing GMP. Its aim is to harmonize inspection practice and GMP standards and develop mutual confidence between member jurisdictions.	Patel and Chotai (2011)
Current	Continuous Harmonization	Regulatory bodies, such as those in the European Union, constantly revise directives to keep within the frames of PIC/S and WHO requirements and to incorporate the latest scientific and technological improvements.	Kinderman (2020)

Table 11.2 Comparison of preventive and reactive approaches in quality control.

	Preventive approach (Core of GMP/HACCP)	Reactive approach (traditional quality control)	References
Features	• Implement Hazard Analysis and Critical Control Points (HACCP) systems • Conduct regular equipment maintenance and calibration • Establish supplier quality assurance programs • Develop and enforce standard operating procedures (SOPs) • Invest in employee training on food safety and quality control	• Conduct product testing and quality checks post-production • Implement recall procedures for contaminated or defective products • Respond to customer complaints and address issues as they arise • Perform root cause analysis after incidents occur • Develop crisis management plans for potential quality issues	(Blackburn, 2003, pp. 3–19; Griffith & Redmond, 2009; Jarvis, 2014; Meghwal et al., 2017; Owusu-Apenten & Vieira, 2022, pp. 217–236)
Benefits	• Reduces the likelihood of contamination or product defects • Enhances brand reputation and consumer trust • Minimizes costly product recalls and waste	• Allows for immediate action on detected problems • Can be less resource-intensive in the short term	(Covarrubias et al., 2022; Sharma et al., 2023)
Challenges	• Requires significant upfront investment in systems and training • May slow down production processes initially	• Increases the risk of contaminated or defective products reaching consumers • May lead to costly recalls and damage to brand reputation • Can result in regulatory fines and legal issues	(Memon et al., 2015; Noor Hasnan et al., 2022, Sharma et al., 2023)

This same spirit of collaboration extends beyond the factory floor. The collaborative method between international bodies also acts as a useful way of facilitating appropriate exchange of data among regulatory agencies and contributes to the generation of GMP that is comprehensive and global in nature. As a result of identifying best practices, solving common issues and creating effective systems, the participating authorities boost the quality and safety of products across various markets and regions (Okpala & Korzeniowska, 2023).

Best practice at a beverage industry is generally recognized to involve a well-balanced combination of proactive and reaction measures at enterprise level but leans more toward the proactive measures (Meghwal et al., 2017). In particular, the best practice is implemented by setting up an effective strategy of prevention as the major instrument to protect the quality of products; having reliable reactive approaches to deal with unanticipated problems; ensuring ongoing process modification based on numbers and feedback created by the preventative and responsive measures; and conducting regular quality control and risk management policy checks and updates.

This emphasis on prevention stems from a simple truth: the field of beverage safety is perhaps the most critical factor in the beverage industry, as it impacts the health of the consumer directly, as well as to their well-being, subjectively. The stakes are incredibly high. As far as dirty or otherwise unacceptable drink is suspected to trigger a significant malady, epidemic, or even death, a supervisor and the entire corporate structure are compelled to guarantee security at every single point of the manufacturing procedure (Sharma et al., 2023). A relentless focus on food safety also secures customers, bolsters consumer integrity in the brand, ensures legal compliance, and anchors sustainable business prosperity in a highly competitive market. In order to deal with these imperatives, beverage companies should set out an effective, documented food hazard management system that has the ability to predict hazards at all levels of production. Principles of such a system are careful hygiene levels, constant training of the employees and the supplier management. Also, well-designed policy must contain effective traceability systems and recall procedures (Memon et al., 2015). In enabling fast detection and recall of potentially dangerous products, such measures reduce the chances of widespread public-health outbreaks and save the reputation and finances of stakeholders.

Of all these hazards, microbiological hazards and spoilage in the beverage industry are the most important and prominent threats, and the effects offered are both on quality and shelf life of products as well as their safety. A variety of microorganisms, namely bacteria, yeasts, and molds can penetrate beverages during many stages of production, and change the nutritional profile, flavor perception and appearance. These contaminants could be due to raw materials, equipment, or inadequate sanitization. Pathogenic bacteria pose a direct threat to consumer health, while non-pathogenic spoilage microorganisms like lactic-acid bacteria and yeasts ruin the quality of the products by producing gases, sediments and off-flavors (Xu et al., 2020). The adequacy of the protection of beverages during production and distribution relies on hazard analysis critical control point (HACCP) regimes in conjunction with more expansive good manufacturing practices (GMP) (Blackburn, 2003, pp. 3–19; Bortoletto et al., 2018). The key factors, common organisms, and control measures for these hazards are detailed in Table 11.3.

In addition to microbes, other aspects of quality in beverage production both on chemical and physical grounds are a number of factors that define the safety of the business product, its flavor, look and the experience that will be encountered by the consumer. One of the major concerns is the quality of water in which certain amounts of minerals, pH, and microorganisms can largely affect the flavor, quality, and stability of the water. The quality of raw material is also of great importance; the producer should be sure of the predictability of the ingredients, whether the ingredients contain a contaminant or adulterant, and must incorporate adequate storage and handling of the ingredients to prevent degradation.

There is also a risk in processing and operational risks to quality in terms of temperature control, filtration efficiency and proper mixing or homogenization. Physical processes tend to combine with possible chemical reactions, including oxidation of which gives off-flavors, color change, enzyme reaction disrupting stability, and unwanted fermentation. In addition to this, packaging interactions may affect the product by migrating the chemicals, being denaturing due to exposure to sunlight, or penetration of oxygen. All these directly affect stability of the drink and its freshness, which may cause the growth of microorganisms in storage, the sedimentation or separation of the drink components, and the loss of gases in the carbonated beverages.

Table 11.3 Spoilage microorganisms in the beverage industry: characteristics, effects, and GMP controls.

Beverage type	Spoilage microorganisms	Key microbial characteristics & spoilage markers	Spoilage signature (effects on quality)	Relevant GMP focus area	References
Fruit juices (acidic, e.g., apple, orange)	*Alicyclobacillus acidoterrestris*	**Spore-former; Thermo-acidophilic** (survives pasteurization, grows at low pH). **Marker:** Guaiacol.	Produces **guaiacol**, leading to "antiseptic," "smoky," or "medicinal" off-flavors. Minimal visible spoilage (no gas).	**Process Control** (Validating kill-steps for spores). **Material Management** (Testing raw ingredients, e.g., concentrate).	Aadil et al. (2019)
Carbonated soft drinks (high sugar, low pH)	*Zygosaccharomyces bailii*	**Osmotolerant** (survives high sugar/ Brix). **Preservative-resistant** (can grow in the presence of benzoates and sorbates).	Ferments sugars, producing **CO_2** and ethanol. Leads to package swelling/explosion, sediment, haze, and "yeasty" off-flavors.	**Sanitation** (Targeted cleaning of a resistant organism). **Process Control** (Controlling preservative levels, pH, and water activity).	Nwaiwu and Ibekwe (2017)
Beer (brewing)	*Lactobacillus* & *Pediococcus* spp. (Lactic Acid Bacteria)	**Hop-resistant** (some strains). **Markers:** Lactic acid; Diacetyl.	Produces **lactic acid** (sourness). Produces **diacetyl** ("buttery" or "butterscotch" off-flavor). Causes haze/ turbidity.	**Sanitation** (Aggressive CIP/SIP of lines and tanks). **Process Control** (Yeast management; sterile filtration).	Xu et al. (2020)
Wine	*Brettanomyces/ Dekkera* spp. (Yeast)	**Ethanol-tolerant**. **Markers:** 4-ethylphenol (4-EP); 4-ethylguaiacol (4-EG).	Produces volatile phenols: **4-EP:** "Band-aid," "stable," "barnyard" aroma. **4-EG:** "Smoky," "spicy" aroma.	**Sanitation** (Deep cleaning of barrels and equipment). **Process Control** (SO_2 management; filtration).	Aadil et al. (2019), pp. 1–38; Blackburn (2003), pp. 3–19

Continued

Table 11.3 Spoilage microorganisms in the beverage industry: characteristics, effects, and GMP controls.—cont'd

Beverage type	Spoilage microorganisms	Key microbial characteristics & spoilage markers	Spoilage signature (effects on quality)	Relevant GMP focus area	References
Dairy-based beverages (e.g., UHT milk)	*Bacillus cereus* *Pseudomonas* spp.	**Spore-former** (B. cereus); survives UHT. **Psychrotrophic** (Pseudomonas); grows at refrigeration temps, produces heat-stable enzymes.	B. cereus: "Sweet curdling," bitterness. Pseudomonas: Produces heat-stable **lipases** and **proteases** causing rancidity and bitterness, even after pasteurization.	**Material Management** (Cold chain integrity; raw milk quality). **Process Control** (Validating UHT). **Personnel & Training**.	Nyokabi et al. (2021); Phiri et al. (2021)
Bottled water	*Pseudomonas aeruginosa* *Aeromonas* spp.	**Biofilm-formers**. (Often introduced from source water or bottling environment).	Forms **biofilms** (slime) in equipment and bottles. Can cause off-odors, cloudiness, and potential health risks.	**Facility/Equipment Design** (Hygienic design to prevent harborage). **Process Control** (Ozonation, UV treatment). **Sanitation**.	Shachman (2004)
Spirits (e.g., cachaça)	*Lactobacillus* spp. Wild Yeasts	(Contamination during fermentation). **Markers:** Ethyl carbamate; Acrolein.	Inconsistent fermentation. Production of hazardous chemical contaminants like **ethyl carbamate** (a carcinogen) and **acrolein**.	**Process Control** (Controlling fermentation parameters; distillation cuts). **GMP Implementation**.	Bortoletto et al. (2018)
Traditional fermented beverages	*Escherichia coli* *Staphylococcus aureus*	**Pathogens** (not spoilage organisms). **Markers:** Presence indicates fecal or human contamination.	**Direct public health hazard**; potential for foodborne illness. (Product may or may not appear spoiled).	**Personnel & Training** (Critical importance of personal hygiene). **Sanitation** (Handwashing; potable water use).	Byakika et al. (2019)

Finally, the product also has to meet the expectations of the consumers in terms of sensory properties and this means that it has to be consistent in terms of flavor, aroma, mouthfeel, and control of color (clear or turbid). The manufactures also need to make sure the nutritional content is in line with label legislations and assertions especially on vitamin and mineral retention. Last but not least, some stringent measures are required to avoid certain safety risks such as contaminants such as heavy metals, pesticide residues, mycotoxins, allergens control as to avoid cross-contamination and proper labeling. The following issues ought to be addressed through high quality standards, good manufacturing practice, and testing at production (Aadil et al., 2019, pp. 1–38; Patra et al., 2019).

To further underscore a key point from this list, in the beverage sector, a qualitative status of water is a steward in the production of products regarding safety, tastes, and integrity of the products (Shachman, 2004). In the case of optimal water quality, producers will be able to achieve high regulatory requirements and match the consumer expectations. On the other hand, any contamination or impurities in water can essentially change the sense of a beverage as well as its visual impact and even its long-time quality. The water can also be of bad quality and favors microbiological growth, scale formation and increases the rate of corrosion in process equipment thus increasing the cost of operation and endangering human life. To reduce such risks, beverage companies devote considerable funds to extremely specialized treatment technology and strict quality-control procedures, which guarantee targeted pH, mineral content, and microbial purity (Cantor, 2009). For the industry to thrive, by being water quality conscious, it is able to both protect its image and give water-quality conscious advantages to their products, as well as command confidence and brand identity among their consumers.

The specific risks a manufacturer faces also depend on the beverage category, as risk profiles depend on, and differ due to shifting consumer preferences, evolving regulatory framework and dynamic market conditions. A more stringent examination of alcoholic beverages is caused by the ever-changing social views, the increased laws and even health issues. Society is growing more health-conscious and, in a number of jurisdictions, the types of ingredients used to make carbonated soft drinks face carbonated soft drink sugar-tax regimes that affect consumer decisions based on purchasing behaviors (Nwaiwu & Ibekwe, 2017). There is a continuing argument over the marketing practices as well as caffeine levels of energy beverages. Substitutes made of plants would require special attention toward the flavor, texture and nutrition sufficiency; functional drinks should comprehensively prove themselves to be healthy. Beyond the liquid itself, there has also been the focused attention on the packaging materials (mainly plastics), and other sources of water. Sustainability obligations, novel consumer demands, and possible weaknesses within supply-chains must be-kept under scrutiny across all types of products to guarantee sustainability and value to the market over the long-term.

To manage these market-facing risks, a comprehensive process of consumer education is required so that the enterprises can outline the unique benefits and add value to their merchandize. Businesses inevitably have to face communicative issues that are connected with the perception and anticipation of product sustainability. The first approach would be to implement packaging innovation, that is, using recyclable/biodegradable material to address the issue with sustainability, and other material costs may be reduced in the long run (Samuel et al., 2019). Additionally, the three-way partnership between food scientists, nutritionists, and sustainability professionals is essential in the development of commodities that meet consumer tastes and selection toward flavor, nutrition and environmental conservation.

This brings the discussion back to the central theme: the beverage industry depends on the application of current good manufacturing practices (cGMP), a term emphasizing that practices must be dynamic and evolve with technology as a way of ensuring the products in terms of safety, quality, and consistency. These regulatory bodies include the U.S. Food and Drug Administration which develops these fundamental standards by defining what is required of the production, processing, packaging, and storage of beverages. Aspects of process involving facility design, maintenance of machines, employee training, quality-control procedures are also part of cGMP elements of production (Dong & Doneski, 2023). Compliance with these standards reduces possible risks of contamination, guarantees the maintenance of hygiene requirements as well as the traceability of the material and products. As a result, cGMP reduces product alerts, enhances consumer trust and contributes to regulatory regulation and to the intensification of efficiency. With the development of the industry, it is essential to be educated and able to react to cGMP regulations to maintain competitiveness and meet increasing customer standards of high-quality, safety of goods. Observed audits and inspections ensure manufacturers of beverages produce their products according to the cGMP requirements. These assessments ensure that a suitable protocol is implemented in every production phase and point out any possible areas of the improvement. The long-term benefits to the organizations adhering to cGMP are the reduced cost of production, increased product consistency and increased brand name (Kumar Sharma & Kumar Pandey, 2025).

Finally, it is crucial to understand how GMP relates to other quality systems. GMP and HACCP are complementary, although different systems that have been used collectively to support food safety and quality in manufacturing activities (Owusu-Apenten & Vieira, 2022, pp. 217–236). GMP gives a basis to be followed which is characterized by fundamental procedural, facility design, equipment maintenance and personal hygiene requirements all which are aimed at the creation of safe food products (Blackburn, 2003, pp. 3–19). Adding to this foundation of GMP, HACCP provides a structured, scientific approach to the identification, assessment and control of specific risks across a production cycle, with a key focus on those parts of the production process (Critical Control Points) where risks are most easily mitigated or eliminated through competent risk management. By taking a combination of these two frameworks, collectively they provide a comprehensive framework in which food safety can be allocated to, where GMP provides the overall infrastructure that is required in order to implement HACCP successfully. In short, one cannot effectively implement HACCP without first having robust GMPs in place. This collaborative tie bolsters the effectiveness of regulatory observation, which raises the quality of products and safeguards the customer. This therefore means that successful application of HACCP in combination with GMP requires a thorough understanding of the production process as well as the hazards at every point of production. With the help of the critical control points identification and the creation of an adequate monitoring protocols, the HACCP helps to proactively manage the hazard and intervene almost instantly in cases related food safety issues. This preventive attitude can not only increase efficiency in operation, minimize waste and boost the consumer confidence in the food sector, but also enhance the overall protection of the food supply (Owusu-Apenten & Vieira, 2022, pp. 217–236). This hierarchical relationship is illustrated in Fig. 11.1.

Building upon this introductory overview, this chapter will embark on a detailed exploration of the principles, implementation, and oversight of Good Manufacturing Practices within the beverage sector. It will first dissect the core principles of GMP, providing practical analysis of quality management, sanitation, facility design, personnel training, documentation, and material control.

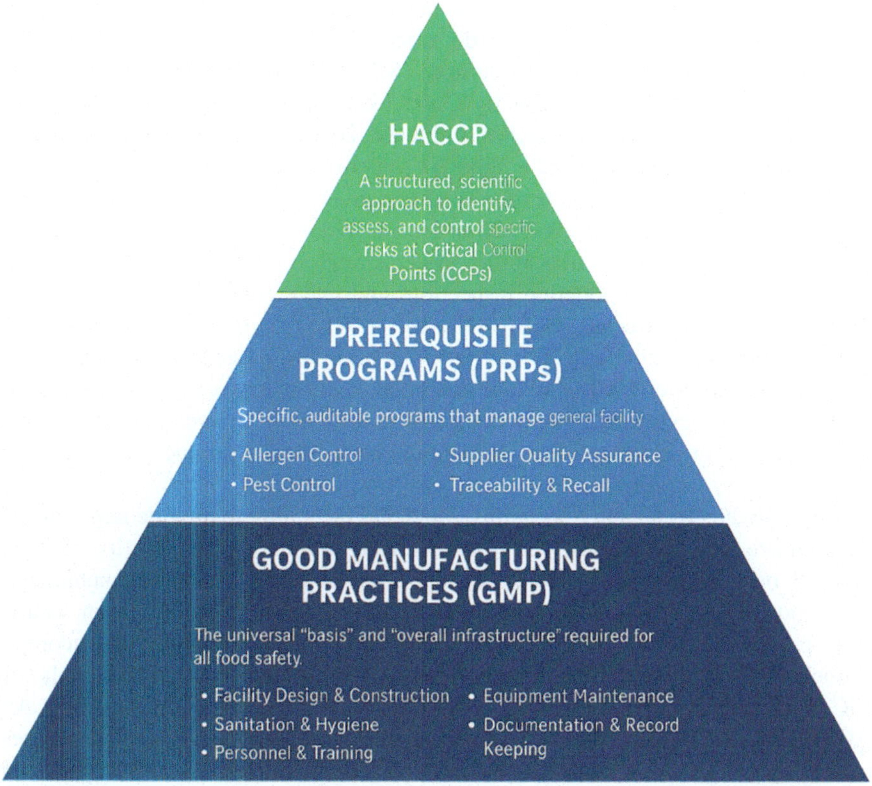

FIGURE 11.1

Tiered structure of food safety systems: GMP, PRPs and HACCP.

Following this, the chapter will navigate the complex global regulatory landscape, comparing the frameworks of key international and national bodies such as Codex Alimentarius, ISO, the FDA, and EFSA. Finally, to provide a real-world perspective, the chapter will analyze common non-conformances and implementation challenges, offering insight into how beverage companies can bridge the gap between regulatory requirements and day-to-day operational reality.

11.2 Principles of good manufacturing practices

11.2.1 Core objectives of good manufacturing practices

Good Manufacturing Practices (GMP) in the beverage sector seeks mostly to guarantee throughout all phases of manufacture consistent product quality, safety, traceability, and operational efficiency. GMP demands a well-ordered material management system under which each raw material and packing element is compliant with specifications, clearly marked with reference codes, kept under hygienic and regulated conditions to prevent cross contamination or deterioration, and isolated for inspection and testing (Blanchfield, 2005; Jarvis, 2014). By guaranteeing all delivered supplies satisfy established criteria and safety standards with appropriate documentation and due diligence upon receipt (Jarvis, 2014), the adoption of Supplier Quality Assurance (SQA) policies further supports this goal. With methods in place to avoid contamination by Good Manufacturing Practices, Standard Operating Procedures, and validated cleaning approaches (Lelieveld, 2016), maintaining GMP standards depends on hygiene control, building design, and equipment sanitation alongside.

Another main goal of GMP is the creation of strong process design and control systems enabling the production of safe, premium drinks within specific requirements. This covers the creation of documented operating procedures, traceability systems, and organized surveillance of key control points (Jarvis, 2014). With preproduction inspections and intermediate product validations assuring deviations are found and corrected swiftly (Brown, 2009), manufacturing operations have to be traceable and all equipment should be able of reaching accuracy, precision, and process consistency. One other important aspect of GMP is on the microbial safety by preventing contamination of pathogens like Listeria monocytogenes, Salmonella and E. coli or by processing techniques like heat treatment, acidification or drying to obtain the desired shelf life and product characteristics (Brown, 2009).

GMP ensures product recall and traceability which has the ability to provide importance for public health and minimize economic losses. The system is ready to immediately identify, isolate and recall the substandard or defective goods from the supply chain (Jarvis, 2014; Blanchfield, 2005, pp. 324–347). Supported by lot coding, electronic systems like RFID and blockchain, and paperwork documenting product origin, movement, and storage circumstances, traceability encompasses both backward tracking to raw material sources and forward tracking to distribution channels (PRODUCT IDENTIFICATION AND TRACEABILITY, 2018; ELECTRONIC IDENTIFICATION AND DIGITAL TRACEABILITY TECHNIQUES, 2018). Designated teams must start recall processes in crisis; communicate effectively with regulatory agencies; and guarantee that only authorized statements are used during public disclosures (Jarvis, 2014).

GMP's fundamental goals all come down to guaranteeing food safety, preserving product integrity, and preserving consumer trust by way of regulated material flow, certified manufacturing processes, and responsive recall systems. These techniques taken together protect public health while promoting corporate sustainability and regulatory compliance.

11.2.2 Key principles

11.2.2.1 Quality management

Quality Management deals with the ensuring product integrity, consumer health and the credibility of various beverages like water, fruit juices, dairy products, carbonated beverages, alcoholic beverages etc being a critical and complicated system. Microbiological risks, chemical degradation, and physiological instability are three major quality-related problems the sector confronts. Out of this Microbial contamination is very crucial as beverages being rich in sugars, acids and other nutrients provide a suitable environment for growth of spoilage organisms including bacteria, yeasts and molds (Patra et al., 2019). Microbial suppression depends mostly on temperature management by freezing, pasteurization, and nonthermal methods. Proper quality management, nevertheless, encompasses thorough sanitizing practices including standard operating procedures (SOPs) and sanitating standard operating procedures (SSOPs) beyond processing (Aadil et al., 2019, pp. 1–38). Forming a preventive rather than reactive quality assurance system, these are incorporated with GMP and HACCP guidelines (Meghwal et al., 2017).

Other than the microbial contamination chemical degradation like lipid oxidation, enzymatic browning and Maillard sections influence the shelf life and sensory properties of these beverages. These reactions yield rancidity, off flavors, nutrient loss as see in degradation of vitamins and PUFA, formation of dangerous intermediates like acrylamide and 5-hydroxymethylfurfural (Aadil et al., 2019, pp. 1–38). A major worry in milk-based drinks and those rich in unsaturated fats is lipid oxidative rancidity, which causes unpleasant volatile compound generation even at parts per billion (ppb) levels. Furthermore, influencing texture and customer acceptability, protein oxidation can lead to undesired alterations in emulsification, solubility, and water holding capacity. Beverages packed in different containers which range from clear to colored light exposure adds to the complexity of the quality assurance as photooxidation reaction of light sensitive ingredients like riboflavin, chlorophyll and carotenoids can induce chemical changes which further leads to flavor degradation and nutrient loss as seen prominently in dairy based and fruit-based beverages. Light causes terpenes and riboflavin degradation in alcoholic beverages stored in green colored bottles leading to off-flavors and color changes as reported by Aadil et al. (2019). Water treatment is another fundamental cornerstone of beverage quality control. Most non-alcoholic drinks mostly comprise water, which is also very important in the formulation methods as well as equipment cleaning. Thus, it directly affects the microbial, sensory and physicochemical properties of the final product. Contaminates which are commonly seen include suspended solids, algae, trihalomethanes, iron, sulfates and dissolved organic matter can vary the taste, pH balance and be a source of other hazards. Hence to remove these and make it sensorially and microbiological acceptable industries have developed sophisticated water treatment techniques like Ozonization, chlorination and UV treatment (Cantor, 2009; Font-Ribera et al., 2017; Garfí et al., 2016; Shachman, 2004). Beyond the technical structure, quality should be seen in a bigger conceptual and contextual context.

Quality is a dynamic, complex idea that affects and is shaped by economic activity, consumer expectations, and product distinctiveness, according to Okpala and Korzeniowska (2020). It is not only a stationary scientific term. This calls for continuous adjustments in quality methods by beverage manufacturers to meet changing consumer needs and legal requirements. From raw material intake to final packaging, a strong quality management system (QMS) should include regular product evaluation, real-time monitoring, recordkeeping, and traceability. The aim is to build a failsafe system whereby flaws are discovered and fixed at their root rather than in postproduction (Patra et al., 2019). This calls for integrating sensory testing, instrumental analysis, and biochemical assessments to monitor consistency in appearance, flavor, texture, and nutritional composition. Furthermore, needing training of personnel, method validation, and instrument calibration to ensure with strong confidence each production batch fulfills the specified criteria (Salgar et al., 2023).

Ultimately, the goals of quality management in the beverage industry are to build trust, ensure health, and provide consumers with safe, high-value products.

11.2.2.2 Sanitation

Sanitation, being an important aspect of Good Manufacturing Practices, guarantees the safety of the food and the quality in the beverage industry. Derived from the Latin word sanitas, it represents health. With respect to processing food, sanitation means establishing and maintaining a clean and healthy environment in the industry (Marriott et al., 2018). Sanitation in the industry aims to provide safe and healthy products by eliminating biological, chemical or physical contaminants; limiting the microbial growth and guaranteeing the product is treated, processed and stored in a clean environment under healthy personnel. The core of this program is based on scientific principles to achieve the objectives. According to Jarvis (2014) to maintain the hygiene and preserve the product integrity it is necessary to avoid environmental sources of contamination that is, microbes, foreign materials, personnel and their possessions. Personal hygiene, suitable protective clothing and limited movement in the risk zones can prevent the cross contamination within the industry.

Sanitary design concepts should be included in the equipment and infrastructure when constructing fresh beverage facilities or modernizing existing ones. This approach prevents microbial harborage sites, facilitates efficient cleaning, and enhances product safety by reducing the risk of foodborne illnesses and potential recalls (Lelieveld et al., 2014). A strong sanitation program includes regularly cleaning and sanitizing all equipment and facility surfaces, including HVAC systems. For example, clean and sanitized coils in heating and cooling units prevent airborne microbial contamination and improve energy efficiency, potentially reducing maintenance costs by up to 20%.

Sanitation procedures in the beverage industry are particularly crucial when cleaning-in-place (CIP) systems are used. These systems allow tanks and pipework to be cleaned without dismantling, essential in beverage operations where manual cleaning is impractical or unsafe. Cleaning typically involves using detergents to remove soil and residues, then disinfection using heat (e.g., 82°C for 30 s) or chemical agents. Heat can be sufficient, but chemical disinfectants are more frequently utilized because of their affordability and usefulness (CLEANING AND SANITATION, 2018).

The sanitation process consists of four fundamental stages: wetting and penetration of cleaning agents into soil and surfaces, chemical reaction and removal of organic and mineral soils, prevention of soil redeposition, and microbial disinfection (Holah, 2014). These processes rely on the interplay of four critical factors—mechanical (kinetic) energy, chemical energy, thermal energy, and time. For example, pressure washing and automated scrubbing apply mechanical energy, while the temperature and duration of cleaning processes influence their effectiveness. In some cases, extended contact time allows for lower concentrations of chemicals or reduced mechanical force, such as in soak-tank cleaning operations (Fryer & Christian, 2005, pp. 468–496).

Another fundamental idea is keeping an eye on sanitation efficacy. Quality control staff must regularly assess the cleaning results through visual inspections, microbiological swabs, ATP bioluminescence, rinse water testing, and in-process or final goods inspections. These steps assist in identifying any lingering contamination compromising product safety and guarantee that hygienic criteria are continuously fulfilled. Cleaning supplies must be handled and stored safely to avoid unintentional contamination or abuse (CLEANING AND SANITATION, 2018).

Adequate sanitation promotes operational effectiveness, preserves beverage quality and shelf life, and strengthens food safety management systems. In the beverage industry, it is both a legal necessity and a cornerstone of quality control.

11.2.2.3 Personnel and training

Since staff and training directly impact the safety, hygienic conditions, and overall quality of the final product, they are crucial components of Good Manufacturing Practices (GMP) in the beverage industry. The behavior and awareness of the workers are essential to the ongoing application of GMP.

When handling and producing beverages, staff must exercise good hygiene to avoid physical, chemical, and biological contamination (Shenvi et al., 2021). Thus, well-designed training programs are needed to guarantee that workers at all levels have the information and abilities needed to carry out their duties under GMP standards.

The personnel chosen for food and beverage processing must have the proper education, training, experience, and, if relevant, technical or professional qualifications. Blanchfield (2005) asserts that their duties and responsibilities must be precisely specified and recorded, ideally in job descriptions. Beyond qualifications, cleanliness and tidiness indicate a person's likely adherence to hygienic procedures. The significance of worker fit extends beyond hiring; ongoing assessment and bolstering of employee engagement are equally critical. For instance, if employment is terminated or morale is low, the potential risks to product quality or safety due to disinterest or negligence must be considered and mitigated.

Training must be ongoing and should start with induction during recruitment, followed by frequent refreshers to ensure compliance with updated protocols and regulations. Jarvis (2014) emphasized the need for training to reflect best practices grounded in national or international standards rather than relying on assumptions or outdated methods. All employees—including production, quality control, maintenance, and cleaning staff—must receive relevant training to carry out their tasks effectively. Training records must be maintained, and regular assessments should be conducted to evaluate knowledge retention and implement GMP practices.

Effective training programs must be targeted, practical, and tailored to the specific roles of the trainees. Griffith and Redmond (2009) highlight that training should be delivered within a hazard and risk framework using job-relevant examples, free from jargon, and in a language the trainees understand. Trainers must be credible, respected, and capable of motivating staff, identifying potential barriers to implementation and proposing solutions. Training should address what needs to be done and explain why ensuring food safety and quality is necessary.

Having a strong organizational culture that expects and discourages GMP compliance is equally important. Documentation is crucial for documenting procedures and facilitating traceability, both of which are critical components of an effective training program; according to De Silva (2020) and (Salgar et al., 2023) state that to guarantee regulatory alignment, training needs to be tailored to the task the employee is assigned and incorporate the most recent GMP updates. Manufacturing environments are more resilient and safety-conscious when industries invest in organized and ongoing training to empower employees and ensure excellent product quality.

11.2.2.4 Facility design and construction

In the beverage industry, ensuring consumer safety and product quality is paramount. GMP involve properly designing, installing, and maintaining facilities and equipment. These physical infrastructures are essential for preventing contamination and avoiding operational inefficiencies. The overall quality, safety, and hygiene are managed, maintained, and designed.

Facilities for the production of beverages directly impact a beverage product's overall quality, safety, and hygiene. The production of beverages must be carefully designed in terms of layout and construction to facilitate hygienic operations. Buildings should be planned, modified, and maintained to safeguard the materials and products from deterioration, contamination, or cross-contamination (Blanchfield, 2005, pp. 324–347). In support of this, Jarvis (2014) points out that to reduce the possibility of contamination from outside sources, facilities should bar ordinary staff from accessing processing sections. The plant layout should enable a logical flow of materials, from raw ingredient intake to final product packaging and dispatch, without intersecting with waste disposal or non-sanitary operations.

Construction materials play an equally vital role. All walls, floors, and ceilings must be made of smooth, non-absorbent, and easy-to-clean materials (Holah, 1992). The most contaminated area in a processing plant, the flooring, must resist wear and tear, slippage, and microbial growth. As highlighted by H.L.M. Lelieveld (2016), flooring in wet or greasy areas should be rough enough to prevent accidents but also impervious and easily cleanable to maintain hygiene. Walls must be cleaned with repeated cleaning, exposure to heat, and chemical agents used in sanitation, while ceilings should be designed to avoid dust accumulation and dripping.

Environmental control in beverage production areas is essential for product safety and personnel comfort. According to Pradeep et al. (2021), Proper Heating, Ventilation, and Air conditioning (HVAC) systems are necessary to manage airflow, prevent condensation, and control temperature and humidity, directly impacting microbial growth and product stability. Air handling units must be designed to prevent contamination from external air and reduce the risk of airborne particles entering clean zones.

Also, utilities must have sufficient supply and quality, such as compressed air and drinkable water. For all cleaning, processing, and ingredient uses, a potable water supply is essential, according to H.L. M. (Lelieveld., 2016); the facility's design must also include sewage and waste disposal systems to effectively manage sanitary sewage and process waste, reducing the possibility of environmental pollution and insect attraction.

The equipment used in beverage manufacturing must be appropriately designed for its intended use and should comply with hygienic design principles. According to Costa et al. (2013), Food-grade equipment should consider construction materials, geometry, surface finish, seals, and joints to minimize microbial niches and facilitate cleaning. For instance, equipment surfaces must be smooth and corrosion-resistant, particularly when they come into contact with beverages. Sharp corners, crevices, and open joints should be avoided to reduce contamination risks.

Blanchfield (2005) also points out that any changes to machinery, operations, or process parameters must consider GMP implications. Equipment should be easy to clean and sanitize, accessible for inspection and maintenance, and resistant to the conditions under which it operates (e.g., pressure, temperature, acidity). Heat exchangers, widely used in pasteurizing and sterilizing beverages, must be designed to ensure efficient thermal performance while minimizing fouling and pressure drops, as (Holah, 1992) discussed.

Beverage facilities are frequently separated into zones according to hygiene risk to prevent cross-contamination. Aseptic filling rooms and bottling are high-risk locations that must be physically isolated from low-risk sectors. HVAC systems should be zoned appropriately to guarantee that air pressure differentials stop pollutants from moving from low-risk to high-risk zones. Jarvis (2014) adds that areas for storing and processing high-risk materials should be segregated from general operations to uphold hygiene standards.

In addition, all doors and windows must be designed to prevent pest entry and environmental ingress. Doors should be self-closing or fitted with plastic strip curtains, and windows must be made of shatterproof materials with insect screens, where applicable. Adequate lighting, protected by shatter-resistant covers, is necessary to allow effective cleaning and inspection.

Additionally, as Halkjær-Knudsen (2016) suggested, risk assessment should be integrated into facility and equipment design phases to balance GMP and biosafety requirements. Active planning promotes long-term operational sustainability and reduces the need for expensive retrofitting.

11.2.2.5 Documentation and record keeping

Recordkeeping and documentation are both integral parts of Good Manufacturing practices in any beverage industry. They provide us with a complete picture of both the past and the current manufacturing processes, which act as a foundation, supporting the robust quality management system. They also favor us in planning for the future and making decisions. The visibility brought about by the quality assurance systems through proper paperwork ensures compliance with the regulations and supports the production of safe and high-quality beverages.

Khoja et al. (2019) recommend that manufacturers keep reliable, thorough and verifiable records in any of the forms, such as photographic media, paper-based, or electronic, as part of GMP. Examples of such paperwork include requirements for materials, production methods and control protocols. This sort of paperwork helps investigators and enables personnel to make educated decisions regarding batch releases by offering a defined audit trail. Often, looking at these papers and records during their inspections, regulatory inspectors evaluate a facility's adherence to GMP standards. Moreover, keeping compliance requires good document management: preparation, release, use, storage, retrieval, and disposal.

As per Blanchfield (2005), good documentation is an essential element of GMP and is particularly critical in carrying out a suitably functioning HACCP system. Documentation serves multiple purposes: defining policies, materials, operations, activities, control measures, and products; recording and communicating necessary information throughout the manufacturing process; reducing the risk of errors caused by oral communication; and forming a vital part of the audit trail needed to trace the history of all components involved in producing the final beverage product. The documentation system should make it practicable to track the complete history of each batch, including the use and disposal of raw materials, intermediates, and finished products. Documents generally fall into four main categories: those that outline policies, those that describe requirements, instructions, and procedures, those that set out schedules or programs to be completed, and those requiring entries before, during, or after production to record events. A failure to maintain appropriate records and documentation undermines the effectiveness of GMP.

Jarvis (2014) adds that manufacturers must maintain adequate records to demonstrate GMP compliance. The quality system should specify the storage duration for each document and the storage method, which may be in paper, microfiche, or electronic format. The three major documentation types typically cover quality and operational systems, personnel and production programs, and production and quality records.

According to Salgar et al. (2023), Consistent instruction of operators in document procedures is essential. Throughout the production process, records must be kept, either digitally or manually, to confirm that all guidelines and instructions have been followed. This will guarantee that the beverage is consistent in quantity and quality. Every departure from accepted procedures needs to be recorded and carefully examined. In order to ensure precise product storage and retrieval, manufacturing and distribution records must offer full traceability for every batch. A recall system should also be implemented to make removing any batch from sale or distribution easier if needed. It is essential to assess any product-related complaints, determine the underlying reasons for quality flaws and put corrective measures in place to address the problems and stop them from reoccurring. For a detailed breakdown of the specific records involved in this process, Table 11.4 provides examples of the documentation required to adhere to GMP standards.

Table 11.4 Examples of documentation required to adhere to GMP (Jarvis 2014).

Area of activity	Documentation
Quality assurance	Quality policy statement, approved at the board level
	Ingredient specifications
	Supplier Quality Assurance and purchase contracts
	Specifications for intermediate, bulk and finished products
	Quality assurance and quality control procedures
	Laboratory protocols and reporting systems
	Housekeeping and pest control procedures
	Audit records of suppliers and contract packers
	New product development system requirements and procedures
	Independent audit requirements and records
	Customer and official complaint records
	Legislative requirements for products and processes
Operational management	Production programs
	Plant operating procedures
	Manufacturing procedures
	Machine operator instructions
	Cleaning procedures and instructions
	Health and safety information
	Plant maintenance schedules
	Logistic and transportation records
	Organization charts and reporting relationships
Personnel programs	Employment records
	Training programs for permanent and temporary employees
	Employee training records
Signed production quality records	Sources of ingredients, raw materials and packaging, lot numbers, receipt and usage dates, and so on
	Process data, including readings from gauges and other instruments, temperature record charts, and so on
	Data relating to weight and volume of packaged product
	Quality and environmental audit reports
	Records of cleaning, sanitization, and monitoring
	Laboratory records for ingredients, intermediate and finished products, process water, in-line cleaning, and so on
	Production and laboratory audit records
	Records of quarantined products and their eventual fate
	Records of all reused and reworked materials
	Records of product recall, with reports on packaging, storage, sanitation, and so on

11.2.2.6 Design of material management

Material management is vital in optimizing profitability and ensuring consistent quality in the beverage industry. Efficient handling of materials—from inventory control to vendor relationships—contributes to economic performance and supports sustainability goals, particularly through waste reduction and improved packaging design (Asaolu et al. 2012; Samuel et al., 2019). One essential component of material management is hygiene control. It includes things like cleaning procedures, equipment sanitation, and facility architecture. SOPs, GMPs, and efficient cleaning techniques are used to control these elements and reduce the danger of contamination (H.L.M. Lelieveld, 2016). As Blanchfield (2005) outlined, each ingredient and packaging material must comply with its respective specifications, and every delivery or batch should be traceable via a reference code linking it to storage, processing, and laboratory records. To ensure that every batch can be accurately traced to its raw ingredients and associated laboratory data, deliveries are quarantined upon arrival and inspected, sampled, and tested by the food control manager before release. Errors can be prevented with proper identification and storage procedures. Additionally, safety is improved by pre-treating and separating non-compliant or useless materials. Raw materials must be stored hygienically and in specified conditions with controlled temperature and humidity, and stock rotation must be observed unless otherwise authorized. The weighing and measuring of ingredients—whether manual or automated—should be carried out using calibrated equipment of suitable precision, and all operations must be recorded in batch manufacturing records to avoid errors such as omissions or double additions.

Packaging materials must also adhere to strict specifications that ensure protection, compatibility, and regulatory compliance. Their identity should never be compromised, and any material unfit for use must be marked and quarantined for disposal. As with ingredients, packaging should be released only after inspection and approval, and its issues from stores must follow documented and authorized procedures. To prevent cross-contamination or mislabeling, operators must confirm that the correct packaging is used for each product, especially when multiple products or versions are manufactured. Obsolete or incorrectly dated packaging should be removed from production areas to avoid accidental use. Jarvis (2014) further emphasizes that a well-defined Supplier Quality Assurance (SQA) procedure is critical, detailing specifications, tolerances, labeling, and traceability for all materials, including potable water. Suppliers must be regularly audited, and any non-conformance must be reported and addressed. Just-in-time deliveries, while efficient, must still include certificates of compliance and be verified upon arrival. Brown (2009) highlights the importance of designated delivery areas that facilitate rapid unloading while maintaining temperature stability and minimizing contamination risks. These areas should allow direct movement of materials to storage and be equipped for inspection and cleaning. Materials delivered unpacked must be handled with clean equipment, and disinfection of outer packaging might be necessary when moving into high-hygiene zones. Storage areas must be tailored for different materials (ambient, chilled, frozen, or low-humidity), with reliable monitoring and record systems, and layouts should allow FIFO stock rotation and clear traceability.

Additionally, preparation and processing areas must be organized to prevent recontamination, and temperature drops must be carefully controlled before sterilization or pasteurization. According to Blackburn (2003), raw materials can introduce microbiological hazards; hence, microbiological testing is often required to confirm the absence of pathogens or verify that specifications are met. Even when not identified as Critical Control Points (CCPs), such controls fall under GMP or Good Hygiene Practices (GHP). They are vital for preventing the introduction of contaminants through raw ingredients. A well-designed material management system in the beverage industry—spanning raw material intake to final packaging—forms the foundation of a safe, traceable, and GMP-compliant manufacturing process.

11.2.2.7 Process design and control

Implementing Good Manufacturing Practices (GMP) in the beverage industry requires a strong foundation in process design and control. These factors improve operational effectiveness and regulatory compliance while guaranteeing the steady production of safe, high-quality products. Manufacturers face increased contamination risks, product inconsistencies, and inefficiencies without a reliable design and control system, leading to food safety incidents and economic losses.

Effective process design establishes the groundwork for producing beverages consistently meeting quality standards. It considers raw material characteristics, equipment limitations, and critical processing parameters. A well-controlled process must accommodate variations in raw materials while delivering a uniform final product. Additionally, it must include built-in preventive measures to manage microbiological, chemical, and physical hazards, which are especially critical in beverage production due to their vulnerability to spoilage and microbial contamination (Brown, 2009).

Each stage must be carefully managed and monitored throughout the production process—from raw material intake to packaging and storage. Important variables like flow rates, processing time, pH, and temperature must be verified and optimized. According to Jarvis (2014), preproduction checks are crucial for confirming that the equipment is clean and working and that the right supplies and labels are available before operations begin. When the standard procedure is broken, corrective action should be taken immediately. To guarantee compliance and traceability, all corrective activities must be appropriately documented. For example, in thermally processed beverages, failure to maintain correct heat treatment can lead to the survival of heat-resistant pathogens like *Clostridium botulinum* or spoilage organisms such as *Bacillus* species. Hence, identifying and strictly managing Critical Control Points (CCPs) is essential to ensure that the required heat treatment is both adequate and consistent (LABUZA and FU, 1995).

The process design must ensure compatibility between product formulation and processing conditions in beverages that use alternative preservation methods, such as acidification, drying, or modified atmosphere packaging (MAP). For instance, acidified beverages must achieve uniform pH distribution to effectively inhibit microbial growth, while MAP must be evaluated to prevent conditions that favor anaerobic pathogen development (Brown, 2009).

Moreover, process design supports GMP principles related to facility layout, equipment design, and hygienic zoning, all of which help prevent cross-contamination during manufacturing (Bakri Jali et al., 2016).

Detailed operating procedures and instructions, a critical part of process control, help standardize operations across the production line. According to Jarvis (2014), clear and regularly updated guidelines are essential for understanding. Training operators on these procedures reduces human errors and enhances product quality.

Process design and control are not one-time tasks but require continuous monitoring and improvement. As new ingredients, technologies, or market trends emerge, processes must be reviewed and updated to maintain safety and quality. Tools like predictive microbiology and Time/Temperature

Integrators (TTIs) help anticipate microbial responses under various storage conditions and improve product safety during distribution (LABUZA and FU, 1995).

11.2.2.8 Product recall and traceability

Product recall and traceability are essential to implement Good Manufacturing Practices (GMP) in the beverage industry, ensuring product safety, legality, and quality while minimizing financial losses and protecting brand integrity (Memon et al., 2015). A comprehensive traceability system enables manufacturers to trace products from the source of raw materials through the production process and finally to the consumer (PRODUCT IDENTIFICATION AND TRACEABILITY, 2018). Product history, production schedules, handling circumstances, ownership at different phases, and even provenance criteria like cultivation method and geographic origin must all be documented via a strong information system. Recalls can be caused by quality flaws, life-threatening risks, or non-compliance with regulations, making these systems critical (Jarvis, 2014. *Good Manufacturing Practice*).

Companies must have a predefined recall strategy supported by written procedures and a trained crisis management team to handle such crises effectively. This team, comprising representatives from production, legal, commercial, distribution, and technical sectors, must act under clearly defined authority, especially when facing accidental contamination or intentional sabotage (Blanchfield, 2005; Jarvis, 2014). Recalls should be executed quickly and precisely, supported by lot identification and batch tracking to avoid excessive product withdrawal. Product name, size, identifying marks, defect details, urgency level, and consumer helpline numbers must be communicated to stakeholders and the public when necessary (Blanchfield, 2005, pp. 324–347).

Modern approaches to traceability employ electronic identification techniques, such as Optical Character Recognition (OCR), Radio Frequency Identification (RFID), and blockchain, which enhance real-time tracking and offer added assurance of product authenticity and compliance (ELECTRONIC IDENTIFICATION AND DIGITAL TRACEABILITY TECHNIQUES (2018)). In order to monitor factors like temperature, which are particularly important in cold-chain management, these digital solutions interact with sensor technologies and expedite recall procedures. Implementing traceability presents difficulties for the beverage industry, especially for sectors that deal with bulk or continuous processing. However, optimizing production batch sizes and traceability granularity has been shown to reduce the impact of recalls on shareholder profits and overall company performance (Gunawan et al., 2017; Memon et al., 2015).

Recall triggers may originate from several places—consumer complaints, regulatory bodies, retailers, or even internal audits—and procedures must be executable at any given moment, both during working hours and otherwise. Crisis plans are also needed to consider the risk of bioterrorism, contamination by disgruntled staff, or other sabotage risks, which require additional physical and procedural security within the facility (Blanchfield, 2005; Jarvis, 2014).

11.3 Regulatory frameworks in the beverage sector

The beverage industry has an elaborate system of regulatory measures that consist of regulations, rules, and guidelines, which have been intended to safeguard consumers and maintain quality and safety of products (Kotsanopoulos & Arvanitoyannis, 2017). The framework and standards cover all the dimensions of beverage manufacturing, distribution and selling such as the specifications of ingredients to be used, labeling requirements, the packaging requirements and the quality-control measures. The most important job of implementation and enforcement lies in the hands of agencies like the US Food and Drug Administration (FDA) (Grazal & Earl, 1997) and Food Safety and Standards Authority of India (FSSAI) in India, and internationally through bodies like the Codex Alimentarius Commission which sets and expands international standards which are then reflected at country level as regulation (Kotsanopoulos & Arvanitoyannis, 2017). In order to meet the requirements of commitments, the manufacturers have to monitor and handle intense testing, heavy documentation, and strictly follow meticulous production guidelines. Regulatory frameworks are the most dynamic functions because as consumers and their scientific knowledge evolve, the regulatory environment will change accordingly to accommodate the responses to any new issues such as sugar, artificial ingredients, and environmental practices. As consumer preferences and scientific understanding evolve, regulatory frameworks in the beverage sector continue to adapt, addressing emerging concerns such as sugar content, artificial additives, and environmental sustainability (Lehto et al., 2017).

11.3.1 Codex Alimentarius and WHO/FAO guidelines

The Codex Alimentarius was created in May 1963 by the Food and Agricultural Organization (FAO) and the World Health Organization (WHO) and is considered to be the key international organisation and its mandate is to establish standards of foods that are applicable to the beverage industry (Kotsanopoulos & Arvanitoyannis, 2017). It is charged with the responsibilities of protecting the population health, developing food-safety procedures, and encouraging fair trading practices across the globe. The Codex offers sector advice in the labeling, additives, contaminants, and hygiene needs in the beverage sector. In addition to these, they also provide details like the individual limits of heavy-metals, microbiological tolerances and maximum residues of the pesticide materials. An example is the specific standard for patulin, a mycotoxin found in apple juice, for which Codex has set a maximum limit of 50 μg/kg to prevent health risks associated with microbial contamination in fallen fruit (Codex Alimentarius Commission. 2003).

11.3.2 ISO standards relevant to beverage GMP (e.g., ISO 22000; ISO 9001)

As regards the existing scholarship, compliance with internationally accepted practices is necessary in order to achieve the safety of the products, quality control exercises, and legal conformity within the beverage industry (Kotsanopoulos & Arvanitoyannis, 2017). Among guiding principles, in this framework, it is important to point at ISO 22000 and ISO 9001.

The ISO 22000 forms the main part of food-safety management systems, which provides a methodical, preventive solution that could be applied across entire food-and-beverage chain (Chen et al., 2020). The standard can be implemented by combining HACCP principles and prerequisite programs (PRPs) so risks associated with raw-material sourcing to delivery of the final product can be identified, assessed, and controlled (Blackburn, 2003, pp. 3–19; Owusu-Apenten & Vieira, 2022, pp. 217–236). The ISO 22000 has global acceptance and will enable the strengthening of the internal safety standards and at the same time meets internally standardized operating requirements, something crucial in the current global market. For instance, in the carbonated soft drink (CSD) industry, ISO 22000 implementation specifically targets acid-tolerant spoilage yeasts such as *Zygosaccharomyces* spp., prioritizing rigorous prerequisite programs (PRPs) over the thermal processing steps typically used in juice production (Alhasani, 2026).

As suitable to various industries, ISO 9001 presents an auxiliary structure to the quality-management systems (QMS). Its focus on the satisfaction of the customers, standardization of processes, continuous improvement, and regulatory compliance make it so important to the beverage GMP (Kotsanopoulos & Arvanitoyannis, 2017). By integrating the ISO 9001 in its daily routine operations, manufacturers will be in a position to maintain quality in every functional process, such as purchasing, production, packaging, and delivering, and this will lead to better operation and increase consumer confidence (International Organization for Standardization, 2015).

The key to successful execution of these standards is organizational devotion to systematic documentation, reporting, internal and external auditing and specific employee training, as well as constant testing of performance (Kotsanopoulos & Arvanitoyannis, 2017; Patel & Chotai, 2011). Inherently, ISO-based systems help to develop a proactive safety and quality culture, other than a reactive stance of compliance. It is aso noteworthy that safety evaluations for food additives used in beverages are underpinned by risk assessments conducted by the Joint FAO/WHO Expert Committee in Food Additives (JECFA), which provides the scientific basis for international maximum permitted levels (Joint FAO/WHO Expert Committee on Food Additives, 2017).

Besides, ISO 22000 and/or ISO 9001 certification is another source of competitive advantage. There is high demand of third-party certification by many international retailers, importers and institutional buyers as a pre-condition to purchase (Kotsanopoulos & Arvanitoyannis, 2017). As a result, beverage companies that invest in these standards not only reduce the risk of food safety incidents and regulatory penalties but also strengthen their competitiveness in both domestic and international markets (Chen et al., 2020).

11.3.3 United States—FDA CFR title 21 part 117 (FSMA), TTB (alcohol)

U.S. Food and Drug Administration (FDA) Code of Federal Regulations (CFR) Title 21 Part 117 generally known as Food Safety Modernization Act (FSMA) has a wide sweep of impact on beverage industry, including alcoholic beverages regulated by Alcohol and Tobacco Tax and Trade Bureau (TTB) (Grazal & Earl, 1997). Although TTB assumes the major role in controlling the production, labeling, and distribution of alcohol beverages, the FSMA framework of FDA reaches some parts of alcohol manufacture, especially in parts where TTB authority does not run. Operators are therefore left with the burden of sorting the authority of the two agencies together with meeting the requirements of the FDA as well as the TTB. Such bi-directional regulatory setting requires thorough understanding of food safety foundation, hazard analysis, and preventive mediums of beverage manufacturing operations (Blackburn, 2003, pp. 3–19). Specifically for fruit juices, producers must adhere to the specialized Juice HACCP regulation (21 CFR Part 120), which mandates a 5-log reduction of the most resistant pathogen (e.g., E. coli O157:H7 in apple juice), a requirement that operates in tandem with broader FSMA preventive controls (FDA, 2018). The broader regulatory framework governing food additives is codified in 21 CFR Parts 170–199, which sets out permitted substances for direct addition to food for human consumption (Food and Drug Administration, 2023a). Alongside this, the FDA maintains the GRAS (Generally Recognized as Safe) substances inventory, which provides an additional regulatory pathway for substances with established safety profiles (Food and Drug Administration, 2023b). Requirement of complying with FSMA makes beverage companies undertake thorough risk analysis and warm preventive measures, and to keep minute records of their food safety proceedings. This involves the classification of any risks that may occur along the production line, creation of critical control points as well as developing some monitoring procedures to maintain the safety of products (Blackburn, 2003, pp. 3–19). Constant employee awareness, control check-ups and continual refinement of food safety programs are essential elements of attaining conformity to both FDA and TTB regulations in the beverage industry.

11.3.4 European Union—EFSA regulations and Hygiene Package

The government regulation mechanism in the European Union to govern beverage industry is dictated by EU Hygiene Package and European Food Safety Authority (EFSA) (Grazal & Earl, 1997). EFSA has been commissioned to carry out risk assessment and publish scientific opinion on safety issues related to food (Lehto et al., 2017) and the Hygiene Package provides regulations which sets the standards aimed at maintaining safety along the chain. These rules cover various asserts of the manufacture of the drinks, including hygiene routine, risk analysis and critical control points (HACCP) (Blackburn, 2003, pp. 3–19), tracing, and labeling specification. Beverage companies are to meet strict requirements as to the origin of ingredients used, the process they go through, the packaging, and even storage. In addition, regular controls and audits are required to check compliance and keep the levels of safety high (Kotsanopoulos & Arvanitoyannis, 2017). Going further, the EU has more regulations in alcoholized drinks, fruit juice and bottled water to deal with the reputable safety requirements of each product category item. Adherence to EU food safety law is essential to beverage sector in order to achieve access to market and consumer trust. The regulation includes the enforcement of the sourcing of ingredients; the practices used in manufacturing processes and the labeling and packaging. Failure may attract fines, recall of the product and tainting of the reputation (Memon et al., 2015).

In order to be compliant, companies adopt the use of a complete management quality system and hire food-safety experts in addition to working with industry experts. Numerous corporate organizations also come up with voluntary guidelines that express their desire to excel. This offensive measurement allows organizations to manage changes in the regulations, reduce the risks of non-conformity and become leaders in food safety assurance and quality.

11.3.5 India—FSSAI regulations and BIS standards

The beverage industry in India is governed through a two-part regulation system with the Food Safety and Standards Authority in India (FSSAI) and the Bureau of Indian Standards (BIS), as the regulatory bodies. The FSSAI is mandated with food safety and the duty to regulate food and beverage production, storage, distribution, sales and imports under the Food Safety and Standards Act of 2006. It sets a standard that relates to additives and contaminants and the requirements of compulsory labeling; the most recent update to the food additives regulatory framework being the Food Safety and Standards (Food Additives) Fourth Amendment Regulations (Food Safety and Standards Authority of India, 2022), At the same time, the BIS develops and implements quality specifications on a broad spectrum of features of the products such as the content of beverages, packaging materials, hygiene, and environmental concerns. The adherence to the regulations of FSSAI and the guidelines of BIS are both inevitable in ensuring the safety of products, quality assurance and protection of consumers. This is a two-tier regulatory framework which is supposed to maintain high quality standards in Indian beverages as well as integrate the practice within the country with the international best practices. The cooperation of the BIS with the FSSAI offers a unified regulation framework which covers all the stages of the production and distribution of the beverages. Such co-operation reduces the regulatory loopholes thus it ensures the consumers keep on consuming products of same quality and safety. In addition, the twinning paradigm brings forth unending innovation and accompaniment of better performance as manufacturers endeavor toward the attainment and even exceeding of the high demands of the two agencies. An illustrative example of this regulatory specificity is the FSSAI's creation of the "Carbonated Fruit Beverage" category, which mandates a minimum fruit juice content (e.g., 5% for lemon and 10% for other fruits) to clearly distinguish value-added agricultural products from synthetic aerated waters (Food Safety and Standards Authority of India, 2022).

11.3.6 Other regional authorities—China (SAMR), Canada (CFIA), Australia (FSANZ)

China's State Administration for Market Regulation (SAMR) oversees food safety, product quality, and market competition (Liu, 2014). SAMR was established in 2018 as part of a government restructuring effort with the aim to streamline regulatory processes. The agency has broad authority to enforce food safety laws, conduct inspections, and also issue recalls for non-compliant products. SAMR works in conjunction with other Chinese government bodies to ensure comprehensive food safety oversight across the nation (Liu, 2014).

The Canadian Food Inspection Agency (CFIA) in Canada is the main agency that controls the safety and nutrition value of foods. CFIA develops and enforces standards to preserve human health, health of the animals, plant health, as well as conduct regular inspections, run food-safety programs, and take other interventions when the specified standards are violated. Another mandate of the CFIA deals with the monitoring of harmonized food recalls (Kotsanopoulos & Arvanitoyannis, 2017).

Food Standards Australia New Zealand (FSANZ) develops and enforces the Australia New Zealand Food Standards Code that defines food safety, food composition, and food labeling standards. FSANZ is workable with other governmental entities where the evidence-based risk management and assessment are utilized to achieve and maintain food-safety levels and population health (Kotsanopoulos & Arvanitoyannis, 2017). The national code is implemented through an inspection program, complaint investigation, advice and education by the state and territory regulatory agencies. Additionally, the country has a system of coordinated actions that handle the appearance of the foodborne sickness and other food-safety crises.

A comprehensive summary of these international organizations and their quality standards is provided in Table 11.5.

A particularly complex area of international regulation involves food additives. While some standards are harmonized, the specific legal frameworks, approval processes, and permitted uses differ significantly across regions, as detailed in Tables 11.6 and 11.7.

11.4 Nonconformances of good manufacturing practices

11.4.1 Non-conformance of GMP

Good manufacturing practices (GMP) form the basis for the food safety systems in the beverage industry, as it is important in guaranteeing cleaning and manufacturing conditions that are not met properly by many small and medium enterprises (SMEs). This noncompliance with GMP is a result of

Table 11.5 International organisations and quality standards.

Region/ Country	Regulatory body/Standard	Scope/Key requirements	References
International	Codex Alimentarius (WHO/FAO)	Global food safety guidelines, additives, labeling, hygiene, and contaminants	Codex Alimentarius Commission (2023)
	Codex STAN 193-1995	MLs for contaminants and toxins in food and feed	Codex Alimentarius Commission (2023)
	ISO (International Organization for Standardization)	ISO 22000: Food Safety Management System ISO 9001: Quality Management System	International Organization for Standardization (2015, 2018)
USA	FDA (Food and Drug Administration)	Beverage ingredients, packaging, labeling, GMP, HACCP under FSMA	U.S. Food and Drug Administration (2018)
	USDA	Organic certification, some juice standards	U.S. Department of Agriculture & Agricultural (2000)
	TTB	Alcoholic beverage formulation, labeling, and taxes	Alcohol and Tobacco Tax and Trade Bureau (2020)
European Union	EFSA	Scientific risk assessment of food and beverages	European Food Safety Authority (2002)
	EC Regulations	Reg. 852/2004 (hygiene), 1333/2008 (additives), 1169/2011 (labeling) Reg. No. 110/2008 Definition, description, labeling and geographical indications of spirit drinks, Reg. No 1881/2006 MLs for certain contaminants in foodstuffs	European Commission (2004, 2008, 2011)
Canada	CFIA	Inspection, compliance, bilingual labeling	Canadian Food Inspection (2019)
	Health Canada	Nutrient standards, food additive approvals, MLs for various chemical contaminants	Health Canada, Food and Drug Regulations (2022)
India	FSSAI	Mandatory product registration, labeling, ingredient & additive compliance	Food Safety and Standards Authority of India (2022)
China	SAMR/NHC	GB standards, food safety, labeling, contamination limits GB 4789.25-2024: National Food Safety Standard Microbiological Testing Alcohol, Beverages, Frozen Drinks Sampling and Testing Processing	State Administration for Market Regulation & National Health Commission (2022)
Japan	MHLW/FSC	Positive list for additives, JAS standards, safety assessment	Ministry of Health Labour and Welfare Japan (2018)

Table 11.5 International organisations and quality standards.—cont'd

Region/ Country	Regulatory body/Standard	Scope/Key requirements	References
Australia/NZ	FSANZ	Allergen disclosure, ingredient regulation	Food Standards Australia New Zealand (2023)
		Food Standards Code: Std. 2.6 Non-alcoholic beverages, Std. 2.7 Alcoholic beverages.	Food Standards Australia New Zealand (2023)
Middle East	GSO + Local Ministries	Halal certification, Codex-based safety standards	Gulf Standardization Organization (2020)
Africa	National bodies + ARSO	Import/export inspection, Codex-aligned rules	African Organisation for Standardisation (2016)
South America	INVIMA (Colombia), ANVISA (Brazil)	Additives, microbiological safety, labeling in local languages	Agência Nacional de Vigilância Sanitária (2019)

many factors, including a lack of training, insufficient managerial monitoring, financial restrictions and insufficient understanding. The noncompliances seen include poor personal hygiene, insufficient paperwork, insufficient cleaning and maintenance, lack of operational control, and unhygienic design considerations as seen in the SMEs (Najah et al., 2020). This increases the probability of the defects in the beverage compromising the quality of the food, and sometimes an outbreak of foodborne illness. It becomes the responsibility of the beverage industry to identify the sources of nonconformity and understand the underlying causes in order to maintain compliance with GMP and improve food safety (Noor Hasnan et al., 2022; Meghwal et al., 2017). These common underlying causes of GMP failure are categorized and illustrated in Fig. 11.2.

11.4.1.1 Inadequate sanitary design and facilities

Insufficient sanitary design and facilities are one of the most common GMP nonconformances seen in various beverage industry. The factors that brought about these were financial constraints prohibiting adequate facility investment, lack of understanding and poor knowledge of hygienic design needs. Inadequacy in maintaining personal cleanliness has been reported in yoghurt processing (Cusato et al., 2013), surup manufacturing (Ndiaye et al., 2018), sweet potato puree processing (Malavi et al., 2018), fermented cereal beverages (Byakika et al., 2019), and milk production and processing (Nyokabi et al., 2021; Phiri et al., 2021).

For example, Malavi et al. (2018) reports on gloves and paper towels not provided; Cusato et al. (2013) windows without mosquito screens; and Purwantiningrum et al. (2018) inappropriate wall materials such as plaited bamboo mats. The absence of handwashing stations close to production zones (Bakri Jali et al., 2016) and inadequate design and flow in syrup manufacturing operations Ndiaye et al. (2018) have raised contamination risks.

This was a direct effect of poor training, lack of oversight and insufficient supply of hygiene supplies. In a sweet potato puree processing plant, it was seen that 57% of the people did not wash their hands during production (Malavi et al., 2018); milk producers sometimes dried their hands using

Table 11.6 Comparative table of food additive regulatory frameworks.

Regulatory element	European union (EU)	United States (US)	India (FSSAI)	Codex alimentarius (international)	References
Regulatory authority	European Commission (EC); European Food Safety Authority (EFSA)	U.S. Food and Drug Administration (FDA)	Food Safety and Standards Authority of India (FSSAI)	Codex Alimentarius Commission; Joint FAO/WHO Expert Committee on Food Additives (JECFA)	Codex Alimentarius Commission (2003), European Food Safety Authority (2002), U.S. Food and Drug Administration (FDA) (2018), Alimentarius (1995), Food Safety and Standards Authority of India (2022)
Legal instruments	Regulation (EC) No. 1333/2008 on food additives; Reg. (EC) No. 231/2012 on specifications	Federal Food, Drug, and Cosmetic Act; 21 CFR Parts 170–199, 73–74, 182–184	Food Safety and Standards (Food Products Standards and Food Additives) Regulations, 2011	Codex STAN 192-1995 (General Standard for Food Additives - GSFA); Codex Procedural Manual	European Commission (2008), European Commission (2011), Codex Alimentarius Commission (2003), Food Safety and Standards Authority of India (2011)
Regulatory model	Positive list system: additives are authorized only per specified food category	Dual system: GRAS (Generally Recognized as Safe) and Food Additive Petition (FAP)	Positive list system; regulations specify additive limits by food category	Positive list model using INS (International Numbering System) and Maximum Permitted Levels (MPLs)	European Food Safety Authority (2002), U.S. Food and Drug Administration (FDA) (2018); Food Safety and Standards Authority of India (2011)
Approval process	Scientific dossier submitted to EFSA → safety evaluation → Commission authorization → inclusion in Annex II	GRAS self-determination or notification; alternatively, FAP submission → FDA review → CFR listing	Application reviewed by Scientific Panel on Food Additives → risk assessment → publication in Gazette	JECFA conducts risk assessment → Codex Committee endorsement → GSFA update	European Food Safety Authority (2002), Joint FAO/WHO Expert Committee on Food Additives (2017), Codex Alimentarius Commission (1995)

Categorization of additives	Sweeteners, colors, preservatives, emulsifiers, stabilisers, thickeners, etc.	Certified and exempt color additives, GRAS substances, and food additives	INS-based additive classes (e.g., stabilizers, emulsifiers, preservatives)	Unified by INS code: acidity regulators, antioxidants, emulsifiers, etc.	European Food Safety Authority (2002); Codex Alimentarius Commission (1995)
Public additive listings	Annexe II (authorized uses and limits); E-number classification	21 CFR 172 (additives), 182–184 (GRAS), 73–74 (colors)	Appendix A: food category-wise permissible INS additives	GSFA tables (Codex STAN 192-1995); FAO online portal	European Commission (2008); Codex Alimentarius Commission (1995); Food Safety and Standards Authority of India (2011)
Labeling norms	Functional class + E-number or name (e.g., "E211 - Sodium Benzoate")	Common name: specific warnings for phenylketonurics (e.g., aspartame)	Functional class + INS number (e.g., "Preservative INS 211")	Functional class + INS code per GSFA guidelines	European Commission, 2008; Codex Alimentarius Commission, 1995; Food Safety and Standards Authority of India (2011)
Permitted limits/ Maximum levels	Defined per category in mg/kg or mg/L; based on ADI and exposure data	Minimum effective level; some CFR-defined limits; GMP applies otherwise	Listed in Appendix A with quantitative thresholds (mg/kg or mg/L)	MPLs as per GSFA; ADI values determined by JECFA risk assessments	U.S. Food and Drug Administration (FDA), 2018; Codex Alimentarius Commission, 1995; Food Safety and Standards Authority of India, 2011
Color additives	E100–E199 (e.g., E150d—Caramel IV); only EU-approved colors allowed	FD&C certified colors (e.g., FD&C Red No. 40) and exempt natural colors	Natural and synthetic colors identified by INS codes (e.g., INS 160b)	INS numbers with JECFA-evaluated toxicology (e.g., INS 160a—β-carotene)	Food and Drug Administration (2023b), Food Safety and Standards Authority of India (2022), Joint FAO/WHO Expert Committee on Food Additives (2017)

Continued

Table 11.6 Comparative table of food additive regulatory frameworks.—cont'd

Regulatory element	European union (EU)	United States (US)	India (FSSAI)	Codex alimentarius (international)	References
Sweeteners	E950–E968 (e.g., E951 Aspartame; E955 Sucralose)	Approved GRAS sweeteners (e.g., Sucralose, Stevia, Aspartame)	Permitted sweeteners (e.g., INS 951, 955, 960) in defined limits	INS-coded non-nutritive and nutritive sweeteners (e.g., INS 960—Steviol glycosides)	Food and Drug Administration (2023a), Codex Alimentarius Commission (1995); Food Safety and Standards Authority of India (2011)
Preservatives	E200–E299 (e.g., E211—Sodium Benzoate, E202—Potassium Sorbate)	GRAS or CFR-specified (e.g., Sodium Benzoate in 21 CFR 172.175)	INS 211, 202 used in permissible beverage categories	Codex MPLs for preservatives (e.g., INS 211—up to 600 mg/L in carbonated drinks)	European Commission, 2008; Codex Alimentarius Commission, 1995; Food Safety and Standards Authority of India (2011), Food and Drug Administration (2023b)
Stabilisers/ Thickeners	E400–E499 (e.g., E415—Xanthan Gum; E401—Sodium Alginate)	GRAS-listed (e.g., Carrageenan, Xanthan Gum)	INS 415, 401, etc. as per food category permissions	INS 415, 401 listed in GSFA with JECFA safety validation	European Commission (2008); Food Safety and Standards Authority of India (2011), Food and Drug Administration (2023b), Joint FAO/ WHO Expert Committee on Food Additives (2017)
Public transparency tools	EU Additives Database; EFSA scientific opinions	eCFR portal, GRAS Notification Inventory, FDA Federal Register	FSSAI Gazette notifications and regulatory portal	FAO GSFA Online database; Codex Circular Letters	European Food Safety Authority (2002); Codex Alimentarius Commission (1995); Food Safety and Standards Authority of India (2011)

Reevaluation & risk monitoring	EFSA systematic re-evaluation program; ADI revision and exposure updates	Post-market surveillance; GRAS reassessment by FDA as needed	Scientific panel reviews; stakeholder consultation, and expert meetings	Periodic JECFA re-evaluations; Codex Committee consultations	European Food Safety Authority (2002); Codex Alimentarius Commission (1995); Food Safety and Standards Authority of India (2011), (Joint FAO/WHO Expert Committee on Food Additives, 2017)
Examples of approved additives in beverages	Citric Acid (E330), Sodium Benzoate (E211), Caramel Color (E150d)	Citric Acid (GRAS), FD&C Yellow No. 5, Potassium Sorbate	Citric Acid (INS 330), Sunset Yellow (INS 110), Sodium Benzoate (INS 211)	Citric Acid (INS 330), Benzoates (INS 211), Natural Colors (e.g., INS 160a)	European Commission (2008); Codex Alimentarius Commisson (1995); Food Safety and Standards Authority of India (2011), Food and Drug Administration (2023b)

Table 11.7 Comparative Table of Food Additives permitted by different food authorities.

Additive	FDA (USA)	FSSAI (India)	EU (European union)	References
Lecithin (INS 322)	Generally Recognised as Safe (GRAS); no specific limit specified.	Permitted up to 1500 mg per 100g in formulated supplements for children.	Permitted under Good Manufacturing Practice (GMP); no specific maximum limit specified.	FDA: 21 CFR §184.1400 (GRAS). Food and Drug Administration, 2023b), FSSAI: (Food Products Standards and Food Additives) Regulations, 2011, Appendix A, INS 322. (Food Safety and Standards Authority of India, 2011) EU: Regulation (EC) No 1333/2008, Annex II, E322 (European Commission, 2008)
Mono- and diglycerides (INS 471)	GRAS; no specific limit specified.	Permitted up to 500 mg per 100g in formulated supplements for children.	Permitted under GMP; no specific maximum limit specified.	FDA: 21 CFR §184.1505 (GRAS). (Food and Drug Administration, 2023b) FSSAI: FSS (Food Products Standards and Food Additives) Regulations, 2011, Appendix A, INS 471. (Food Safety and Standards Authority of India, 2011) EU: Regulation (EC) No 1333/2008, Annex II, E471 (European Commission, 2008)
Citric acid (INS 330)	GRAS; no specific limit specified.	Permitted under GMP; no specific maximum limit specified.	Permitted under GMP; no specific maximum limit specified.	FDA: 21 CFR §184.1033 (GRAS). (Food and Drug Administration, 2023b) FSSAI: FSS Regulations, 2011, Appendix A, INS 330. (Food Safety and Standards Authority of India, 2011) EU: Regulation (EC) No 1333/2008, Annex II, E330; (European Commission, 2008)
Sodium benzoate (INS 211)	Permitted up to 0.1% (1000 ppm) in beverages.	Permitted up to 200 ppm in beverages.	Permitted up to 150 mg/L in non-alcoholic flavored drinks.	FDA: 21 CFR §184.1733 (GRAS; max 0.1% in food). (Food and Drug Administration, 2023b) FSSAI: FSS Regulations, 2011, Appendix A, INS 211. (Food Safety and Standards Authority of India, 2011) EU: Regulation (EC) No 1333/2008, Annex II, E211 (EFSA ANS Panel, 2016)
Potassium sorbate (INS 202)	Permitted up to 0.1% (1000 ppm) in beverages.	Permitted up to 300 ppm in beverages.	Permitted up to 300 mg/L in non-alcoholic flavored drinks.	FDA: 21 CFR §182.3640 (GRAS). (Food and Drug Administration, 2023b) FSSAI: FSS Regulations, 2011, Appendix A, INS 202. (Food Safety and Standards Authority of India, 2011) EU: Regulation (EC) No 1333/2008, Annex II, E202 (EFSA FAF Panel, 2019)

Aspartame (INS 951)	Permitted up to 0.5% (5000 ppm) in certain beverages.	Permitted up to 600 ppm in carbonated water.	Permitted up to 600 mg/L in soft drinks.	FDA: 21 CFR §172.804 (Food and Drug Administration, 2023a) FSSAI: FSS Regulations, 2011, Appendix A, INS 951 (Food Safety and Standards Authority of India, 2011). EU: Regulation (EC) No 1333/2008, Annex II, E951 (EFSA ANS Panel, 2013)
Acesulfame K (INS 950)	Permitted up to 0.5% (5000 ppm) in certain beverages.	Permitted up to 350 ppm in carbonated water.	Permitted up to 350 mg/L in soft drinks.	FDA: 21 CFR §172.800 (Food and Drug Administration, 2023a) FSSAI: FSS Regulations, 2011, Appendix A, INS 950 (Food Safety and Standards Authority of India, 2011). EU: Regulation (EC) No 1333/2008, Annex II, E950 (European Commission, 2008)
Sucralose (INS 955)	Permitted up to 0.5% (5000 ppm) in certain beverages.	Permitted up to 300 ppm in carbonated water.	Permitted up to 300 mg/L in soft drinks.	FDA: 21 CFR §172.831 (Food and Drug Administration, 2023a). FSSAI: FSS Regulations, 2011, Appendix A, INS 955 (Food Safety and Standards Authority of India, 2011). EU: Regulation (EC) No 1333/2008, Annex II, E955 (European Commission, 2008)
Caramel color (INS 150a-d)	Permitted under GMP; no specific maximum limit specified.	Permitted under GMP; no specific maximum limit specified.	Permitted under GMP; no specific maximum limit specified.	FDA: 21 CFR §73.85 (Food and Drug Administration, 2023b). FSSAI: FSS Regulations, 2011, Appendix A, INS 150a–d (Food Safety and Standards Authority of India, 2011); EU: Regulation (EC) No 1333/2008, Annex II, E150a–E150d (European Commission, 2008)
Sunset yellow FCF (INS 110)	Permitted up to 0.02% (200 ppm) in beverages.	Permitted up to 100 ppm in beverages.	Permitted up to 100 mg/L in beverages.	FDA: 21 CFR §74.705 (Food and Drug Administration, 2023a). FSSAI: FSS Regulations, 2011, Appendix A, INS 110. (Food Safety and Standards Authority of India, 2011) EU: Regulation (EC) No 1333/2008, Annex II, E110; (EFSA ANS Panel, 2014)

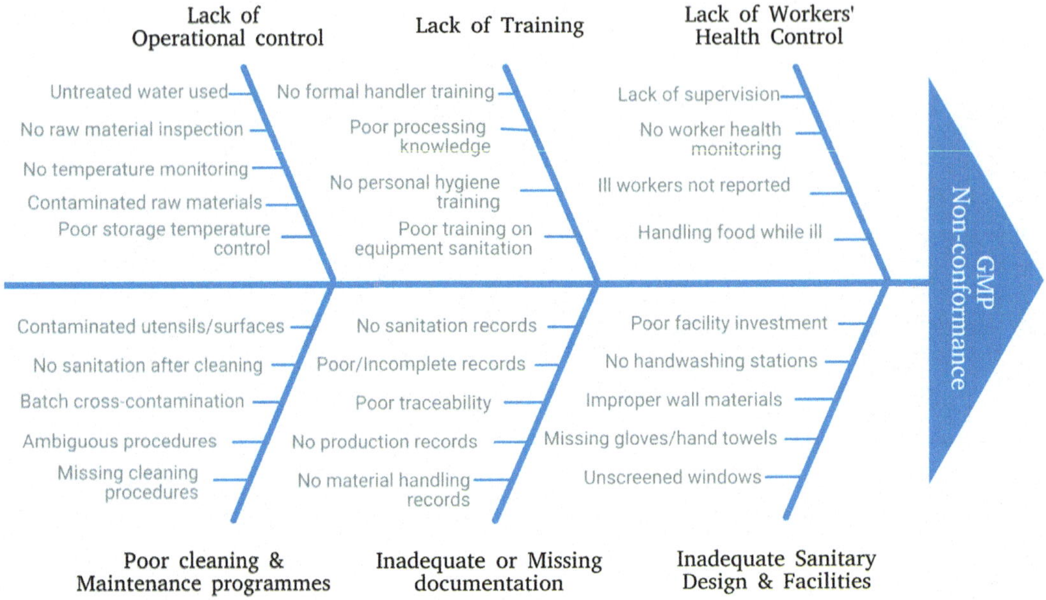

FIGURE 11.2

Root causes of GMP nonconformance in beverage SMEs.

reusable towels or not at all (Nyokabi et al., 2021). This made the products susceptible to microbial contamination like *Staphylococcus aureus* and E. coli carried from hands to foods, hence presenting a significant microbial safety hazard.

11.4.1.2 Inadequate or missing documentation

Documentation methods were sometimes absent or not properly kept in milk processing, yoghurt, and sweet potato puree (Cusato et al., 2013; Nyokabi et al., 2021; Malavi et al., 2018). Records on missing cleaning, cleanliness, maintenance, temperature monitoring, and material handling were among those faults that covered. Milk processors, for example, had little or no production records, therefore making it difficult to follow sources of contamination (Nyokabi et al., 2021). The sweet potato puree processing (Malavi et al., 2018) did not record sanitation procedures. Traceability, operating consistency, and the capacity for quick response to quality or safety events suffered from this dearth of paperwork.

11.4.1.3 Poor cleaning and maintenance programmes

As seen from the past, the beverage industry does not uphold its superiority in cleaning and maintenance techniques. As reported by Cusato et al. (2013), yoghurt manufacturers missed chemical detection guidelines and cleaning procedures. Malavi et al. (2018) found that utensils and surfaces got contaminated with microorganisms as a result of inadequate hygiene during the preparation of sweet potato puree. Cross-contamination between batches was evident in fermented cereal beverages due to insufficient cleaning (Byakika et al., 2019). Lack of sanitation after cleaning resulted in a risk of infection, as seen by Phiri et al. (2021) in the milk processing unit. Unsatisfactory training, ambiguous cleaning processes, and insufficient resources led to microbiological dangers and reduced cleanliness in the finished goods.

11.4.1.4 Lack of operational control

Untreated water, insufficient raw material inspection and lack of temperature monitoring were among the major operational control issues. Safety was compromised as reported by Malavi et al. (2018) by using water for washing and as an ingredient in sweet potato puree processing, which was not treated. Similarly, Nyokabi et al. (2021) and Phir et al. (2021) reported the usage of untreated water in milk processing units. Yoghurt manufacturers failed to control the storage temperature resulting in spoilage of many products and failed to identify them (Cusato et al., 2013). Contaminated raw materials like flour and water were reportedly being used in fermented cereal beverages (Byakika et al., 2019). This nonconformity was a direct result of a lack of supervision, expertise, and resources, leading to microbial contamination and product quality deterioration.

11.4.1.5 Lack of training

Lack of training is a persistent problem in the beverage industry. Formal training in cleanliness, sanitation, and recordkeeping was usually not conducted (Ndiaye et al., 2018; Phiri et al., 2021). Milk handlers, for instance, in the milk processing unit were not properly trained on personal hygiene, and equipment sanitation was reported by Phiri et al. (2021). Similarly, units that handled fermented beverages had poor food processing training, resulting in safety problems and contamination (Byakika et al., 2019). This lack of training fueled improper execution of Good Manufacturing Practices (GMP) and promoted hazardous handling techniques.

11.4.1.6 Lack of workers' health control

Monitoring the health of workers plays an important role in implementing good manufacturing practices in food and beverage industries, which were found to be absent in milk processing units and fermented cereal beverage companies (Byakika et al., 2019; Phiri et al., 2021). Since there were no reporting or inspections of workers' food, it may have been handled when they were ill. The main factors contributing to this included a lack of supervision, along with limited financial resources. The consequences of this were a higher risk of disease transmission from workers to food, limiting the safety and consumers' trust.

11.5 Conclusion

Good Manufacturing Practices (GMP) and regulatory standards in the beverage industry plays an important role in ensuring safety of products, quality of products and consumer confidence on products. A strict approach to GMP requirements, procedures, and regulations assists the manufacturers to keep the desired production quality, reduce the risk of contamination, and be able to comply with the legal challenges. These are operations which deal with all the extension of production in the way the facilities are designed, equipment is preserved, training of personnel and the quality control measures. Food safety concerns are likely to become a new trend as the beverage industry continues to change, so it is pertinent to keep up to date with new regulations. Those organizations that focus on the GMP provisions and regulatory compliance are safeguarding the health of the people and improving their image and competitiveness on the international market. Finally, effective assimilation of the GMP practices and regulatory evaluation in beverage manufacturing operations leads to overall growth and sustainability of the industry. Implementing extensive training of staff at every organization level is essential in ensuring GMP and regulatory compliance is kept on a steady level. Such programs ought to entail not only the technical know-how in the manufacture of the beverages, but they should also take note of the significance of the culture of food safety and personal accountability in provision of quality and safety of the products. Frequent evaluations and auditing should be made to make sure there is something that can be done better and that the practices of the company are up-to-date according to the best practices observed in the industry and regulatory demands. Also, when using technology and information analysis, a company can greatly increase the efficiency of tracking and strengthening its GMP compliance. Comprehensive tracking systems, automated control of production quality, and real-time control regarding the critical control points may offer a great deal of the knowledge related to the production efficiency and possible safety-related drawbacks. Following these innovations in technology will enable the beverage manufacturers to be ahead of the problems, streamline their operations and show case their desire to supply their customers with safe and quality beverages all over the world.

References

Aadil, R. M., Madni, G. M., Roobab, U., Ur Rahman, U., & Zeng, X. A. (2019). *Quality control in beverage production: An overview quality control in the beverage industry: Volume 17: The science of beverages*. Pakistan: Elsevier. https://doi.org/10.1016/B978-0-12-816681-9.00001-1

African Organisation for Standardisation. ARS 53:2016 General principles of food hygiene: Code of practice. ARSO Food Safety Standards Framework. ARSO. https://www.arso-oran.org.

Agência Nacional de Vigilância Sanitária, (ANVISA).. Resolução da Diretoria Colegiada – RDC No. 329/2019: Food Additives. ANVISA. http://portal.anvisa.gov.br.

Alcohol and Tobacco Tax and Trade Bureau. (2020). Beverage Alcohol Manual: A Practical Guide (Vol. 1–3). U. S. Department of the Treasury. https://www.ttb.gov/other-alcohol/beverage-alcohol-manual

Alhasani, K. (2026). The Possibility of Applying Quality Management In Projects According to The Requirements of The Specification (ISO10006:2017). *Warith Scientific Journal*.

Asaolu, T. O., Agorzie, C. J., & Unam, J. M. (2012). Agorz materials management : An effective tool for optimizing profitability in the Nigerian food and beverage manufacturing industry. *Journal of Emerging Trends in Economics and Management Sciences, 3*, 25–31.

Bakri Jali, M., Abdul Ghani, M., & Md Nor, N. (2016). The confusion of design and facilities in good manufacturing practice requirements among industries in Malaysia. *Environment-Behaviour Proceedings Journal, 1*(3), 156–167. https://doi.org/10.21834/e-bpj.v1i3.361

Blackburn, C.d. W. (2003). *Microbiological analysis and food safety management: GMP and HACCP systems detecting pathogens in food*. United Kingdom: Elsevier. https://doi.org/10.1533/9781855737044.1.3

Blanchfield, J. R. (2005). *Good manufacturing practice (GMP) in the food industry*. Elsevier BV. https://doi.org/10.1533/9781845690533.3.324. This chapter copyright © Institute of Food Science & Technology.

Bortoletto, A. M., Silvello, G. C., & Alcarde, A. R. (2018). Good manufacturing practices, hazard analysis and critical control point plan proposal for distilleries of cachaça. *Scientia Agricola, 75*(5), 432–443. https://doi.org/10.1590/1678-992x-2017-0040

Brown, M. (2009). Safe process design and operation. In *Foodborne pathogens* (pp. 431–480). Elsevier. https://doi.org/10.1533/9781845696337.1.431

Byakika, S., Mukisa, I. M., Byaruhanga, Y. B., Male, D., & Muyanja, C. (2019). Influence of food safety knowledge, attitudes and practices of processors on microbiological quality of commercially produced traditional fermented cereal beverages, a case of Obushera in Kampala. *Food Control, 100*, 212–219. https://doi.org/10.1016/j.foodcont.2019.01.024

Canadian Food Inspection, Agency. (2019). *Safe Food for Canadians Regulations (SOR/2018-108). Government of Canada*. https://laws-lois.justice.gc.ca/eng/regulations/SOR-2018-108/.

Cantor, A. F. (2009). *Water distribution system monitoring*. CRC Press. https://doi.org/10.1201/9781439800539

Chen, H., Liu, S., Chen, Y., Chen, C., Yang, H., & Chen, Y. (2020). Food safety management systems based on ISO 22000:2018 methodology of hazard analysis compared to ISO 22000:2005. *Accreditation and Quality Assurance, 25*(1), 23–37. https://doi.org/10.1007/s00769-019-01409-4

CLEANING AND SANITATION. (2018). In *Food and drink – Good manufacturing practice* (pp. 173–182). Wiley. https://doi.org/10.1002/9781119388494.ch21

Codex Alimentarius Commission. (2003). *Code of practice for the prevention and reduction of patulin contamination in apple juice and apple juice ingredients in other beverages (CAC/RCP 50-2003)*. World Health Organization/Food and Agriculture Organization.

Codex Alimentarius Commission. (1995, revised 2023). General Standard for Food Additives (CXS 192-1995). Annex Tables 1–3 (additive-specific maximum use levels). FAO/WHO. https://www.fao.org/gsfaonline/docs/CXS_192e.pdf

Costa, C. A., Luciano, M. A., & Pasa, A. M. (2013). Guiding criteria for hygienic design of food industry equipment. *Journal of Food Process Engineering, 36*(6), 753–762. https://doi.org/10.1111/jfpe.12044

Covarrubias, C. E., Rivera, T. A., Soto, C. A., Deeks, T., & Kalergis, A. M. (2022). Current GMP standards for the production of vaccines and antibodies: An overview. *Frontiers in Public Health, 10*. https://doi.org/10.3389/fpubh.2022.1021905

Cusato, S., Gameiro, A. H., Corassin, C. H., Sant'ana, A. S., Cruz, A. G., Faria, J. D. A. F., & De Oliveira, C. A. F. (2013). Food safety systems in a small dairy factory: Implementation, major challenges, and assessment of systems' performances. *Foodborne Pathogens and Disease, 10*(1), 6–12. https://doi.org/10.1089/fpd.2012.1286

De Silva, T. (2020). Good Manufacturing Practice (GMP). In *Handbook of food preservation* (pp. 1003–1016). CRC Press. https://doi.org/10.1201/9780429091483-64

Doneski, L., & Dong, M. W. (2023). Current good manufacturing practice (cGMP): An overview for the analytical chemist. *LCGC North America, 41*(10), 416–421. https://doi.org/10.56530/lcgc.na.qh7467g7

EFSA ANS Panel. (2013). Scientific opinion on the re-evaluation of aspartame (E 951) as a food additive. *EFSA Journal, 11*(12), 3496. https://doi.org/10.2903/j.efsa.2013.3496.

EFSA ANS Panel. (2014). Scientific opinion on the reconsideration of the temporary ADI and refined exposure assessment for Sunset Yellow FCF (E 110). *EFSA Journal, 12*(7), 3765. https://doi.org/10.2903/j.efsa.2014.3765.

EFSA ANS Panel. (2016). Scientific opinion on the re-evaluation of benzoic acid (E 210), sodium benzoate (E 211), potassium benzoate (E 212) and calcium benzoate (E 213) as food additives. *EFSA Journal, 14*(3), 4433. https://doi.org/10.2903/j.efsa.2016.4433.

EFSA FAF Panel. (2019). Scientific opinion on the follow-up of the re-evaluation of sorbic acid (E 200) and potassium sorbate (E 202) as food additives. *EFSA Journal, 17*(3), 5625. https://doi.org/10.2903/j.efsa.2019.5625.

Electronic identification and digital traceability techniques. (2018). Electronic identification and digital traceability techniques. In *Food and drink – Good manufacturing practice* (pp. 125–128). Wiley. https://doi.org/10.1002/9781119388494.ch16

European Commission. (2004). Regulation (EC) No 852/2004 of the European Parliament and of the Council on the hygiene of foodstuffs. *Official Journal of the European Union, L, 139*, 1–54. https://eur-lex.europa.eu/eli/reg/2004/852/oj.

European Commission. (2008). Regulation (EC) no 1333/2008 of the European parliament and of the council on food additives. *Official Journal of the European Union, L354*, 16–33.

European Commission. (2011). Regulation (EU) No 1169/2011 of the European Parliament and of the Council on the provision of food information to consumers. *Official Journal of the European Union, L, 304*, 18–63. https://eur-lex.europa.eu/eli/reg/2011/1169/oj.

European Food Safety Authority. (2002). Regulation (EC) No 178/2002 of the European Parliament and of the Council laying down the general principles and requirements of food law, establishing EFSA. *Official Journal of the European Union, L, 31*, 1–24. https://eur-lex.europa.eu/eli/reg/2002/178/oj.

Font-Ribera, L., Cotta, J. C., Gómez-Gutiérrez, A., & Villanueva, C. M. (2017). Trihalomethane concentrations in tap water as determinant of bottled water use in the city of Barcelona. *Journal of Environmental Sciences, 58*, 77–82. https://doi.org/10.1016/j.jes.2017.04.025

Food and Drug Administration. (2023a). *Food additives permitted for direct addition to food for human consumption. Code of federal regulations, Title 21 (21 CFR parts 170–199)*. U.S. Government Publishing Office. https://www.ecfr.gov/.

Food and Drug Administration. (2023b). *Generally Recognized as Safe (GRAS) substances inventory*. U.S. Department of Health & Human Services. https://www.fda.gov/.

Food Safety and Standards Authority of India. (2011). Food Safety and Standards (Food Products Standards and Food Additives) Regulations, 2011. Gazette of India, Extraordinary, Part III, Sec. 4 (August 1, 2011). https://www.fssai.gov.in/cms/regulations.php

Food Safety and Standards Authority of India. (2022). *Food safety and standards (food additives) fourth amendment regulations, 2022*. FSSAI.

Food Standards Australia New, Zealand. (2023). *Australia New Zealand Food Standards Code, Standard 2.6.2: Non-alcoholic beverages and brewed soft drinks. FSANZ.* https://www.legislation.gov.au/Series/F2015L00447.

Fryer, P. J., & Christian, G. K. (2005). *Improving the cleaning of heat exchangers handbook of hygiene control in the food industry*. United Kingdom: Elsevier Inc.. https://doi.org/10.1533/9781845690533.3.468

Garfí, M., Cadena, E., Sanchez-Ramos, D., & Ferrer, I. (2016). Life cycle assessment of drinking water: Comparing conventional water treatment, reverse osmosis and mineral water in glass and plastic bottles. *Journal of Cleaner Production, 137*, 997–1003. https://doi.org/10.1016/j.jclepro.2016.07.218

Grazal, J. G., & Earl, D. S. (1997). EU and FDA GMP regulations: Overview and comparison. *The Quality Assurance Journal, 2*(2), 55–60. https://doi.org/10.1002/(sici)1099-1786(199706)2:2<55::aid-qaj35>3.0.co;2-x

Griffith, C., & Redmond, E. (2009). Good practice for food handlers and consumers. In *Foodborne pathogens* (pp. 518–543). Elsevier. https://doi.org/10.1533/9781845696337.1.518

Gulf Standardization Organization. GSO 2055-1:2015, Halal Food: General Requirements. GSO. https://www.gso.org.sa.

Gunawan, I., Vanany, I., & Widodo, E. (2017). IEEE computer society Indonesia the influence of traceability system practice to product recall capability in bulk food industry: Observation and interview. In *IEEE International Conference on Industrial Engineering and Engineering Management* (pp. 1688–1692). https://doi.org/10.1109/IEEM.2017.8290179

Halkjær-Knudsen, V. (2016). Designing a facility with both good manufacturing practice (GMP) and biosafety in mind: Synergies and conflicts. *Applied Biosafety, 12*(1), 7–16. https://doi.org/10.1177/153567600701200102

Health Canada. (2022). Food and Drug Regulations (C.R.C., c. 870). Government of Canada. https://laws-lois.justice.gc.ca/eng/regulations/C.R.C.,_c._870/

Heir, R. S. (1994). Good Manufacturing Practice: An Historical Overview and Actual Status. *Drug Information Journal, 28*(4), 341–349. https://doi.org/10.1177/009286159402800408.

Holah, J. T. (1992). Industrial Monitoring: Hygiene in Food Processing. In L. F. Melo, T. R. Bott, M. Fletcher, & B. Capdeville (Eds.), *NATO ASI Series: 223. Biofilms Science and Technology*. Dordrecht: Springer. https://doi.org/10.1007/978-94-011-1824-8_57.

Holah, J. T. (2014). Cleaning and disinfection practices in food processing. In *Hygiene in food processing* (pp. 259–304). Elsevier. https://doi.org/10.1533/9780857098634.3.259

International Organization for Standardization. (2018). ISO 22000:2018 food safety management systems. https://www.iso.org/standard/65464.html

International Organization for Standardization. (2015). ISO 9001:2015: Quality management systems, Requirements (5th ed.). ISO. https://www.iso.org/standard/62085.html

Jarvis, B. (2014). Good manufacturing practice. In *Encyclopedia of food microbiology* (pp. 106–115). Elsevier. https://doi.org/10.1016/B978-0-12-384730-0.00149-X

Joint FAO/WHO Expert Committee on Food Additives. (2017). *Evaluation of certain food additives: Eighty-fourth report*. WHO Technical Report Series 1000.

Khoja, S. S., Patel, L. J., Khoja, S., Panjwani, K. R., & Ray, J. (2019). Review on good documentation practice in pharmaceutical manufacturing unit as per european union GMP Chapter-4 on documentation. *Pharma, 7*(1), 1. https://doi.org/10.29161/pt.v7.i1.2019.1

Kinderman, D. (2020). The challenges of upward regulatory harmonization: The case of sustainability reporting in the European union. *Regulation & Governance, 14*(4), 674–697. https://doi.org/10.1111/rego.12240

Kotsanopoulos, K. V., & Arvanitoyannis, I. S. (2017). The role of auditing, food safety, and food quality standards in the food industry: A review. *Comprehensive Reviews in Food Science and Food Safety, 16*(5), 760–775. https://doi.org/10.1111/1541-4337.12293

Kumar Sharma, A., & Kumar Pandey, A. (2025). Quality assurance in the herbal drug industry under current good manufacturing practices (CGMP). *International Journal of Innovative Science and Research Technology*, 2099–2102. https://doi.org/10.38124/ijisrt/25apr1144

Labuza, T. P., & Fu, B. (1995). Use of time/temperature integrators, predictive microbiology, and related technologies for assessing the extent and impact of temperature abuse on meat and poultry products. *Journal of Food Safety, 15*(3), 201–227. https://doi.org/10.1111/j.1745-4565.1995.tb00134.x

Lehto, S., Buchweitz, M., Klimm, A., Straßburger, R., Bechtold, C., & Ulberth, F. (2017). Comparison of food colour regulations in the EU and the US: A review of current provisions. *Food Additives & Contaminants: Part A, 34*(3), 335–355. https://doi.org/10.1080/19440049.2016.1274431

Lelieveld, H. L. M., Mostert, M. A., & Curiel, G. J. (2014). Hygienic design of food processing equipment. In *Hygiene in food processing* (pp. 91–141). Elsevier. https://doi.org/10.1533/9780857098634.2.91

Lelieveld, H. L. M. (2016). *Handbook of hygiene control in the food industry.* Elsevier. https://doi.org/10.1016/C2014-0-01825-4

Liu, X. (2014). International perspectives on food safety and regulations – A need for harmonized regulations: Perspectives in China. *Journal of the Science of Food and Agriculture, 94*(10), 1928–1931. https://doi.org/10.1002/jsfa.6646

Malavi, D. N., Muzhingi, T., & Abong, G. O. (2018). Good manufacturing practices and microbial contamination sources in Orange fleshed sweet potato puree processing plant in Kenya. *International Journal of Food Science, 2018.* https://doi.org/10.1155/2018/4093161

Marriott, N. G., Wes Schilling, M., & Gravani, R. B. (2018). *Sanitation and the food industry* (pp. 1–17). Springer Nature. https://doi.org/10.1007/978-3-319-67166-6_1

Meghwal, M., Heddurshetti, U., & Biradar, R. (2017). *Good manufacturing practices for food processing industries: Principles and practical applications food technology: Applied research and production techniques* (pp. 4–28). India: Apple Academic Press.

Memon, M. S., Lee, Y. H., & Mari, S. I. (2015). Analysis of traceability optimization and shareholder's profit for efficient supply chain operation under product recall crisis. *Mathematical Problems in Engineering*, 2015. https://doi.org/10.1155/2015/896239

Ministry of Health, Labour and Welfare (Japan). (2018). Food Sanitation Act (Act No. 233 of 1947, as revised 2018). MHLW. https://www.mhlw.go.jp/english/policy/health/sl-food/

Najah, Z., Lestari, G. D., Diwan, A. M., Dzikribillah, M. D., & Febriansah, M. R. (2020). Good Manufacturing Practices (GMP) in small enterprise of milkfish satay. *Food ScienTech Journal, 2*(2), 104. https://doi.org/10.33512/fsj.v2i2.10398.

Ndiaye, N. A., Cissé, M., Bonne, R., Sene, B., Kane, N. C., & Montet, D. (2018). Application of a facilitating HACCP system using two innovative methods for the production of hibiscus syrup by a Senegalese small and medium business (SMBs). *International Food Research Journal, 25*(1), 376–382.

Noor Hasnan, N. Z., Basha, R. K., Amin, N. A. M., Ramli, S. H. M., Tang, J. Y. H., & Aziz, N. A. (2022). Analysis of the Most frequent nonconformance aspects related to good manufacturing practices (GMP) among small and medium enterprises (SMEs) in the food industry and their main factors. *Food Control, 141*. https://doi.org/10.1016/j.foodcont.2022.109205

Nwaiwu, O., & Ibekwe, V. (2017). Assessment of HACCP Safety System and Good Manufacturing Practices in a Multi-product Soft Drink Bottling Plant. *Current Journal of Applied Science and Technology, 24*(3), 1–12. Article no.CJAST.37310.

Nyokabi, S., Luning, P. A., de Boer, I. J. M., Korir, L., Muunda, E., Bebe, B. O., Lindahl, J., Bett, B., & Oosting, S. J. (2021). Milk quality and hygiene: Knowledge, attitudes and practices of smallholder dairy farmers in central Kenya. *Food Control, 130*. https://doi.org/10.1016/j.foodcont.2021.108303

Okpala, C. O. R., & Korzeniowska, M. (2020). Concept, content, and context perspectives of quality of agrofood products: Reflections on some consumer decision-making-purchase scenarios. *Frontiers in Nutrition, 7*. https://doi.org/10.3389/fnut.2020.578941

Okpala, C. O. R., & Korzeniowska, M. (2023). Understanding the relevance of quality management in agro-food product industry: From ethical considerations to assuring food hygiene quality safety standards and its associated processes. *Food Reviews International, 39*(4), 1879–1952. https://doi.org/10.1080/87559129.2021.1938600

Owusu-Apenten, R., & Vieira, E. (2022). *Food safety management, GMP & HACCP*. Springer Science and Business Media LLC. https://doi.org/10.1007/978-3-030-65433-7_10

Patel, K. T., & Chotai, N. P. (2011). Documentation and records: Harmonized GMP requirements. *Journal of Young Pharmacists, 3*(2), 138–150. https://doi.org/10.4103/0975-1483.80303

Patra, S., Choudhary, R., Madhuri, R., & Sharma, P. K. (2019). *Quality control of beverages for health safety: Starting from laboratory to the point-of-care detection techniques quality control in the beverage industry: Volume 17: The science of beverages* (pp. 39–83). India: Elsevier. https://doi.org/10.1016/B978-0-12-816681-9.00002-3

Phiri, B. S. J., Sakumona, M., Hang'ombe, B. M., Fetsch, A., & Schaarschmidt, S. (2021). The traditional dairy value chain in Zambia and potential risk factors to microbiological food safety. *Food Control, 124*. https://doi.org/10.1016/j.foodcont.2021.107885

Pradeep, A. D., Vivekanandhan, R., Rameshkumar, T., & Sangaravadivel, P. (2021). Design of Hvac system for beverage industry. *IOP Conference Series: Materials Science and Engineering, 1059*(1), Article 012063. https://doi.org/10.1088/1757-899x/1059/1/012063

PRODUCT IDENTIFICATION AND TRACEABILITY. (2018). In *Food and drink – Good manufacturing practice* (pp. 115–120). Wiley. https://doi.org/10.1002/9781119388494.ch14

Purwantiningrum, I., Widyhastuty, W., Christian, J., & Sari, N. (2018). Assessment of good manufacturing practice for small scale food industry in Malang region, East Java, Indonesia. *IOP Conference Series: Earth and Environmental Science, 131*(1), Article 012028. https://doi.org/10.1088/1755-1315/131/1/012028

Salgar, J. B., Bais, S. K., & Savant, P. S. (2023). Review on current good manufacturing practice. *International Journal of Advanced Research in Science, Communication and Technology*, 689–703. https://doi.org/10.48175/ijarsct-7933

Samuel, A. U., Oyawale, F., & I Fayomi, O. S. (2019). Effects of waste management in beverage industries: A perspective. *Journal of Physics: Conference Series, 1378*(2), Article 022048. https://doi.org/10.1088/1742-6596/1378/2/022048

Shachman, M. (2004). *The soft drinks companion*. CRC Press. https://doi.org/10.1201/9780203492123

Sharma, A., Gamta, V., & Luthra, G. (2023). The importance of good manufacturing practices (GMP) in the healthcare industry. *Journal of Pharmaceutical Research International, 35*(18), 75–90. https://doi.org/10.9734/jpri/2023/v35i187394

Shenvi, A., Kamath K, K., Subrahmanyam, E. V. S., & Shabaraya, A. R. (2021). Significance of personnel hygiene practices in pharmaceutical industry. *International Journal of Drug Regulatory Affairs, 9*(4), 1–5. https://doi.org/10.22270/ijdra.v9i4.493

State Administration for Market Regulation & National Health Commission. (2022). *GB 4789.25-2024: National Food Safety Standard, Microbiological Examination of Food: Examination of Alcohol, Beverages, and Frozen Drinks*. Standardization Administration of China.

U.S. Department of Agriculture, Agricultural Marketing Service. (2000). National Organic Program (7 CFR Part 205). https://www.ecfr.gov/current/title-7/subtitle-B/chapter-I/subchapter-M/part-205

U.S. Food and Drug Administration (FDA). (2018). *Guidance for industry: Juice HACCP and the FDA food safety modernization act*. Center for Food Safety and Applied Nutrition.

Xu, Z., Luo, Y., Mao, Y., Peng, R., Chen, J., Soteyome, T., Bai, C., Chen, L., Liang, Y., Su, J., Wang, K., Liu, J., & Kjellerup, B. V. (2020). Spoilage lactic acid bacteria in the brewing industry. *Journal of Microbiology and Biotechnology, 30*(7), 955–961. https://doi.org/10.4014/jmb.1908.08069

Index

'*Note:* Page numbers followed by "f" indicate figures, "t" indicate tables'.

A

D

G

H

N

Q

R

S

T

Printed and bound by CPI Group (UK) Ltd, Croydon, CR0 4YY
14/09/2026
02216410-0011